Dentistry
for the
Child
and
Adolescent

Dentistry
for the
Child
and
Adolescent

RALPH E. McDONALD, DDS, MS
Dean Emeritus and Professor Emeritus
of Pediatric Dentistry
Indiana University School of Dentistry
Indianapolis, Indiana

DAVID R. AVERY, DDS, MSD
Ralph E. McDonald Professor and Director
of Pediatric Dentistry
Indiana University School of Dentistry
James Whitcomb Riley Hospital for Children
Indianapolis, Indiana

JEFFREY A. DEAN, DDS, MSD
Associate Professor of Pediatric Dentistry and Orthodontics
Director, Advanced Education Program in Pediatric Dentistry
Acting Chair, Department of Oral Facial Development
Indiana University School of Dentistry
James Whitcomb Riley Hospital for Children
Indianapolis, Indiana

EIGHTH EDITION

with 710 illustrations

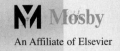

Mosby
An Affiliate of Elsevier

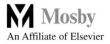

An Affiliate of Elsevier

11830 Westline Industrial Drive
St. Louis, Missouri 63146

NOTICE

Dentistry is an ever-changing field. Standard safety precautions must be followed, but as new
research and clinical experience broaden our knowledge, changes in treatment and drug therapy
may become necessary or appropriate. Readers are advised to check the most current product
information provided by the manufacturer of each drug to be administered to verify the
recommended dose, the method and duration of administration, and contraindications. It is the
responsibility of the licensed prescriber, relying on experience and knowledge of the patient, to
determine dosages and the best treatment for each individual patient. Neither the publisher nor
the authors assume any liability for any injury and/or damage to persons or property arising from
this publication.

Previous editions copyrighted 1969, 1974, 1978, 1983, 1988, 1994, 2000

Library of Congress Cataloging-in-Publication Data

Dentistry for the child and adolescent / [edited by] Ralph E. McDonald, David R. Avery,
    Jeffrey A. Dean.—8th ed.
        p. ; cm.
    Includes bibliographical references and index.
    ISBN 0-323-02450-5
      1. Pedodontics. 2. Youth—Dental care. I. McDonald, Ralph E., 1920- II. Avery, David
R. III. Dean, Jeffrey A., D.D.S.
      [DNLM: 1. Dental Care for Children. 2. Pediatric Dentistry—methods. WU 480 D4145 2004]
    RK55.C5D44 2004
617.6'45—dc22   2003068648

Executive Editor: Penny Rudolph
Senior Developmental Editor: Jaime Pendill
Publishing Services Manager: Patricia Tannian
Senior Project Manager: Anne Altepeter
Book Design Manager: Gail Morey Hudson

Printed in the United States of America

Last digit is the print number: 9 8 7 6 5 4 3 2 1

Contributors

CHRISTOPHER EDWARD BELCHER, MD
Director
Pediatric Infectious Diseases
Infectious Diseases of Indiana
Indianapolis, Indiana

DAVID BIXLER, DDS, PhD
Professor Emeritus of Oral Facial Genetics
    and Medical and Molecular Genetics
Indiana University
Indianapolis, Indiana

DAVID T. BROWN, DDS, MS
Professor, Department of Restorative Dentistry
Indiana University School of Dentistry
Indianapolis, Indiana

DAVID A. BUSSARD, DDS, MS
Assistant Clinical Professor of Oral and Maxillofacial
    Surgery
Indiana University School of Dentistry
Private Practice of Oral and Maxillofacial Surgery
Indianapolis, Indiana

ROBERT L. CREEDON, DDS
Professor Emeritus
Department of Pediatrics/Dentistry
College of Medicine, University of Cincinnati
Director, Division of Pediatric Dentistry (retired)
Department of Pediatrics
Cincinnati Children's Hospital Medical Center
Cincinnati, Ohio

ROBERT J. CRONIN, Jr., DDS, MS
Professor and Director, Graduate Division
Department of Prosthodontics
The University of Texas Health Science Center at
    San Antonio Dental School
San Antonio, Texas

MURRAY DOCK, DDS, MSD, RPh
Associate Professor
Department of Pediatrics
College of Medicine, University of Cincinnati
Director, Residency Program in Pediatric Dentistry
Division of Pediatric Dentistry
Cincinnati Children's Hospital Medical Center
Cincinnati, Ohio

ROBERT J. FEIGAL, DDS, PhD
Professor and Chair, Department of Preventive
    Sciences
School of Dentistry, University of Minnesota
Minneapolis, Minnesota

DONALD J. FERGUSON, DMD, MSD
Professor and Chair, Department of Orthodontics
Director, Advanced Orthodontic Training
    Program
Henry M. Goldman School of Dental Medicine
Boston University
Boston, Massachusetts

CHARLES J. GOODACRE, DDS, MSD
Dean and Professor, Department of Restorative
    Dentistry, School of Dentistry
Loma Linda University
Loma Linda, California

ANN PAGE GRIFFIN, BA
Clinical Associate Professor
Department of Family Medicine
East Carolina University
Greenville, North Carolina
Faculty Associate, Department of Pediatric
    Dentistry
College of Dentistry, University of Tennessee
Memphis, Tennessee

LEE M. HARRISON, Jr., DDS, MS
Clinical Associate Professor
Department of Pediatric Dentistry
School of Dentistry, Louisiana State University
New Orleans, Louisiana
Private Practice of Pediatric Dentistry
Shreveport, Louisiana

JAMES K. HARTSFIELD, Jr., DMD, MS, MMedSci, PhD
Professor and Director of Oral Facial Genetics
Professor of Orthodontics
Department of Oral Facial Development
School of Dentistry, Indiana University
Professor, Department of Medical and Molecular
    Genetics
School of Medicine, Indiana University
President, Meridian Orthodontics, PC
Indianapolis, Indiana

ROBERTA A. HIBBARD, MD
Professor, Department of Pediatrics
School of Medicine, Indiana University
Indianapolis, Indiana

RANDY A. HOCK, MD, PhD
Medical Director
Department of Pediatric Hematology/Oncology and
    Pediatric Hospice
St. Vincent Children's Hospital
Indianapolis, Indiana

DONALD V. HUEBENER, DDS, MS, MAEd
Professor, Plastic and Reconstructive Surgery
Department of Surgery, School of Medicine
Washington University, St. Louis, Missouri
Professor, Pediatric Dentistry
School of Dental Medicine
Southern Illinois University
Alton, Illinois

CHRISTOPHER V. HUGHES, DMD, PhD
Associate Professor and Chair
Department of Pediatric Dentistry
Henry M. Goldman School of Dental Medicine
Boston University
Boston, Massachusetts

JAMES E. JONES, DMD, MSD, PhD, EdD
Dean and Professor, School of Health Sciences
Indiana University Purdue University—
  Fort Wayne
Fort Wayne, Indiana
Professor of Pediatric Dentistry
Indiana University School of Dentistry
Indianapolis, Indiana

GEORGE E. KRULL, DDS
Private Practice of Pediatric Dentistry
Clarkston, Michigan

JOHN T. KRULL, DDS
Assistant Professor of Pediatric Dentistry
Indiana University School of Dentistry
Private Practice of Orthodontics
Indianapolis, Indiana

THOMAS H. LAPP, DDS, MS
Clinical Assistant Professor of Oral and Maxillofacial
  Surgery
Indiana University School of Dentistry
Private Practice of Oral and Maxillofacial
  Surgery
Indianapolis, Indiana

JASPER L. LEWIS, Jr., DDS, MS
Clinical Assistant Professor, Department
  of Pediatric Dentistry, College of
  Dentistry
University of Tennessee
Memphis, Tennessee
Clinical Professor, Department of Surgery
Chief of the Division of Dentistry
Clinical Assistant Professor
Department of Family Medicine
School of Medicine, East Carolina University
Private Practice of Pediatric Dentistry
Greenville, North Carolina

JAMES L. McDONALD, Jr., PhD
Professor of Oral Biology
Associate Dean for Dental Education
Indiana University School of Dentistry
Indianapolis, Indiana

JOHN S. McDONALD, DDS, MS, FACD
Volunteer Professor
Departments of Surgery and Anesthesia
Volunteer Associate Professor
Department of Pediatrics
Division of Pediatric Dentistry
College of Medicine, University of Cincinnati
Cincinnati, Ohio
Private Practice of Oral and Maxillofacial
  Pathology/Head and Neck Pain
Cincinnati, Ohio

DALE A. MILES, DDS, MS, FRCD(C)
Professor of Oral and Maxillofacial Radiology
Associate Dean for Clinical Affairs and
  Faculty Development
Arizona School of Dentistry and Oral Health
Mesa, Arizona

B. KEITH MOORE, PhD
Professor and Director of Dental Materials
  Graduate Program
Indiana University School of Dentistry
Indianapolis, Indiana

EDWIN T. PARKS, DMD, MS
Professor of Oral Pathology,
Medicine and Radiology
Indiana University School of Dentistry
Indianapolis, Indiana

ALAN MICHAEL SADOVE, MD
James Harbaugh Endowed Professor of
  Plastic Surgery
Indiana University School of Medicine
Chief, Plastic Surgery
James Whitcomb Riley Hospital for Children
Indianapolis, Indiana

BRIAN J. SANDERS, DDS, MS
Associate Professor of Pediatric Dentistry
Indiana University School of Dentistry
Director, Clinic Pediatric Dentistry
James Whitcomb Riley Hospital for Children
Indianapolis, Indiana

AMY D. SHAPIRO, MD
Medical Director
Indiana Hemophilia and Thrombosis Center, Inc.
Indianapolis, Indiana

GEORGE K. STOOKEY, MSD, PhD
Distinguished Professor Emeritus of Preventive and
  Community Dentistry
Indiana University School of Dentistry
Indianapolis, Indiana

JAMES A. WEDDELL, DDS, MSD
Associate Professor of Pediatric Dentistry
Indiana University School of Dentistry
James Whitcomb Riley Hospital for Children
Indianapolis, Indiana

GERALD Z. WRIGHT, DDS, MSD, FRCD(C)
Professor Emeritus
The University of Western Ontario
London, Ontario, Canada
Secretary General,
International Association of Paediatric Dentistry

KAREN M. YODER, MSD, PhD
Associate Professor and Director of Community
  Dentistry
Indiana University School of Dentistry
Indianapolis, Indiana

Preface

The eighth edition of *Dentistry for the Child and Adolescent* presents current diagnostic and treatment recommendations based on research, clinical experience, and current literature. This newest edition follows the same basic structure and format of the previous seven editions. The contributors who joined us in preparation of this latest revision express a coordinated philosophy in the approach to the most modern concepts of dentistry for the child and adolescent. The information contained herein is relevant to the contemporary science and practice of pediatric dentistry. This textbook is designed to help undergraduate dental students and postdoctoral pediatric dental students provide efficient and superior comprehensive oral health care to infants, children, teenagers, and medically compromised individuals. It also provides experienced dentists with reference information regarding new developments and techniques.

Chapter 2, Child Abuse and Neglect, includes an up-to-date overview of this topic and management of documentation and reporting requirements. In addition, the chapter contains several new photographs to help illustrate this societal problem. Chapter 5, Radiographic Techniques, includes new information on the use of digital radiography in pediatric dentistry. Chapter 6, Clinical Genetics for the Dental Practitioner, has a new lead author and provides updated information in several topic areas, particularly in genetic influence on external apical root resorption associated with orthodontic treatment. Theories relating to the molecular biology of tooth eruption are provided in Chapter 9. Chapter 10, Dental Caries in the Child and Adolescent, has been reformatted and presents much new information to reflect contemporary knowledge and management of the disease as well as an increased emphasis on early childhood caries. Chapter 13, Local Anesthesia for the Child and Adolescent, has been expanded to include a section on anxiety control, pain, and the use of analgesics in pediatric dentistry. Chapter 14, Pharmacologic Management of Patient Behavior, has a new lead author and has been thoroughly reviewed and updated to provide the latest information regarding sedation techniques for children. Chapter 17, Pit and Fissure Sealants and Preventive Resin Restorations, has undergone a major revision; a new co-author has provided fresh illustrations for the chapter as well. Chapter 18, Restorative Dentistry, provides an increased emphasis on the latest restorative materials and in particular on the "alternative restorative technique." Treatment modalities for pulp therapy and trauma have been incorporated in Chapters 19 and 21 that utilize the new science and information associated with molecular biology, in an attempt to maintain the vitality of the tissues associated with these treatments whenever possible. Chapter 23, Dental Problems of Children with Disabilities, and Chapter 24, Management of the Medically Compromised Patient, have been updated and revised to include information regarding the dental management of patients with sickle cell anemia. The latest information on the incorporation of early orthodontic treatment has been added to Chapter 27, Management of the Developing Occlusion, and a new co-author has helped with Chapter 28, Multidisciplinary Team Approach to Cleft Lip and Palate Management. In particular, the protocols developed by the American Cleft Palate–Craniofacial Association have been incorporated. And finally, Chapter 29, Practice Management, has been revised significantly and Chapter 30, Community Oral Health, has been completely rewritten.

Ralph E. McDonald
David R. Avery
Jeffrey A. Dean

Acknowledgments

A textbook can be planned and written only with the supportive interest, encouragement, and tangible contributions of many people. Therefore, it is a privilege to acknowledge the assistance of others in the preparation of this text. First of all, we would like to thank the many authors and co-authors who have made this eighth edition possible. Donna Bumgardner and Elizabeth Holsapple provided manuscript preparation and valuable editorial assistance. Mark Dirlam, Kyla Jones, Tom Meador, and Terry Wilson provided assistance with new illustrations. Our excellent library staff was eager to help in any way possible, and the assistance of Susan Beane, Janice Cox, Amy Edwards, Sue Hutchinson, and Kirk Smith is much appreciated. We also gratefully acknowledge the professional staff at Elsevier who has provided valuable assistance and superb guidance in the publication of this eighth edition; special thanks to Penny Rudolph, executive editor; Jaime Pendill, senior developmental editor; and Anne Altepeter, senior project manager.

The faculties of pediatric dentistry and other disciplines at Indiana University have contributed substantially to this work in many ways. We truly appreciate their willingness to share information relevant to scientific accuracy of the manuscripts. In particular, we gratefully acknowledge Drs. Michael Baumgartner, Howard Eigen, Margherita Fontana, Richard Gregory, Michelle Howenstine, Vanchit John, Gopal Krishna, Chris Miller, John Rau, Paul Walker, and Susan Zunt. Many pediatric dentistry postdoctoral students and auxiliary staff have also assisted in numerous ways. The encouragement and support of all members of our families sustained our resolve to complete this task when it seemed that it would not get done. We extend our heartfelt thanks to all who played a role in helping us bring this project to a successful conclusion.

Contents

1

Examination of the Mouth and Other Relevant Structures

RALPH E. McDONALD

DAVID R. AVERY

JEFFREY A. DEAN

CHAPTER OUTLINE

A dentist is traditionally taught to perform a complete oral examination of the patient and to develop a treatment plan from the examination findings. Then the dentist makes a case presentation to the patient or parents, outlining the recommended course of treatment. This process should include the development and presentation of a prevention plan that outlines an ongoing comprehensive oral health care program for the patient and establishment of the "dental home."

The plan should include recommendations designed to correct existing oral problems (or halt their progression) and to prevent anticipated future problems. It is essential to obtain all relevant patient and family information, to secure parental consent, and to perform a complete examination before embarking on this comprehensive oral health care program for the pediatric patient. *Anticipatory guidance* is the term often used to describe the discussion and implementation of such a plan with the patient and/or parents. The American Academy of Pediatric Dentistry has published guidelines concerning the periodicity of examination, preventive dental services, and oral treatment for children as summarized in Fig. 1-1.

Each pediatric patient should be given an opportunity to receive complete dental care. The dentist should not attempt to decide what the child, parents, or third-party agent will accept or can afford. If parents reject a portion or all of the recommendations, the dentist has at least fulfilled the obligation of educating the child and the parents about the importance of the recommended procedures. Parents of even moderate income will usually find the means to have oral health care completed if the dentist explains to them that the child's future oral health and even general health are related to the correction of oral defects.

INITIAL PARENTAL CONTACT WITH THE DENTAL OFFICE

The parent usually makes the first contact with the dental office by telephone. This initial conversation between the parent and the office receptionist is very important. It provides the first opportunity to attend to the parent's concerns by pleasantly and concisely responding to questions and by offering an office appointment. The receptionist must have a warm, friendly voice and the ability to communicate clearly. The receptionist's responses should assure the parent that the well-being of the child is the chief concern.

The information recorded by the receptionist during this conversation constitutes the initial dental record for the patient. Filling out a patient information form is a convenient method of collecting the necessary initial information (see Fig. 29-2). Additional discussion of the initial communication with parents is presented in Chapter 29.

THE DIAGNOSTIC METHOD

Before making a diagnosis and developing a treatment plan, the dentist must collect and evaluate the facts associated with the patient's or parents' chief concern and any other identified problems that may be unknown to the patient or parents. Some pathognomonic signs may lead to an almost immediate diagnosis. For example, obvious gingival swelling and drainage may be associated with a single, badly carious primary molar. Although the collection and evaluation of these associated facts are performed rapidly, they provide a diagnosis only for a single problem area. On the other hand, a comprehensive diagnosis of all the patient's problems or potential problems may sometimes need to be postponed until more urgent conditions are resolved. For example, a patient with necrotizing ulcerative gingivitis or a newly fractured crown needs immediate treatment, but the treatment will likely be only palliative, and further diagnostic and treatment procedures will be required later.

The importance of thoroughly collecting and evaluating the facts concerning a patient's condition cannot be overemphasized. Moskow and Barr[1] have described several examination methods that aid the dentist in this process.

The following list of methods is based largely on their chapter "Examination of the Patient" in *Current Therapy in Dentistry:*

- Medical and dental history taking
- Inspection
- Palpation
- Auscultation
- Exploration
- Radiography
- Percussion
- Transillumination
- Vitality tests
- Study casts
- Laboratory tests
- Photography

In certain unusual cases all of these diagnostic aids may be necessary to arrive at a comprehensive diagnosis. Certainly no oral diagnosis can be complete unless the diagnostician has evaluated the facts obtained by medical and dental history taking, inspection, palpation, exploration (if teeth are present), and often imaging (radiographs, etc.). For a more thorough review of evaluation of the dental patient, the reader is referred to the chapter by Glick, Siegel, and Brightman in the textbook *Burket's Oral Medicine.*

Guidelines on Periodicity of Examination, Preventive Dental Services, Anticipatory Guidance, and Oral Treatment for Children, Revised May 2000

Birth-12 Months
1. Complete the clinical oral assessment and appropriate diagnostic tests to assess oral growth and development and/or pathology.
2. Provide oral hygiene counseling for parents, guardians, and caregivers, including the implications of the oral health of the caregiver.
3. Remove supra- and subgingival stains or deposits as indicated.
4. Assess the child's systemic and topical fluoride status (including type of infant formula used, if any, and exposure to fluoridated toothpaste), and provide counseling regarding fluoride. Prescribe systemic fluoride supplements if indicated, following assessment of total fluoride intake from drinking water, diet, and oral hygiene products.
5. Assess appropriateness of feeding practices, including bottle feeding and breast-feeding, and provide counseling as indicated.
6. Provide dietary counseling related to oral health.
7. Provide age-appropriate injury prevention counseling for orofacial trauma.
8. Provide counseling for non-nutritive oral habits (e.g., digit, pacifiers).
9. Provide diagnosis and required treatment and/or appropriate referral for any oral diseases or injuries.
10. Provide anticipatory guidance for parent/guardian.
11. Consult with the child's physician as indicated.
12. Based on evaluation and history, assess the patient's risk for oral disease.
13. Determine interval for periodic reevaluation.

12-24 Months
1. Repeat birth to 12-month procedures every 6 months or as indicated by the individual patient's needs/susceptibility to disease.
2. Review patient's fluoride status, including any child care arrangements that may affect systemic fluoride intake and provide parental counseling.

3. Provide topical fluoride treatments every 6 months or as indicated by the individual patient's needs.

2-6 Years
1. Repeat 12- to 24-month procedures every 6 months or as indicated by the individual patient's needs/susceptibility to disease. Provide age-appropriate oral hygiene instructions.
2. Complete a radiographic assessment of pathology and/or abnormal growth and development, as indicated by the individual patient's needs.
3. Scale and clean the teeth every 6 months or as indicated by the individual patient's needs.
4. Provide topical fluoride treatments every 6 months or as indicated by the individual patient's needs.
5. Provide pit and fissure sealants for primary and permanent teeth as indicated by the individual patient's needs.
6. Provide counseling and services (athletic mouth guards) as needed for or ofacial trauma prevention.
7. Provide assessment/treatment or referral of developing malocclusion as indicated by the individual patient's needs.
8. Provide diagnosis and required treatment and/or appropriate referral for any oral disease, habits, or injuries as indicated.
9. Assess speech and language development, and provide appropriate referral as indicated.

6-12 Years
1. Repeat 2- to 6-year procedures every 6 months or as indicated by the individual patient's needs/susceptibility to disease.
2. Provide substance abuse counseling (e.g., smoking, smokeless tobacco).

12-18 Years
1. Repeat 6- to 12-year procedures every 6 months or as indicated by the individual patient's needs/susceptibility to disease.
2. At an age determined by the patient, parent, and dentist, refer the patient to a general dentist for continuing oral care.

FIG. **1-1.** General oral health care guidelines for children.

PRELIMINARY MEDICAL AND DENTAL HISTORY

It is important for the dentist to be familiar with the medical and dental history of the pediatric patient. Familial history may also be relevant to the patient's oral condition and may provide important diagnostic information in some hereditary disorders. Before the dentist examines the child, the dental assistant can obtain sufficient information to provide the dentist with knowledge of the child's general health and can alert the dentist to the need for obtaining additional information from the parent or the child's physician. The form illustrated in Fig. 1-2 can be completed by the parent. However, it is more effective for the dental assistant to

ask the questions informally and then to present the findings to the dentist and offer personal observations and a summary of the case. The questions included on the form will also provide information about any previous dental treatment.

Information regarding the child's social and psychologic development is important. Accurate information reflecting a child's learning, behavioral, or communication problems is sometimes difficult to obtain initially, especially if the parents are aware of their child's developmental disorder but are reluctant to discuss it. Behavior problems in the dental office are often related to the child's inability to communicate with the dentist and to follow instructions. This inability may be attributable to a learning disorder. An indication of learning

DATE_____

Child's name_____ Sex_____ Birth date_____ Place of birth_____
           Last, first, nickname

Date of last medical examination _____ Child's physician/pediatrician _____ Telephone_____

Physician's address _____

MEDICAL HISTORY

GROWTH AND DEVELOPMENT Any learnig, behavioral, excessive nervousness, or communication
problems?   No ( )   Yes ( )
Has child had psychological counseling or is counseling being considered for the near future?   No ( )   Yes ( )
Were there any complications during pregnancy or was child premature at birth?   No ( )   Yes ( )
Any problems with physical growth?   No ( )   Yes ( )

CENTRAL NERVOUS SYSTEM Any history of cerebral palsy, seizures, convulsions, fainting, or loss of
consciousness?   No ( )   Yes ( )
Any history of injury to the head?   No ( )   Yes ( )
Any sensory disorders? (Seeing, Hearing)   No ( )   Yes ( )

CARDIOVASCULAR SYSTEM Any history of congenital heart disease, heart murmur, or heart damage
from rheumatic fever?   No ( )   Yes ( )
Has any heart surgery been done or recommended?   No ( )   Yes ( )
Any history of chest pains or high blood pressure?   No ( )   Yes ( )

HEMATOPOIETIC AND LYMPHATIC SYSTEMS Has your child ever had a blood transfusion or blood
products transfusion?   No ( )   Yes ( )
Any history of anemia or sickle cell disease?   No ( )   Yes ( )
Does your child bruise easily, have frequent nosebleeds, or bleed excessively from small cuts?   No ( )   Yes ( )
Is your child more susceptible to infections than other children are?   No ( )   Yes ( )
Is there any history of tender or swollen lymph nodes or glands?   No ( )   Yes ( )

RESPIRATORY SYSTEM Any history of pneumonia, cystic fibrosis, asthma, shortness of breath, or difficulty in breathing?   No ( )   Yes ( )

GASTROINTESTINAL SYSTEM Any history of stomach, intestinal or liver problems?   No ( )   Yes ( )
Any history of hepatitis or jaundice?   No ( )   Yes ( )
Any history of eating disorders, such as anorexia nervosa or bulimia (binge/purge)?   No ( )   Yes ( )
Any history of unintentional weight loss?   No ( )   Yes ( )

GENITOURINARY SYSTEM Any history of urinary tract infections, bladder or kidney problems?   No ( )   Yes ( )
Is the patient pregnant or possibly pregnant?   No ( )   Yes ( )

ENDOCRINE SYSTEM Any history of diabetes?   No ( )   Yes ( )
Any history of thyroid disorders or other glandular disorders?   No ( )   Yes ( )

SKIN Any history of skin problems?   No ( )   Yes ( )
Any history of cold sores (herpes) or canker sores (aphthae)?   No ( )   Yes ( )

EXTREMITIES Any limitations of use of arms or legs?   No ( )   Yes ( )
Any arthritis, joint bleeding, joint replacements or other joint problems?   No ( )   Yes ( )
Any problems with muscle weakness or muscular dystrophy?   No ( )   Yes ( )

ALLERGIES Is your child allergic to any medication?   No ( )   Yes ( )
Any hay fever, hives, or skin rashes caused by allergies?   No ( )   Yes ( )
Any other allergies?   No ( )   Yes ( )

MEDICATIONS OR TREATMENTS Is your child currently taking any medication (prescription or non-
prescription medicine)?   No ( )   Yes ( )
If yes, Medication(s)   Dose   Times per day
_____   _____   _____
_____   _____   _____
_____   _____   _____

Has your child ever recieved radiation therapy (x-ray treatments) or is it planned?   No ( )   Yes ( )
Has your child ever recieved chemotherapy or is it planned?   No ( )   Yes ( )

HOSPITALIZATIONS
Has your child been hospitalized?
Hospital   (1)_____   (2)_____   (3)_____
Date   _____   _____   _____
Reason   _____   _____   _____

FIG. **1-2.** Form used in completing the preliminary medical and dental history.   *Continued*

disorders can usually be obtained by the dental assistant while asking questions about the child's learning process; for example, asking a young school-aged child how he or she is doing in school is a good lead question. Remember, though, to keep the questions age-appropriate to the child.

A notation should be made if a young child has been hospitalized previously for general anesthetic and surgical procedures. Shaw has reported that hospitalization and a general anesthetic procedure can be a traumatic psychologic experience for a preschool child and may sensitize the youngster to procedures that will

IMMUNIZATIONS: Is your child presently protected by immunization against

DPT: diphtheria, whooping cough (pertussis), tetanus?	No ( )	Yes ( )
IPV: polio or poliomyelitis?	No ( )	Yes ( )
MMR: measles (rubeola), mumps, and German measles (rubella)?	No ( )	Yes ( )
Hib (*Haemophilus b*)?	No ( )	Yes ( )
Pneumococcal pneumonia?	No ( )	Yes ( )
Hepatitis B	No ( )	Yes ( )

PLEASE CHECK ANY OF THE ILLNESSES THAT YOUR CHILD HAS NOW, HAS RECENTLY BEEN EXPOSED TO, OR HAS HAD IN THE PAST:

	Now	Exposed	Past
• Chickenpox (varicella)	☐	☐	☐
• Earache (otitis)	☐	☐	☐
• Eye infection (conjunctivitis)	☐	☐	☐
• German measles or 3-day measles (rubella)	☐	☐	☐
• Glandular fever or mono (infectious mononucleosis)	☐	☐	☐
• HIV/AIDS	☐	☐	☐
• Lead poisoning	☐	☐	☐
• Measles (rubella)	☐	☐	☐
• Mumps (parotitis)	☐	☐	☐
• Scarlet fever (scarlatina)	☐	☐	☐
• Sore throat (tonsillitis or pharyngitis)	☐	☐	☐
• Substance abuse, alcoholism, drug addiction	☐	☐	☐
• Tuberculosis	☐	☐	☐
• Upper respiratory infection (URI), or common cold (pharyngitis, rhinitis, sinusitis, or tonsillitis)	☐	☐	☐
• Venereal disease (genital herpes, gonorrhea, syphilis or other)	☐	☐	☐

DENTAL HISTORY

Does your child have a toothache or other immediate dental problem?	No ( )	Yes ( )
Has your child ever had a toothache?	No ( )	Yes ( )
Has your child had any injury to the mouth, teeth or jaws (fall, blow, etc.)?	No ( )	Yes ( )
Is this your child's first dental visit? If no:	No ( )	Yes ( )

Date: Dentist: Reason:

Has your child ever had an unfavorable dental experience?	No ( )	Yes ( )
Is (was) your child nourished by nursing beyond one year of age? If yes:	No ( )	Yes ( )

Check: Breast_____ Nursing bottle_____ Both_____ ,and to what age?_____

Does your child fail to eat a well-balanced diet? If yes, what foods or food groups are not adequate?	No ( )	Yes ( )

_____

Does (or has) your child have (or had) sucking habit beyond one year of age? If yes:	No ( )	Yes ( )

Check: Thumb(s)_____ Finger(s)_____ Pacifier_____ Other:_____

Does (or has) your child have (or had) any other oral habits beyond one year of age? If yes:	No ( )	Yes ( )

Check: Lip biting_____ Mouth breathing,_____ Nail biting_____ Teeth grinding_____ Other_____

Does (or has) your child have (or had) difficulty opening his or her mouth, or does the child's jaw sometimes lock or stick in a certain position?	No ( )	Yes ( )
Does (or has) your child have (or had) popping or clicking noises or pain during chewing or yawning?	No ( )	Yes ( )
Does (or has) your child have (or had) frequent headaches or pain in or about the ears, eyes, or cheeks?	No ( )	Yes ( )

DENTAL DISEASE PREVENTION

How often does your child brush?_____ times per_____	No ( )	Yes ( )
Does your child use dental floss?	No ( )	Yes ( )
Does someone assist your child with brushing and cleaning the teeth?	No ( )	Yes ( )
Does someone inspect for thoroughness after the procedure?	No ( )	Yes ( )
Does your child use a fluoride toothpaste?	No ( )	Yes ( )
Has your child ever had a fluoride treatment?	No ( )	Yes ( )
Has your child ever taken fluoride supplement or vitamins with fluorides?	No ( )	Yes ( )

DRINKING WATER SOURCE

City water supply_____ Name of city_____

Private well or other than city_____ Has a fluoride analysis been done?_____

Date of analysis_____ Fluoride content_____

▶ Signature (Parent or guardian)   ▶ Student Signature

DENTIST'S COMMENTS:

Medical consultation recommended? No_____ Yes_____ Date requested_____

Purpose for consultation:_____

SEMIANNUAL REVIEW OF MEDICAL-DENTAL HISTORY: If history remains essentially unchanged, sign below

Date_____ Parent_____ Student_____

Date_____ Parent_____ Student_____

Date_____ Parent_____ Student_____

A new history form should be completed at least every 2 years.

FIG. **1-2, cont'd**, Form used in completing the preliminary medical and dental history.

be encountered later in a dental office.[2] If the dentist is aware of previous hospitalization and the child's fear of strangers in clinic attire, the necessary time and procedures can be planned to help the child overcome the fear and accept dental treatment.

Occasionally, when the parents report significant disorders, it is best for the dentist to conduct the medical and dental history interview. When the parents meet with the dentist privately, they are more likely to discuss the child's problems openly and there is less chance for misunderstandings regarding the nature of the disorders. In addition, the dentist's personal involvement at this early time strengthens the confidence of the parents. When there is indication of an acute or chronic systemic disease or anomaly, the dentist should consult the child's physician to learn the status of the condition, the long-range prognosis, and the current drug therapy.

Current illnesses or histories of significant disorders signal the need for special attention during the medical and dental history interview. In addition to consulting the child's physician, the dentist may decide to record additional data concerning the child's current physical condition, such as blood pressure, body temperature, heart sounds, height and weight, pulse, and respiration. Before treatment is initiated, certain laboratory tests may be indicated and special precautions may be necessary. A decision to provide treatment in a hospital and possibly under general anesthesia may be appropriate.

The dentist and the staff must also be alert to identify potentially communicable infectious conditions that threaten the health of the patient and others as well. Knowledge of the current recommended childhood immunization schedule is helpful. It is advisable to postpone nonemergency dental care for a patient exhibiting signs or symptoms of acute infectious disease until the patient has recovered. Further discussions of management of dental patients with special medical, physical, or behavioral problems are presented in Chapters 2, 3, 14, 15, 23, 24, and 28.

The pertinent facts of the medical history can be transferred to the oral examination record (Fig. 1-3) for easy reference by the dentist. A brief summary of important medical information serves as a convenient reminder to the dentist and the staff, because they refer to this chart at each treatment visit.

The patient's dental history should also be summarized on the examination chart. This should include a record of previous care in the dentist's office and the facts related by the patient and the parent regarding previous care in another office. Information concerning the patient's current oral hygiene habits and previous and current fluoride exposure helps the dentist develop an effective dental disease prevention program for the patient. For example, if the family drinks well water, a sample may be sent to a water analysis laboratory to determine the fluoride concentration.

CLINICAL EXAMINATION

Most facts needed for a comprehensive oral diagnosis in the young patient are obtained by a thorough clinical and radiographic examination. In addition to examining the structures in the oral cavity, the dentist may in some cases wish to note the patient's size, stature, gait, or involuntary movements. The first clue to malnutrition may come from observing a patient's abnormal size or stature. Similarly, the severity of a child's illness, even if oral in origin, may be recognized by observing a weak,

unsteady gait of lethargy and malaise as the patient walks into the office. All relevant information should be noted on the oral examination record (see Fig. 1-3), which becomes a permanent part of the patient's chart.

The clinical examination, whether the first examination or a regular recall examination, should be all inclusive. The dentist can gather useful information while getting acquainted with a new patient. Attention to the patient's hair, head, face, neck, and hands should be among the first observations made by the dentist after the patient is seated in the chair.

The patient's hands may reveal information pertinent to the comprehensive diagnosis. The dentist may first detect an elevated temperature by holding the patient's hand. Cold, clammy hands or bitten fingernails may be the first indication of abnormal anxiety in the child. A callused or unusually clean digit suggests a persistent sucking habit. Clubbing of the fingers or a bluish color in the nail beds suggests congenital heart disease that may require special precautions during dental treatment.

Inspection and palpation of the patient's head and neck are also indicated. Unusual characteristics of the hair or skin should be noted. The dentist may observe signs of head lice (Fig. 1-4), ringworm (Fig. 1-5), or impetigo (Fig. 1-6) during the examination. Proper referral is indicated immediately, since these conditions are contagious. After the child's physician has supervised the treatment to control the condition, the child's dental appointment may be rescheduled. If a contagious condition is identified but the child also has a dental emergency, the dentist and the staff must take appropriate precautions to prevent spread of the disease to others while the emergency is alleviated. Further treatment should be postponed until the contagious condition is controlled.

Variations in size, shape, symmetry, or function of the head and neck structures should be recorded. Abnormalities of these structures may indicate various syndromes or conditions associated with oral abnormalities.

TEMPOROMANDIBULAR EVALUATION

In 1989, Okeson and others[3] published a special report on temporomandibular disorders in children. The authors indicated that, although several studies include children 5 to 7 years of age, most observations have been made on the young adolescent. Studies have placed the findings into the categories of symptoms or signs—those reported by the child or parents and those identified by the dentist during the examination.

One should evaluate temporomandibular joint (TMJ) function by palpating the head of each mandibular condyle and observing the patient while the mouth is

ORAL EXAMINATION RECORD

Patient _____ Birth date _____ Chart _____ Date
           LAST   FIRST   NICKNAME

MEDICAL HISTORY SUMMARY
Last history completed _____
Current medical status and medications:

DENTAL HISTORY SUMMARY
Date of: Last exam _____ Last radiographs F.M. _____ B.W. _____ Other _____

Appliances: _____ Last cemented _____
Describe any present problem:

Past treatment summarized:

EXTRA-ORAL FINDINGS
Head
Neck
Face
Lips
Hands

INTRA-ORAL FINDINGS
Palate and oropharynx
Airway
Tongue and floor of mouth
Buccal mucosa
Frena
Gingivae and periodontium

PLAQUE SCORE
Today's score ☐   Last score ☐

OCCLUSION REVIEW

FACIAL PROFILE: _____
MOLAR RELATIONSHIP:
  PERMANENT R   L   PRIMARY
    Unerupted ☐ ☐   (Terminal plane) R   L
    End to end ☐ ☐   Straight   ☐ ☐
    Class   __ __   Mes. step   ☐ ☐
                        Dist. step   ☐ ☐
                        Primate space   ☐ ☐

CANINE RELATIONSHIP: R   L
  Class   __ __
INCISOR RELATIONSHIP:
  Overjet   ___ mm.
  Overbite   ___ %
  Openbite   ___ mm.
MIDLINE: Normal ☐ Deviates ☐
  Maxilla   R ☐ L ☐ mm. ___
  Mandible   R ☐ L ☐ mm. ___
  Mandibular shift No ☐ Yes ☐
    R ☐ L ☐ Ant. ☐ mm. ___
ARCH LENGTH: (general impression)
  Maxilla   Mandible
    Adequate   ☐   Adequate   ☐
    Inadequate ☐   Inadequate ☐
ERUPTION SEQUENCE AND TIMING: Normal ☐
or Describe:

TMJ AND FUNCTION:
Opening path:
  Normal Deviated _____
Closing path:
  Normal Deviated _____
Opening: ___ mm.
  Normal Limited _____
Joint Sounds:
  None   Left   Right
  Opening   _____   _____
  Closing   _____   _____
  Crepitus _____   _____
Muscle Tenderness: None _____
Tongue Function: Normal _____

CROSSBITES:

ORAL HABITS:

SUPERNUMERARY TEETH/CONGENITALLY MISSING TEETH:

ECOPTIC ERUPTION:

OTHER ANOMALIES:

ANALYSIS RECOMMENDED: No ☐   Yes ☐

FIG. **1-3.** Chart used to record the oral findings and the treatment proposed for the pediatric patient.

closed (teeth clenched), at rest, and in various open positions (Fig. 1-7, *A* and *B*). Movements of the condyles or jaw that are not smoothly flowing or deviate from the expected norm should be noted. Similarly, any crepitus that may be heard or identified by palpation, or any other abnormal sounds, should be noted. Sore masticatory muscles may also signal TMJ dysfunction. Such deviations from normal TMJ function may require further evaluation and treatment. There is a consensus (American Academy of Pediatric Dentistry, Reference

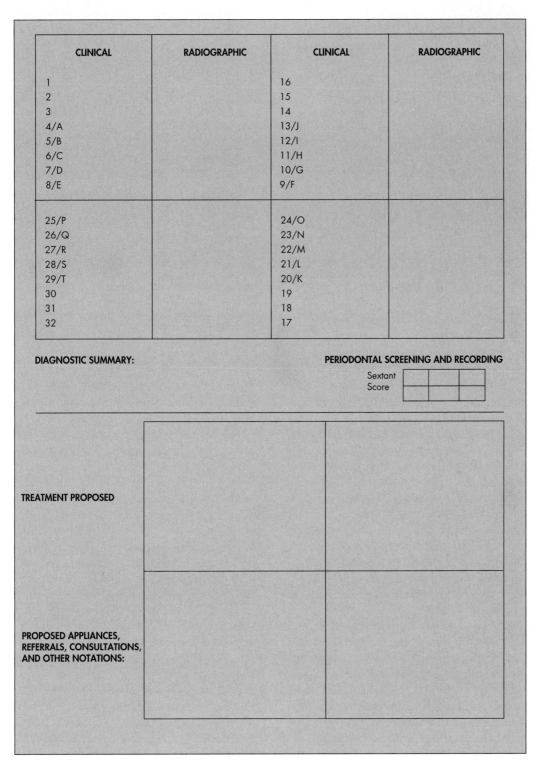

CLINICAL	RADIOGRAPHIC	CLINICAL	RADIOGRAPHIC
1		16	
2		15	
3		14	
4/A		13/J	
5/B		12/I	
6/C		11/H	
7/D		10/G	
8/E		9/F	
25/P		24/O	
26/Q		23/N	
27/R		22/M	
28/S		21/L	
29/T		20/K	
30		19	
31		18	
32		17	

DIAGNOSTIC SUMMARY:

PERIODONTAL SCREENING AND RECORDING

Sextant
Score

TREATMENT PROPOSED

PROPOSED APPLIANCES,
REFERRALS, CONSULTATIONS,
AND OTHER NOTATIONS:

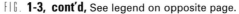

FIG. **1-3, cont'd,** See legend on opposite page.

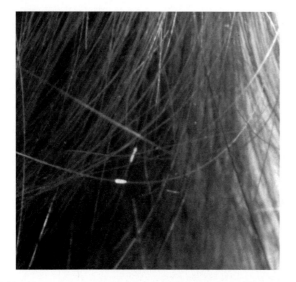

FIG. **1-4.** Evidence of head lice infestation. Usually the insects are not seen, but their eggs, or nits, cling to hair filaments until they hatch. *(Courtesy Dr. Hala Henderson.)*

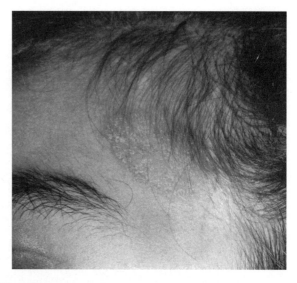

FIG. **1-5.** Lesion on forehead above left eyebrow is caused by ringworm infection. Several fungal species may cause the lesions on various areas of the body. The dentist may identify lesions on the head, face, or neck of a patient during a routine clinical examination. *(Courtesy Dr. Hala Henderson.)*

Manual 2002-2003) that temporomandibular disorders in children can be managed effectively by the following conservative and reversible therapies: patient education, mild physical therapy, behavioral therapy, medications, and occlusal splints.[4]

Discussion of the diagnosis and treatment of complex TMJ disorders goes beyond the scope of this text. However, information on this subject is available from many sources. We suggest Okeson's *Management of Temporomandibular Disorders and Occlusion* (2003) as an excellent textbook in this subject area.

The extraoral examination continues with palpation of the patient's neck and submandibular area (Fig. 1-7, *C* and *D*). Again, deviations from normal, such as unusual tenderness or enlargement, should be noted and follow-up tests performed or referrals made as indicated.

If the child is old enough to talk, speech should be evaluated. The positions of the tongue, lips, and paraoral musculature during speech, while swallowing, and while at rest may provide useful diagnostic information.

The intraoral examination of a pediatric patient should be comprehensive. There is a temptation to look first for obvious carious lesions. Certainly controlling carious lesions is important, but the dentist should first evaluate the condition of the oral soft tissues and the status of the developing occlusion. If the soft tissues and the occlusion are not observed early in the examination, the dentist may become so engrossed in charting carious lesions and in planning for their restoration that other important anomalies in

the mouth are overlooked. Any unusual breath odors and abnormal quantity or consistency of saliva should also be noted.

The buccal tissues, lips, floor of the mouth, palate, and gingivae should be carefully inspected and palpated (Fig. 1-8). The use of the periodontal screening and recording program (PSR) is often a helpful adjunct in children. PSR is designed to facilitate early detection of periodontal diseases with a simplified probing technique and minimal documentation. Clerehugh and Tugnait[5] recommend initiation of periodontal screening in children following eruption of the permanent incisors and the first molars. They suggest routine screening in these children at the child's first appointment and at regular recare appointments so that periodontal problems are detected early and treated appropriately. Immunodeficient children are especially vulnerable to early loss of bone support.

A more detailed periodontal evaluation is occasionally indicated even in young children. Periodontal disorders of children are discussed further in Chapter 20.

The tongue and oropharynx should be closely inspected. Enlarged tonsils accompanied by purulent exudate may be the initial sign of a streptococcal infection, which can lead to rheumatic fever. When streptococcal throat infection is suspected, immediate referral to the child's physician is indicated. In some cases it may be helpful to the physician and

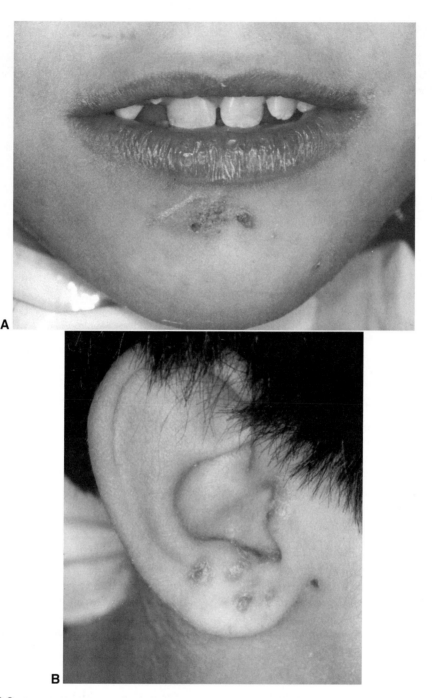

FIG. **1-6.** Characteristic lesions of impetigo, on the lower face **(A)** and on the right ear **(B)**. These lesions occur on various skin surfaces, but the dentist is most likely to encounter them on upper body areas. The infections are of bacterial (usually streptococcal) origin and generally require antibiotic therapy for control. The child often spreads the infection by scratching the lesions. *(Courtesy Dr. Hala Henderson.)*

convenient for the dentist to obtain a throat culture specimen while the child is still in the dental office, which contributes to an earlier definitive diagnosis of the infection. The diagnosis and treatment of soft tissue problems are discussed throughout this book, especially in Chapters 7, 8, and 20.

After thoroughly examining the oral soft tissues, the dentist should inspect the occlusion and note any dental or skeletal irregularities. The dentition and resulting occlusion may undergo considerable change during childhood and early adolescence. This dynamic developmental process occurs in all three planes of

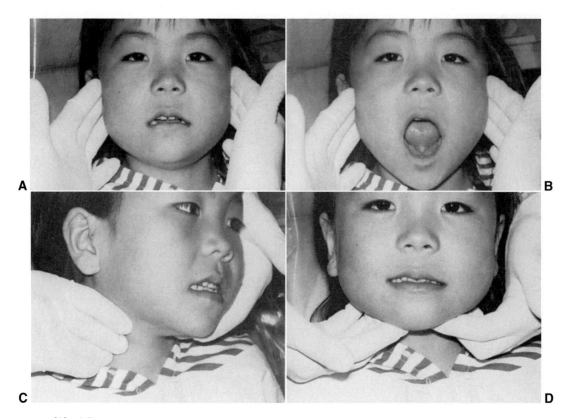

FIG. **1-7. A** and **B,** Observation and palpation of temporomandibular joint function. **C** and **D,** Palpation of the neck and submandibular areas.

space, and with periodic evaluation the dentist can intercept and favorably influence undesirable changes. Monitoring of the patient's facial profile and symmetry; molar, canine, and anterior segment relationships; dental midlines; and relation of arch length to tooth mass should be routinely included in the clinical examination. More detailed evaluation and analysis are indicated when significant discrepancies are found during critical stages of growth and development. Diagnostic cast and cephalometric analyses may be indicated relatively early in the mixed dentition stage and sometimes in the primary dentition. Detailed discussions of analyses of developing occlusions and interceptive treatment recommendations are presented in Chapters 25 through 27.

Finally, the teeth should be inspected carefully for evidence of carious lesions and hereditary or acquired anomalies. The teeth should also be counted and identified individually to ensure recognition of supernumerary or missing teeth. Identification of carious lesions is important in patients of all ages but is especially critical in young patients because the lesions may progress rapidly in early childhood caries if not controlled. Eliminating the carious activity and restoring the teeth as needed will prevent pain and the spread of infection

and also contribute to the stability of the developing occlusion.

If the dentist prefers to perform the clinical examination of a new pediatric patient before the radiographic and prophylaxis procedures, it may be necessary to correlate radiographic findings or other initially questionable findings with the findings of a second brief oral examination. This is especially true when the new patient has poor oral hygiene. Detailed inspection and exploration of the teeth and soft tissues cannot be performed adequately until the mouth is free of extraneous debris.

During the clinical examination for carious lesions each tooth should be dried individually and inspected under a good light. A definite routine for the examination should be established. For example, a dentist may always start in the upper right quadrant, work around the maxillary arch, move down to the lower left quadrant, and end the examination in the lower right quadrant. Morphologic defects and incomplete coalescence of enamel at the base of pits and fissures in molar teeth can often be detected readily by visual and explorer examination after the teeth have been cleaned and dried. The decision as to whether to place a sealant or to restore a defect depends on the patient's

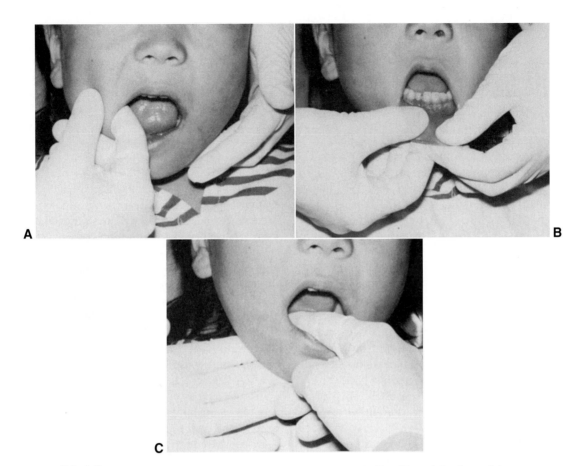

FIG. **1-8.** Inspection and palpation of the buccal tissues **(A)**, the lips **(B)**, and the floor of the mouth **(C)**.

history of dental caries, the parents' or patient's acceptance of a comprehensive preventive dentistry program (including dietary and oral hygiene control), and the patient's dependability in returning for recare appointments.

In patients with severe dental caries, caries activity tests and diet analysis may contribute to the diagnostic process by helping to define specific etiologic factors. These procedures probably have an even greater value in helping the patient or parents understand the carious disease process and in motivating them to make the behavioral changes needed to control the disease. The information provided to the patient or parents should include instruction in plaque control and the appropriate recommendations for fluoride exposure. Dental caries susceptibility, the caries disease process, caries activity tests, diet analysis, and caries control are discussed in Chapter 10. Plaque control procedures and instructions are presented in detail in Chapter 11.

The dentist's comprehensive diagnosis depends on the completion of a number of procedures but requires a thorough, systematic, and critical clinical examination. Any deviation from the expected or desired size, shape,

color, and consistency of soft or hard tissues should be described in detail. The severity of associated problems and their causes must be clearly identified to the parents or the patient before success of a comprehensive oral health care program can be expected.

During the initial examination and also at subsequent appointments, the dentist and auxiliaries should be alert to signs and symptoms of child abuse and neglect. Because of the increasing prevalence of these problems and the important role the dentist can play in detecting their signs and symptoms, Chapter 2 has been devoted to this subject.

UNIFORM DENTAL RECORDING

Many different tooth charting systems are currently in use, including the universal system illustrated in the hard tissue examination section of Fig. 1-3. This system of marking permanent teeth uses the numbers 1 to 32, beginning with the upper right third molar (No. 1) and progressing around the arch to the upper left third molar (No. 16), down to the lower left third molar (No. 17), and around the arch to the lower right third molar (No. 32). The primary teeth are identified in the universal system by the first 20 letters of the alphabet, A through T.

The Fédération Dentaire International Special Committee on Uniform Dental Recording has specified the following basic requirements for a tooth charting system:

1. Simple to understand and teach
2. Easy to pronounce in conversation and dictation
3. Readily communicable in print and by wire
4. Easy to translate into computer input
5. Easily adaptable to standard charts used in general practice

The committee found that only one system, the two-digit system, seems to comply with these requirements. According to this system, the first digit indicates the quadrant and the second digit the type of tooth within the quadrant. Quadrants are allotted the digits 1 to 4 for the permanent teeth and 5 to 8 for the primary teeth in a clockwise sequence, starting at the upper right side; teeth within the same quadrant are allotted the digits 1 to 8 (primary teeth, 1 to 5) from the midline backward. The digits should be pronounced separately; thus the permanent canines are teeth one-three, two-three, three-three, and four-three.

In the "Treatment Proposed" section of the oral examination record (see Fig. 1-3), the individual teeth that require restorative procedures, endodontic therapy, or extraction are listed. Gingival areas requiring follow-up therapy are also noted. A check mark can be placed beside each listed tooth and procedure as the treatment is completed. Additional notations concerning treatment procedures completed and the date are recorded on supplemental treatment record pages.

RADIOGRAPHIC EXAMINATION

When indicated, radiographic examination for children must be completed before the comprehensive oral health care plan can be developed, and subsequent radiographs are required periodically to allow detection of incipient carious lesions or other developing anomalies.

A child should be exposed to dental ionizing radiation only after the dentist has determined the radiographic requirement, if any, to make an adequate diagnosis for the individual child at the time of the appointment.

Obtaining isolated occlusal, periapical, or bite-wing films is sometimes indicated in very young children (even infants) because of trauma, toothache, suspected developmental disturbances, or proximal caries. Carious lesions appear smaller on radiographs than they actually are.

As early as 1967, Blayney and Hill[6] recognized the importance of diagnosing incipient proximal carious lesions with the appropriate use of radiographs. If the pediatric patient can be motivated to adopt a routine of good oral hygiene supported by competent supervision, many of these initial lesions will be arrested.

Radiographic techniques for the pediatric patient are described in detail in Chapter 5.

EARLY EXAMINATION

Historically, dental care for children has been designed primarily to prevent oral pain and infection, the occurrence and progress of dental caries, the premature loss of primary teeth, the loss of arch length, and the development of an association between fear and dental care. The dentist is responsible for guiding the child and parent, resolving oral disorders before they can affect health and dental alignment, and preventing oral disease. The goals of pediatric dental care therefore are primarily preventive. The dentist's opportunity to conduct an initial oral examination and parental consultation during the patient's infancy is a key element in achieving and maintaining these goals.

Some dentists, especially pediatric dentists, like to counsel expectant parents before their child is born. They consider it appropriate to discuss with expectant mothers the importance of good nutrition during pregnancy and practices that can influence the expected child's general and dental health.

It is also appropriate to inquire about medication the expectant mother is taking. It is known that the prolonged ingestion of tetracyclines may result in discolored, pigmented, and even hypoplastic primary teeth.

The expectant mother should be encouraged to visit her dentist and to have all carious lesions restored. The presence of active dental caries and accompanying high levels of *Streptococcus mutans* can lead to transmission by the mother to the infant and may be responsible for the development of carious lesions at a very early age.

It is not intended that the pediatric dentist should usurp the responsibility of the expectant mother's physician in recommending dietary practices, but instead that the dentist should reinforce good nutritional recommendations provided by medical colleagues.

INFANT DENTAL CARE

In 2002 the American Academy of Pediatric Dentistry revised the guidelines on infant oral health care.

The infant oral health care visit should be seen as the foundation on which a lifetime of preventive education and dental care can be built to help assure optimal oral health into childhood. Oral examination, anticipatory guidance including preventive education, and appropriate therapeutic intervention for the infant can enhance the opportunity for a lifetime of freedom from preventable oral disease.

RECOMMENDATIONS:

1. Infant oral health care begins ideally with prenatal oral health counseling for parents. An initial oral evaluation visit should occur within 6 months of the eruption of the first primary tooth and no later than 12 months of age.
2. At the infant oral evaluation visit, the dentist should do the following:
   a. Record a thorough medical and dental history, covering the prenatal, perinatal, and postnatal periods
   b. Complete a thorough oral examination
   c. Assess the patient's risk of developing oral and dental disease, and determine an appropriate interval for periodic reevaluation based on that assessment
   d. Discuss and provide anticipatory guidance regarding dental and oral development, fluoride status, nonnutritive oral habits, injury prevention, oral hygiene, and effects of diet on dentition
3. Dentists who perform such services for infants should be prepared to provide therapy when indicated or should refer the patient to an appropriately trained individual for necessary treatment.

Thus it is appropriate for a dentist to perform an oral examination for an infant of any age, even a newborn, and an examination is recommended anytime the parent or physician calls with questions concerning the appearance of an infant's oral tissues. Even when there are no known problems, the child's first dental visit and oral examination should take place by at least 1 year of age. This early dental visit enables the dentist and parents to discuss ways to nurture excellent oral health before any serious problems have had an opportunity to develop. An adequate oral examination for an infant is generally quite simple and very brief, but it may be the important first step toward a lifetime of excellent oral health.

Some dentists may prefer to "preside" during the entire first session with the infant and parents. Others may wish to delegate some of the educational aspects of the session to auxiliary members of the office staff and then conduct the examination and answer any unresolved questions. In either case, it is sometimes necessary to have an assistant available to help hold the child's attention so that the parents can concentrate on the important information being provided.

It is not always necessary to conduct the infant oral examination in the dental operatory, but it should take place where there is adequate light for a visual examination. The dentist may find it convenient to conduct the examination in the private consultation room during the initial meeting with the child and the parents. The examination procedures may include only direct observation and digital palpation. However, if primary molars have erupted or if hand instruments may be needed, the examination should be performed in an area where instrument transfers between the dental assistant and the dentist may proceed smoothly.

The parents should be informed before the examination that it will be necessary to gently restrain the child and that it is normal for the child to cry during the procedure. The infant is held on the lap of a parent, usually the mother. This direct involvement of the parent provides emotional support to the child and allows the parent to help restrain the child. Both parents may participate or at least be present during the examination.

The dentist should make a brief attempt to get acquainted with the infant and to project warmth and caring. However, many infants and toddlers are not particularly interested in developing new friendships with strangers, and the dentist should not be discouraged if the infant shuns the friendly approach. Even if the child chooses to resist (which is common and normal), only negligible extra effort is necessary to perform the examination procedure. The dentist should not be flustered by the crying and resistant behavior and should proceed unhurriedly but efficiently with the examination. The dentist's voice should remain unstrained and pleasant during the examination. The dentist's behavior should reassure the child and alleviate the parents' anxiety concerning this first dental procedure.

One method of performing the examination in a private consultation area is illustrated in Fig. 1-9, *A*. The dentist and the parent are seated face to face with their knees touching. Their upper legs form the "examination table" for the child. The child's legs straddle the parent's body, which allows the parent to restrain the child's legs and hands. An assistant is present to record the dentist's examination findings as they are dictated and to help restrain the child if needed. If adequate space is available in the consultation area, the approach illustrated in Fig. 1-9, *B*, may prove useful. The dental assistant is seated at a desk or writing stand near the child's feet. The dental assistant and the parent are facing the same direction side by side and at a right angle to the direction the dentist is facing. The dental assistant is in a good position to hear and record the dentist's findings as they are dictated, even if the child is crying loudly. These positions (see Fig. 1-9) are also convenient for demonstrating oral hygiene procedures to the parents.

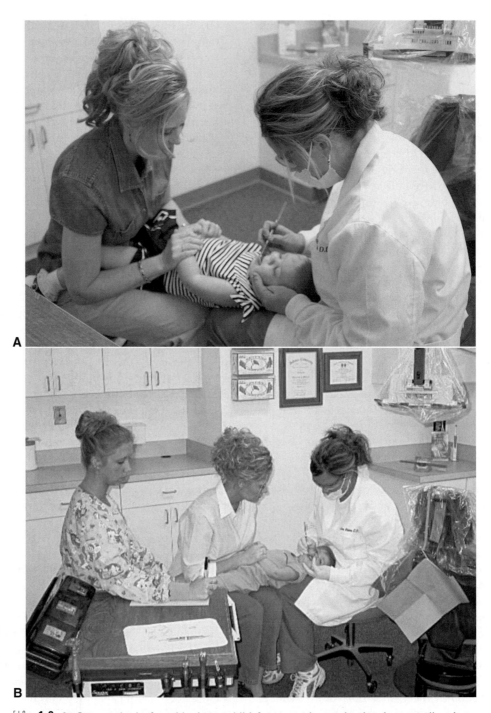

FIG. **1-9. A,** One method of positioning a child for an oral examination in a small, private consultation area. The dental assistant is nearby to record findings. **B,** If space allows three people to sit in a row, this method may be used to make it easier for the dental assistant to hear the findings dictated by the dentist. The dental assistant also helps restrain the child's legs.

The positions of the dentist, parent, child, and dental assistant during the examination at the dental chair are illustrated in Fig. 1-10. The dental assistant is seated higher to permit good visibility and to better anticipate the dentist's needs. The assistant is also in a good position to hear and record the dentist's findings. The parent and the dental assistant restrain the child's arms and legs. The child's head is positioned in the bend of the parent's arm. The dentist establishes a chairside position so that not only the dentist's hands but also the lower arms and abdomen may be available for support of the child's head if necessary.

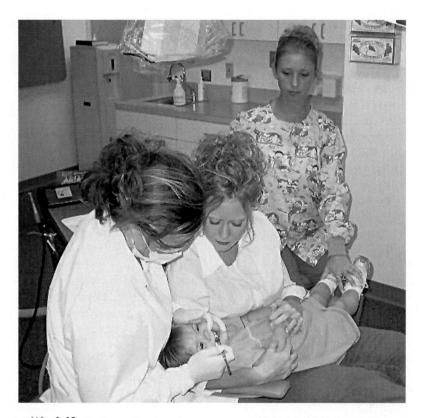

FIG. **1-10.** Oral examination of a very young child in the dental operatory.

The infant oral examination may often be performed by careful direct observation and digital palpation. The dentist may need only good lighting for visibility and gauze for drying or debriding tissues. Sometimes a tongue depressor and a soft-bristled toothbrush are also useful. At other times, as previously mentioned, the dentist will want the complete operatory available. The examination should begin with a systematic and gentle digital exploration of the soft tissues without any instruments. The child may find this gentle palpation soothing, especially when alveolar ridges in teething areas are massaged. The digital examination may help relax the child and encourage less resistance. If hand instruments are needed, the dentist must be sure to have a stable finger rest before inserting an instrument into the child's mouth.

Although there is little or no effective communication between the dentist and patient, the child realizes at the conclusion of the examination that nothing "bad" happened. The child also realizes that the procedure was permitted by the parents, who remained and actually helped with the examination. The child will not hold a lasting grudge against anyone, and the experience will not have a detrimental effect on future behavior as a dental patient. On the contrary, our experiences suggest that such early examinations followed by regular recall examinations often contribute to the youngsters'

becoming excellent dental patients without fear at very young ages. These children's chances for enjoying excellent oral health throughout life are also enhanced.

DETECTION OF SUBSTANCE ABUSE

It is within the scope of pediatric dentistry to be concerned with life-threatening habits and illnesses such as alcoholism and drug addiction that may occur in the older child.

Rosenbaum[7,8] has reported that abusers in the teen years and younger are as common as adult addicts. Drug abuse problems interact directly with the dental care of a patient. Obtaining and maintaining a satisfactory history is important. The office health questionnaire, as presented in this chapter, must be worded to allow the patient or parent to give some indication of a drug problem. It is often difficult to detect addiction from casual observation. Therefore input from the patient giving an indication of addiction is needed. At subsequent visits, the dentist must also consider changes in the general health history as well as answers to specific questions.

It is also important to know if the patient is taking drugs at the time of the dental visit because there could be an interaction with drugs that may be given in the dental office, for example, nitrous oxide. If the patient is under the influence of an abused substance, dental treatment should be postponed until a time when the patient is not "high."

Symptoms of substance abuse may include depression, feelings of inadequacy, frustration, helplessness, immaturity, self-alienation, poor object relations, and major deficiencies in ego structure and functioning. Heavy drug users tend to have poor impulse control. Hygiene in general and oral hygiene specifically are frequently neglected by those with a drug problem. In addition, because a patient is taking drugs that affect normal thought processes, the pain from untreated dental conditions may be masked. This combination of factors results in a patient with very little dental interest who is practicing unsatisfactory prevention. The result is increased oral disease.

Identification of substance abusers is difficult, even for an experienced observer. There are specific clues, however, that can be sought when one is attempting to draw general conclusions. Abrupt changes in behavior are common, as are signs of depression and moodiness. Interest in the opposite sex often decreases. Without any apparent consumption of alcohol, a drug-addicted person can appear intoxicated. There may be a desperate need for money, as well as a loss of appetite and loss of weight. The presence of scars along veins could be indicative of drug injection. Addicts frequently wear long-sleeved shirts, regardless of the weather, in an effort to cover identifying scars.

In a group of addicted patients the following traits have been observed: deviant social background, school dropout, prostitution, broken relationships, inability to retain a job, low self-esteem, and impulsive behavior. Histories of hepatitis, poor diet, craving for sweets, venereal disease, and blackouts were reported.

In the past when many dentists thought about substance abuse, they envisioned the use of marijuana, alcohol, or amphetamines. Substances abused by children and adults today cover a much wider spectrum; they include solvents, inhalants, narcotics, stimulants, sedatives, hallucinogens, tranquilizers, and tobacco, perhaps the most addictive of all.

Hillis[9] reports that drug and alcohol abuse has changed from a personal adult problem to a medical, social, economic, and political issue. She raises this question:

Ten years ago would you have expected to visit a third-grade class in your community and find little boys in Cub Scout uniforms and little girls in jumpers learning about drugs that even adults cannot handle? This scene is both terrifying and encouraging: terrifying in that drugs are such a problem that even third graders must be prepared to deal with them, and encouraging in that we finally are fighting back to prevent drugs from taking any more of our children.

MacDonald[10] reports that experimentation is a normal adolescent learning tool, but when combined with normal adolescent curiosity and fearlessness, it may be dangerous. Tobacco smoking is an example of a common teenage experiment. By their senior year, approximately one fourth, or 27.5%, of one class studied smoked daily.

ETIOLOGIC FACTORS IN SUBSTANCE ABUSE

Drug abuse in young people can be traced to many causes, the most important of which is considered to be rebellion against parents and society. Other factors may include a need to forget the pressures of daily living, a desire for pleasure, and a need to conform to the group with which young people want to be associated. Through drugs young people obtain a momentary feeling of independence and power because they have disobeyed the rules of their parents and society. The satisfaction gained through rebelling against parents can give adolescents a reinforcing motive for persisting in drug abuse.

Children of wealthy parents are increasingly recognized as a high-risk group for the development of such traits as narcissism, poor impulse control, poor tolerance of frustration, depression, and poor coping ability. Therefore it is not surprising that a large number of children within this group use drugs to cope with frustrations, boredom, anxiety, and depression.

Pallikkathayil and Tweed describe young drug users, especially those who are extensively involved in drug use, as less conforming than their peers, more tolerant of deviant behavior, and more likely to have a history of delinquent behavior before beginning to use drugs.[11] In general, drug users have been found to be less interested in formal education, less involved in organized activities such as athletics, and less likely to have well-defined goals than youngsters who do not use drugs. Adolescents who use drugs heavily have been described as manifesting more psychologic problems than nonusers do. Significantly higher percentages of nonusers of drugs reported close relationships with their parents. Drug users are more often found to experience broken homes or the loss of a parent.

SPECIFIC SUBSTANCES AND FREQUENCY OF USE

Amphetamines are often used to ward off sleepiness, curb appetite, and relieve depression. Repeated consumption of these drugs results in the development of tolerance.

Benson[12] has reported on the course and outcome of drug abuse in relation to medical and social conditions in select groups of young drug abusers in Sweden. Abuse of cannabis predominated 2 to 1 over abuse of heavier drugs. In addition, emergency department data show that the use of the amphetamine derivative MDMA (ecstasy) in conjunction with marijuana increased from 8 cases in 1990 to 796 cases in 1999 (National Institute on Drug Abuse, http://www.drugabuse.gov). Black[13] found that glue sniffing among adolescents was increasing in the United Kingdom, where it had rarely been reported before 1970. It has been a problem longer than that in the United States, where 7% to 12% of high school pupils reportedly have tried it at least once, with about 4% sniffing regularly. In the United Kingdom glue sniffing is now common among young people in inner-city areas, and it is suggested that these impoverished youngsters substitute it for alcohol. Glue sniffers are young adolescents, more often boys (although girls are increasingly represented), whose families have most of the marks of inner-city deprivation, such as poverty, overcrowding, unemployment, and delinquency. Most of these youth do not live with both of their natural parents. A small amount of glue is squeezed onto a rag or into a small bag and inhaled. The effect is sometimes enhanced by encasing the head in a larger plastic bag. Mild intoxication is produced and lasts for about 30 minutes.

Coulehan and others[14] described the prevalence of gasoline sniffing and lead toxicity in Navaho Indian adolescents. Gasoline sniffing is the deliberate deep inhalation of gasoline vapors to achieve an altered mental state. Fifteen to 20 breaths may be sufficient to produce euphoria, ataxia, and disorientation lasting 5 or 6 hours. More massive exposure to these volatile hydrocarbons can lead to acute central nervous system depression and loss of consciousness, coma, and death. Adolescents who sniff gasoline tend to have other behavioral problems as well, including failure of school courses, suspension from school, and a record of being arrested. They are also more likely to use other drugs.

Inhalation abuse of various toxic agents continues to be a significant health problem among the younger members of our society. King, Smialek, and Troutman[15] reported on the sudden death of adolescents resulting from the inhalation of typewriter correction fluid. A report describes four cases of sudden death in adolescents associated with recreational sniffing of typewriter correction fluid. The solvents used in most of these fluids are 1,1,1-trichloroethane and trichloroethylene, which are known to induce potentially fatal arrhythmias. Sniffing typewriter correction fluid poses a significant and underappreciated danger to the lives of these young abusers. Typewriter correction fluid, marketed as Liquid Paper, Wite-Out, and Sno-Paque,

and commonly referred to as "white-out," is a readily available, inexpensive agent now being used by teenagers to obtain a rapid "high." The observation of dried white or colored chalky residue on the hands or face could be a clue to the presence of these volatile chemicals in the body.

Since the early 1970s there has been a great resurgence in the use of all forms of smokeless tobacco in the United States. Sales of smokeless tobacco have increased about 11% each year, with an estimated 22 million users in the United States.

Current advertising implies that smokeless tobacco habits are innocuous and safe; however, there is mounting evidence that the use of smokeless tobacco has the potential for causing cancer of the oral cavity, pharynx, larynx, and esophagus. A review of the medical and dental literature has identified many cases of cancer directly associated with smokeless tobacco use. Smokeless tobacco can produce significant effects on the soft and hard tissues of the mouth, including bad breath, discolored teeth and restorations, excessive wear, abrasion of the incisal and occlusal surfaces of the teeth, decreased ability to taste and smell, gingival recession, advanced periodontal destruction of the hard and soft tissues, leukoedema and erythema of the soft tissues, leukoplakia, and cancer. Smokeless tobacco can also pose a health hazard in certain medically compromised persons because its use results in increased blood pressure.

Suppose the dentist identifies a person who needs help. What can be done? Unless the dentist is exceptionally well qualified to handle problems of addiction, the answer is direct or indirect referral to a treatment center. If the person expresses a need, the dentist may directly inform that person or the parents about agencies in the area that provide assistance. However, addicts may react defensively, even with hostility, if a direct approach is used.

As with any problem related to general or dental health, preventive efforts must begin with the young. Children at a very young age need to be helped to develop a positive self-image, a sense of self-worth, and a separate identity.

SUICIDAL TENDENCIES IN CHILDREN AND ADOLESCENTS

During the examination of the child the pediatric dentist should be alert to signs and symptoms of suicidal tendencies. How prevalent is suicide in the young child and adolescent? According to Dr. Pamela Cantor, who spoke at the thirty-ninth annual meeting of the American Academy of Pediatric Dentistry (1986), suicide is now an epidemic, with the rate having increased 125% in the 30-year period from 1950 to 1980.[16] There is one adolescent suicide in the United States every 90 minutes and one attempted suicide every minute. The notion to kill oneself may be entrenched in early childhood and influenced by the society in which we live. There is evidence from many sources that suicide is second only to accidents as a cause of death among teenagers.

In 1980, 6000 teenagers killed themselves and an estimated 400,000 adolescents attempted suicide. MacDonald[17] has credited Dr. Perihan Rosenthal, head of child and adolescent psychiatry at Beth Israel Hospital in Newark, Ohio, with identifying the phenomenon of child suicide in 1979. Since then she has seen 30 suicidal children under 6 years of age. The youngest diagnosed was $2\frac{1}{2}$ years of age. Children under 13 years of age really do not have a firm grasp of what death means. The young child is still caught up in thinking that death can be partial or reversible. Young children will attempt suicide with the means available to them—jumping out of a window, running into traffic, or jumping in front of a car.

Suicidal tendencies follow a pattern and background that can be observed by the astute professional or parent. According to the American Academy of Child Psychiatry, an estimated 10% of children in the United States suffer depression before 12 years of age. Depression in young people has been clearly linked to suicidal tendencies. It is important to be alert to the signs of suicidal tendencies, which are most often observed in the following individuals: one who is a female and a firstborn; one who shows depression with the addition of a second child; one who is very dependent on the mother but would be likely to experience parental conflicts during adolescence; one residing in a household in which there are struggles, conflicts, or divorce; one from a household in which the father is away from home a lot and, when present, is often overly critical; and one who feels that "the world would be better off without me." In addition, such tendencies may be seen in a girl who spends almost all of her time with a boyfriend and expects him to fill the role of an absent father; if the boyfriend rejects her, suicide or attempted suicide is frequent. Among those who are unable to derive satisfaction from living, who grow up too fast, who have low self-esteem and are bored with life, and who "keep things inside" and will not ask for help, suicide is also a problem. Some of the direct and indirect causes of suicide in children and adolescents according to Dr. Cantor are related to violence in the media, availability of guns, decreased employment opportunities for young people, alcohol and drug habits resulting in depression, and societal attitudes that teens are an inconvenience.[16] It should be recognized that the pediatric dentist and the orthodontist are in a unique position to recognize early warning signs of adolescent suicide. Loochtan and Cole[18] surveyed 1000 practicing orthodontists and 54 department chairs of postdoctoral programs. Of those surveyed, 50% had had at least one patient attempt suicide and 25% had had a young patient actually commit suicide.

INFECTION CONTROL IN THE DENTAL OFFICE

The dental team is exposed to a wide variety of microorganisms in the saliva and blood of their patients. These may include hepatitis B virus, herpes simplex viruses, cytomegalovirus, measles virus, mumps virus, chickenpox virus, human immunodeficiency virus type 1, *Mycobacterium tuberculosis*, streptococci, staphylococci, and numerous others that can infect the respiratory tract. Because it is impossible to identify all of those patients who may harbor dangerous microorganisms in their mouths, it is necessary to use standard precautions and practice infection control procedures routinely to avoid spread of disease. The following infection control procedures as described by Miller and Palenik[19] are based on those recommended for dentistry by the American Dental Association and by the Centers for Disease Control and Prevention (CDC) in the Public Health Service of the U.S. Department of Health and Human Services:

- Always obtain a thorough medical history, as discussed previously in this chapter, and include questions about medications, current illnesses, hepatitis, unintentional weight loss, lymphadenopathy, oral soft tissue lesions, or other infections.
- Clean all reusable instruments in an ultrasonic cleaner or washer/disinfector. Wear heavy rubber gloves, mask, and protective clothing and eyewear to protect against puncture injuries and splashing.
- Sterilize all reusable instruments that penetrate or come into contact with oral tissues or that become contaminated with saliva or blood. Metal or heat-stable instruments should be sterilized in a steam autoclave, a dry heat oven, or an unsaturated chemical vapor sterilizer. Heat-sensitive items may require up to 10 hours' exposure time for sterilization in a liquid chemical agent approved by the U.S. Food and Drug Administration as a disinfectant/sterilant, followed by rinsing with sterile water. High-level disinfection may be accomplished by submersion in the disinfectant/sterilant chemical for the exposure time recommended on the product label, followed by rinsing with water.
- Monitor the use and functioning of the sterilizer by using spore tests routinely (e.g., weekly for most dental offices). Chemical indicators may be used on the outside of packs.

- Insist that gloves be worn during all patient treatment procedures and when touching items contaminated with blood or saliva during operatory cleanup.
- Wear a surgical mask and protective eyewear when splatter or an aerosol of the patient's saliva or blood may be generated during treatment.
- Wear a protective gown or uniform when skin or clothing is likely to be soiled with blood or saliva. This attire should be changed at least daily or when visibly soiled.
- Use protective covers such as clear plastic wrap or paper backed with an impervious coating to protect operatory surfaces that are difficult to disinfect (e.g., light handles or x-ray unit heads).
- Use rubber dams whenever possible, along with high-speed evacuation, to reduce splatter and aerosols.
- Require vaccination against hepatitis B for all members of the dental team (dentists, hygienists, assistants, laboratory technicians). Blood tests should be given after vaccination to confirm response to the vaccine.
- Perform hand washing between patient contacts (after removing gloves) and after touching objects that may be contaminated with blood or saliva. An antimicrobial surgical hand scrub should be performed before gloving for surgical procedures. Hand washing with an antimicrobial or a plain, mild, nonirritating liquid soap is appropriate for examinations and nonsurgical procedures.
- Perform waste disposal functions in a way that protects those who must handle the waste. Use puncture-resistant containers marked with a biohazard label to dispose of needles, scalpel blades, and other sharp instruments immediately after use at chairside. To prevent needle stick injuries, needles should not be recapped by hand, bent, or broken before disposal. Nonsharp, regulated waste (e.g., cotton rolls or gauze pads saturated with blood or saliva) must be placed in sealed, sturdy, impervious bags to prevent leakage and marked as a biohazard through labeling or color coding. Liquid wastes may be poured down a drain connected to a sanitary sewer system.
- Place biopsy specimens in a sturdy container with a tight lid to prevent leaking during transport. Care should be taken not to contaminate the outside of the container.
- Clean and then disinfect contaminated operatory surfaces between patients. Wipe down the surfaces with absorbent toweling and disinfect with a 1:10 dilution of household bleach (for nonmetal surfaces) or with an Environmental Protection Agency–registered chemical germicide (e.g., an iodophor or phenolic).
- Use heat sterilization for all handpieces and air-water syringe tips before reuse. Water-cooled handpieces and the syringe should be activated and flushed with water for 3 minutes at the beginning of the day and for 30 seconds after completing care on each patient. They should be cleaned and sterilized according to the manufacturer's directions.
- Clean and disinfect impressions and intraoral appliances before handling, adjusting, or sending them to a dental laboratory. They should also be cleaned and disinfected when they are received from the dental laboratory and before placement in the patient's mouth. It is important to consult with the manufacturer of the dental material regarding disinfection procedures. In addition, the most recent Centers for Disease Control Guidelines for Infection Control in Dental Health Care Settings—2003 update and revise previous guidelines and consolidate recommendations from other relevant CDC guidelines as well as those of other major infection control organizations.[20] The document contains a review of the scientific evidence regarding dental infection control issues as well as consensus, evidence-based recommendations.

BIOFILM

A recent development in infection control involves microbial biofilm production inside the waterlines of dental units. The American Dental Association has stated that the microbiologic quality of dental unit water needs to be improved, and it has set a goal for dental unit manufacturers to make available dental units that will deliver treatment water with no more than 200 colony-forming units per milliliter (cfu/ml). Although municipal water supplies commonly are found to have an average of 5 to 50 cfu/ml, studies in the United States have shown the concentration of microorganisms in dental unit water to be from 20,000 to 500,000 cfu/ml. Currently, the options for improving dental unit water quality include use of separate water containers with periodic disinfection of the waterlines, use of in-line microbial filters, chemical or ultraviolet treatment of the water, and use of sterilizable water delivery systems. Research and development is ongoing in this area to verify the effectiveness of current approaches and to investigate new systems that may improve water quality.

EMERGENCY DENTAL TREATMENT

All too often a patient's initial dental appointment is prompted by an emergency situation. The diagnostic procedures necessary for an emergency dental appointment have already been outlined in this chapter. However, the emergency appointment tends to focus on and resolve a single problem or a single set of related problems rather than provide a comprehensive oral diagnosis and management plan for the patient. Once the emergency problem is under control, the dentist should offer comprehensive services to the patient or parents.

The remainder of this book presents information for dentists and dental students to augment their diagnostic and management skills in providing oral health care services to children and adolescents during both emergency and preplanned dental visits.

REFERENCES

1. Moskow BS, Barr CE: Examination of the patient. In Goldman HM and others, editors: *Current therapy in dentistry,* vol 4, St Louis, 1970, Mosby.
2. Shaw O: Dental anxiety in children, *Br Dent J* 139:134-139, 1975.
3. Okeson JP and others: Temporomandibular disorders in children, *Pediatr Dent* 11(12):325-333, 1989.
4. American Academy of Pediatric Dentistry: Guideline on acquired temporomandibular, *Pediatr Dent (supplemental issue: reference manual 2002-2003)* 24:103-104, 2002.
5. Clerehugh V, Tugnait A: Diagnosis and management of periodontal diseases in children and adolescents, *Periodontol 2000* 26:146-168, 2001.
6. Blayney JR, Hill IN: Fluorine and dental caries, *J Am Dent Assoc* 74:233-302, 1967.
7. Rosenbaum CH: Dental precautions in treating drug addicts: a hidden problem among teens and preteens, *Pediatr Dent* 2:94-96, 1980.
8. Rosenbaum CH: Did you treat a drug addict today? *Int Dent J* 31:307-312, 1981.
9. Hillis N: Epidemic, *J Med Assoc Ga* 74:239-241, 1985.
10. MacDonald DI: Drugs, drinking and adolescence, *Am J Dis Child* 138:117-125, 1984.
11. Pallikkathayil L, Tweed S: Substance abuse: alcohol and drugs during adolescence, *Nurs Clin North Am* 18:313-321, 1983.
12. Benson G: Course and outcome of drug abuse and medical and social conditions in selected young drug abusers, *Acta Psychiatr Scand* 71:48-66, 1985.
13. Black D: Glue sniffing, *Arch Dis Child* 57:893-894, 1982.
14. Coulehan JL and others: Gasoline sniffing and lead toxicity in Navajo adolescents, *Pediatrics* 71:113-117, 1983.
15. King GS, Smialek JE, Troutman WG: Sudden death in adolescents resulting from the inhalation of typewriter correction fluid, *JAMA* 253:1604-1606, 1985.
16. Cantor P: Adolescent suicide: who are they? How can we help? Unpublished paper presented at the thirty-ninth annual meeting of the American Academy of Pediatric Dentistry, Colorado Springs, Colo, 1986.
17. MacDonald S: *Suicidal children: from diapers to depression,* Fort Myers, Fla, March 3, 1986, News Press.
18. Loochtan RM, Cole RM: Adolescent suicide in orthodontics: results of a survey, *Am J Orthod Dentofacial Orthop* 1010:180-187, 1991.
19. Miller CH, Palenik CJ: *Infection control and management of hazardous materials for the dental team,* ed 2, St Louis, 1998, Mosby.
20. Centers for Disease Control and Prevention: Guidelines for Infection Control in Dental Health Care Settings—2003, *MMWR* 52(RR17):1-16, 2003.

SUGGESTED READINGS

American Academy of Pediatric Dentistry: Infant oral health care, *Pediatr Dent (supplemental issue: reference manual 2002-2003)* 24:47, 2002.

American Academy of Pediatric Dentistry: Periodicity of examination, preventive dental services, anticipatory guidance and oral treatment for children, *Pediatr Dent (supplemental issue: reference manual (2002-2003)* 24:52-53, 2002.

Depaola LG and others: A review of the science regarding dental unit waterlines, *J Am Dent Assoc* 133(9):1199-1206, 2002.

Glick M, Siegel MA, Brightman VJ: Evaluation of the dental patient: diagnosis and medical risk assessment. In Greenberg MS, Glick M, editors: *Burket's oral medicine, diagnosis and treatment,* ed 10, Hamilton, Ontario, 2003, BC Decker.

Okeson JP: *Management of temporomandibular disorders and occlusion,* ed 5, St Louis, 2003, Mosby.

Palenik CJ: Strategic planning for infection control, *J Contemp Dent Pract* 1(4):103, 2000.

2

Child Abuse and Neglect

ROBERTA A. HIBBARD

BRIAN J. SANDERS

Child abuse and neglect affect millions of children in the United States each year. Health care and dental professionals are in unique positions to identify the possibly abused child and must be knowledgeable in the recognition, documentation, treatment, and reporting of suspected child abuse cases. To appropriately intervene, professionals must be willing to consider abuse or neglect as a possibility—if it is not considered, it cannot be diagnosed. This chapter includes a discussion of the types of child maltreatment frequently encountered, the clinical presentation and management of such issues, and the documentation and reporting of suspected child abuse.

IS IT CHILD ABUSE?

Child abuse and neglect encompass a variety of experiences that are threatening or harmful to the child and are the result of acts of commission or omission on the part of a responsible caretaker. This includes physical or mental injury, sexual abuse, and negligent treatment or maltreatment of a child less than 18 years of age by a person responsible for the child's welfare. Many gray areas exist in the determination of threat or harm, and disagreements about the "abusive" nature of some experiences are common. No one individual is responsible for "deciding" what is abuse or neglect. Identification, treatment, and intervention are the tasks of professionals from multidisciplinary backgrounds working together to provide care and evaluation in the best interests of the child.

Maltreatment is not always willful; that is, the harm or injury inflicted is not always the intent of the act. Anger expressed actively or passively against the child is often unplanned, but nonetheless can result in significant injury or death. Education and prevention efforts may teach parents to redirect their actions and explore more appropriate discipline techniques and ways to manage anger or frustration.

PHYSICAL ABUSE

Physical abuse is often the most easily recognized form of child abuse. The battered child syndrome was initially described by Kempe et al in 1962 and elaborated further by Kempe and Helfer in 1972 as the clinical picture of physical trauma or failure to thrive in which the explanation of injury was not consistent with the severity and type of injury observed.[1,2] These injuries are inflicted and not accidental; some result from punishment that is inappropriate for the child's age, condition, or level of development. Some result from a parent's frustration and lack of control in acting out anger. Physical abuse is usually recognized by the pattern of injury and/or its inconsistency with the history related. Bruises, welts, fractures, burns, and lacerations are commonly inflicted physical injuries. Approximately 50% of physical abuse results in facial and head injuries that could be recognized by the dentist; 25% of physical abuse injuries occur in or around the mouth.

SEXUAL ABUSE

Sexual abuse and *sexual misuse* are frequently interchanged terms that denote any sexually stimulating activity that is inappropriate for the child's age, level of cognitive development, or role within the family. Many definitions incorporate the desire for sexual gratification on the part of one of the participants. In the spectrum of child sex play, sexual experimentation, and parent-child physical-sexual contact, it may be difficult to distinguish normal behavior from lustful intrusion. Sexually abusive acts may range from exhibitionism or kissing to fondling, intercourse, pornography, or rape. Trauma to the mouth may result from sexual contact.

NEGLECT

Inattention to the basic needs of a child, such as food, clothing, shelter, medical care, education, and supervision, may constitute neglect. While physical abuse tends to be episodic, neglect tends to be chronic. Determination of neglect also depends on the child's age and level of development as it may relate to periods of time without supervision, the parents' whereabouts, parental intention, and responsibilities of the child when the child is not supervised or not attending school. The American Academy of Pediatric Dentistry defines dental neglect as "willful failure of parent or guardian to seek and follow through with treatment necessary to ensure a level of oral health essential for adequate function and freedom from pain and infection."[3] Level of medical and dental care, adequate nutrition, and adequate food and clothing must be considered in light of cultural and religious differences, poverty, community requirements and standards, and the impact of such neglect on the physical well-being of the child.

EMOTIONAL ABUSE

Emotional abuse has been a concern for many years, but definitions and standards for identifying such abuse have been extremely difficult to establish. It is often difficult to demonstrate the direct or causal link between emotional and verbal abuse, and harm to the child. Such harm is usually seen as abnormal behaviors or mental health problems that are multifactorial in origin. Emotional and verbal abuse involve interactions or lack of interactions on the part of the caretaker that inflict damage on the child's personality, emotional well-being, or development. It must be an identifiable act or omission that has demonstrable harm to the child and generally occurs in various ways over a prolonged period. Continuous isolation, rejection, degradation, terrorization, corruption, exploitation, or denial of affection are examples of behaviors that frequently have damaging effects on the child.

FACTITIOUS DISORDER BY PROXY

Perhaps the most difficult form of child maltreatment to identify and treat is a factitious disorder—factitious disorder by proxy, Munchausen syndrome by proxy, or pediatric condition falsification. These are conditions in which the perpetrator (usually the mother) relates a fictitious history, produces false signs or symptoms, and fabricates illnesses in the child that result in extensive medical evaluations, testing, and often prolonged hospitalizations. The fabrication may be deliberate to gain medical attention, the result of parental psychosis, or simply fraudulent to obtain money or services. Because health care providers are often dependent on the parental history of the child's illness, it takes some time for the practitioner to realize the inconsistencies and possibly fabricated or exaggerated nature of the complaints. These children present with persistent and recurrent illnesses that cannot be explained, signs and symptoms that do not make sense clinically, and problems that are rare, unusual, or bizarre. The bizarre nature of many of these cases makes them almost unbelievable to professionals involved, and an unbelieving social and legal system has considerable difficulty protecting a child.

LEGAL REQUIREMENTS

Every state has legal statutes requiring that suspected child abuse or neglect be reported to authorities. Statutes vary somewhat from state to state regarding detailed definitions of child abuse and neglect, but all states mandate that health care providers (including dentists) report child abuse or neglect when it is suspected. It is important to emphasize that one is required to report suspicions of child abuse and one need not have proof. It is the job of social and legal authorities to determine whether abuse has occurred and what intervention is legally necessary.

WHO IS ABUSED?

Children from all walks of life may be victims of child abuse or neglect—no age, race, gender, or socioeconomic level is spared. Statistics on child abuse reflect only those cases known or suspected, and all studies struggle with the component of the unknown. Approximately 50% to 65% of child maltreatment encompasses neglect and 25% involves physical abuse; sexual abuse and emotional abuse account for the majority of the remaining cases. Children who are victims of one form of maltreatment often are maltreated in other ways as well.

Sociodemographic characteristics of maltreated children vary somewhat by type of abuse or neglect. The average age of identification of maltreatment victims is 7.4 years; 49% are male; and 68% are white, 21% are black, and 11% belong to other ethnic groups. Females are slightly overrepresented as abuse victims because sexual abuse is more prevalent among females. The youngest children (infants to 2 years) tend to be neglected most often and sexually or emotionally abused least often. Older children (12 to 17 years) are the least neglected, but the most sexually and emotionally abused; they are physically abused slightly more than average. Family characteristics overrepresented among families of maltreated children and therefore considered risk factors include female head of family, receipt of public assistance and thus lower income, presence of more children in the home, and presence of spousal abuse, drug or alcohol abuse, or significant health or economic stresses. Risk factors play a role, but ultimately every child is a potential victim.

IDENTIFICATION OF POSSIBLE CHILD ABUSE

As stated earlier, child abuse and neglect are not identified if they are not considered as a diagnostic possibility. One must be willing to consider the diagnosis of abuse to make the diagnosis. A number of characteristics of the child, parent, or story given to explain the child's condition may lead a professional to suspect child maltreatment.

Indicators of child abuse and neglect are those signs or symptoms that should raise one's suspicions of the possibility of child maltreatment. The presence of such indicators does not "prove" maltreatment. Many of the signs or symptoms are nonspecific and may be present for a variety of reasons—child abuse is only one of those reasons. Indicators of abuse and neglect often depend on the child's age and developmental level and vary with the child's experiences and resiliency.

PHYSICAL INDICATORS

Situations raising the strongest suspicions and the most easily recognized maltreatment cases are those in which the pattern of injury is not consistent with the account explaining it. For example, a 3-month-old (nonambulatory) child is not going to sustain a spiral femur fracture from crawling. A bruise in the shape of a handprint on the cheek does not result from a fall down the stairs (Fig. 2-1). Accounts from two or more individuals (such as parents or a parent and child) that conflict with each other or that change over time are also very suspicious. Any significant injury that is reportedly "unwitnessed" should raise concerns of possible abuse.

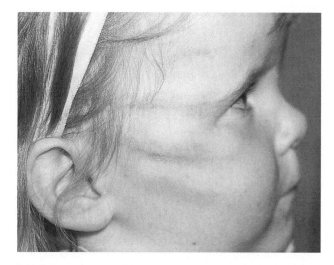

FIG. **2-1.** Bruise in the shape of a handprint on the cheek. *(From Hobbs CJ and Wynne JM: Physical signs of child abuse: a colour atlas, ed 2, WB Saunders [Harcourt Publishers Limited], London, 2001.)*

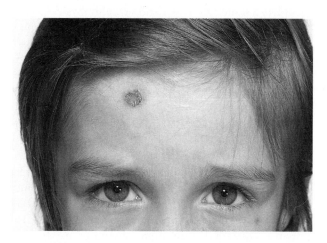

FIG. **2-2.** Intentional cigarette burn. *(From Hobbs CJ and Wynne JM: Physical signs of child abuse: a colour atlas, ed 2, WB Saunders [Harcourt Publishers Limited], London, 2001.)*

Physical indicators of child maltreatment tend to be somewhat more objective but must also be considered with the history. Unexplained bruises or welts in places not routinely subject to the child's rough-and-tumble lifestyle are those that become suspicious. Shin bruises and forehead bumps are expected in toddlers; bruises in the small of the back or torso are not. Unexplained injuries on the face, mouth, or lips; bruises clustering to form regular patterns or reflecting the shape of an article used to inflict the injury; and scattered significant bruises on different surface areas at various stages of healing are all very suspicious. Similarly, unexplained fractures of the head, multiple fractures in varying stages of healing, injuries to growth centers in the bone, and fractures in children younger than 2 years of age should raise concerns. Such injuries can be unintentional, but a clear explanation must be sought. Skull fractures may result from a fall from table to floor, but accompanying severe retinal hemorrhages or subdural hematoma with brain injury makes that explanation untenable. Burns are another form of recognizable child abuse; intentional cigarette (Fig. 2-2) and immersion burns should be readily distinguishable from accidental splash burns.

BEHAVIORAL INDICATORS

Significant behavioral changes often linked to child maltreatment include withdrawal, depression, poor school performance, regression in developmentally appropriate behavior, acting out, clinginess, and somatic complaints. Young maltreated children may show inappropriate affection toward others or may be extremely wary and distant in social interactions. Many children demonstrate affection toward an abusive parent; this should not be construed as evidence against maltreatment. Children who are afraid to go home, are frightened by their parents, or report injury by caretakers should be taken seriously. Extensive lists can be found describing behavioral indicators of possible maltreatment. These should be considered in light of the child's entire clinical history and presentation and not in isolation. When good explanations for such behaviors are not found, maltreatment is an appropriate consideration.

Behavioral indicators also may be present in caretakers. Lack of concern or inappropriately high levels of concern in relation to the severity of the child's injury are not unusual observations. Parents may be defensive and hostile when questioned or may refuse hospitalization and testing for the child. The explanation for the injury may be inconsistent with the pattern or the child's abilities, or the explanation may change when the perpetrator realizes that the first story is not believed. Poor judgment, jealousy or extreme protectiveness, child abandonment, violent behavior, or erratic behavior (which suggests drug or alcohol use, or psychiatric illness) are other clues to possible maltreatment.

Other indications of possible child abuse or neglect include a delay in seeking medical care for obvious injury, repeated ingestions of harmful substances, repeated hospitalizations, doctor or emergency department shopping, or excessive use of medical care for an apparently well child. Children whose basic needs for medical and dental care, food, clothing, shelter, or education are not being met may be victims of neglect.

EVALUATION

Trauma to the orofacial structures is a frequent manifestation of child abuse. Studies have indicated that the incidence is as high as 50% in child physical abuse.

The dentist who suspects child abuse or neglect needs to complete a thorough dental and general physical examination. Because abusive parents do not always show the same caution when visiting the dentist as when visiting the physician, the dental practitioner may be the first person to identify the abused child. Therefore the dentist must learn to recognize an abused child and make the appropriate referral.

Any evaluation requires a medical history and physical examination. The combination of information is what influences or creates the suspicion of possible child maltreatment. The history should be a complete dental and medical history. Details regarding any trauma should be complete and obtained separately from more than one source (i.e., parent and child) if possible. Open-ended questions should be used; those with a yes-no response must be avoided. Details should include who witnessed the injury and who was with the child when it occurred, where the child and supervising adults were, and what exactly happened. Questions should include how and when the incident occurred. A description of present and past injuries, as well as the child's developmental abilities, may be helpful. Once enough information is obtained that the dentist is suspicious of child abuse or neglect, detailed questioning should be suspended.

COMMUNICATION WITH THE PATIENT

Professionals who are identifying and reporting suspected child maltreatment will have to talk to children in most circumstances to clarify a possible suspicion. They should not, however, be conducting investigative interviews of children to learn all the details or sort out the truthfulness of comments. A suggested guideline is the following: if based on your knowledge and experience you have reason to believe the child may have been abused or neglected, report it. Further detailed interviewing by a noninvestigating professional is neither necessary nor appropriate; that is the job of child protective service agencies. If, however, the child is talking and wants to disclose more, it is appropriate to listen and provide support.

PHYSICAL EXAMINATION

The examination of the patient by a dentist should include the entire body that is exposed without undressing the child. The examination begins before the patient is even back in the operatory. Observe the patient's posture, gait, and clothing. The dental staff should be trained in recognizing abuse and neglect so that they may alert the dentist of their suspicions. Inappropriate dress may be an indication of neglect and/or abuse. For example, a child who appears with a long-sleeved shirt in the middle of the hot summer may be dressed in this manner to cover old injuries. The child's behavior may

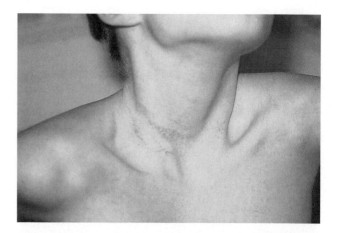

FIG. **2-3.** Attempted strangulation marks on the neck of an adolescent. *(From Hobbs CJ and Wynne JM: Physical signs of child abuse: a colour atlas, ed 2, WB Saunders [Harcourt Publishers Limited], London, 2001.)*

also be inappropriate. A lack of spontaneous smiling and avoidance of eye contact may be indicators, as is being overly watchful and vigilant.

The dentist should start the examination at the top, beginning with the hair and scalp, and systematically work down. Alopecia without an underlying medical cause may be an indicator of malnutrition or hair pulling. Continue the examination by looking at the nose and nasal septum. A deviated septum or clotted blood may be an indicator of previous trauma. Look for any periorbital ecchymosis, ptosis, and deviated or unequal pupils, which indicate significant facial trauma. In cases of suspected head trauma, a neurologic assessment (history and physical) by the dentist can help so that the child receives the immediate attention that is necessary. If any question exists of possible abnormality, the child should be referred to a pediatrician or neurosurgeon familiar with child abuse as soon as possible.

Any bruise in the shape of an object, such as a belt, looped cord, handprint, or hanger, should alert the practitioner to inflicted trauma. The varying color of bruises should be particularly noted to identify the several stages of resolution that would indicate ongoing trauma. The neck should be examined for evidence of rope burns or bruises (Fig. 2-3) that may indicate attempted strangulation. Severe shaking can result in large bruises on the back of the neck that may also indicate brain damage. Physical trauma to the child's chest or ribs may elicit a painful response from the child if a lifting motion is used to slide the child up to the top of the dental chair during the examination. The presence of adult bite marks (Fig. 2-4) may be a sign of physical abuse, sexual abuse, or neglect. They may also be

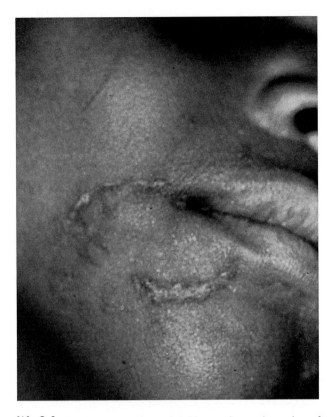

FIG. **2-4.** The presence of an adult bite mark may be a sign of physical or sexual abuse or neglect. *(Courtesy American Society of Dentistry for Children.)*

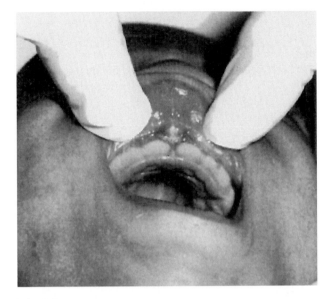

FIG. **2-5.** Torn frenulum from blunt force trauma to mouth. Upon further investigation, this child was found to have 17 fractures.

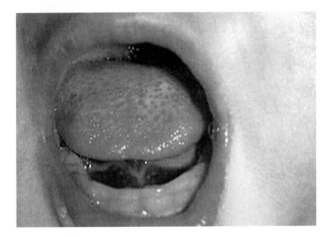

FIG. **2-6.** Sublingual hemorrhage in an infant with signs of genital and abdominal trauma.

helpful in identifying the abuser. They need to be clearly documented and photographs taken, if possible, at the time they are first observed, since they tend to fade rapidly. A forensic dentist or bite mark expert should be consulted as soon as possible when adult bite marks are suspected. Any visible patterns of injury should be photographed if possible; most law enforcement agencies will dispatch a photographer if requested in child abuse cases.

On completion of the general physical examination, the dentist should examine the teeth and supporting structures. Note any missing teeth or previously traumatized teeth (avulsions, luxations, intrusions, or fractures) and pay especially close attention to any soft tissue injuries. The mandible should be examined for any deviation on opening, range of motion, trismus, and occlusion at rest. The maxilla should also be examined for any mobility indicating a facial fracture. Bleeding under the tongue may indicate a fracture of the body of the mandible.

Note the condition of the maxillary labial frenum and the lower lingual frenum. A torn maxillary frenum on a child who is too young to walk indicates possible trauma to the mouth from a slap, fist blow, or forced feeding. A torn lingual frenum could be indicative of sexual abuse or forced feeding (Figs. 2-5 and 2-6).

Bruising or petechia of the soft and hard palate may indicate sexual abuse in the form of oral penetration (Fig. 2-7). If any evidence of infection or ulceration is noted, specimens should be cultured for evidence of a sexually transmitted disease, such as gonorrhea, syphilis, or venereal warts. The child who presents with extensive, untreated dental caries, untreated infection, or dental pain may be considered a victim of physical neglect because the parents are not attending to the child's basic medical needs. Before filing a report, the dentist should determine if the failure to provide dental

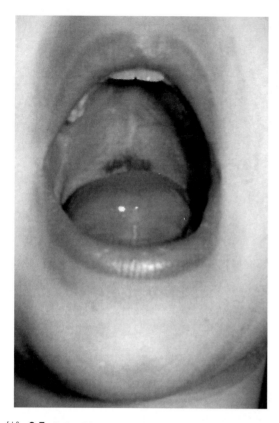

FIG. **2-7.** Palatal hemorrhage from oral-genital contact.

care is willful or due to a lack of awareness or finances. Taking a good medical and dental history and making repeated attempts to obtain appropriate treatment for the child will help sort out these issues. A call to a child protective service agency is indicated if repeated attempts to address the cause of the dental neglect are not met with success, because dental neglect can cause significant pain, discomfort, and possible disability.

MANAGEMENT: DOCUMENTATION AND REPORTING

Clinical and medicolegal management of suspected child abuse and neglect involve several basic steps: medical and dental management, documentation (including photographs), and reporting.

As health care professionals, dentists should be especially sensitive to the need for protecting children from abuse or neglect. They must, of course, treat dental injuries. It is also important for dentists to know that they are legally mandated to report suspected child abuse or neglect. Reporting is initiated simply with a telephone call to the appropriate child protective service agency. The telephone call initiates a response by appropriately trained professionals, but the dentist should follow the call with a written report. Dentists are mandated to report based on "reasonable suspicion,"

and they are not responsible for any further investigation. Cases of abuse and neglect are often resolved without litigation, and the reporting dentist will not necessarily be called to testify even if the case goes to court.

TREATMENT

Any medical or dental treatment that is indicated by the child's condition should be provided. A referral for a complete pediatric history taking and physical examination will assist in identifying and treating other possibly associated conditions (failure to thrive, anemia, and so on). Medical evaluation should include assessment for medical conditions that can mimic or be confused with child abuse. A young child (younger than 18 months to 2 years) who has suffered a fracture should be examined by means of a skeletal survey to detect other fractures; children with bruising need to be examined for possible blood clotting disorders.

DOCUMENTATION

All data collected in the medical history and physical examination must be documented in a complete and objective manner. Pertinent positive and negative findings should be included. Actual comments and behaviors should be recorded; opinions about those behaviors should be avoided. For visible injuries, photographs should be taken if possible. The child's name and the date of the photograph should be included in the picture. Most law enforcement officials will take photographs if requested to do so when suspected child abuse is reported. When suspected maltreatment is reported to authorities, the time, date, and method of reporting (phone or written report) should be documented in the medical and dental record.

REPORTING

The dentist is obligated by law to report suspected findings of child abuse to the appropriate authorities, that is, child protective service agencies and/or law enforcement officials. Failure to do so may result in the filing of civil or criminal charges against the dentist. With increased public awareness and inclusion of courses on child abuse in the dental curriculum, ignorance of the laws of child abuse is not an acceptable excuse.

PARENTAL CONCERNS

In most situations, parents should be told of the concerns about possible child abuse or neglect and the legal requirement to report it to local authorities. Health care professionals should not make any accusations about who may have caused the harm. Simple statements such as the following should be used: "Based on my training, I am concerned that this injury could not have happened this way. Because of this, I am required by law to make a report to Child Protective Services."

In those situations in which a child is suspected to have been significantly harmed in the home, in which the parent is expected to be violent, or in which possible retribution against the child for having told is a concern, it may be more prudent to contact authorities and have them present to protect the child before parents are told. The dental professional has *no* legal obligation to inform parents that abuse or neglect is suspected or will be reported; some situations may best be handled by not telling them at the time a report is filed.

The major concern must be for the welfare of the patient, and any concerns about losing a patient from a practice should be secondary. Individuals are protected from civil and criminal liability if the report is made in good faith. When the dentist's action is presented to parents as motivated by concern for the child and by an attitude of "let's figure out what is going on," many parents are eventually appreciative and will continue to seek support and care from the reporting professional.

There should be no reluctance on the part of the dentist to report suspected child abuse because of concern that it will require a great deal of time. In most cases after the initial report has been filed no further involvement is necessary on the part of the dentist, and few cases require a court appearance. It is possible to report suspected child abuse anonymously, but it is preferred that you give your name so that the agency can contact you if there are any further questions.

OBLIGATION OF THE DENTIST

The privileged quality of communication between the caretakers or the patient and the practitioner is not grounds for excluding evidence in a judicial proceeding resulting from a report or for failing to make a report as required by law. Strict confidentiality of records is maintained. Reports and any other information obtained in reference to a report are confidential and available only to persons authorized to examine them by the juvenile code. Some state statutes stipulate that a mandated reporter who fails to make a report when abuse or neglect is suspected may be liable for proximate damages caused by the failure to report. Criminal liability is another possibility.

The health care professional must remember that it is suspicions of child abuse or neglect that must be reported; proof is not required. It is the responsibility of child protective service agencies and law enforcement officials to investigate suspicions and determine if intervention is necessary. The health care professional can assist by providing as much information as possible through communication and coordination. Investigating professionals cannot do their jobs if the health care professional does not share detailed information regarding why the suspicions exist. Health care professionals unhappy with the outcome of system intervention

(e.g., that nothing was done) are usually those who would not or did not provide the information available that would assist authorities in making the best informed decisions. If the health care professional feels that a bad decision is being made, a follow-up phone call to the assigned caseworker or caseworker's supervisor to clarify concerns and interventions is appropriate. Many misperceptions exist about what interventions are possible legally. Communication and coordination can improve everyone's knowledge and understanding about a child's needs and what can be done to meet them.

Child abuse and neglect are identifiable in the dental office. Knowledgeable practitioners must be able and willing to identify, document, and report suspicions of child maltreatment. Awareness of local child protective community resources and professionals can facilitate interaction with the legal system and improve the ability to appropriately protect abused or neglected children.

REFERENCES

1. Kempe CH et al: *The battered child syndrome, JAMA* 181:17-24, 1962.
2. Kempe C, Helfer R: *Helping the battered child and his family,* Philadelphia, 1972, JB Lippincott.
3. American Academy of Pediatric Dentistry: Definition of dental neglect, *Pediatr Dent* 24(7):6, 2002-2003.

SUGGESTED READINGS

American Dental Association Council on Dental Practice: *The dentist's responsibility in identifying and reporting child abuse,* Chicago, 1987, The Association.

Becker DB, Needleman HL, Kotelchuck M: Child abuse and dentistry: orofacial trauma and its recognition by dentists, *J Am Dent Assoc* 97:24-28, 1978.

Blain SM: Abuse and neglect as a component of pediatric treatment planning, *J Calif Dent Assoc* 19(9):16-24, 1991.

Brassard MR, Germain R, Stuart N: *Psychological maltreatment of children and youth,* New York, 1987, Pergamon Press.

Bross D et al, editors: *The new child protection team handbook,* New York, 1988, Garland Publishing.

Burgess AW et al: *Sexual assault of children and adolescents,* Lexington, Mass, 1978, DC Heath.

Carrotte PV: An unusual case of child abuse, *Br Dent J* 168:444-445, 1990.

Croll TP, Menna VJ, Evans CA: Primary identification of an abused child in a dental office: a case report, *Pediatr Dent* 3:339-342, 1981.

Croll TP et al: Rapid neurologic assessment and initial management for the patient with traumatic dental injuries, *J Am Dent Assoc* 100:530-534, 1980.

Daro D: *Confronting child abuse: theory, policy and practice,* New York, 1987, Free Press.

Davis GR, Domoto PK, Levy RL: The dentist's role in child abuse and neglect, *J Dent Child* 46:185-192, 1979.

Davis MJ, Vogel L: Neurological assessment of the child with head trauma, *J Dent Child* 62:93-96, 1995.

Faller K, editor: *Social work with abused and neglected children: a manual of interdisciplinary practice,* New York, 1981, Free Press.

Giangrego E: Child abuse: *recognition and reporting, Spec Care Dentist* 6:62-67, 1986.

Golden MH, Samuels MP, Southall DP: How to distinguish between neglect and deprivational abuse, *Arch Dis Child* 88: 105-107, 2003.

Indiana State Department of Health, Division of Maternal and Child Health: Child abuse and neglect identifying and reporting for the health care provider, 1991.

Kempe C, Helfer R: *Helping the battered child and his family,* Philadelphia, 1972, JB Lippincott.

Kittle PE, Richardson DS, Parker JW: Two child abuse/child neglect examinations for the dentist, *J Dent Child* 48:175-180, 1981.

Malecz RE: Child abuse, its relationship to pedodontics: a survey, *J Dent Child* 46:193-194, 1979.

Myers JE, Wendell PD: *Child abuse reporting legislation in the 1980s,* Denver, 1987, The American Humane Association.

Needleman HL: Orofacial trauma in child abuse: types, prevalence, management and the dental profession's involvement, *Pediatr Dent* 8:71-80, 1986.

Perspectives on child maltreatment in the 80's, DHHS Pub No (OHDS) 84-30338, Washington, DC, US Department of Health and Human Services, National Center on Child Abuse and Neglect.

Sanger RG, Bross DC: *Clinical management of child abuse and neglect,* Chicago, 1984, Quintessence Publishing.

Saxe MD, McCourt JW: Child abuse: a survey of ASDC members and diagnostic data assessment for dentists, *J Dent Child* 58:361-366, 1991.

Sheridan MS: The deceit continues: an updated literature review of Munchausen syndrome by proxy, *Child Abuse Negl* 27: 431-451, 2003.

Sidebotham P, Golding J, ALSPAC Study Team: Child maltreatment in the "children of the nineties." A longitudinal study of parental risk factors, *Child Abuse Negl* 25:1177-1200, 2001.

Stanley RT: Child abuse—what's a dentist to do, *Ohio Dent J* 55(9):16-27, 1981.

Wissow LS: Child abuse and neglect, *N Engl J Med* 332(21): 1425-1431, 1995.

3

Nonpharmacologic Management of Children's Behaviors

GERALD Z. WRIGHT

The foundation of practicing dentistry for children is the ability to guide them through their dental experiences. In the short term, this ability is a prerequisite to providing for their immediate dental needs. More long-lasting beneficial effects also can result when the seeds for future dental health are planted early in life. A professional goal is to promote positive dental attitudes and improve the dental health of society. Logically, children are keys to the future.

A major difference between the treatment of children and the treatment of adults is the relationship. Treating adults generally involves a one-to-one relationship, that is, a dentist-patient relationship. Treating a child, however, usually relies on a one-to-two relationship among dentist, pediatric patient, and parents or guardians. Fig. 3-1, which illustrates this relationship, is known as the *pediatric dentistry treatment triangle*. Recently, society has been centered in the triangle. Management methods acceptable to society and the litigiousness of society have been factors influencing treatment modalities. Note that the child is at the apex of the triangle and is the focus of attention of both the family and the dental team. Although mothers' attitudes have been shown to significantly affect their children's behaviors in the dental office, the roles of families have been changing, and the entire family environment must be considered. Because changes are constantly occurring within each personality, one must remember that there is an ever-changing, dynamic relationship among the corners of the triangle—the child, the family, and the dental team. The arrows placed on the lines of communication also remind us that communication is reciprocal.

The importance of this unifying concept will become evident as management techniques are described.

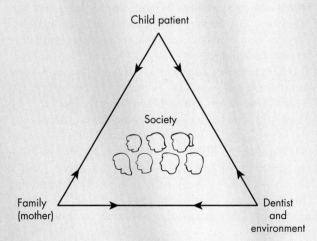

FIG. **3-1.** The pediatric treatment triangle illustrates basic relationships in pediatric dentistry.

However, this concept also serves as a means for organizing the present chapter, whose goal is to discuss the nonpharmacologic approaches to managing children's behavior in dentistry.

PEDIATRIC DENTAL PATIENTS

Child development involves the study of all areas of human development from conception through young adulthood. It involves more than physical growth, which often implies only an increase in size. Development implies a sequential unfolding that may involve changes in size, shape, function, structure, or skill.

Over the years, numerous child development theories have evolved. Summarizing them, Alpern stated that the most important general principle concerning development is that human development is not unitary.[1] He contended that there were several relatively important aspects of child development and that no single aspect could be used to assess development. He cautioned about relating to children through a single developmental label and suggested that a basic appreciation of child development knowledge could be helpful to the dentist.

Early child development study linked changes to specific chronologic ages. The initial work gathered age norms for physiologic developmental tasks. Eventually personality description principles also evolved. One of the pioneering and most notable groups, headed by Arnold Gesell, was at Yale University. Some of the typical personality characteristics related to specific chronologic ages that have relevance to dentistry are listed in Box 3-1. They can help guide management strategies. For example, if the dentist knows the limitation of a 2-year-old's vocabulary, it becomes apparent that communication must occur through the sense of touch and voice modulation rather than through the spoken word. Recognizing also the close symbiotic relationship with parents, dentists generally try to keep the parent-child pair intact.

Relating personality characteristics to chronologic ages has led to some interesting labeling. For example, a noncompliant 2-year-old often is referred to as in the stage of the *terrible twos*. Dentists sometimes refer to such children as being in the *precooperative stage*. Unfortunately, this has led in some instances to using the age of the child, rather than the child's ability, as a reason for noncompliance.

The broad area of physical development involves changes that occur in children's size, strength, motor coordination, functioning of body systems, and so forth. Thus the child's total physical growth and efficiency from the moment of conception until adulthood is termed *physical development*. Because a child's physical development is relatively independent of other major areas of development, subareas of physical development

BOX 3-1   Age-Related Psychosocial Traits and Skills for 2- to 5-Year-Old Children*

TWO YEARS

Geared to gross motor skills, such as running and jumping
Likes to see and touch
Very attached to parent
Plays alone; rarely shares
Has limited vocabulary; shows early sentence formation
Becoming interested in self-help skills

THREE YEARS

Less egocentric; likes to please
Has very active imagination; likes stories
Remains closely attached to parent

FOUR YEARS

Tries to impose powers
Participates in small social groups
Reaches out—expansive period
Shows many independent self-help skills
Knows "thank you" and "please"

FIVE YEARS

Undergoes a period of consolidation; deliberate
Takes pride in possessions
Relinquishes comfort objects, such as a blanket or thumb
Plays cooperatively with peers

*Based on the work of Dr. A. Gesell.

TABLE 3-1   Average Age and Age Range of Selected Physical Developmental Milestones

DEVELOPMENTAL TASK	AVERAGE AGE	NORMAL RANGE
Focuses on light	2 wk	1-4 wk
Lies on stomach, lifts chin	3 wk	1-10 wk
Birth weight doubles	6 mo	5-7 mo
Rolls from back to stomach	7 mo	5½ -11 mo
Sits alone	7 mo	6-11 mo
Stands with support	10 mo	7½ -14 mo
Stands alone	13½ mo	9-18 mo
Walks alone	14 mo	10-20 mo
Bowel control attained	18 mo	1-2½ yr
First menstruates	12 yr, 9 mo	10-17 yr

have to be relatively independent. A child's coordination cannot be judged by physical size, nor is physical strength related to dental development.

Relating physical changes to specific chronologic ages led to the establishment of developmental milestones that became a means of assessing individual children. Some of the classic developmental milestones are shown in Table 3-1. From these milestones, ranging from infancy through early childhood, two pieces of information are derived: (1) the average age at which a child acquires particular skills and (2) the normal range of ages at which a skill is acquired. A general principle is that, the earlier a skill emerges, the narrower is the range. On the other hand, developmental tasks tend to occur with wider ranges of normality as age increases. For the dentist, this holds practical importance. For example, consider the task of teaching children how to floss their teeth. Because the ability to floss occurs later in life (9 to 12 years of age), there is a wide performance range. Knowing the general developmental principle reminds the clinician to consider the ability or readiness of the individual to perform a given task.

Another area that has received great attention from psychologists is the socialization of children. As with physical development, age-specific skills have been derived for social development; these take into account both interpersonal relationships and independent functioning skills. Some of the key personality characteristics already have been identified in Box 3-1.

An important process for dentists is the child's growth toward independent functioning. For their survival, infants are dependent on others to clothe, feed, and nurture them. As children grow and their ability to care for themselves improves, they gain social independence. Recognizing that the change from functional dependency to functional autonomy is a normal process in social development can assist the dentist. Many young children, who lack digital dexterity, want to brush their own teeth. Parents, on the other hand, understand the lack of digital skills and often insist on attending to their children's oral health care. Appreciating that this tug-of-war is a normal part of social maturation allows the dentist to intercede and make appropriate conciliatory recommendations.

Intellectual development is probably the area most comprehensively studied, beginning in the early 1900s with the work of Alfred Binet.[2] The method that he employed quantified mental abilities in relation to chronologic age. It led to the concept of the IQ (intelligence quotient), which was measured by tasks examining memory, spatial relationships, reasoning, and a variety of other primary mental skills. By determining the average age required to pass each task, he derived age norms. This enabled an examiner to determine a child's mental age based on performance. For health care providers, viewing children in terms of their mental ages can be a helpful approach.

TABLE 3-2	Intelligence Quotient (IQ) Classification Guide	
IQ RANGE	**GENERAL CLASSIFICATION**	**PERCENT OF POPULATION**
140 and up	Very superior	0.5
120-139	Superior	2.5
110-119	High average	14
90-109	Average	60
80-89	Low average	12
70-79	Borderline impaired	7
69 and below	Mentally retarded	4

TABLE 3-3	American Association of Mental Deficiency Classification Schema	
IQ RANGE*	**CLASSIFICATION**	**PRACTICAL DESCRIPTION**
52-68	Mild	Can be educated in special classes to gain elementary school–level academic skills
36-51	Moderate	Can be trained to perform self-help skills and to achieve sheltered workshop employment
20-35	Severe	Abilities typically limited to simple language usage and the mastery of basic self-help skills
19 and below	Profound	Consistent custodial care required

IQ, Intelligence quotient.
*Based on Stanford-Binet intelligence test scores.

The IQ formula used by Binet was the following:

$$IQ = \frac{\text{Mental age}}{\text{Chronologic age}} \times 100$$

Thus a child who performs tasks accomplished by a 10-year-old and who has the chronologic age of 8 years has an IQ of 125 ($10/8 \times 100 = 125$). Quantification of intelligence has led to various classification guides. Table 3-2 shows the IQ ranges, the descriptive general terms, and the relative populations fitting into each category. An understanding of the levels of mental retardation can be helpful in treating young patients. Table 3-3 shows four IQ ranges and provides practical descriptions of the various groups.

Since the time of Binet, more than 300 tests have been devised to measure intellectual development. The best known and best standardized of these tests are the Wechsler intelligence scales as included in the text by Anastasi.[3] These are individualized tests, as opposed to group tests, and separate forms of the test are available for preschoolers (Wechsler Preschool and Primary Scale of Intelligence, or WPPSI), children (Wechsler Intelligence Scale for Children-Revised, or WISC-R), and adults (Wechsler Adult Intelligence Scale, or WAIS). The IQ scores that result indicate probable current levels of intellectual functioning for that person and have a high degree of reliability and validity.

At best, scores from all such tests, even the highly standardized ones, are only estimates and may not be a fair appraisal for a given child on a given day. The younger the child, the less reliable the test scores. The more delayed the child, the less reliable the test scores. The more an individual's cultural and educational opportunities differ from the norm, the less reliable and valid that test is for that individual. However, the information from psychometric assessments can alert a dentist to the possibility that a child may need an individualized approach in the dental office, as well as elsewhere.

The environment is such a crucial factor in the development of a human being that it can be discussed as an independent factor only on the theoretic level. The fact that each child appears to have a characteristic temperament from his or her earliest age has been suggested by Sigmund Freud and by Gesell and Ilg.[4,5] In recent years, however, some psychiatrists and psychologists have emphasized the influence of the child's early environment when discussing the origin of human personality. Whether personality is developed by "nature" (genetic influence) or "nurture" (environmental influence) is an age-old, unresolved question. However, if these two influences are in harmony, healthy development of the child can be expected; if they are dissonant, behavioral problems are almost sure to ensue.

VARIABLES INFLUENCING CHILDREN'S DENTAL BEHAVIORS

A fearful or anxious child who anticipates an unpleasant visit is more likely to have such an experience than is a child who has a low level of fear or anxiety. Anxiety or fearfulness affects a child's behavior and, to a large extent, determines the success of a dental appointment. The various schools of psychologic thought agree that anxiety is a personality trait, but they have various opinions concerning the origin of this trait. By the same token, dentistry has had some difficulty identifying the stimuli that lead to misbehavior in the dental office, although several variables in children's backgrounds have been related to it.

Maternal Anxiety. In past years, it has been customary for mothers, more often than fathers, to accompany children to the dental office. For this reason, the effect of maternal anxiety on children's dental visits has received considerable attention in the dental literature. Although in the near future this topic might be renamed "parental anxieties," at the moment such a change would be premature.

With few exceptions, most investigations indicate a significant correlation between maternal anxiety and a child's cooperative behavior at the first dental visit. High anxiety on the part of parents tends to affect their children's behavior negatively. Although the scientific data reveal that children of all ages can be affected by their mothers' anxieties, the effect is greatest with those under 4 years of age. This might be anticipated because of the child-parent symbiosis that begins in infancy and gradually diminishes.

Medical History. The importance of the medical history, a highly complex variable, has been debated over the years. Some pediatric dentists believe that it has little bearing on a child's behavior in the dental office, whereas others consider it a major factor affecting children's cooperation. There is general agreement, however, that children who view medical experiences positively are more likely to be cooperative with the dentist. The emotional quality of past visits rather than the number of visits is significant.

Pain experienced during previous medical visits is another consideration in a child's medical history. The pain may have been moderate or intense, real or imaginary. Nonetheless, parental beliefs about past medical pain also are significantly correlated with their children's cooperative behavior in the dental environment. Study also has shown that previous surgical experiences adversely influence behavior at the first dental visit, but this was not the case in subsequent visits.

Awareness of Dental Problem. Some children may approach their dentist knowing that they have a dental problem. The problem may be as serious as a chronic dental abscess or as simple as extrinsic staining of the dentition. However, there is a tendency toward negative behavior at the first dental visit when the child believes that a dental problem exists. Such behavior may be the result of apprehension transmitted to the child by a parent. The significance of the variable provides the dentist with a good reason for educating the parents about the value of arranging a child's first dental visit before there are any dental problems.

CLASSIFYING CHILDREN'S COOPERATIVE BEHAVIOR

Numerous systems have been developed for classifying the behavior of children in the dental environment. An understanding of them holds more than academic interest. The knowledge of these systems can be an asset

to the dentist in several ways: it can assist in directing the management method, it can provide a means for systematically recording behaviors, and it can assist in evaluating the validity of current research.

Wright's clinical classification places children in three categories[6]:

- Cooperative
- Lacking in cooperative ability
- Potentially cooperative

During examination of a child, the cooperative behavior of the patient is taken into account because it is a key to rendering treatment. Most children seen in the dental office cooperate. Cooperative children are reasonably relaxed. They have minimal apprehension. They may be enthusiastic. They can be treated by a straightforward, behavior-shaping approach. When guidelines for behavior are established, they perform within the framework provided.

In contrast is the child lacking in cooperative ability. This category includes very young children with whom communication cannot be established and of whom comprehension cannot be expected. Because of their age, they lack cooperative abilities. Another group of children who lack cooperative ability is those with specific debilitating or disabling conditions. The severity of the child's condition prohibits cooperation in the usual manner. At times, special behavior management techniques are employed for these children. Although their treatment is accomplished, immediate major positive behavioral changes cannot be expected. Characteristically, the nomenclature applied to a potentially cooperative child is *behavior problem*. This type of behavior differs from that of children lacking cooperative ability because these children *have* the capability to perform cooperatively. This is an important distinction. When a child is characterized as potentially cooperative, clinical judgment is that the child's behavior can be modified; that is, the child can become cooperative.

The dental literature is filled with descriptions of potentially cooperative patients. Moreover, the adverse reactions have been given specific labels, such as uncontrolled, defiant, timid, tense-cooperative, and whining. Dentists often use these labels because they convey, in as few words as possible, the essence of the clinical problem.

Another system, which has been used in behavioral science research, is referred to as the Frankl Behavioral Rating Scale.[7] The scale divides observed behavior into four categories, ranging from definitely positive to definitely negative. Following is a description of the scale:

Rating 1: Definitely Negative. Refusal of treatment, forceful crying, fearfulness, or any other overt evidence of extreme negativism.

Rating 2: Negative. Reluctance to accept treatment, uncooperativeness, some evidence of negative attitude but not pronounced (sullen, withdrawn).

Rating 3: Positive. Acceptance of treatment; cautious behavior at times; willingness to comply with the dentist, at times with reservation, but patient follows the dentist's directions cooperatively.

Rating 4: Definitely Positive. Good rapport with the dentist, interest in the dental procedures, laughter and enjoyment.

Although the Frankl method of classification has been a popular research tool, it also lends itself to a shorthand form that can be used for recording children's behavior in the dental office. One can identify those children displaying a positive cooperative behavior by jotting down + or ++. Conversely, uncooperative behavior can be noted by – or – –. A shortcoming of this method is that the scale does not communicate sufficient clinical information regarding uncooperative children. If a child is judged as –, the user of this classification system must qualify as well as categorize the reaction. By recording "–, tearful," a better description of the clinical problem is made.

THE FUNCTIONAL INQUIRY

Before the dentist treats children, medical and dental histories are usually obtained. However, a functional inquiry, from a behavioral viewpoint, also should be conducted. During the inquiry, there are two primary goals: (1) to learn about patient and parental concerns and (2) to gather information enabling a reliable estimate of the cooperative ability of the child. Coupling the findings from the functional inquiry with the clinical experience, the dentist is in a much better position to meet the patient's needs and to apply appropriate management strategies to treat individual pediatric patients than by simply proceeding inadequately informed.

Usually, functional inquiries are conducted in two ways: (1) by a paper and pencil questionnaire completed by the parent and (2) by direct interview of child and parent. In some offices one method may predominate, whereas in others both techniques are used. Each method has specific merits.

Written questionnaires can be important tools for gaining information, because probing questions can uncover critical facts about child-rearing practices in the home, a child's school experiences, or the patient's developmental status. Four questions with clinical relevance that can be added to history forms are listed in Box 3-2.

The responses to these questions, originally from behavioral science research, can alert the clinician to a potential behavioral problem. If a parent responds negatively to more than one question, the chance of

BOX **3-2**	Clinically Relevant Questions That Can Be Added to History Forms

	(CIRCLE ONE)
How do you think your child has reacted to past medical procedures?	Very well Moderately well Moderately poorly Very poorly
How would you rate your own anxiety (fear, nervousness) at this moment?	High Moderately high Moderately low Low
Does your child think there is anything wrong with his or her teeth, such as a chipped tooth, decayed tooth, gum boil?	Yes No
How do you expect your child to react in the dental chair?	Very well Moderately well Moderately poorly Very poorly

encountering a behavior problem rises considerably. An unlimited list of questions could, of course, be prepared for paper and pencil questionnaires, but from the dentist's viewpoint, a lengthy list is impractical.

Most practicing dentists recognize the merits of personal contact with parents. For the personal interview to serve as an efficient functional inquiry tool, a structured framework is necessary. The paper and pencil questionnaire is a starting point. It provides general information or clues and helps guide the personal interview. Consider the following question:

Do you consider your child to be (check one):

___ advanced in learning?
___ progressing normally?
___ a slow learner?

If the parent has indicated that the child is a slow learner, more factual information is necessary. A leading question in the personal interview might be, "What school does your child attend?" A child may attend a special education class or a special school. Knowledge of the child's class or special school can offer a clue about the functional level of the patient. There is no limit to the depth of the personal interview, but if it is to be efficient, questioning must be thoughtful. Other avenues that can be explored include rewards and consequences used in the home environment. These provide insight into the type of behavior management techniques that would be acceptable to a parent.

PARENTS OF PEDIATRIC PATIENTS

From the moment of their children's birth, parents shape children's behaviors by selective encouragement and discouragement of particular behaviors, by their disciplinary techniques, and by the amount of freedom they allow. In early years, at least, it is mainly from parents that children learn what they are supposed to do and what behavior is forbidden.

Because North America is a cultural mosaic, understanding parents' dental behaviors is not always easy. Dental attitudes may be deeply rooted. Differences are revealed in intercountry studies. For example, consider digital sucking, a habit with dental relevance. Examining schoolchildren in Sweden, Larsen found a 12% prevalence of the habit, whereas Golden recorded a 56% prevalence in Israeli children residing on a kibbutz.[8,9]

The socioeconomic status of parents also has some bearing on their acceptance of management methods. Fields, Machen, and Murphy had 67 parents view videotapes of children's treatments and rate their acceptability of the techniques.[10] Although most parents favored commonly used behavior-shaping methods, socioeconomic status correlated negatively with the use of general anesthesia. Those in the higher socioeconomic group frowned on the use of general anesthesia. The reduced approval may result from the fact that the higher social group was more enlightened about the associated risks.

Societal changes in the latter part of the twentieth century have created dynamics that can indirectly affect the behavior of children in dental offices. For example, a center of social policy reported that one in ten children lives in a household not headed by a parent. Often these children are brought to dental offices by caretakers or child care workers who are unfamiliar with the children's histories. Reconstituted or blended families, same-sex families, and single-parent families all present with their special sets of circumstances. Considering 218 children of teenaged mothers from birth to 5 years, Stier et al found them at greater risk for maltreatment than children of older mothers.[11]

Generalizations have been made, such as that future-oriented, conscientious, middle-class parents tend to seek dental care readily and cooperatively, and that they accept brushing and dental checkups as a matter of course. These generalizations must be approached cautiously. The dental team must recognize the individuality of parents. Some parents from the middle or upper socioeconomic strata may be well meaning and realize the importance of dentistry yet fail to follow through. Sometimes these parents are too busy with their everyday lives to cooperate with oral hygiene programs or even to bring the child to the dental office. Generalizations do not always hold true.

Despite the acknowledged importance of the parental role in the pediatric treatment triangle and the necessity of gaining parental cooperation, it is only recently that the dental literature has provided dentists with advice for dealing with parents. Good information can be gleaned from three studies by Fields, Machen, and Murphy, Murphy, Fields, and Machen, and Lawrence et al in which parents were shown videotaped scenes of different management techniques.[10,12,13] Four of the techniques were tell-show-do, positive reinforcement, voice control, and the use of a mouth prop. The six other techniques included various types of restraint methods, sedation, and general anesthesia. The techniques in this latter group were judged unacceptable by parents in the first two studies and acceptable by parents participating in the third study. The methodologic difference in the third study was the verbal explanation given to parents before showing them the videotapes. A comparison of these studies points out the importance of communicating with parents. Parents of pediatric patients often require understanding and have to be led through their children's dental experiences. We live in a litigious society, and it is critical to develop rapport with parents.

Casamassimo and Wilson reported on a survey of diplomates of the American Board of Pediatric Dentistry.[14] Most diplomates indicated that there has been a change in parental demographics. There are more single parents, increased mobility, and more dual-income families. The findings from this report found that children's behaviors in dental offices were strongly related to parenting styles, preferences, and demands. Failure of parents to set limits on their children's behaviors was the main parental child-rearing problem. They also found that parental expectations often were unattainable.

Dentists in practice have to anticipate these types of problems and learn to deal with them. The diplomates suggested several methods of coping with parent's and children's behaviors; however, one recommendation, the improvement of communication, dwarfed all others in frequency. Communication can mean many things, but in this instance it refers to the dentist's getting his or her message across to the parents and having them working with the dentist.

STRATEGIES OF THE DENTAL TEAM

A primary objective during dental procedures is to lead children step by step so that they develop a positive attitude toward dentistry. Fortunately, most children progress easily and pleasantly through their dental visits without undue pressure on themselves or the dental team. These successes can be attributed to a number of factors, such as a child's confident personality, a parent's proper preparation of the child for the appointment, or a dental team's excellent communicative skills. On the other hand, some children's dental office experiences cause anxiety and the beginning of a negative dental attitude. Sometimes these controllable but apprehensive children are managed without medication, provided that appropriate nonpharmacologic psychologic techniques are employed.

Because management techniques are used daily and come naturally to many persons, their importance is sometimes overlooked or they are taken for granted. This increases the potential for avoidable behavior problems. However, fully understanding and consciously implementing strategies can lead to recognizable improvements in child management skills. Although this section heightens awareness of various techniques commonly used in dental offices today, it should be regarded as only a start to the study of behavior management strategies.

PREAPPOINTMENT BEHAVIOR MODIFICATION

Psychologists have developed many techniques for modifying patients' behaviors by using the principles of learning theory. These techniques are called *behavior modification.* Usually they are thought about in conjunction with dentist-patient intraoperatory relationships. However, *preappointment behavior modification,* as it is used here, refers to anything that is said or done to positively influence the child's behavior before the child enters a dental operatory. The merit of this strategy is that it prepares the pediatric patient and eases the introduction to dentistry. It has received a great deal of attention because the first dental visit is crucial in the formation of the child's attitude toward dentistry. If the first visit is pleasant, it paves the road for future successes.

Several methods of preappointment behavior modification are recognized. Films or videotapes have been developed to provide a model for the young patient. The goal is to have the patient reproduce behavior exhibited by the model. On the day of the appointment, or perhaps at a previous visit, the new pediatric patient views the presentation.

Most modeling studies indicate that there is merit in introducing children to dentistry in this way, but not all studies show statistically improved cooperative behavior on the part of the children. The lack of replication may be the result of differences in experimental design, dental teams, or videotapes or films. It suggests a necessity for careful videotape or film selection for office use.

Preappointment behavior modification can also be performed with live patient models such as siblings, other children, or parents. Many dentists allow young children into the operatory with parents to preview the dental experience. Because the observing child likely will be initiated into dental care with a dental examination, a parent's recall visit offers an excellent modeling opportunity. On these occasions many young children climb into the dental chair after their parents' appointments. These previews should be selected carefully. Young children are sometimes frightened by loud noises, as from a high-speed handpiece.

The merits of modeling procedures, commonly using audiovisual or live models, are recognized by psychologists. Rimm and Masters summarized them as follows: (1) stimulation of new behaviors, (2) facilitation of behavior in a more appropriate manner, (3) disinhibition of inappropriate behavior due to fear, and (4) extinction of fears.[15] These procedures offer the practicing dentist some interesting ways to modify children's behavior before their dental visit.

Another behavior modification method involves preappointment mailings. Precontact with the parent can provide directions for preparing the child for an initial dental visit and therefore can increase the likelihood of a successful first appointment. Precontact offers a practical approach for teaching parents of new pediatric dental patients how to prepare their children for a first dental visit. Beneficial effects were demonstrated in a controlled study by Wright, Alpern, and Leake.[16] Children seemed better prepared by their mothers, and the dentist saw more cooperative pediatric patients. Almost all parents understood the letter's contents, acknowledged the dentist's thoughtfulness, and welcomed the concern for the proper presentation to their children. A similar letter is offered in Fig. 3-2.

Dentists using preappointment mailings should be selective. Correspondence has run the gamut from the simplest welcoming letter to a bombardment of mailings. Numerous mailings cause a reversal in parental attitude. Overpreparation could confuse a parent or provoke anxiety.

FUNDAMENTALS OF BEHAVIOR MANAGEMENT

Behavior management involves the total dental health team. Indeed, many dental auxiliaries are invaluable when it comes to dealing with children. All of the personnel have a stake in guiding a child through the dental experience.

Over the years, behavior management has meant different things to different people. In 1895 McElroy wrote, "Although the operative dentistry may be perfect, the appointment is a failure if the child departs in tears."[17] This was the first mention in dental literature of measuring the success or failure of a child's appointment by anything other than technical proficiency. Pediatric dentistry has progressed since that time, and a

Dear Parent:

Children who have pleasant dental appointments when they are very young are likely to have a favorable outlook toward dental care throughout life. The first appointment is very important in this attitude formation. That is the reason I am writing to you.

At our first appointment we will examine your child's teeth and gums and take any necessary x-ray films. For most children this will be an interesting and even happy occasion. All the people on our staff enjoy children and know how to work with them, but you, parents, play an important role in getting children started with a good attitude toward dental care. One of the useful things that you can do is to be completely natural and easygoing when you tell your child about the appointment with the dentist. This approach enables children to view their dental visit as an opportunity to meet some new people who want to help them stay healthy.

Your cooperation is appreciated. Remember, good general health depends partly on the development of good habits, such as sensible eating, sleeping routines, and exercise. Dental health also depends on good habits, such as proper toothbrushing, regular dental visits, and a good diet. We will have a chance to further discuss these points during your child's appointment.

Sincerely,

FIG. **3-2.** Letter currently used in clinical practice to assist parents in preparing children for first dental visit. *(Adapted from Wright GZ, Alpern GD, Leake JL: ASDC* J Dent Child *40:265-271, 1973.)*

currently adopted definition is the following:

Behavior management is the means by which the dental health team effectively and efficiently performs treatment for a child and, at the same time, instills a positive dental attitude.

Effectively in this definition refers to providing high-quality dental care. Efficient treatment is a necessity in private practice today. Quadrant dentistry, or perhaps half-mouth dentistry, using auxiliary personnel is vital in delivering efficient service to children. Finally, the development of a pediatric patient's positive attitude is an integral part of this definition. In the past many practitioners have considered "getting the job done" to be behavior management. The current definition suggests a great deal more.

What has been omitted from the definition of behavior management also is interesting. There is no mention of any specific techniques or modalities of treatment. The definition allows the exercise of individuality. The challenge to the dentist is to satisfy the elements of the definition as frequently as possible and as safely as possible for each child in a dental practice.

Although various methods in managing pediatric dental patients have evolved over the years, certain practices and concepts remain fundamental to good behavior management. These are basic to establishing good dental team–pediatric patient relationships. These

practices increase the chances for success when dealing with children. They should be considered inviolate. The following fundamentals of behavior management center on the attitude and integrity of the entire dental team.

Positive Approach. There is general agreement that the attitude or expectations of the dentist can affect the outcome of a dental appointment. The child will respond with the type of behavior expected. In essence, the child fulfills the dentist's prophecy. Thus positive statements increase the chances of success with children. They are more effective than thoughtless questions or remarks. To obtain success with children, it is important to anticipate success.

Team Attitude. Personality factors such as warmth and interest that can be conveyed without a spoken word are critical when dealing with children. A pleasant smile tells a child that an adult cares. Children respond best to a natural and friendly attitude. Often this can be conveyed immediately to the pediatric patient through a casual greeting. Children also can be made to feel comfortable in the dental office by the use of nicknames, which can be placed on a patient's record. Noting school accomplishments or extracurricular activities such as Cub Scouts, baseball, hockey, or other hobbies helps in initiating future conversations and demonstrates a friendly, caring attitude to a pediatric patient.

Organization. Plans in the dental office have many dimensions, beginning, for example, with the reception area. Who summons the new patient? The dentist, the dental assistant, the dental hygienist, or the receptionist? If a child creates a disturbance in the reception area, who will deal with the problem? Each dental office must devise its own contingency plans, and the entire office staff must know in advance what is expected of them and what is to be done. Such plans are key features of many pediatric dental offices because they increase efficiency and contribute to successful dental staff–pediatric patient relationships. Also, a well-organized, written treatment plan must be available for the dental office team. Delays and indecisiveness can build apprehension in young patients.

Truthfulness. Unlike adults, most children see things as either "black" or "white." The shades between are difficult for them to discern. To youngsters the dental health team is either truthful or not. Because truthfulness is extremely important in building trust, it is a fundamental rule for dealing with children.

Tolerance. A seldom-discussed concept, tolerance level varies from person to person. It refers to the dentist's ability to rationally cope with misbehaviors while maintaining composure. Recognizing individual tolerance levels is especially important when dealing with children. As well as varying from person to person, tolerance levels fluctuate for a given individual. For example, an upsetting experience at home can affect the clinician's mood in the dental office. Some people are in a better frame of mind early in the morning, whereas the coping abilities of others improve as the day progresses. Thus afternoon people should instruct receptionists not to book children with behavior problems the first thing in the morning. Learning to recognize factors that overtax tolerance levels is another fundamental, since it prevents loss of self-control.

Flexibility. Because children are children, lacking in maturity, the dental team must be prepared to change its plans at times. A child may begin fretting or squirming in the dental chair after half an hour, and the proposed treatment may have to be shortened. On the other hand, a dentist may plan an indirect temporary pulp treatment, but because the child is difficult, the plan may have to be altered to complete treatment at a single session. Many dentists, following accepted four-handed dentistry practices, work at the 11 o'clock or 12 o'clock position. Treatment of small children may demand a change in operating position. Thus the dental team must be flexible as the situation demands.

COMMUNICATING WITH CHILDREN

Several effective communication techniques can be suggested. These key points are guidelines, not inflexible rules, for in the unpredictable world of dealing with children, one must always be prepared to improvise as the situation requires.

Establishment of Communication. Previous editions of this textbook have stated that the first objective in the successful management of the young child is to establish communication. It is generally agreed that involving a child in a conversation not only enables the dentist to learn about the patient but also may relax the youngster. There are many ways of initiating verbal communication, and the effectiveness of these approaches differs with the age of the child. Generally, verbal communication with younger children is best initiated with complimentary comments, followed by questions that elicit an answer other than yes or no.

Establishment of the Communicator. Members of the dental team must be aware of their roles when communicating with a pediatric patient. Generally the dental assistant talks with the child during the transfer from reception room to operatory and during preparation of the child in the dental chair. When the dentist arrives, the dental assistant usually takes a more passive role, since the child can listen to only one person at a time. It is important that communication occur from a single source. When both dentist and dental assistant provide directions, the result may be a response that is undesirable simply because the child becomes confused.

Message Clarity. Communication is a complex, multisensory process. It includes a transmitter, a medium, and a receiver. The dentist or dental health team is the transmitter, the spoken word frequently is the medium, and the pediatric patient is the receiver. The message must be understood in the same way by both the sender and the receiver. As Chambers indicates, there has to be a "fit" between the intended message and the understood one.[18]

Very often, to improve the clarity of messages to young patients, dentists use euphemisms to explain procedures. For pediatric dentists, euphemisms or word substitutes are like a second language. Examples of word substitutes that can be used to explain procedures to children are given in Box 3-3.

It is important to be careful in selecting words and phrases used to indoctrinate the new pediatric dental patient, because for the young child, language labels are the basis for many generalizations. The classic example is the language label for "doctor," which confuses many youngsters. This is known as *mediated generalization.* Eventually, as a result of experiences, the child learns that the "dentist doctor" is different from the "physician doctor" and that the physician's office and the dentist's office are different environments. The process of sorting out such differences is referred to as *discrimination.*

Voice Control. Throughout the dental literature, reference is made to *voice control.* It is difficult to describe this effective communicative technique using

BOX 3-3   Word Substitutes for Explaining Procedures to Children

DENTAL TERMINOLOGY	WORD SUBSTITUTES
rubber dam	rubber raincoat
rubber dam clamp	tooth button
rubber dam frame	coat rack
sealant	tooth paint
topical fluoride gel	cavity fighter
air syringe	wind gun
water syringe	water gun
suction	vacuum cleaner
alginate	pudding
study models	statues
high speed	whistle
low speed	motorcycle

the written word. Sudden and firm commands are used to get the child's attention or to stop the child from whatever is being done. Monotonous, soothing conversation is supposed to function like music set to a mood. In both cases what is heard is more important because the dentist is attempting to influence behavior directly, not through understanding.

Although dentists have always recognized the merit of properly employing voice control when children's behaviors have been disruptive, Greenbaum et al have given it scientific credence.[19] Considering the use of loud commands as a punishment technique, they compared the effects of loud and normal voice commands given to 40 children with potential behavior problems. Their findings demonstrated that loud commands reduced disruptive behaviors.

The theory of Chambers is that voice control is most effective when used in conjunction with other communications.[18] A sudden command to "stop crying and pay attention" may be a necessary preliminary measure for future communication. The same message spoken in a foreign language probably would be equally effective in stopping disruptive patient behavior that is preventing communication. Used properly in correct situations, voice control is an effective management tool.

Multisensory Communication. In verbal communications, the focus is on *what* to say or *how* it is said. However, nonverbal messages also can be sent to patients or received from them. Body contact can be a form of nonverbal communication. The dentist's simple act of placing a hand on a child's shoulder while sitting on a chairside stool conveys a feeling of warmth and friendship. Greenbaum et al found that this type of physical contact helped children to relax, especially those 7 to 10 years of age.[19]

Eye contact is also important. The child who avoids it often is not fully prepared to cooperate. Apprehension can be conveyed without a spoken word. Detecting a rapid heartbeat or noticing beads of perspiration on the face are observations that alert the dentist to a child's nervousness. When the dentist talks to children, every effort should be made not to tower above them. Sitting and speaking at eye level allows for friendlier and less authoritative communications.

Problem Ownership. In difficult situations, dentists sometimes forget that they are dealing with children. They begin by sending "you" messages. For example, "You must sit still!" These are negative messages and only undermine the rapport between a pediatric patient and dentist. "You" messages carry the implication that the child is wrong. An alternative is to send "I" messages. These messages establish the focus of the problem, such as "I can't fix your teeth if you don't open your mouth wide." This is one of the techniques discussed by Wepman and Sonnenberg that is particularly well suited to increase the flow of information between the dentist and the pediatric patient.[20] These techniques are incorporated into the Parent Effectiveness Training Program, which was popularized in the early 1970s.

Active Listening. Listening also is important in the treatment of children. However, listening to the spoken words may be more important in dealing with the older child than it is in dealing with the younger child, for whom attention to nonverbal behavior often is more crucial. Active listening is the second step in encouraging the kind of genuine communication cited by Wepman and Sonnenberg.[20] The patient is stimulated to express feelings, and the dentist does the same, as necessary processes in communication.

Appropriate Responses. Another principle in communicating with children is that "the response should be appropriate to the situation." The appropriateness of the response depends primarily on the extent and nature of the relationship with the child, the age of the child, and evaluation of the motivation of the child's behavior. An inappropriate response would be a dentist's displaying extreme displeasure with an anxious young child on the first visit when there has been insufficient time to establish a good rapport. On the other hand, if a dentist has made inroads with a child, who then displays unacceptable behavior, a dentist may well express disapproval without losing personal control. The response is then appropriate.

BEHAVIOR SHAPING

Behavior shaping is a common nonpharmacologic technique. It is a form of behavior modification; hence, it is based on the established principles of social learning. By definition, it is that procedure which very slowly develops behavior by reinforcing successive approximations of the desired behavior until the desired behavior comes to be. Proponents of the theory hold that most behavior is learned and that learning is the establishment of a connection between a stimulus and a response. For this reason, it is sometimes called *stimulus-response (S-R) theory.*

When shaping behavior, the dental assistant or dentist is teaching a child how to behave. Young children are led through these procedures step by step. They have to be communicative and cooperative to absorb information that may be complex for them. The following is an outline for a behavior-shaping model:

1. State the general goal or task to the child at the outset.
2. Explain the necessity for the procedure. A child who understands the reason is more likely to cooperate.
3. Divide the explanation for the procedure. Children cannot always grasp the overall procedure with a single explanation; consequently, they have to be led through the procedure slowly.
4. Give all explanations at a child's level of understanding. Use euphemisms appropriately.
5. Use successive approximations. More than four decades ago, Addelston formalized a technique that encompasses several concepts from learning theory.[21] It was called the *tell-show-do (TSD) technique.* Since its introduction in 1959, it has remained a cornerstone of behavior management. TSD is a series of successive approximations. It is a component of behavior shaping that should be routinely used by all members of the dental team who work with children. Dental assistants, dental hygienists, and dentists should demonstrate various instruments step by step before their application by telling, showing, and doing. When the dentist works intraorally, a pediatric patient should be shown as much of the procedure as possible. Only when the child has a view of the procedures being undertaken are successive approximations being performed properly (Fig. 3-3).
6. Reinforce appropriate behavior. Be as specific as possible, because specific reinforcement is more effective than a generalized approach. This advice is supported by the clinical research of Weinstein et al, who studied dentists' responses to children's behavior and found that immediate and specific reinforcements were most consistently followed by reductions in children's fear-related behaviors.[22]
7. Disregard minor inappropriate behavior. Ignored minor misbehavior tends to extinguish itself when it is not reinforced.

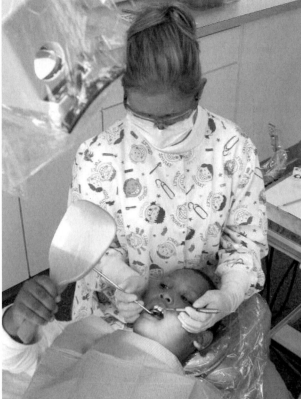

FIG. **3-3.** Child views intraoral procedure with hand mirror. If mirror blocks light to oral cavity, smaller mirror is used. With fiberoptic handpieces, blockage of light is not a problem.

Behavior shaping is regarded as a learning model. A general rule about learning models is that *the most efficient learning models are those that follow the learning theory model most closely.* Deviations from the model create less efficiency in terms of learning. One way to improve consistency in this area is to record various clinical sessions with pediatric patients, using a tape recorder or videotape system, and then to review the tapes, keeping in mind the basics of the behavior-shaping learning model.

Although TSD is similar to behavior shaping, the two differ. As well as demanding the reinforcement of cooperative behavior, behavior shaping also includes the need to retrace steps if misbehavior occurs. For example, if a child is shown an instrument and looks away, the dentist must revert to the explanatory portion of the procedure. Behavior shaping requires that the "desired behavior" be observed along the way. If the dentist proceeds along the sequential steps and begins performing treatment when the desired behavior is not present, there is deviation from the learning model and a greater likelihood of increased misbehavior.

RETRAINING

Children who require retraining approach the dental office displaying considerable apprehension or negative behavior. The demonstrated behavior may be the result of a previous dental visit or the effect of improper parental or peer orientation. Determining the source of the problem is obviously helpful, for then the problem can be avoided through another technique or deemphasized, or a distraction can be used. These ploys begin the retraining program, which eventually leads to behavior shaping.

When encountering negative behavior, the dentist should always have in mind that an objective is to build a new series of associations in the child's mind. If a child's expectation of being hurt is not reinforced, a new set of expectations is learned. The dentist can be trusted! The child develops a new perception of the dental office and a new relationship to dentistry. Unacceptable behavior learned previously becomes extinguished. It is critical to remember that *the stimulus must be altered to elicit a change in the response.*

Individuals respond to stimuli to which they have been preconditioned. If the original stimulus and the new one are very similar, then the response will be similar. This is known as *stimulus generalization.* If a child has had an unpleasant experience in the dental office and then is taken to a different office where there is a different dentist and an entirely different staff and surroundings, the child still tends to generalize that an unpleasant event will occur in this new dental office. There are enough similar stimuli to produce this response. To offset the generalization, the dental team must demonstrate a "difference." This is one of the reasons why the use of nitrous oxide–oxygen sedation often works when retraining children. It offers a difference.

AVERSIVE CONDITIONING

The behavior modification method of aversive conditioning is also known as *hand-over-mouth exercise,* or by the acronym *HOME.* Its purpose is to gain the attention of a highly oppositional child so that communication can be established and cooperation obtained for a safe course of treatment. The technique fits the rules of learning theory: maladaptive acts (screaming, kicking) are linked to restraint (hand over mouth), and cooperative behavior is related to removal of the restriction and the use of positive reinforcement (praise).

It is important to stress that aversive conditioning is not used routinely but as a method of last resort, usually with children 3 to 6 years of age who have appropriate communicative abilities. Levitas emphasizes that for the very young, the immature, those with physical disabilities, or those who have mental or emotional disabilities, this behavioral approach is unacceptable.[23]

In recent years concern has been shown about the use of aversive conditioning. Some dentists have characterized the technique as punishment. Surveys of pedodontic diplomates in 1972 and 1981, however, demonstrated acceptance by a substantial portion of the profession. In both instances more than 80% of the pediatric dentists indicated that they used aversive therapy at times. Inquiring into acceptance of the technique by dental educators, Davis and Rombom obtained similar results; 83% of the respondents taught aversive conditioning in advanced training programs.[24] Some parents, too, have disapproved of the technique, and another concern has been a legal one. Bowers points out that acceptance of aversive conditioning by the dental profession is not an absolute assurance of the legality of the technique and that until a court rules on its legitimacy there remains some degree of uncertainty.[25] He also contends that the dentist who uses aversive conditioning in accordance with the standards of the prudent dentist in the locale and who obtains the requisite consent to treatment should not fear liability for battery or malpractice.

Aversive conditioning can be a safe and effective method of managing a child with an extremely difficult behavior problem. However, any departure from the accepted application of aversive conditioning may expose the dentist to liability. Those dentists or dental students who contemplate using it should consult detailed writings beforehand. Hagan et al strongly suggest that dentists also should be aware of the acceptability of the technique in their practice location.[26]

PRACTICAL CONSIDERATIONS

Some procedural aspects of dental practice help to guide children through their dental experiences successfully. Like many of the techniques described previously, they have evolved over the years without experimental testing. Nevertheless, these practical considerations form an integral part of present-day dental practice. They also would be fruitful areas for future research.

Scheduling. Children are bundles of energy. Lacking the patience of adults, many children become restless and tired when faced with long delays in a reception area. This should be taken into account when designing an office schedule. A good general rule is that a child should not be kept waiting in the reception area and that every effort should be made to be on time.

Morning appointments have been suggested for children. It is a practice that has guided scheduling in many dental offices. The suggestion was based on the facts that children are more alert and the dental team is fresher in the morning. Many dentists also believe that when age groups are kept together (preschoolers in the morning and older children in the afternoon), the peer group has a positive influence, with children serving as models for each other. Another advantage is that the dental office may run more smoothly with less psychologic change of pace.

Sometimes expediency rather than a realistic evaluation of a child's behavior may predispose the dentist toward morning appointments for preschool children. Frequently it is easier to persuade parents to take younger children out of nursery school or kindergarten than to arrange morning appointments for elementary or junior high school children. From a behavioral standpoint, other factors seem important when deciding the appointment time. Patient-related concerns include patient age, presence of a handicapping condition, and need for any sedation. The dentist's attitude also is important. Some dentists avoid seeing children with behavior problems first thing in the morning. A policy regarding scheduling should be formulated by the dentist, and scheduling should not be left to chance.

Another scheduling concern has been appointment length. Historically, writers have agreed that the nature of childhood precludes giving the sustained attention that may be required for long dental visits. Generally, a long visit is defined as any period in excess of half an hour. Most of these views were expressed more than 30 years ago, and appointments have increased in duration. Improved technology, the application of time and motion studies by efficiency experts, and the current trend toward quadrant or half-mouth dentistry have altered contemporary practices. Whether this affects children adversely remains a question for researchers. In Lenchner's study, the behavior of 43 children between 3 and 5½ years of age who were undergoing operative dentistry was examined in both short and long appointments.[27] Short appointments ranged from 16 to 30 minutes, whereas longer appointments were 48 to 125 minutes. The investigator found no significant difference in children's behavior during long dental appointments compared with shorter ones. On the other hand, Getz and Weinstein, studying videotapes of 36 children between 3 and 5 years of age who were undergoing restorative treatment, found the opposite.[28] The longer the restorative phase, the greater the likelihood of a stress-fear reaction. Thus current evidence on appointment duration is divided.

Parent-Child Separation. Excluding the parent from the operating room can contribute toward development of positive behavior on the part of the child. Over the years, Starkey has been one of the strongest advocates of separation of the child from the parent during treatment and has suggested that the policy of requiring the parent to remain in the reception room could be justified for many of the following reasons[29]:

- The parent often repeats orders, which creates an annoyance for both the dentist and the pediatric patient.
- The parent injects orders, becoming a barrier to development of rapport between the dentist and the child.
- The dentist is unable to use voice intonation in the presence of the parent because he or she may be offended.
- The child divides attention between the parent and dentist.
- The dentist divides attention between the parent and child.

There are other reasons for advocating a separation policy. Most dentists probably are more relaxed and comfortable when the parent remains in the reception area. Perhaps they then do not feel that they are "performing with an audience." As a consequence of their more relaxed manner, their actions are likely to have more positive effects on many children's behaviors.

When an office policy is formed, remember that many dentists who exclude parents from the operatory make exceptions. A parent can be a major asset in supporting and communicating with a disabled child, often providing important information and interpretation. Another important exception relates to age. Very young children (those who have not reached the age of understanding and full verbal communication) have a close symbiotic relationship with parents; consequently, they usually are accompanied by them. The age factor was studied by Frankl, Shiere, and Fogels, who investigated the effect of a parent's presence in the operatory.[7] In their study the intact group (parent present with child) reacted more favorably than the separated group. It should be noted that children 3½ to 4 years of age appeared to benefit most from the parent's presence. Those older than 4 years demonstrated similar levels of response to dental care regardless of parental presence. Thus dentists who contemplate admitting only parents of infants and toddlers to the operatory might consider extending the age level somewhat.

The separation procedure warrants serious consideration. The dentist must develop an office policy, notify the office staff of it, and assume responsibility to train office personnel in reception room strategies. In this age of accountability, the dentist may also have to explain the policy to a parent. Establishment of the policy therefore should be based on a rationale that takes into account the benefits and drawbacks resulting from separation as well as the dentist's personal views.

Because some dentists become tense when parents are present and others enjoy having parents in the operatory, to some extent an office policy becomes an individual decision.

Tangible Reinforcements. Giving gifts to children has become a fact of commercial life in North America. There is general agreement on the merit of this practice in the dental office, for gift giving can serve as a reward. If the gift has a dental significance (such as a toothbrush kit), so much the better. In these situations the gift is also used as a reinforcement for dental health.

Various trinkets in a toy chest should be used as tokens of affection for children, not as bribes. Finn made the following distinction between rewards and bribes: "A bribe is promised to induce the behavior. A reward is recognition of good behavior after completion of the operation, without previously implied promise."[30] The gift-giving practice can have spectacular results. Many children who seem tense during operative procedures suddenly perk up on completion and scurry for a gift. These gifts provide a pleasant reminder of the appointment.

Dental Attire. Because fears are transferable from one situation to another, dentists have had some concern about wearing child-friendly apparel. If a child had poor experiences previously (whether with a physician or a barber), it is possible that these fears could be generalized to the dental situation, since a uniform can be common to all. Similarly, children who have been exposed to prior surgical procedures might be frightened by a face mask. Investigating this potential problem, Siegel et al suggested that wearing a mask during dental treatment represents a minimal stressor for the young child but recommended introducing the child to the dental environment and experience without the use of a protective mask.[31]

Opinions have differed on the relative importance of the dental team's attire. Research evidence from psychiatry and nursing has indicated few pervasive differences associated with the clothing worn. Similarly, research in dentistry has indicated that there were no significant preferences by patients. On the other hand, a survey of the Association of Pedodontic Diplomates suggested that enough children react unfavorably to white uniforms that many pediatric dentists have taken to wearing colored clothing.

Wearing apparel conceivably can influence both patients and professional staff. Less formal attire undoubtedly will have a beneficial effect on some children. It could also aid the staff by contributing toward a more natural and casual attitude. On the other hand, there are those who feel that street clothing might affect their professional image. Because conclusive evidence is lacking, it could be said that a dentist's attire remains a personal decision. Today, many practitioners and their staff have opted for wearing colorful scrubs and clinic gowns.

LIMITATIONS

Children today differ from those of 20 or 30 years ago. The child begins school earlier. Through the media, the child is more aware than children were years ago. We hear more of children facing poverty, experiencing learning disorders, and developing poor coping skills, and are more aware of children with eating disorders and drug usage. Children also have legal and social advocates who have influenced management techniques. Limitations on the dentist exist today that were unheard of previously.

Parenting also has changed. Much of the behavioral science research was done with traditional families in the 1960s and 1970s. Single-parent homes were less common, and terms such as *reconstituted families* and *partner relationships* were unknown. What about the child-rearing practices in these families? Two decades ago, when "father" came to the office, it usually meant that the child had a behavior problem and "father" was the enforcer. If a child misbehaved, the father might have spanked the child. Today, this is unacceptable in many families. With both parents working in many homes, it is not unusual for a father to accompany a child to the dental office. Have parental expectations changed in the dental office? Yes. This chapter discussed the reasons why parents might be excluded from the operatory, but it also urged reviewing the policy periodically. Years ago parents did not expect to enter the operatory. Currently, more and more parents insist on their right to accompany their child. Societal changes influence our management methods, and there is a need to review past research carefully and assess its applicability to the present.

The dentist has societal limitations, too, and they are changing approaches to management. Years ago the HOME technique might have been used to subdue a 3-year-old so that the dentist could perform an examination. This chapter did not describe the technique in detail because in today's society the dentist must have informed consent before using the HOME technique. It is also mandatory to be well trained in the use of the technique. Indeed, Carr et al report that the majority of pediatric dentists they surveyed use less aversive techniques (e.g., parents in the operatory, etc.) and had decreased or discontinued use of controversial techniques like HOME because of parental influences and legal and ethical concerns.[32] Dental students rarely have the opportunity to use the technique. Because dental practitioners are encouraged to perform behavior management consistent with their educational training and clinical experience, the technique may not belong in the armamentarium of most general practitioners.

The corners of the pediatric treatment triangle have been changing rapidly, and this influences the practice of dentistry for children. Recognizing these changing times, the Clinical Affairs Committee of the American Academy of Pediatric Dentistry has produced guidelines for behavior management.[33] The techniques recommended in this chapter conform to these guidelines. However, there are limitations to written standards; these standards change. Dental students and dentists must remember to keep abreast of the times in this highly dynamic area.

REFERENCES

1. Alpern GD: Child development: basic concepts and considerations. In Wright GZ: *Behavior management in dentistry for children*, Philadelphia, 1975, WB Saunders.
2. Binet A: New methods for the diagnosis of the intellectual level of subnormals, *L'Année Psycholgique* 12:191-244, 1905.
3. Anastasi A: *Psychological testing*, New York, 1976, Macmillan.
4. Freud S: *The problem of anxiety*, New York, 1936, WW Norton and Co. Originally published in 1923 in German.
5. Gesell A, Ilg FL: *Child development: an introduction to the study of human growth*, New York, 1949, Harper & Row.
6. Wright GZ: *Behavior management in dentistry for children*, Philadelphia, 1975, WB Saunders.
7. Frankl SN, Shiere FR, Fogels HR: Should the parent remain in the operatory? *J Dent Child* 29:150-163, 1962.
8. Larsen E: Dummy and fingersucking, *Sven Tandlak Tidskr* 64:667, 1971.
9. Golden A: Patterns of child rearing in relation to thumbsucking, *Br J Orthod* 5:81-85, 1978.
10. Fields HW Jr, Machen JB, Murphy MG: The acceptability of various behavior management techniques relative to types of treatment, *Pediatr Dent* 6:199-203, 1984.
11. Stier DM et al: Are children born to young mothers at increased risk of maltreatment? *Pediatrics* 91:642-648, 1993.
12. Murphy ML, Fields HW Jr, Machen, JB: Parental acceptance of pediatric dentistry behavior techniques, *Pediatr Dent* 6: 193-198, 1984.
13. Lawrence SM et al: Parental attitudes toward behavior management techniques in pediatric dentistry, *Pediatr Dent* 13:151-155, 1991.
14. Casamassimo P, Wilson S: Effects of changing US parenting styles on dental practice: perceptions of diplomates of the American Board of Pediatric Dentistry, *Pediatric Dent* 24: 18-22, 2002.
15. Rimm DC, Masters JC: *Behavior therapy: techniques and empirical findings*, New York, 1974, Academic Press.
16. Wright GZ, Alpern GD, Leake JL: The modifiability of maternal anxiety as it relates to children's cooperative dental behavior, *J Dent Child* 40:265-271, 1973.
17. McElroy CM: Dentistry for children, *Calif Dent Assoc Trans*, p 85, 1895.
18. Chambers DW: Behavior management techniques for pediatric dentists: an embarrassment of riches, *J Dent Child* 44:30-34, 1977.
19. Greenbaum PE et al: Dentist's reassuring touch: effects on children's behavior, *Pediatr Dent* 15:20-24, 1993.
20. Wepman BJ, Sonnenberg EM: Effective communication with the pedodontic patient, *J Pedod* 2:316-321, 1979.
21. Addelston HK: Child patient training, *Fortn Rev Chic Dent Soc* 38:7-9, 27-29, 1959.
22. Weinstein P et al: The effect of dentists' behaviors on fear-related behaviors in children, *J Am Dent Assoc* 104:32-38, 1982.
23. Levitas TC: HOME—hand over mouth exercise, *J Dent Child* 41:178-182, 1974.
24. Davis MJ, Rombom HM: Survey of the utilization and rationale for hand-over-mouth (HOM) and restraint in post-doctoral pedodontic education, *Pediatr Dent* 1:87-90, 1979.
25. Bowers LT: The legality of using hand-over-mouth exercise for management of child behavior, *J Dent Child* 49:257-265, 1982.
26. Hagan PP et al: The legal status of informed consent for behavior management techniques in dentistry, *Pediatr Dent* 6:204-208, 1984.
27. Lenchner V: The effect of appointment length on behavior of the pedodontic patient and his attitude toward dentistry, *J Dent Child* 33:61-74, 1966.
28. Getz T, Weinstein P: The effect of structural variables on child behavior in the operatory, *Pediatr Dent* 3:262-266, 1981.
29. Starkey PE: Training office personnel to manage children. In Wright GZ: *Behavior management in dentistry for children*, Philadelphia, 1975, WB Saunders.
30. Finn SB: *Clinical pedodontics*, ed 4, Philadelphia, 1973, WB Saunders.
31. Siegel LJ et al: The effects of using infection-control barrier techniques on young children's behavior during dental treatment, *J Dent Child* 59:17-22, 1992.
32. Carr KR et al: Behavior management techniques among pediatric dentists practicing in the southeastern United States, *Pediatr Dent* 21:347-353, 1999.
33. American Academy of Pediatric Dentistry: Guidelines for behavior management, *Pediatr Dent (supplemental issue: reference manual 2002-2003)* 24:68-74, 2002.

SUGGESTED READINGS

Baghdadi ZD: Principles and application of learning theory in child patient management, *Quintessence Int* 32:135-141, 2002.

Dummett CO, Adair SM: Workshop on practical and cost-effective issues of behavior management, *Pediatr Dent* 21: 470-471, 1999.

Greenbaum PE et al: Dentist's voice control: effects on children's disruptive behaviors, *Health Psychol* 9:546-558, 1990.

Molinari GE, DeYoung AK: Non-pharmacologic behavior management techniques used with pediatric dental patients, *J Mich Dent Assoc* 84:30-33, 2002.

Nainar SM: Profile of pediatric dental literature: thirty-year time trends (1969-1998), *J Dent Child* 68:388-390, 2001.

Wright GZ, Starkey PE, Gardner DE: *Child management in dentistry*, Bristol, 1987, IOP Publishing.

4

Development and Morphology of the Primary Teeth

RALPH E. McDONALD

DAVID R. AVERY

This chapter presents a brief review of the development of the teeth. An accurate chronology of primary tooth calcification is of clinical significance to the dentist. It is often necessary to explain to parents the time sequence of calcification in utero and during infancy. The common observation of tetracycline pigmentation, developmental enamel defects, and generalized hereditary anomalies can be explained if the calcification schedule is known. A brief discussion of the morphology of the primary teeth is also appropriate before considering restorative procedures for children.

A much more complete review is available in the reference texts on oral histology, dental anatomy, and developmental anatomy listed at the end of the chapter. Furthermore, contemporary scientists are rapidly gaining knowledge of tooth development at the molecular level. We suggest that readers with a special interest in the molecular events of tooth development study the listed references by Ferguson et al and Sahlberg et al, and an extensive review article by Smith.[1-5]

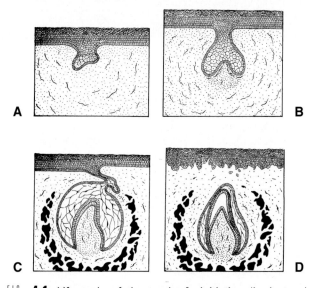

FIG. **4-1.** Life cycle of the tooth. **A,** Initiation (bud stage). **B,** Proliferation (cap stage). **C,** Histodifferentiation and morphodifferentiation (bell stage). **D,** Apposition and calcification. *(Adapted from Schour I, Massler M: Studies in tooth development: the growth pattern of human teeth,* J Am Dent Assoc *27:1785, 1940.)*

LIFE CYCLE OF THE TOOTH

INITIATION (BUD STAGE)

Evidence of development of the human tooth can be observed as early as the sixth week of embryonic life. Cells in the basal layer of the oral epithelium proliferate at a more rapid rate than do the adjacent cells. The result is an epithelial thickening in the region of the future dental arch that extends along the entire free margin of the jaws. This thickening is called the *primordium of the ectodermal portion of the teeth* and what results is called the *dental lamina.* At the same time, 10 round or ovoid swellings occur in each jaw in the position to be occupied by the primary teeth.

Certain cells of the basal layer begin to proliferate at a more rapid rate than do the adjacent cells (Fig. 4-1, *A*). These proliferating cells contain the entire growth potential of the teeth. The permanent molars, like the primary teeth, arise from the dental lamina. The permanent incisors, canines, and premolars develop from the buds of their primary predecessors. The congenital absence of a tooth is the result of a lack of initiation or an arrest in the proliferation of cells. The presence of supernumerary teeth is the result of a continued budding of the enamel organ.

PROLIFERATION (CAP STAGE)

Proliferation of the cells continues during the cap stage. As a result of unequal growth in the different parts of the bud, a cap is formed (Fig. 4-1, *B*). A shallow

invagination appears on the deep surface of the bud. The peripheral cells of the cap later form the outer and inner enamel epithelium.

As with a deficiency in initiation, a deficiency in proliferation results in failure of the tooth germ to develop and in less than the normal number of teeth. Excessive proliferation of cells may result in epithelial rests. These rests may remain inactive or become activated as a result of an irritation or stimulus. If the cells become partially differentiated or detached from the enamel organ in their partially differentiated state, they assume the secretory functions common to all epithelial cells, and a cyst develops. If the cells become more fully differentiated or detached from the enamel organ, they produce enamel and dentin, which results in an odontoma (see Fig. 7-5) or a supernumerary tooth. The degree of differentiation of the cells determines whether a cyst, an odontoma, or a supernumerary tooth develops (see Figs. 27-50 to 27-52).

HISTODIFFERENTIATION AND MORPHODIFFERENTIATION (BELL STAGE)

The epithelium continues to invaginate and deepen until the enamel organ takes on the shape of a bell (Fig. 4-1, *C*). It is during this stage that there is a differentiation of the cells of the dental papilla into odontoblasts and of the cells of the inner enamel epithelium into ameloblasts.

Histodifferentiation marks the end of the proliferative stage as the cells lose their capacity to multiply. This stage is the forerunner of appositional activity. Disturbances in the differentiation of the formative cells of the tooth germ result in abnormal structure of the dentin or enamel. One clinical example of the failure of ameloblasts to differentiate properly is amelogenesis imperfecta (see Fig. 7-31). The failure of the odontoblasts to differentiate properly, with the resultant abnormal dentin structure, results in the clinical entity dentinogenesis imperfecta (see Fig. 7-28).

In the morphodifferentiation stage the formative cells are arranged to outline the form and size of the tooth. This process occurs before matrix deposition. The morphologic pattern of the tooth becomes established when the inner enamel epithelium is arranged so that the boundary between it and the odontoblasts outlines the future dentinoenamel junction. Disturbances and aberrations in morphodifferentiation lead to abnormal forms and sizes of teeth. Some of the resulting conditions are peg teeth, other types of microdontia, and macrodontia.

APPOSITION

Appositional growth is the result of a layerlike deposition of a nonvital extracellular secretion in the form of a tissue matrix. This matrix is deposited by the formative cells, ameloblasts, and odontoblasts, which line up along the future dentinoenamel and dentinocemental junction at the stage of morphodifferentiation. These cells deposit the enamel and dentin matrix according to a definite pattern and at a definite rate. The formative cells begin their work at specific sites referred to as *growth centers* as soon as the blueprint, the dentinoenamel junction, is completed (Fig. 4-1, *D*).

Any systemic disturbance or local trauma that injures the ameloblasts during enamel formation can cause an interruption or an arrest in matrix apposition, which results in enamel hypoplasia (see Fig. 7-16). Hypoplasia of the dentin is less common than enamel hypoplasia and occurs only after severe systemic disturbances (see Fig. 7-15).

CALCIFICATION

Calcification (mineralization) takes place following matrix deposition and involves the precipitation of inorganic calcium salts within the deposited matrix. The process begins with the precipitation of a small nidus about which further precipitation occurs. The original nidus increases in size by the addition of concentric laminations. There is an eventual approximation and fusion of these individual calcospherites into a homogeneously mineralized layer of tissue matrix. If the calcification process is disturbed, there is a lack of fusion of the calcospherites. These deficiencies are not readily identified in the enamel, but in the dentin they are evident microscopically and are referred to as *interglobular dentin.*

EARLY DEVELOPMENT AND CALCIFICATION OF THE ANTERIOR PRIMARY TEETH

Kraus and Jordan have found that the first macroscopic indication of morphologic development occurs at approximately 11 weeks in utero.[6] The maxillary and mandibular central incisor crowns appear identical at this early stage as tiny, hemispheric, moundlike structures.

The lateral incisors begin to develop morphologic characteristics between 13 and 14 weeks. There is evidence of the developing canines between 14 and 16 weeks. Calcification of the central incisor begins at approximately 14 weeks in utero, with the maxillary central incisor slightly preceding the lower central. The initial calcification of the lateral incisor occurs at 16 weeks and of the canine at 17 weeks.

It is interesting to note that the developmental dates listed precede by 3 to 4 weeks the dates that appear in the chronology of the human dentition, as developed by Logan and Kronfeld.[7] This observation has been confirmed by Lunt and Law.[8]

EARLY DEVELOPMENT AND CALCIFICATION OF THE POSTERIOR PRIMARY TEETH AND THE FIRST PERMANENT MOLAR

The maxillary first primary molar appears macroscopically at 12½ weeks in utero. Kraus and Jordan[6] have observed that as early as 15½ weeks the apex of the mesiobuccal cusp may undergo calcification. At approximately 34 weeks the entire occlusal surface is covered by calcified tissue. At birth, calcification includes roughly three fourths of the occlusal gingival height of the crown.

The maxillary second primary molar also appears macroscopically at about 12½ weeks in utero. There is evidence of calcification of the mesiobuccal cusp as early as 19 weeks. At birth, calcification extends occlusogingivally to include approximately one fourth of the height of the crown.

The mandibular first primary molar initially becomes evident macroscopically at about 12 weeks in utero. Calcification may be observed as early as 15½ weeks at the apex of the mesiobuccal cusp. At birth, a completely calcified cap covers the occlusal surface.

The mandibular second primary molar also becomes evident macroscopically at 12½ weeks in utero. According to Kraus and Jordan, calcification may begin at 18 weeks.[6] At the time of birth the five centers have coalesced and only a small area of uncalcified tissue remains in the middle of the occlusal surface. There are sharp conical cusps, angular ridges, and a smooth occlusal surface, all of which indicate that calcification of these areas is incomplete at birth. Thus there is a calcification sequence of central incisor, first molar, lateral incisor, canine, and second molar.

The work of Kraus and Jordan would indicate that the adjacent second primary and the first permanent molars undergo identical patterns of morphodifferentiation but at different times and that the initial development of the first permanent molar occurs slightly later. Their excellent research has also shown that the first permanent molars are uncalcified before 28 weeks of age; at any time thereafter calcification may begin. Some degree of calcification is always present at birth.

MORPHOLOGY OF INDIVIDUAL PRIMARY TEETH

MAXILLARY CENTRAL INCISOR

The mesiodistal width of the crown of the maxillary central incisor is greater than the cervicoincisal length.

Developmental lines are usually not evident in the crown; thus the labial surface is smooth. The incisal edge is nearly straight even before abrasion becomes evident. There are well-developed marginal ridges on the lingual surface and a distinctly developed cingulum (Figs. 4-2 and 4-3). The root of the incisor is cone shaped with tapered sides.

MAXILLARY LATERAL INCISOR

The outline of the maxillary lateral incisor is similar to that of the central incisor, but the crown is smaller in all dimensions. The length of the crown from the cervical to the incisal edge is greater than the mesiodistal width. The root outline is similar to that of the central incisor but is longer in proportion to the crown.

MAXILLARY CANINE

The crown of the maxillary canine is more constricted at the cervical region than are the incisors, and the incisal and distal surfaces are more convex. There is a well-developed sharp cusp rather than a relatively straight incisal edge. The canine has a long, slender, tapering

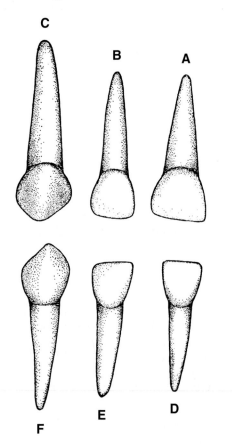

FIG. **4-2.** Primary right anterior teeth, labial aspect. **A,** Maxillary central incisor. **B,** Maxillary lateral incisor. **C,** Maxillary canine. **D,** Mandibular central incisor. **E,** Mandibular lateral incisor. **F,** Mandibular canine. *(From Ash MM, Nelson SJ: Wheeler's dental anatomy, physiology, and occlusion, ed 8, Philadelphia, 2003, WB Saunders.)*

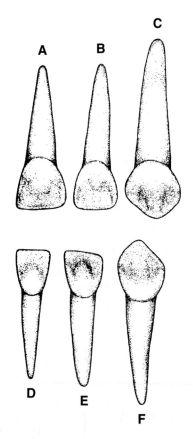

FIG. **4-3.** Primary right anterior teeth, lingual aspect. **A,** Maxillary central incisor. **B,** Maxillary lateral incisor. **C,** Maxillary canine. **D,** Mandibular central incisor. **E,** Mandibular lateral incisor. **F,** Mandibular canine. *(From Ash MM, Nelson SJ: Wheeler's dental anatomy, physiology, and occlusion, ed 8, Philadelphia, 2003, WB Saunders.)*

root that is more than twice the length of the crown. The root is usually inclined distally, apical to the middle third.

MANDIBULAR CENTRAL INCISOR

The mandibular central incisor is smaller than the maxillary central, but its labiolingual measurement is usually only 1 mm less. The labial aspect presents a flat surface without developmental grooves. The lingual surface presents marginal ridges and a cingulum. The middle third and the incisal third on the lingual surface may have a flattened surface level with the marginal ridges, or there may be a slight concavity. The incisal edge is straight, and it bisects the crown labiolingually. The root is approximately twice the length of the crown.

MANDIBULAR LATERAL INCISOR

The outline of the mandibular lateral incisor is similar to that of the central incisor but is somewhat larger in all dimensions except labiolingually. The lingual surface may have greater concavity between the marginal ridges. The incisal edge slopes toward the distal aspect of the tooth.

MANDIBULAR CANINE

The form of the mandibular canine is similar to that of the maxillary canine, with a few exceptions. The crown is slightly shorter, and the root may be as much as 2 mm shorter than that of the maxillary canine. The mandibular canine is not as large labiolingually as its maxillary opponent.

MAXILLARY FIRST MOLAR

The greatest dimension of the crown of the maxillary first molar is at the mesiodistal contact areas, and from these areas the crown converges toward the cervical region (Figs. 4-4 to 4-6).

The mesiolingual cusp is the largest and sharpest. The distolingual cusp is poorly defined, small, and rounded. The buccal surface is smooth, with little evidence of developmental grooves. The three roots are long, slender, and widely spread.

MAXILLARY SECOND MOLAR

There is considerable resemblance between the maxillary primary second molar and the maxillary first permanent molar. There are two well-defined buccal

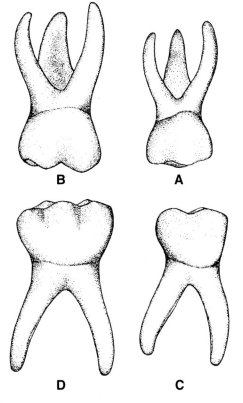

FIG. **4-4.** Primary right molars, buccal aspect. **A,** Maxillary first molar. **B,** Maxillary second molar. **C,** Mandibular first molar. **D,** Mandibular second molar. *(From Ash MM, Nelson SJ: Wheeler's dental anatomy, physiology, and occlusion, ed 8, Philadelphia, 2003, WB Saunders.)*

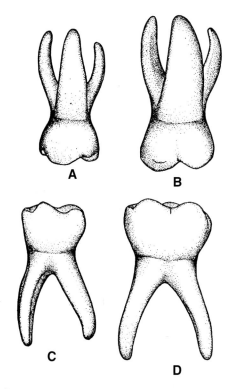

FIG. **4-5.** Primary right molars, lingual aspect. **A,** Maxillary first molar. **B,** Maxillary second molar. **C,** Mandibular first molar. **D,** Mandibular second molar. *(From Ash MM, Nelson SJ: Wheeler's dental anatomy, physiology, and occlusion, ed 8, Philadelphia, 2003, WB Saunders.)*

Roentgen's discovery of the x-ray in 1895 provided one of the most important diagnostic aids in dentistry. Radiographs are essential if we are to treat children successfully. Evidence indicates that, unless carious lesions are discovered early, the primary teeth will not be retained until normal exfoliation.

Early diagnosis of caries prevents the pediatric patient from experiencing dental pain, extraction, and emotional stress. In addition, eruptive or developmental problems can be discovered with the use of radiographic images, and early treatment of these problems may reduce the need for prolonged orthodontic procedures. Some restorative procedures require an accurate registration of the pulpal outline that only a radiograph can reveal.

The selection of appropriate radiographs for the pediatric patient depends on the age of the child, the size of the oral cavity, and the level of patient cooperation. These are determined by a careful clinical examination of the patient before ordering the radiographic survey. The examination determines the need for radiographs and the type to be taken. Ideal technique should expose the patient to a minimum amount of radiation, require as few radiographs as possible, take as little time as possible, and provide a diagnostically accurate examination of the dentition and supporting structures. The child's cooperation is as essential to radiographic examination as is the selection of correct radiographic technique. Both increase the probability of success and reduce additional radiographic exposure.

Dental radiographic equipment can be threatening or can generate curiosity, depending on the child. It is wise to allow the patient to run a hand over the x-ray head and become acquainted with the "camera." The patient might hold one of the films and be shown where it will be placed. If it is a film that requires biting pressure, the patient should be shown how to bite on the film. "Show and tell" will go a long way in gaining cooperation. Careful wording of the description of the procedure is essential to gain patient cooperation. The potential cooperation of many a patient has been lost when the patient hears that you will be "shooting" a couple of films. Imaging the easiest region first may ensure success in other areas. This is particularly important if the child has an exaggerated gag reflex or objects to the placement of the film. The use of topical anesthetic agents may be beneficial in both situations.

The dentist should be patient with the child in obtaining radiographs. Repeated attempts at film placement may be necessary before the actual radiation exposure is made. If the child is uncooperative, firmness, voice control, and tender loving care are often effective. Emotionally, mentally, and physically disabled children require special handling.

RADIATION SAFETY AND PROTECTION

One characteristic of x-radiation is its ability to impart some of its energy to the matter it traverses. If that matter is living tissue, then some biologic injury may occur. Much information about high levels of radiation and subsequent damage is available. The effects of low levels of x-radiation (as used in diagnostic radiology) on biologic systems are virtually unknown. Our assumptions of damage are based on extrapolation of data from high levels to lower levels of radiation.

Still, dental health professionals must be concerned about any risk the patient may encounter during therapy. Concern is focused on three primary biologic effects of low-level radiation: (1) carcinogenesis, (2) teratogenesis (malformations), and (3) mutagenesis. Carcinogenesis and malformations are a response of somatic tissues and in most instances are believed to have a threshold response; that is, a certain amount of radiation is necessary before the response is seen. Mutation may occur as a response of genetic tissue (gonads) to x-radiation and is believed to have no threshold. In general, younger tissues and organs are more sensitive to radiation, with the sensitivity decreasing from the period before birth until maturity. It must also be recognized that far higher doses of radiation can be withstood by localized areas than by the whole body. We know that we live in a world that exposes us to natural background radiation averaging 360 mrem per year (3.60 millisievert) in the United States. Medical and dental radiographic examinations add to that exposure, and so must be ordered judiciously.

With regard to patient protection, evidence has shown that there are critical organs vulnerable to possible development of late effects. These organs should be shielded when possible. These critical organs and the associated adverse biologic effects are the following: (1) the skin (cancer), (2) red bone marrow (leukemia), (3) the gonads (mutation, infertility, and fetal malformations), (4) the eyes (cataracts), (5) the thyroid (cancer), (6) the breasts (cancer), and (7) possibly the salivary glands (cancer).

The practitioner and staff can physically protect the patient and indirectly protect themselves from unnecessary exposure to radiation by the use of correct technique. The most obvious method of protecting the patient is to shield those areas not being evaluated. This is easily accomplished using a lead apron and thyroid collar (Fig. 5-1).

The apron and collar may be incorporated as a single unit or used separately. The apron protects the gonads

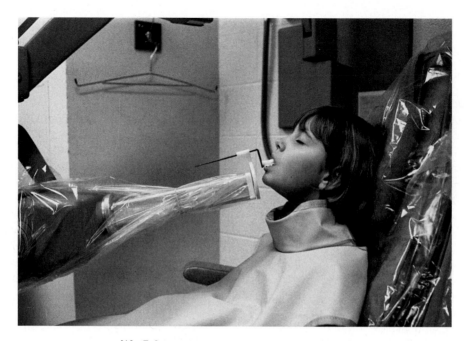

FIG. **5-1.** Lead apron and thyroid collar in place.

and chest from the primary beam and scatter radiation whereas the collar shields the thyroid. This method does not provide complete protection, particularly of the thyroid, but provides a great reduction in exposure. Aprons used in panoramic radiography have a front and back because the source of radiation is from the side and the rear of the patient.

Faster film speeds have contributed most significantly to the reduction in radiation to the patient. Film speeds of the "D," "E," and "F" groups are currently available for intraoral radiography. Faster film also reduces error from patient movement, a consideration with the pediatric patient. Extraoral (panoramic) radiography uses film-screen combinations that also have reduced exposure times. Recently, there has been an increased use of beam-positioning devices (Fig. 5-2) that have virtually eliminated some technical errors, particularly film cone cuts. The length and the shape of the

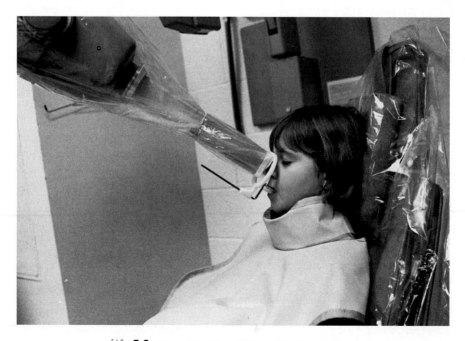

FIG. **5-2.** Use of the Rinn XCP positioning device.

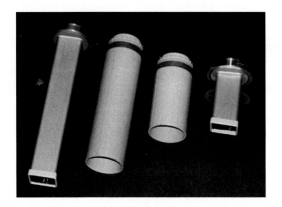

FIG. **5-3.** Rectangular and round cones of various lengths.

cone (Fig. 5-3) have also aided in the reduction of patient radiation exposure. Use of a long rectangular collimator reduces the area unnecessarily exposed to radiation by almost 4 sq in compared with a round collimator. The use of higher kilovolt peak techniques reduces patient exposure to radiation and lowers contrast, thus increasing the number of shades of gray on the film. An additional benefit of using high kilovolt peak technique is that the exposure time is shortened, which potentially reduces retakes caused by patient movement.

Finally, quality control (and thus patient protection) begins in the darkroom. If the darkroom does not function at an optimal level, retakes will be required, necessitating additional patient exposure. The dentist must insist on time-temperature developing and the use of proper-strength chemicals if wet tanks are used. The darkroom should be clean and free of white light (light leaks). If automatic processing is used, chemical parameters must be continuously monitored and the unit must be cleaned weekly.

SELECTION CRITERIA AND RADIOGRAPHIC EXAMINATIONS

The decision to make radiographs is based on a thorough evaluation and examination of the patient. Radiographs should be made only when there is an expectation that disease is present or when an undetected condition left untreated could adversely affect the patient's dental health. Therefore, the decision to use ionizing radiation is based on professional judgment (Table 5-1).

Selection criteria are clinical signs or symptoms that allow the practitioner to identify patients who will benefit from a radiographic examination. Two important considerations when deciding whether to perform a radiographic examination for children are (1) the stage of dentition development and (2) the risk of dental caries.

The criteria for making radiographs, developed in part by the Conference on Radiation Exposure in Pediatric Dentistry, were summarized by Nowak et al[1] as follows.

CRITERIA FOR EXPOSING OF RADIOGRAPHS IN ASYMPTOMATIC CHILDREN

The criteria for exposing radiographs assume that the child is asymptomatic and that the dentist finds no specific clinical indications for radiographic examination. Exceptions to this rule include those conditions in which there is clinical evidence of injury, disease such as caries, pulpal pathosis, delayed or accelerated eruption or exfoliation of teeth, swelling, hemorrhage, pain, or ulceration, or those conditions in which there is a need to evaluate treatment. In such cases, taking appropriate radiographs is indicated to confirm the diagnosis and facilitate and evaluate treatment.

DEVELOPMENT OF THE DENTITION AS CRITERION

Dental radiographs are indicated in the following situations.

Primary Dentition. If the proximal surfaces of the primary teeth cannot be visually and tactilely inspected and the child can be expected to cooperate, then dental radiographs should be made to determine the presence of interproximal caries. If all surfaces of all primary teeth can be examined clinically because of open contact, then radiographs are not indicated.

If the child's behavior is such that obtaining films of adequate diagnostic quality is doubtful, then radiographs should be deferred until behavior improves.

Early Transitional Dentition. (After appearance of permanent first molars or permanent mandibular incisors, or both.) Radiographs are taken to evaluate the presence of interproximal caries, developmental anomalies of teeth, and pathologic conditions of the hard and soft tissues of the mouth, jaws, and associated structures.

Early Permanent Dentition. (After puberty; after patients have achieved most of their adult stature; late adolescence). Radiographs are taken to evaluate the same tissues as in the early mixed dentition and to check the position and developmental status of the third molars.

No other dental radiographs are routinely needed in children. Other radiographs would be prescribed for diagnostic purposes. As an example, diagnostic bitewing radiographs would be taken to detect the presence of interproximal caries if the risk of caries activity were high for that individual. Occlusal caries, detected clinically, and discolored marginal ridges are indications of high risk of caries activity. Periapical films of the canine areas could be taken if these teeth were not clinically palpable by 9 years of age. The dentist must use clinical

TABLE 5-1 | Guidelines for Prescribing Dental Radiographs

PATIENT CATEGORY	CHILD	
	PRIMARY DENTITION (PRIOR TO ERUPTION OF FIRST PERMANENT TOOTH)	TRANSITIONAL DENTITION (FOLLOWING ERUPTION OF FIRST PERMANENT TOOTH)
New patient* All new patients to assess dental diseases and growth and development	Posterior bite-wing examination if proximal surfaces of primary teeth cannot be visualized or probed	Individualized radiographic examination consisting of periapical/occlusal views and posterior bite-wings *or* panoramic examination and posterior bite-wings
Recall patient* Clinical caries or high-risk factors for caries[†]	Posterior bite-wing examination 6-month intervals *or* until no carious lesions are evident	
No clinical caries and no high-risk factors for caries[†]	Posterior bite-wing examination at 12- to 24-month intervals if proximal surfaces of primary teeth cannot be visualized or probed	Posterior bite-wing examination at 12- to 24-month intervals
Periodontal disease or a history of periodontal treatment	Individualized radiographic examination consisting of selected periapical and/or bite-wing radiographs for areas where periodontal disease (other than non-specific gingivitis) can be demonstrated clinically	
Growth and development assessment	Usually not indicated	Individualized radiographic examination consisting of a periapical/occlusal *or* panoramic examination

The recommendations contained in this table were developed by an expert dental panel comprised of representatives from the Academy of General Dentistry, American Academy of Dental Radiology, American Academy of Oral Medicine, American Academy of Pediatric Dentistry, American Academy of Periodontology, and American Dental Association under the sponsorship of the Food and Drug Administration (FDA). The chart is being reproduced and distributed to the dental community by Eastman Kodak Company in cooperation with the FDA.

ADOLESCENT	ADULT	
PERMANENT DENTITION (PRIOR TO ERUPTION OF THIRD MOLARS)	DENTULOUS	EDENTULOUS
Individualized radiographic examination consisting of posterior bite-wings and selected periapicals. A full mouth intraoral radiographic examination is appropriate when the patient presents with clinical evidence of generalized dental disease or a history of extensive dental treatment.		Full mouth intra-oral radiographic examination *or* panoramic examination
Posterior bite-wing examination at 6- to 12-month intervals *or* until no carious lesions are evident	Posterior bite-wing examination at 12- to 18-month intervals	Not applicable
Posterior bite-wing examination at 18- to 36-month intervals	Posterior bite-wing examination at 24- to 36-month intervals	Not applicable
Individualized radiographic examination consisting of selected periapical and/ or bite-wing radiographs for areas where periodontal disease (other than non-specific gingivitis) can be demonstrated clinically		Not applicable
Periapical *or* panoramic examination to assess developing third molars	Usually not indicated	Usually not indicated

*Clinical situations for which radiographs may be indicated include the following:
A. Positive Historical Findings
1. Previous periodontal or endodontic therapy
2. History of pain or trauma
3. Familial history of dental anomalies
4. Postoperative evaluation of healing
5. Presence of implants

B. Positive Clinical Signs/Symptoms
1. Clinical evidence of periodontal disease
2. Large or deep restorations
3. Deep carious lesions
4. Malposed or clinically impacted teeth
5. Swelling
6. Evidence of facial trauma
7. Mobility of teeth
8. Fistula or sinus tract infection
9. Clinically suspected sinus pathology
10. Growth abnormalities
11. Oral involvement in known or suspected systemic disease
12. Positive neurologic findings in the head and neck
13. Evidence of foreign objects
14. Pain and/or dysfunction of the temporomandibular joint
15. Facial asymmetry
16. Abutment teeth for fixed or removable partial prosthesis
17. Unexplained bleeding
18. Unexplained sensitivity of teeth
19. Unusual eruption, spacing, or migration of teeth
20. Unusual tooth morphology, calcification, or color
21. Missing teeth with unknown reason

†Patients at high risk for caries may demonstrate any of the following:
1. High level of caries experience
2. History of recurrent caries
3. Existing restoration of poor quality
4. Poor oral hygiene
5. Inadequate fluoride exposure
6. Prolonged nursing (bottle or breast)
7. Diet with high sucrose frequency
8. Poor family dental health
9. Developmental enamel defects
10. Developmental disability
11. Xerostomia
12. Genetic abnormality of teeth
13. Many multisurface restorations
14. Chemo/radiation therapy

judgment and evaluate such factors as oral hygiene practices, diet, attitude and compliance, fluoride history, alignment of teeth, and morphology of teeth to determine the necessity for, the extent of, and the type and frequency of diagnostic radiographs.

RISK OF THE PATIENT FOR DENTAL CARIES AS CRITERION

A high risk of dental caries may be associated with poor oral hygiene, fluoride deficiency, prolonged nursing (bottle or breast), high-carbohydrate diet, poor family

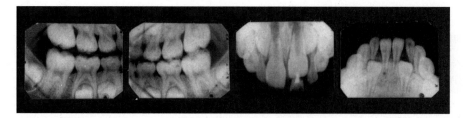

FIG. **5-4.** Four-film series.

dental health, developmental enamel defects, developmental disability and acute or chronic medical history, and genetic abnormality.

The child with a high risk of dental caries should have bite-wing radiographs made as soon as posterior primary teeth are in proximal contact. The age of the patient is not an important variable. If interproximal caries is detected, then follow-up radiographs are indicated semiannually until the child is caries free and therefore is classified as having a low risk for dental caries.

A child who has a low risk for dental caries may be defined as a normal, healthy, asymptomatic patient exposed to optimal levels of fluoride (preferably since birth), who performs daily preventive techniques and consumes a diet with few exposures to retentive carbohydrates between meals. Posterior bite-wing radiographs should be made for the low-risk patient with closed proximal contacts. If no evidence of caries is found, then radiographs may be retaken every 12 to 18 months if primary teeth are in contact or after up to 24 months if permanent teeth are in contact. Bite-wing radiographs may be taken more frequently if the child enters the high-risk category.

The more rapid progression of caries in primary teeth should be considered in determining the time interval between bite-wing radiographs.

TYPES OF FINDINGS ANTICIPATED AS CRITERIA

Bite-wing radiographs are indicated when a clinical examination discloses posterior tooth contact. Bite-wing examinations are recommended at the first clinical evidence of caries. Bite-wing radiographs are usually taken every 12 to 18 months in the absence of dental caries with primary tooth contact or every 24 months with permanent tooth contact.

By the time the first permanent tooth has erupted (posterior or anterior), an anterior occlusal radiograph should be made. This allows detection of conditions such as supernumerary teeth, missing teeth, and dens in dente. A radiographic examination that includes the tooth-bearing areas of the mandible and maxilla is recommended at approximately the time of the early mixed dentition to assess the dental age of the patient

and to aid in the early diagnosis of congenital and developmental anomalies.

The radiographic examination may consist of one of the following: posterior periapical radiographs, panoramic radiograph, or lateral jaw 45-degree projections. Another similar radiographic examination may be made within 2 years after the eruption of the permanent second molars.

To check on growth and development, a cephalometric radiograph may be prescribed by the practitioner who is providing the orthodontic diagnosis or treatment.

RADIOGRAPHIC EXAMINATIONS

When a new patient is seen at the dental office and no previous radiographs are available, it may be necessary to obtain a baseline series of radiographs. Again, we cannot overemphasize that the decision to make a radiographic examination is based on the criteria previously outlined. These examinations include the following.

Four-Film Series. This series consists of a maxillary and mandibular anterior occlusal and two posterior bite-wings (Fig. 5-4).

Eight-Film Survey. This survey includes a maxillary and mandibular anterior occlusal (or periapicals), a right and left maxillary posterior occlusal (or periapicals), right and left primary mandibular molar periapicals, and two posterior bite-wings (Fig. 5-5).

Twelve-Film Survey. This examination includes four primary molar-premolar periapical radiographs, four canine periapical radiographs, two incisor periapical radiographs, and two posterior bite-wing radiographs (Fig. 5-6).

Sixteen-Film Survey. This examination consists of the 12-film survey and the addition of 4 permanent molar radiographs (Fig. 5-7).

COMMONLY USED RADIOGRAPHIC TECHNIQUES

Several techniques are commonly used to radiograph a child's dentition. The technique used depends primarily on the size of the oral cavity, the number of teeth present, and patient cooperation. The procedures

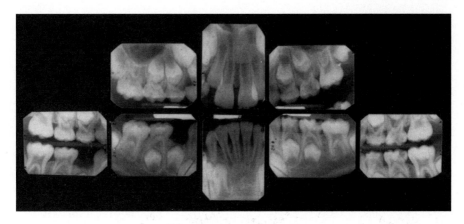

FIG. **5-5.** Eight-film survey.

commonly used by the private practitioner include the following:

1. Bite-wing
2. Periapical
3. Occlusal
4. Panoramic

BITE-WING TECHNIQUE

A No. 0 bite-wing film is usually the most suitable size for the smaller patient. However, some children's mouths are large enough to receive a No. 2 bite-wing film. The head is positioned so that the midsagittal plane is perpendicular and the ala-tragus line is parallel to the floor. The inferior edge of the bite-wing film packet is placed in the floor of the mouth between the tongue and the lingual aspect of the mandible and the bite-tab or positioning device is placed on the occlusal surfaces of the mandibular teeth (Fig. 5-8). The anterior

edge of the film packet is located as far anteriorly as possible in the region of the canine so that the distal aspect of the canine will be recorded. The lower anterior corner of the film packet is bent slightly toward the lingual to facilitate film placement and to decrease possible patient discomfort. The anteroinferior corner of the film packet usually lies near or at the attachment of the lingual frenum in the midline. In addition, the posterosuperior corner may be bent to prevent the gag reflex.

The dentist holds the bite-tab against the occlusal surfaces of the patient's mandibular teeth with an index finger, and the patient is instructed to "close slowly." The finger is rolled out of the way onto the buccal surfaces of the teeth as the patient closes in centric occlusion. The central ray enters through the occlusal plane at a point below the pupil of the eye. The vertical angle is +8 to +10 degrees. The horizontal diameter of the open-end cone is parallel to the end of the bite-tab

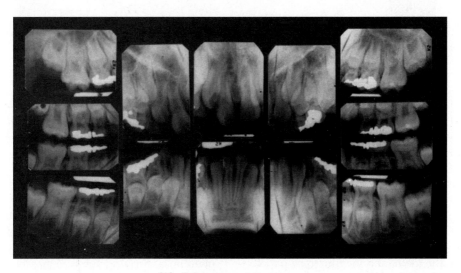

FIG. **5-6.** Twelve-film survey.

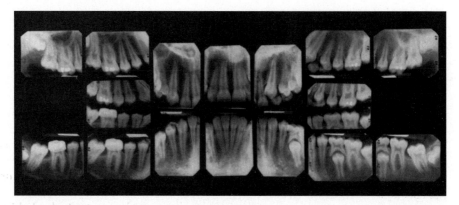

FIG. **5-7.** Sixteen-film survey.

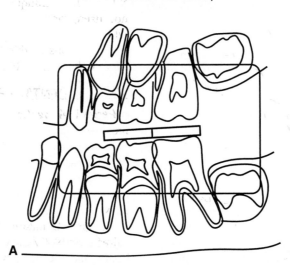

A

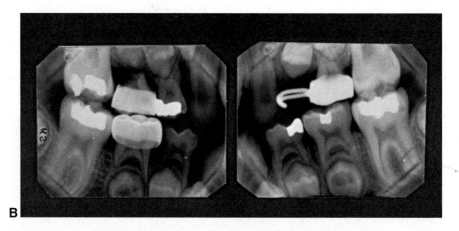

B

FIG. **5-8.** Posterior bite-wing. **A,** Film placement. **B,** Radiograph.

or to the mean tangent of the buccal surfaces of the posterior teeth being radiographed.

PARALLELING TECHNIQUE

In principle the paralleling technique requires the object (long axis of the tooth) and the film to be parallel in all dimensions. To achieve this, the film packet is placed farther away from the object, particularly the maxilla. This tends to magnify the image. This undesirable effect is offset when a longer cone is used, which thus reduces magnification. Use of a longer cone also increases image sharpness by decreasing the penumbra. Striving for true parallelism will enhance image accuracy.

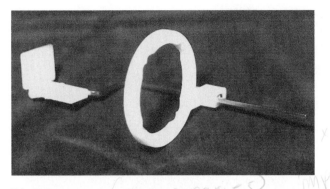

FIG. **5-9.** Rinn XCP positioning devices and film holders cut down to accommodate child patient's mouth.

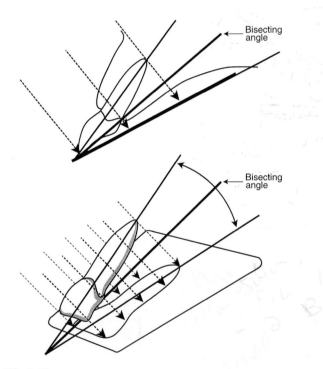

FIG. **5-10.** The bisecting angle. *(Courtesy Mr. Mark Dirlam.)*

Because the film is placed farther away from the object, a film holder is necessary (Fig. 5-9). Some of those holders also have beam-aligning devices to help ensure parallelism and reduce partial exposure of the film; thus unwanted cone cuts are eliminated. For the smaller child, the film holder may need to be reduced in size to accommodate the film and the child's mouth. Film-holding devices with cone alignment guides reduce operator error and thus reduce exposure of the patient to radiation. Because of the shallowness of the child's palate and floor of the mouth, film placement is somewhat compromised. Despite this, the resulting films are quite satisfactory.

BISECTING ANGLE TECHNIQUE

The bisecting angle technique is based on a principle called the *rule of isometry*, which basically states that two triangles are equal if they have two equal angles and a common side. The clinical application of this rule has the central ray directed perpendicularly to a plane that bisects the angle created by the long axis of the tooth and the film (Fig. 5-10). This technique is not as accurate as the paralleling technique and should be used as an accessory technique when paralleling technique is uncomfortable.

Positioning devices and film holders are also available for this technique. If the beam-aligning devices are not used, prescribed head positions are necessary, which may increase operator error. Even though there are limitations to this technique, in some situations it may be the only usable one.

SPECIFIC DENTAL PROJECTIONS

Periapical Technique. There are essentially two methods of taking periapical radiographs: paralleling and bisecting angle techniques. Each has benefits and limitations when used with the pediatric patient. It is not within the scope of this chapter to describe these techniques in detail. Thorough understanding will allow the practitioner to use them to the best advantage in any given situation.

Regardless of which technique is used, film positioning for the two techniques is identical. In general, films are positioned so that all areas of concern can be visualized, and there will usually be multiple views of a particular area. This is beneficial when minor technical errors exclude an area of importance on one film, since it can be visualized on another.

Regional film positions for the maxilla and mandible are identical; that is, film position for the maxillary molar projection is identical to that for the mandibular molar. Therefore only the regional positions are explained (Fig. 5-11). In all cases the identification dot is placed toward the occlusal surface.

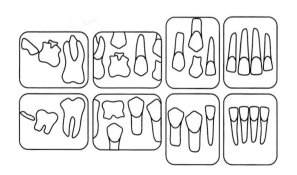

FIG. **5-11.** Positioning landmarks for film placement. *(Courtesy Mr. Mark Dirlam.)*

Molar Projection. The unfolded film packet is positioned so that all of the third molar, the second molar, and all or part of the first molar are recorded. Thus the anterior edge of the film packet is usually located at the mesial contact of the first molar. The plane of the packet should be parallel to the buccal surfaces of the molars.

Premolar or Primary Molar Projection. The packet may be folded anteriorly for relief in the palate or floor of the mouth and positioned so that the first molar, the first and second premolars or first and second primary molars, and the distal surface of the canine are recorded. The film packet is placed parallel to the buccal surfaces of the premolars or primary molars.

Permanent or Primary Canine Projection. The film packet is usually bent, particularly for a younger child, by a long narrow bend of the part of the packet that will be toward the midline. The canine and lateral incisors are to be recorded in their entirety. The film should be positioned so that the central beam of x-rays is parallel to the proximal surfaces of the canine and lateral incisor and therefore perpendicular to the film.

Permanent or Primary Incisor Projection. If the film packet must be folded because of the narrowness of the arch, a $\frac{1}{8}$-inch bend should be made on each edge throughout the entire length of the film that parallels the long axis of the teeth. The film packet is positioned so that the central incisors are centered mesiodistally on the film. The central ray is parallel to the contacts of the proximal surfaces and perpendicular to the film.

Anterior Maxillary Occlusal Technique. In the anterior maxillary occlusal technique, the patient's occlusal plane should be parallel to the floor, and the sagittal plane should be perpendicular to the floor (Fig. 5-12). A No. 2 periapical film is placed in the patient's mouth so that the long axis of the film runs from left to right rather than anteroposteriorly and the midsagittal plane bisects the film. The patient is instructed to bite lightly to hold the film. The anterior edge of the film should extend approximately 2 mm in front of the incisal edge of the central incisors. The central ray is directed to the apices of the central incisors and a centimeter (half-inch) above the tip of the nose and through the midline. The vertical angle is +60 degrees. This film is exposed at the usual setting for maxillary incisor periapical films.

Posterior Maxillary Occlusal Technique. In the posterior maxillary occlusal technique, the patient's occlusal plane should be parallel to the floor, and the sagittal plane should be perpendicular to the floor (Fig. 5-13). A No. 2 periapical film is placed in the patient's mouth so that the long axis of the film is parallel to the floor. The anterior edge of the film should

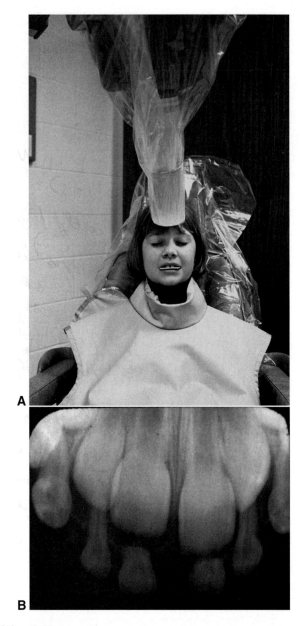

A

B

FIG. **5-12.** Anterior maxillary occlusal. **A,** Technique. **B,** Radiograph.

extend just mesial to the canine. The outer buccal edge of the film should extend approximately 2 mm beyond the primary molar crowns. The patient is instructed to bite lightly to hold the film. The central ray is directed toward the apices of the primary molars as well as interproximally. The vertical angle is +50 degrees. The film is exposed at the usual setting for maxillary premolar periapical films.

Anterior Mandibular Occlusal Technique. The film placement for the anterior mandibular occlusal technique is identical to that for the anterior maxillary

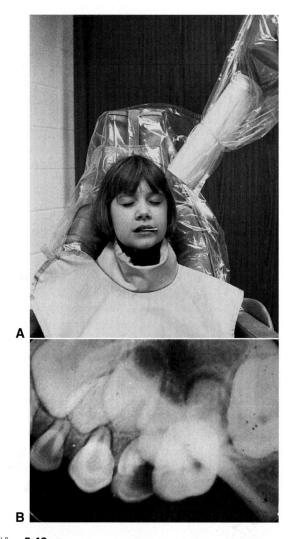

FIG. **5-13.** Posterior maxillary occlusal. **A,** Technique. **B,** Radiograph.

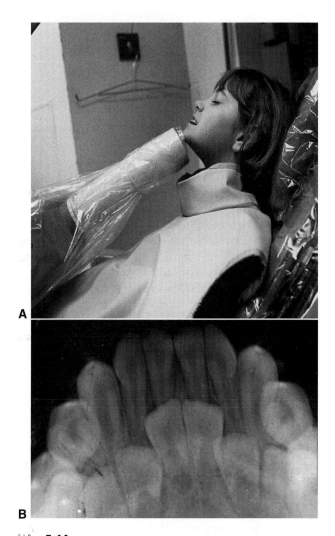

FIG. **5-14.** Anterior mandibular occlusal. **A,** Technique. **B,** Radiograph.

occlusal technique, except that the film must be placed so that the tube side faces the x-ray source (Fig. 5-14). In addition, when the patient occludes on the film, the anterior edge of the film is 2 mm beyond the incisal edge of the lower incisors. The patient's head is positioned so that the occlusal plane is at a −45-degree angle. The cone is then aligned at a −15-degree vertical angle, and the central ray is directed through the symphysis.

PANORAMIC RADIOGRAPHY

Numerous panoramic x-ray units are available to the dental profession. Fig. 5-15 illustrates the use of the Planmeca Proline PM2002 CC panoramic unit (Planmeca). Body-section radiography uses a mechanism by which the x-ray film and the source of the x-rays move simultaneously in opposite directions at the same speed. The reader is directed to textbooks by Langland et al (1989) and Miles et al (1999) for a more definitive discussion of the principles of panoramic imaging.

A panoramic radiographic unit can be used for examination of children. Since the examination is obtained without placement of the film in the mouth, it does not alarm the anxious child who may refuse an intraoral film. Moreover, the young patient may find the movement entertaining or fun. The diversion of being momentarily entertained usually invites cooperation. However, staying completely immobile for 15 seconds may not be possible for some very young children.

Although panoramic radiography is considered a supplement to, rather than a substitute for, the intraoral periapical radiographic series, it does provide excellent

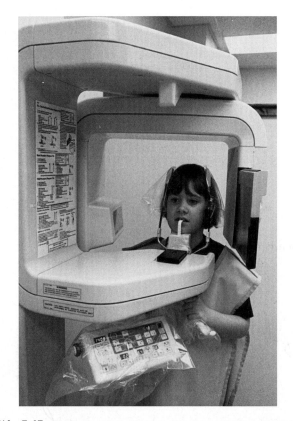

FIG. **5-15.** Patient positioned in a Planmeca Proline PM2002 CC panoramic unit.

coverage of the structures that are viewed during pediatric dental diagnosis. A diagnostic film includes the teeth, the supporting structure, the maxillary region extending to the superior third of the orbit, and the entire mandible including the temporomandibular joint region. Pediatric dentists who have used panoramic radiographic technique have discovered condylar fractures, traumatic cysts, and anomalies that might have gone undetected with the routine periapical series of radiographs (Fig. 5-16).

Panoramic radiology can be valuable when disabled patients are examined if the patient can sit in a chair and hold his or her head in position. It may be necessary to administer relaxants or sedatives to palsied or spastic patients, who are more difficult to control when they are emotionally charged by the dental visit.

The only inherent drawback to panoramic radiography is lack of image detail for diagnosing early carious lesions. Adjunct bite-wing radiographs and selected periapical radiographs are required for that task.

Lateral Jaw Technique. A 5 × 7-inch x-ray film is used for the lateral jaw technique (Fig. 5-17). The film is marked with a right or left lead identification letter placed on the film packet slightly anterior and superior to the central portion of the film. When the film is finally positioned, this letter should be located in the area of the orbit.

The patient's head is positioned so that the occlusal plane is parallel and the sagittal plane is perpendicular to the floor. The long axis of the film, also perpendicular to the floor, rests on the patient's shoulder and against the face. The patient is instructed to rotate the head toward the film until the nose rests against it. Then the chin is raised and the head tilted approximately 15 degrees toward the film. The patient secures the film with the palm of the hand and with fingers extended. The cone is positioned so that the central x-ray beam enters at a point a half-inch behind and

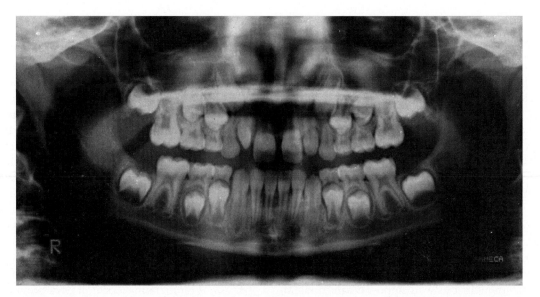

FIG. **5-16.** Panoramic radiograph. Notice the congenitally missing mandibular second premolars.

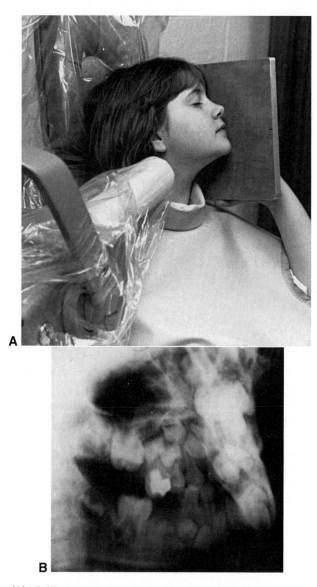

A

B

FIG. **5-17.** Lateral view of jaw. **A,** Technique. **B,** Radiograph.

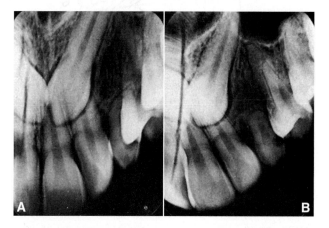

FIG. **5-18.** The buccal object rule. *B,* Buccal; *L,* lingual; *H.A.,* horizontal angle.

FIG. **5-19. A,** Shadow of the maxillary permanent canine is superimposed over the central incisor root. **B,** When the horizontal angle of the x-ray tube is shifted posteriorly, the crown of the unerupted canine appears to move posteriorly. The canine is lingually placed.

below the angle of the mandible on the side opposite the film. The vertical angle is −17 degrees. The central x-ray beam is perpendicular to the horizontal plane of the film.

LOCALIZATION TECHNIQUES

One method of localizing embedded or unerupted teeth uses the buccal object rule, which states that the image of any buccally oriented object appears to move in the opposite direction from a moving x-ray source. On the other hand, the image of any lingually oriented object appears to move in the same direction as a moving x-ray source (Fig. 5-18).

Using this principle for localization, the practitioner makes two radiographs of the unerupted tooth.

The technique consists in positioning the patient's head so that the sagittal plane is perpendicular to the floor and the ala-tragus line is parallel to the floor. An intraoral periapical film is placed in the mouth and then exposed. A second film is placed in the mouth in the same position as the first film, with the patient's head position remaining the same. The second film is then exposed. The vertical angulation should be the same for each exposure. However, the horizontal angle is shifted either anteriorly or posteriorly, depending on the area being examined, for the second view.

Fig. 5-19, *A,* illustrates an unerupted maxillary permanent canine. The shadow of this tooth is superimposed over the central incisor root. When the horizontal angle

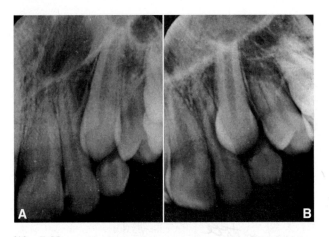

FIG. **5-20. A,** Shadow of the maxillary permanent canine covers a small portion of the lateral incisor root on its distal aspect. **B,** When the horizontal angle of the x-ray tube is shifted posteriorly, the canine appears to move anteriorly. The canine lies buccal to the erupted teeth.

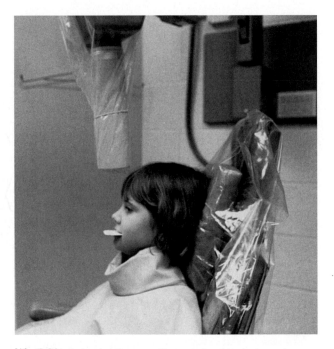

FIG. **5-21.** Cross-section maxillary occlusal technique demonstrating the proper head position and central-ray entry point. The central ray is directed coincidentally with the long axis of the central incisor roots.

of the x-ray tube is shifted posteriorly (Fig. 5-19, *B*), the crown of the unerupted canine also seems to move posteriorly, and the image of the canine crown is no longer superimposed over the central incisor root. If the buccal object rule is applied, it can be seen that the embedded canine is oriented lingually to the erupted teeth.

Fig. 5-20, *A*, illustrates an embedded maxillary permanent canine. The shadow of the crown of this tooth covers a small portion of the lateral incisor root on its distal aspect. When the horizontal angle is shifted posteriorly (Fig. 5-20, *B*), the unerupted crown appears to move anteriorly or in a direction opposite to the

shift of the x-ray source. Thus the unerupted canine is oriented buccally to the erupted teeth.

Another localization technique is the cross-section occlusal radiograph. Depending on the size of the child's mouth, either the adult occlusal or a No. 2 periapical film may be used. To obtain a cross-section occlusal radiograph of the maxilla, the patient's sagittal plane is perpendicular to the floor, and the ala-tragus line is

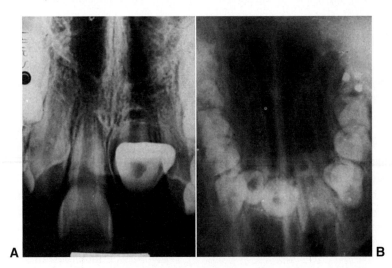

FIG. **5-22. A,** Dilacerated maxillary central incisor. **B,** The crown of the dilacerated central incisor lies labially.

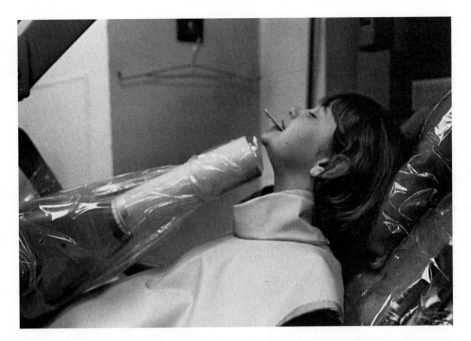

FIG. **5-23.** Cross-section mandibular occlusal technique demonstrating the proper head position and vertical angulation of the x-ray head.

parallel to the floor. The patient is asked to occlude lightly on the film. The central ray is projected through the midsagittal plane and enters the skull 1 cm posterior to bregma. (Bregma is the point at which the sagittal suture meets the coronal suture.) The proper vertical angulation is determined when the central ray is directed through the long axis of the maxillary central incisor roots (Fig. 5-21).

A maxillary central incisor periodical radiograph demonstrating a grossly dilacerated central incisor may be seen in Fig. 5-22, *A.* It is important to determine, before a surgical procedure, if the crown of such a tooth is in a labial or a lingual position. In this instance, the crown is positioned labially (Fig. 5-22, *B*).

The cross-section occlusal film can be employed for localization of anomalies in the mandible. Either the adult occlusal or a No. 2 periapical film can be used. The patient's head is tilted backward sufficiently to direct the central ray through the long axis of the erupted teeth (Fig. 5-23). The patient's head must be tilted on its long axis to accommodate positioning of the x-ray tube. If determination of the buccal or lingual position of an impacted mandibular third molar is desired, the central ray should be projected through the long axis of the mandibular second molar. If it is necessary to localize an unerupted second premolar, the central ray should be directed through the long axis of the first premolar. Fig. 5-24, *A,* reveals an unerupted mandibular premolar that has been displaced by an ossifying fibroma. In Fig. 5-24, *B,* a cross-section occlusal radiograph

demonstrates that the crown of the premolar is lingually placed.

DIGITAL RECEPTORS FOR PEDIATRIC PATIENTS

Digital x-ray systems use solid-state detector technology such as CCD (charge-coupled devices) or CMOS (complementary metal oxide semiconductors) for image acquisition. Most of these systems have electronic wires attached to the sensor. Children under 4 or 5 years of age may not tolerate these wired sensors, may damage the cables because they do not understand the procedure and may "chew" on the cable, or may be more fearful just of the appearance of a wired system. For these reasons a phosphor-based digital x-ray system may be ideal for the pediatric patient. There is one "wireless" solid-state image detector from Schick Technologies, the Schick CDR Wireless sensor (Fig. 5-25). This device has just been introduced to the dental market, so there is not much experience with its use with children as yet.

Photostimulable phosphors (PSPs) or storage phosphors are used for digital imaging for image acquisition. Unlike panoramic or cephalometric screen materials, PSPs do *not* fluoresce instantly to produce light photons. Instead, these materials store the incoming x-ray photon information like a latent image in conventional film-based radiography until the plates are scanned by a laser beam in a drum scanner. The laser scanning excites the phosphor to give up

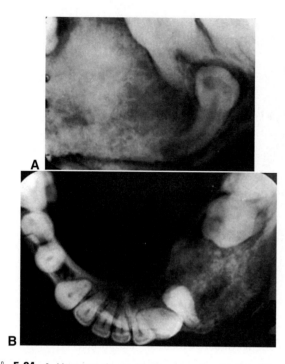

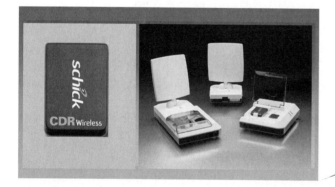

FIG. **5-24. A,** Unerupted mandibular premolar displaced by an ossifying fibroma. **B,** The crown of the unerupted premolar is lingually oriented.

TABLE **5-2** Photostimulable Phosphor Systems			
COMPANY	**SYSTEM**	**PHOSPHOR TYPE**	**RESOLUTION (LP/mm)**
Soredex	Digora	Agfa	>6
AirTechniques	ScanX	Fuji	6-8
Gendex	DenOptix	Fuji	~9

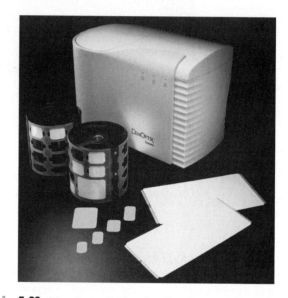

FIG. **5-26.** The Dentsply-Gendex DenOptix phosphor plate scanner.

FIG. **5-25.** The Schick Technologies CDR Wireless system showing the sensor *(left)* and the charging unit and wireless RF antennas *(right).*

the stored energy as an electronic signal, which is then digitized, with various gray levels assigned to points on the curve to create the image information. The currently available phosphor imaging systems (Table 5-2) are from Soredex (Digora), AirTechniques (ScanX) and Gendex (DenOptix).

These phosphor plates have no wire to the computer and resemble intraoral film in every way, including size, thickness, rigidity, and receptor placement. They are soft and flexible much like film, and as with conventional x-ray film techniques, infection control procedures must be employed. The plates must be wrapped, exposed, and unwrapped and then carefully shaken out of the barrier envelope onto a clean surface, wiped with a disinfectant, and fed into the laser scanner. After use, the plates must be exposed to light to eliminate any latent image before they are placed into new barrier envelopes for the next patient. Thus the total time to process each image can take several minutes. Unlike film, however, the plates should *not* be curved or bent, because a permanent defect or artifact will be created in the phosphor coating. The plate would then need to be replaced.

In some machines like the DenOptix system the plates are put into a template holder that is then placed into the drum scanner (Fig. 5-26). After the scanning process is completed, the resultant digital image can then be viewed on a monitor in about 30 seconds to 2.5 minutes depending on the system. This is called analog-to-digital conversion and it is how the phosphor imaging system becomes "digital." The technology is *not* new. This type of signal readout by laser scanning has been used in the laboratory industry

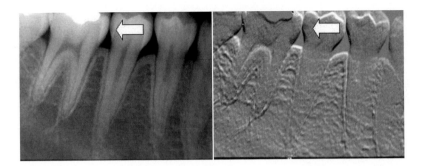

FIG. **5-27.** An interproximal carious lesion on the distal surface of tooth No. 29 *(left)* made more apparent by electronic image processing *(right)*.

for reading biologic fluid samples for decades. This "digital" imaging technique requires two steps to retrieve the final image, just like film. The technique also requires the same two-stage infection control procedures as film. But the final image is digital and can be subjected to electronic image processing to extract disease features more readily for treatment decision making (Fig. 5-27). An excellent explanation of the PSP process appears in the April 2000 issue of *Dental Clinics of North America.*

The advantage of these digital-like phosphors is really in the image processing that can be applied *after* the image is acquired. Although electronic image processing can be performed on conventional x-ray film, the film must first be converted to digital information by scanning the image. Storage phosphors (PSPs) and true digital images from solid-state detectors like CCD and CMOS receptors provide a virtually instantaneous digital image and require no additional data conversion prior to electronic image processing.

If the dentist wishes to employ these digital systems, either solid state or phosphor, he or she must use a good paralleling instrument system and paralleling technique to be successful.

INTERPRETATION

When interpreting radiographs, the dentist must develop a systematic approach so that no areas of the radiographs are missed. No one way is necessarily better than another, provided that the approach is consistently followed. Viewing conditions should be adjusted so that the maximum information can be obtained from the radiographs. The radiographs should be placed in a mount that does not allow light to be transmitted through the periphery, only through the film itself. Other extraneous light from around the mount should also be masked out. It is preferable for the room in which the radiographs are reviewed to have subdued lighting. Finally, it is recommended that a magnifying glass be used. If these viewing

conditions are followed, more information will be obtained, and thus better care will be provided for the patient.

REFERENCE

1. Nowak AJ et al: Summary of the Conference on Radiation Exposure in Pediatric Dentistry, *J Am Dent Assoc* 103:426-428, 1981.

SUGGESTED READINGS

Alcox RW, Jameson WR: Patient exposures from intraoral radiographic examinations, *J Am Dent Assoc* 88:568-579, 1974.

Block AJ, Goepp RA, Mason EW: Thyroid radiation dose during panoramic and cephalometric dental x-ray examinations, *Angle Orthod* 47:17-24, 1977.

Brooks SL, Joseph LP: US Department of Health and Human Services. Basic concepts in the selection of patients for dental x-ray examinations, Food and Drug Administration Pub No 85-8249, Washington, DC, 1985, US Government Printing Office.

Council on Dental Materials, Instruments and Equipment, American Dental Association: Recommendations in radiographic practices, *J Am Dent Assoc* 109:764-765, 1984.

Gibbs SJ et al: Patient risk from intraoral dental radiography, *Dentomaxillofac Radiol* 17:15-23, 1988.

Gibbs SJ et al: Patient risk from rotational panoramic radiograph, *Dentomaxillofac Radiol* 17:25-32, 1988.

Hildebolt CF et al: Dental photostimulable phosphor radiography, *Dent Clin North Am* 44(2):273-299, 2000.

Joseph LP: US Department of Health and Human Services. The selection of patients for x-ray examinations: dental radiographic examinations, Food and Drug Administration Pub No 88-8273, Washington, DC, 1987, US Government Printing Office.

Kasle MJ: Radiograph: cross-fire localization technic, *Dent Surv* 45:29-31, 1969.

Kasle MJ: Radiographic technique for difficult maxillary third molar views, *J Am Dent Assoc* 83:1104-1105, 1971.

Kasle MJ, Langlais RP: *Basic principles of oral radiology*, vol 4, Exercises in dental radiology, Philadelphia, 1981, WB Saunders.

Langland OE et al: *Panoramic radiology*, ed 2, Philadelphia, 1989, Lea & Febiger.

Miles DA et al: *Radiographic imaging for dental auxiliaries*, ed 3, Philadelphia, 1999, WB Saunders.

Myers DR et al: Radiation exposure during panoramic radiography in children, *Oral Surg* 46:588-593, 1978.

National Council on Radiation Protection and Measurements: Dental x-ray protection, Report No 35, Washington, DC, 1970, The Council.

National Council on Radiation Protection and Measurements: Radiation protection in pediatric radiology, Report No 68, Washington, DC, 1981, The Council.

Smith QW et al: Radiation exposure in the dental setting: an update, *Radiol Technol* 55:546, 1983.

Valachovic RW, Lurie AG: Risk-benefit considerations in pedodontic radiology, *Pediatr Dent* 2:128-146, 1980.

White SC, Rose TC: Absorbed bone marrow dose in certain dental radiographic techniques, *J Am Dent Assoc* 98:553-558, 1979.

6

Clinical Genetics for the Dental Practitioner

JAMES K. HARTSFIELD, JR.

DAVID BIXLER

Review of Genetic Principles
CELL DIFFERENTIATION AND DEVELOPMENTAL
  BIOLOGY
CHROMOSOMES
HEREDITARY TRAITS IN FAMILIES
DEVELOPMENTAL BIOLOGY OF ENAMEL
AUTOSOMAL DOMINANT INHERITANCE
AUTOSOMAL RECESSIVE INHERITANCE
X-LINKED OR SEX-LINKED INHERITANCE
    X-Linked Dominant
    X-Linked Recessive
VARIATION IN GENE EXPRESSION
    Penetrance
    Expressivity

MULTIFACTORIAL INHERITANCE
    Multifactorial Inheritance in Human Diseases
**Influence of Genetic Factors on Major Craniofacial,
  Oral, and Dental Conditions**
GENETICS AND DENTAL CARIES
GENETICS AND PERIODONTAL DISEASE
    Early-Onset Periodontitis
GENETICS OF MALOCCLUSION
EXTERNAL APICAL ROOT RESORPTION
GENETICS OF CLEFT LIP AND PALATE

The purpose of this chapter is twofold: to review genetic principles and to mention a few examples of the influence of genetic factors on major craniofacial, oral, and dental conditions. As the basis for relatively rare developmental dysplasias, diseases, and syndromes which show a genetic cause or marked genetic influence becomes known, increasing attention is being paid to those genetic factors that influence (or are associated with) more common conditions. An increased appreciation of how genetic factors interact with environmental (nongenetic) factors to influence growth and pathology will lead to an increased understanding of pathogenesis and the recognition that some groups or individuals may be more susceptible.

Review of Genetic Principles

The genome contains the entire genetic content of a set of chromosomes present within a cell or an organism. Within the genome are genes that represent the smallest physical and functional units of inheritance that reside in specific sites (called loci, or locus for a single location). A gene can be defined as the entire DNA sequence necessary for the synthesis of a functional polypeptide molecule (production of a protein via a messenger RNA intermediate) or RNA molecule (transfer RNA and ribosomal RNA). Genotype generally refers to the set of genes that an individual carries and, in particular, usually refers to the specific pair of alleles (alternative forms of a particular gene) that a person has at a given location (locus) of the genome. In contrast, phenotype is the observable properties and physical characteristics of an individual, as determined by the individual's genotype and the environment in which the individual develops over a period of time.

Remarkable advances in the biochemical techniques that are used to study cell molecular biology and DNA have taken today's researcher to the threshold of understanding the regulation of cell functions. To illustrate, not so long ago DNA analyses were performed on minute amounts (picograms) of DNA. This limitation was necessary because there was so little DNA available for study in the samples. When the DNA polymerase enzyme was discovered that could replicate DNA through the polymerase chain reaction and make it by the gram, this sample problem disappeared. This advance facilitated completion of the human genome project, which resulted not only in definition of a single human genome sequence composed of overlapping parts from many humans, but also in an expanding catalogue of some 1.4 million sites of variation in the human genome sequence. These variations (or polymorphisms) may be used as markers to perform genetic analysis (including analysis of genetic-environmental interaction) in human beings. The genome varies from one individual to the next most often in terms of single base changes of the DNA, called *single nucleotide polymorphisms* (SNPs, pronounced "snips"). The main use of this human SNP map will be to determine the contributions of genes to diseases (or nondisease phenotypes) that have a complex, multifactorial basis.[1]

CELL DIFFERENTIATION AND DEVELOPMENTAL BIOLOGY

It is fascinating that a single fertilized ovum contains within itself the potential for development of the incredibly complicated human organism. Cellular differentiation is a critical component of this developmental process, and aside from the development of antibody diversity, typically occurs in the absence of genetic alteration or mutation. Different types of cells gain their specific identities by using a particular subset of the approximately 30,000 or more genes present within the genome. The types of polypeptides a cell can synthesize include enzymes, which catalyze various activities of cellular metabolism and homeostasis; structural proteins, which form the intracellular and extracellular scaffolding or cellular matrix; and regulatory proteins, which convey signals from the outside of the cell to the nucleus and modulate or control specific gene expression. In a developing embryo, cells reside in a three-dimensional environment and are responsive to signals from themselves (autocrine), from nearby sources (paracrine), and from anatomically distant sources (endocrine). Many of these signals are mediated by soluble molecules (either peptide or nonpeptide in origin) that bind to specific receptors (proteins) that are present on the surface or on the inside of cells. In addition to signals from soluble factors, cells can respond to cell-to-cell or cell-to-extracellular matrix signals.[2]

The action of "turning on" or "turning off" specific genes, referred to as regulation of gene expression, is carefully orchestrated and remains a critical element in determining cell specificity and tissue morphogenesis. Transcription factors bind to DNA and either facilitate or suppress initiation of gene transcription, the most common control point of gene expression. In the development of the craniofacial complex there is increasing evidence for the role of homeobox-containing gene families that encode transcription factors. These then are critical for the control of complex interactions between genes that are subsequently expressed during development.[3]

In summary:

1. The genetic message lies in the DNA itself, which is coded and transmitted from cell generation to cell generation when these DNA molecules are replicated (or duplicated).

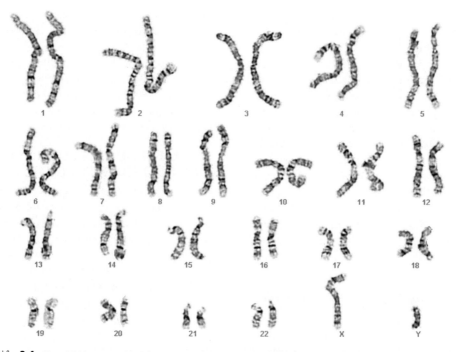

FIG. **6-1.** Banded karyotypes of a normal human male *(left)* and female *(right)*. Group designations according to Denver nomenclature are also indicated. *(Courtesy Cytogenetic Laboratories, Indiana University School of Medicine.)*

2. A given cell type and function is defined by what specific RNA molecules are made from the DNA master. These RNA molecular copies direct protein synthesis in the cell.

3. Transcription factors determine which genes are expressed through the production of the RNA and subsequent protein.

4. Development occurs through the action of specific transcription factors on specific genes that need to be expressed next in time.

CHROMOSOMES

DNA is grouped into units called chromosomes. Humans have 46 chromosomes that contain an estimated 30,000 genes, including numerous duplicates. Of the 46 chromosomes, the sex chromosomes are the X and Y, with the remaining 44 chromosomes referred to as autosomes. Each autosome has a paired mate that is referred to as its homologue. Therefore, with the exception of some of the genes on the X and Y chromosomes in males, there are at least two copies of each gene unless a piece of DNA is deleted. Thus the human chromosome complement consists of 23 pairs of chromosomes (one pair of sex chromosomes and 22 pairs of autosomes).

One area of special interest to the clinician is cytogenetics, the study of chromosomes. This interest has been stimulated by the development of techniques in which cells are grown in culture and the chromosomes are examined under a microscope for changes in size,

shape, and fine structure. This is called *karyotyping*. Fig. 6-1 shows the karyotypes of a normal human male and female. By applying this technique, Lejeune, Turpin, and Gautier demonstrated that the fundamental cause in Down syndrome is the presence of an extra specific chromosome (number 21) in the affected individual's karyotype.[4] When an entire extra chromosome is present, the condition is called a trisomy of the chromosome in question, for example, trisomy 21 for Down syndrome. Fig. 6-2 shows the karyotype of a male who has Down syndrome. The extra chromosome in the group of number 21 and number 22 chromosomes is readily apparent.

Since this report in 1959, many disease states have been shown to be associated with an incorrect chromosome complement. By using this approach with considerable refinement, it was shown that alterations in the fine structure of chromosomes, as well as in their number, could be present. Monosomy of an autosome, or a missing autosomal chromosome, had not been believed to be compatible with life, but several monosomies in live-born children have now been reported. Monosomy of the sex chromosomes can be compatible with life and typically affects development of both internal and external sex organs of the individuals. The best-known example of this is Turner syndrome, which occurs in approximately 1 in every 5000 live female births. These persons are phenotypic females who are usually missing one of the X chromosomes and are

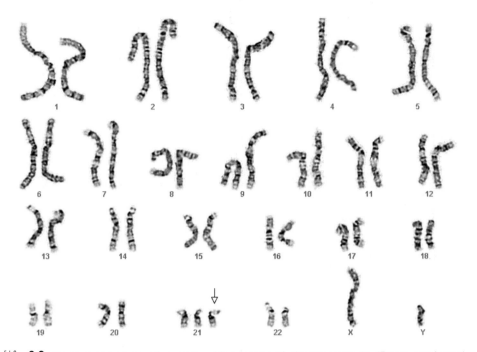

FIG. **6-2.** Banded karyotype of a male with trisomy of chromosome 21 (Down syndrome). *(Courtesy Cytogenetic Laboratories, Indiana University School of Medicine.)*

chromosomally designated as 45,X. Other aberrations of the X chromosome may also cause Turner syndrome. Affected individuals are typically short of stature, lack secondary sex characteristics, and are sterile. The Turner syndrome karyotype is shown in Fig. 6-3. Table 6-1 lists a few of the more common chromosomal aberrations that produce clinical disease, including examples of translocations (the attachment of a broken piece from one chromosome to another, but not homologous, chromosome), and deletions (the absence of a piece of chromosome).

Chromosome abnormalities are an important cause of spontaneous abortion. About 15% of all recognized pregnancies end in spontaneous abortion, and the incidence of chromosome abnormalities in such abortions is greater than 50%. Only 0.3% to 0.5% of all live-born infants have a chromosome abnormality. Clinicians agree that, even though these aberrations are relatively rare, they remain a significant cause of mental and physical abnormalities in humans.

HEREDITARY TRAITS IN FAMILIES

Heritability is the proportion of the total phenotypic variance in a **sample** that is contributed by genetic variance.[5] On an individual basis for a binary trait (i.e., a disease or trait that an individual either has or does not have), heritability is not the proportion of disease or the trait attributable to, or caused by, genetic factors. For a quantitative trait, heritability is not a measure of the proportion of an individual's score attributable to genetic factors.[6] A trait with a heritability of 1 is said to be expressed without any environmental influence, whereas a trait with a heritability of 0.5 has half its variability (from individual to individual) influenced by environmental factors and half by genotypic factors. Values over 1 may occur because the methodology provides an estimate of heritability under several simplifying assumptions that may be incorrect. Still, the estimation of heritability can provide an indication of the relative importance of genetic factors. Confirming that there is a certain degree of genetic influence on a trait is a preliminary step to performing further specific genetic linkage studies (using DNA markers) to determine areas of the genome that appear to be associated with the characteristics of a given trait.[7]

When hereditary traits in families are to be studied, it is convenient to think of three classes of genetically influenced traits. These are (1) monogenic (2) polygenic, and (3) multifactorial. The following summarizes the characteristics of these three classes.

Monogenic traits are traits produced and regulated by a single gene locus. Usually they are relatively rare in the general population (occurrence in fewer than 1 per 1000 individuals). However, if the appearance of an affected person is striking, there may be instant recognition of the disease, as with patients having albinism, achondroplasia, or neurofibromatosis. Monogenetic conditions often occur in families and show transmission

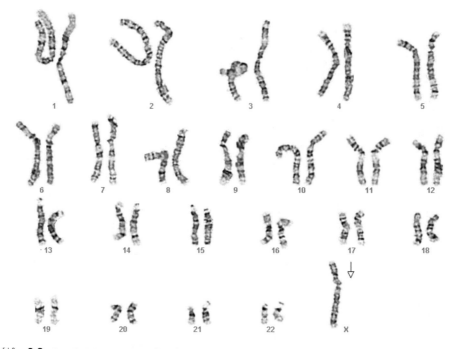

FIG. **6-3.** Banded karyotype of a female with missing X chromosome (Turner syndrome). *(Courtesy Cytogenetic Laboratories, Indiana University School of Medicine.)*

| TABLE **6-1** | A Summary of the More Common Chromosomal Aberrations |

TYPE	SPECIFIC ALTERATION	CLINICAL RESULT
Aneuploidy	Trisomy 21	Down syndrome
	Trisomy 18	Edwards syndrome
	Trisomy 13	Patau syndrome
	Extra X chromosomes	In females: XXX, XXXX, XXXXX syndromes In males: Klinefelter syndrome—XXY, XXXY, and XXXXY
	Monosomy, autosomal	Usually nonviable
	Monosomy, X chromosome	In females: Turner syndrome, 45,X In males: nonviable, 45,Y
Translocation	14/21, 21/21, or 21/22	Translocation carrier (normal phenotype) or Down syndrome
Deletion	Ring chromosome Short arm chromosone No. 5 Philadelphia chromosome (No. 22)	Variable Cri du chat syndrome Chronic myeloid leukemia

characteristics of the mendelian (dominant or recessive) traits.

Polygenic traits, too, are hereditary and typically exert influence over rather common characteristics such as height, skin, and intelligence. This influence takes place through many gene loci collectively asserting their regulation of the trait. Although each gene involved has a minimal effect by itself, the effect of all the genes involved is additive. The associated phenotype is rarely discrete and is most commonly continuous or quantitative. Because these traits show a quantitative distribution of their phenotypes in a population, they do not show mendelian inheritance patterns. Specially developed mathematical models have been devised to analyze such traits in populations, but these are not discussed here. However, it is important to note that the very nature of their control (multiple genes each with a small additive effect) dictates that their environment may readily influence them. Monogenic traits are not readily amenable on a large scale to environmental modification, although there can be variation, presumably secondary to other genetic and environmental factors. By contrast, one can easily think of a dozen environmental factors known to influence height and intelligence quotient.

Finally, the third etiologic group of gene-influenced conditions has been given the name *multifactorial* traits. These traits are controlled by multiple genes but differ significantly from polygenic traits in that control is achieved through an interaction of multiple genes and environmental factors and occurs when a liability threshold is exceeded. Although typically the number of genes involved is many, occasionally a few genes, sometimes only two or three, influence the trait. The effect of these genes on the phenotype is therefore a net effect, not a simple additive one. Furthermore, phenotypic expression approaches that of a discreet mendelian trait and therefore cannot be readily classed as a quantitative trait. Likewise, the effect of a gene influencing the phenotype may not be as great as that of a gene associated with a monogenic trait, but the gene may be referred to as having a major effect. Among the well-known hereditary types of conditions designated as multifactorial are many of the severe nonsyndromic congenital malformations such as cleft lip and palate (CLP), spina bifida-anencephaly, and hip dislocation. More discussion about multifactorial inheritance is given later.

The investigation of human heritable traits usually involves the observation of specific features in a family and the study of that family's pedigree. The affected individual in a family who first brings that family to the attention of the geneticist is called the *proband* or *propositus*. This individual is the index case. Brothers and sisters of the proband are siblings or sibs. Thus, a sibship consists of all the brothers and sisters in a nuclear family unit (parents and their offspring). The clinical appearance in an individual of a given trait, such as eye color or height, is that individual's phenotype, whereas the specific genetic makeup that controls that phenotype is the genotype.

In an earlier section, the point was made that the human chromosome complement has 22 homologous pairs of autosomes and one pair of sex chromosomes. Because of homologue pairing (excluding the X and Y chromosomes in the male), there are at least two copies of each gene, one located at the same position (locus) on each member of the homologous pair. Genes at the same locus on a pair of homologous chromosomes are alleles. When both members of a pair of alleles are identical, the individual is homozygous for that locus. When the two alleles at a specific locus are different, the individual is heterozygous for that locus.

A gene that expresses a particular phenotype in single dose is a dominant gene. If the gene must be present in double dose (homozygous) to express the phenotype, it is a recessive gene. The reader should recognize that it is actually the phenotype that is dominant or recessive and not the gene itself. The terms *dominant gene* and *recessive gene*, though, are commonly used to describe these types of inherited traits in families.

Construction of a pedigree, which is a shorthand method of classifying the family data, conveniently summarizes the family data for the study of inherited traits. The symbols used in constructing a pedigree are shown in Fig. 6-4. The observable inheritance patterns followed by such monogenic traits within families are determined by (1) whether the trait is dominant or recessive, (2) whether the gene is autosomal (on one of the autosomes) or X linked (on the X chromosome), and (3) the chance distribution in the offspring of those genes passed from parents in their gametes (sperm and ova). Pedigree construction is a valuable tool for the clinician who is concerned with the diagnosis of and counseling regarding hereditary traits. Every dentist should be able to construct and interpret a pedigree, because it is a certainty that patients will come to the dentist's office with heritable oral diseases that need diagnosing before treatment is begun.

The simple patterns of monogenic inheritance seen in families are described in the following discussion. Because all the mendelian modes of inheritance are found in the amelogenesis imperfecta (AI) disorders, these are used to illustrate basic genetic principles.

DEVELOPMENTAL BIOLOGY OF ENAMEL

To enable understanding of how molecular biologists are attacking the problem of inherited disorders of teeth, a brief review of dental embryology is needed. The early stages of tooth development are characterized by a budding off of epithelium from the oral epithelium itself into the area of the future alveolar bone. This tooth precursor will give rise to both primary and permanent dentitions in the area (incisor, premolar, etc.). Only the inner layer of the double layer of cells (the inner enamel epithelium) has a functional tooth fate—it gives rise to the enamel. The sequence in which this occurs is now well documented and provides an excellent example of how embryonic tissues differentiate under the influence of adjacent but developmentally different cells. In this case, neural crest cells migrating into the dental lamina area from around the developing neural tube came to lie in an intimate but not touching relationship next to the inner enamel epithelium. These two developmentally different cell layers, inner enamel epithelium (enamel) and neural crest (dentin), are separated by an extracellular matrix.[8] Specific tooth development is then mutually dependent on reciprocal cell-to-cell signaling between these two developmentally different cell layers.[9]

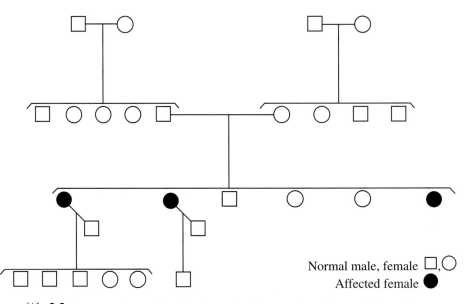

FIG. **6-6.** Autosomal recessive inheritance in pigmented amelogenesis imperfecta.

Normal male, female □,○
Affected female ●

AR-affected child are heterozygotes, it is easy to see that only one out of the four possible combinations of parents' genes results in the homozygous-affected genotype. Hence, the recurrence risk for an affected child in this case is 25%. Note that transmission of the phenotype in a pedigree is horizontal (typically present only in sibs) and not vertical as with a dominant trait.

Of several AR types of AI, the one chosen for discussion here is the pigmented hypomaturation form. In this instance, the genetic defect probably lies in the protein needed in late tooth development to produce a mature, hard, and dense enamel. The defective enamel present is softer than normal but not nearly as soft and easily abraded as in the hypocalcification defect. Remarkably, a brown pigment is found in these outer layers of enamel that are formed last. The nature of this pigment is not known, but it imparts a dark brown, unsightly appearance demanding restorative treatment. A pedigree illustrating AR inheritance of this hypomaturation defect is shown in Fig. 6-6.

X-LINKED OR SEX-LINKED INHERITANCE

Genes on the sex chromosomes are unequally distributed to males and females. This inequality is the result of the following facts: (1) males have one X and one Y chromosome, whereas females have two X chromosomes and (2) the genes active on the Y chromosome are concerned with the development of the male reproductive system. For these reasons, then, males are hemizygous for X-linked genes, meaning that they have only half (or one each) of the X-linked genes. Since females have two X chromosomes, they may be either homozygous or heterozygous for X-linked genes, just as with autosomal genes.

Interesting genetic combinations are made possible by the male hemizygous condition. Because only one gene locus of each kind in the X chromosome is represented in the male, all recessive genes in single dose express themselves phenotypically and thereby behave as though they were dominant genes. On the other hand, XLR genes must be present in double dose (homozygous) in females to fully express themselves. Consequently, full expression of rare XLR diseases in practice is restricted to males and is seen infrequently in females.

To this point we have considered heritable defects in two of the three major types of enamel disorders. The third type—AI, hypoplastic type—shows both autosomal and X-linked modes of inheritance, but only one X-linked type is described here.

X-LINKED DOMINANT

Fig. 6-7 is the pedigree of a family with an X-linked form of AI, hypoplastic type.[13] The clinical features are diagnostic and in some females can be quite striking.

Once again, both dentitions are affected similarly. The surface defect has been described as being granular, lobular, or even pitted. Conceivably, all these different forms of expression are the result of the action of a single gene (or at least its alleles). The enamel is hard but because of its thinness is more susceptible to fracture and abnormal wear. Under the appropriate conditions this trait resembles a hypocalcification defect. However, radiographs quickly resolve this diagnostic problem and show enamel of normal density but with greatly reduced thickness.

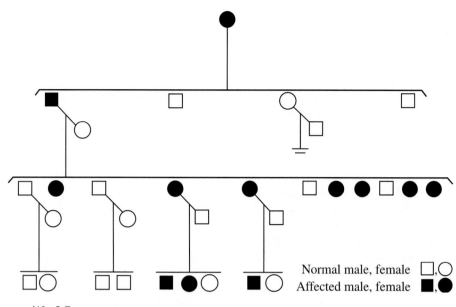

FIG. **6-7.** X-linked dominant inheritance in hypoplastic amelogenesis imperfecta.

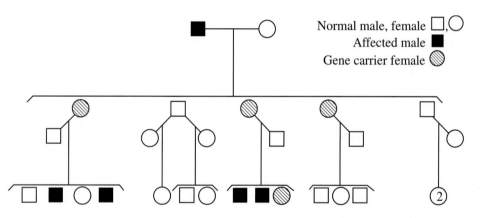

FIG. **6-8.** X-linked recessive inheritance in hypomaturation amelogenesis imperfecta.

X-LINKED RECESSIVE

A pedigree of a family with the X-linked form of enamel hypomaturation is shown in Fig. 6-8. The genetic criteria for diagnosing an XLR trait are summarized as follows:

1. Because the gene cannot be passed from father to son, affected fathers almost never have affected sons. In rare situations, a son could be affected if the mother is a carrier of the XLR trait.
2. All daughters of an affected male receive his X-linked genes. Therefore, affected males transmit the trait to their grandsons through their daughters.
3. The incidence of the trait is much higher in males than in females. This is typified by the disease hemophilia, which is also caused by an XLR gene.

The clinical features of XLR hypomaturation type AI are most striking. The enamel has a somewhat reduced hardness but is not soft. However, the crowns of the teeth look like mountains with snow on them. Hence the name given has been "snow-capped teeth." Radiologically the enamel is hypomature; it shows a lack of contrast between enamel and dentin even though the enamel is of normal thickness.

It should be noted that heterozygous females occasionally show significant clinical expression of a single XLR gene. The reason for this apparent contradiction is the process of X-inactivation, termed *lyonization* after its discoverer, Mary Lyon. This occurs only in females. All female cells have two X chromosomes, but most of the genes on one of the two X chromosomes are inactivated at about the blastula stage of development. This has the effect of making the total number of active, X-linked genes about the same in both males and females. If the female is heterozygous for an X-linked trait, two populations of cells result. One cell population has genes on one X chromosome that are active, while the other cell population has genes on the other X chromosome that are active. When by chance the X chromosome with the deleterious gene is active in a significant proportion of the cells, its expression may be observed in that female. Chance dictates that this imbalance does not occur frequently, but because all females are, by definition of lyonization, mosaic with regard to X-linked traits, phenotypic expression of heterozygous genes may occur in them.

The previous statements concerning the distribution of XLR genes in males and females apply equally as well to XLD genes. The principal difference lies in the fact that when the gene is dominant more females than males will show the trait (see pedigree in Fig. 6-8). Because all XLR genes behave as dominant genes in males, no new criteria are made for their inheritance in males. The following criteria distinguish an XLD trait in families:

1. Affected males must transmit the trait to all of their daughters (as with XLR traits), but all of them are affected, because fathers give their X chromosome to their daughters and their Y chromosome to their sons.
2. Affected males cannot transmit the trait to their sons (just as with XLR traits).
3. Heterozygous females transmit the trait on the average to 50% of their children of both sexes, whereas homozygous-affected females will have only affected children. The latter situation is exceptionally rare for a dominant trait and is practically never observed. Thus, all females affected with a dominantly inherited X-linked trait are considered to be heterozygotes until proven otherwise.

Two points are emphasized here. First, transmission of XLD genes by females follows a pattern indistinguishable from that of autosomal transmission. Thus, these two types of dominant inheritance can be differentiated only by observation of the offspring of affected males. Second, it was noted that XLR disorders are much less common in females than in males. The reverse is true for XLD traits. An XLD trait should appear about twice as often in females as in males, since the former have twice as many X chromosomes as males.

VARIATION IN GENE EXPRESSION

The patterns of inheritance shown in traits determined by genes at a single locus have been presented and discussed. Such patterns, if present, are usually easy to recognize. Unfortunately, many factors may modify the expression of a gene in a family in such a way that a typical monogenic pattern of inheritance is not

discernible. A complete presentation of these modifying factors here is inappropriate, but two concepts related to modification of gene action merit discussion.

PENETRANCE

When a person with a given genotype fails to demonstrate the phenotype characteristic for the genotype, the gene is said to show reduced penetrance. This is a situation most commonly seen with dominant traits. Dentinogenesis imperfecta, an AD trait, is practically 100% penetrant, because all individuals who carry that gene show its phenotype. On the other hand, osteogenesis imperfecta shows incomplete penetrance, because pedigree studies demonstrate individuals who must carry the gene but who do not appear to be affected. Another relevant example is found in the CLP trait. Consider the following family history: a grandfather and his grandson both have CLP but the boy's mother (also the grandfather's daughter) does not. The probability is very high that her son's cleft liability came from his grandfather and therefore was passed through the mother without being expressed as an overt cleft. Possibly the subtle action or predisposition of a clefting gene or genes may be found using measurements of facial structures. Doing so may increase the power of linkage analysis of the predisposing genotype. With the spectacular advances in the understanding of the human genome, we may be able to locate a gene regulating clefting before we know what its action is at the molecular level or how it shows this action as a clinical trait.

EXPRESSIVITY

If a single gene trait can show different phenotypes in the affected members of a kindred, it is said to show variable expressivity. Osteogenesis imperfecta also provides an illustration of variable gene expression. The cardinal signs of this disease are (1) multiple fractures, (2) blue sclera, (3) dentinogenesis imperfecta, and (4) otosclerosis, which results in a hearing deficit. Affected persons in a single family may show any one or a combination of these signs, which illustrates the considerable variation in gene expression. The minimum expression of the gene observed in a family might then be only a blue color to the sclera, which could be unnoticed by the clinician. In this case highly variable gene expression may fade into nonpenetrance.

The craniosynostosis syndromes are AD traits associated with single gene mutations. They also provide good examples of how, even with the strong influence of a single gene, the phenotype can vary markedly. Although it was once thought that a particular mutation in a given gene would always result in a specific syndrome, several identical mutations in the fibroblast growth factor receptor 2 (FGFR2) gene have been found in patients diagnosed with the three different clinical craniosynostosis syndrome entities of Crouzon, Pfeiffer, and Jackson-Weiss syndrome.[14,15]

Another example of the individual variability of these single gene mutation autosomal dominant phenotypes occurred when two individuals in the same family had the classic phenotypes of Pfeiffer and Apert syndrome. In addition, seven other family members had unusually shaped heads and facial appearance reminiscent of Crouzon syndrome.[16] The phenotype may be so variable that this individual may appear to be clinically normal, yet have the same gene mutation associated with Crouzon syndrome in three of his children and two of his grandchildren. Only through the analysis of radiographic measurements was a minimal expression of features suggestive of Crouzon syndrome evident.[17]

MULTIFACTORIAL INHERITANCE

The following features typify multifactorial inheritance, in contrast to monogenic inheritance: (1) multiple genes (polygenes) at different loci are involved in expressing the phenotype, and (2) the phenotype produced is a summation of the effects of polygenes interacting with their environment. The phenotypic result is often a continuously varying spectrum of that trait (e.g., height) rather than presentation as a discrete (trait present or absent) phenotype.

Many common diseases, such as dental caries, have continuous variation with no sharp distinction between normal (average) and abnormal (extremes). However, there may be a specific measurement point beyond which that disease is arbitrarily regarded by the clinician as abnormal.

Multifactorial inheritance is troublesome to analyze genetically; in fact, geneticists often arrive at a diagnosis of multifactorial inheritance for a given trait only after the monogenic forms of inheritance have been considered and found to be unlikely. Certain techniques for studying it have been developed. The simplest is the method of resemblance between relatives, which states that the more closely related two individuals are, the more closely they resemble each other concerning the specific trait in question. It is important to stress, though, the continuous phenotypic variation that is characteristic of inheritance patterns resulting from polygenes.

This issue of continuous variation is emphasized because the most common diseases with which the dentist must deal (i.e., periodontal disease, dental caries, and malocclusion) are multifactorial traits. Only the extremes of variation are readily apparent to the dentist, such as in the child with rampant caries or the adult who is caries free. In this latter instance, if one did not understand the concept of multifactorial inheritance, one might conclude that such individuals represent a discrete

phenotype influenced by a single gene in a mendelian manner. This is frequently not the case.

A most important feature of traits produced by polygenes is that they are susceptible to environmental modification. A phenotype resulting from the concerted action of 100 genes is much more likely to be altered and modified by the existing environment than a trait controlled by only one or even several genes. Still, this does not mean that a trait resulting from only one or even several genes cannot be influenced by environmental factors. The change in phenotype will depend on the individual's ability to respond to the environmental factor, which may be heavily influenced by the same gene(s) originally influencing the phenotype or by other genes.

An example of a polygenic trait that is markedly influenced by environmental factors is dental caries, which is the interaction product of three essential factors: a cariogenic diet, a caries-producing bacterial flora, and a susceptible tooth. These three factors encompass a variety of biologically complicated entities, such as saliva, plaque, tooth matrix formation, and crystallization. It should be easy to see that the development of these complex elements must involve a great number of genes. Environmental modification, such as properly timed systemic fluoride supplementation, produces a considerable alteration in the phenotype without changing the genetic constitution of the individual. The reader can probably think of additional environmental modifications that can produce a greatly altered dental caries experience without changing an individual's genes. Some conditions that we have attributed to a multifactorial inheritance because they tend to occur in particular families may be greatly influenced by a gene or genes that predispose to the condition, depending on what other genetic or environmental factors are involved.

MULTIFACTORIAL INHERITANCE IN HUMAN DISEASES

For many common disorders, such as diabetes and hypertension, and even for the major common congenital malformations (i.e., spina bifida, hydrocephalus, and CLP) there is a definite familial tendency. This is shown by the fact that the proportion of affected near relatives is greater than the incidence in the general population. However, this proportion is much lower than what is expected for a monogenic trait, and the explanation most commonly offered for major congenital malformations is that they are multifactorial traits. As previously stated, one definition of a multifactorial trait is that it represents the summation of the effects of many genes (polygenes) interacting with the environment, hence the term *multifactorial*. Environment is defined as those nongenetic circumstances that render an individual more or less susceptible to a disease state. In contrast to monogenic traits, whose characteristics have been summarized in preceding paragraphs, multifactorial diseases show the following characteristics:

1. Each person has a liability for a given disease, and that liability represents a sum of the genetic and environmental liabilities.
2. The multifactorial-threshold model is a mathematical way of expressing these liabilities. For polygenic traits the model is simply a gaussian curve. As already noted, for multifactorial traits a threshold must be added to allow the continuous polygenic model to be used in describing noncontinuous or discrete traits. For many human congenital malformations, a multifactorial model with threshold is appropriate for describing discrete traits such as CLP. Such a threshold means that all persons with sufficient gene dosage and environmental interaction will be above the threshold of expression and show the cleft lip. Those with less will not show a cleft lip. A graphic representation of this idea is shown in Fig. 6-9.
3. Because of the differing dosage of polygenes in groups that show a specific phenotype (e.g., CLP), the overall incidence of this trait will vary in near relatives of those affected. For example, a dominantly inherited trait has a gene dosage of 1 in 2 (50%). Assuming that several polygenes may be involved in CLP, this figure decreases at least tenfold to about 1% to 5%. Naturally, the incidence in a random population is even lower, or about 1 per 1000. Therefore, increasing gene dosage for a multifactorial trait in a family is associated with an increased incidence of that trait in near relatives of the affected individuals. The nature of this system with a threshold permits large numbers of persons at risk for showing that phenotype (CLP) to carry the liability for clefting without expressing it clinically. Based on current research findings regarding traits that are multifactorial with a threshold, it

appears that it will be difficult to relate these mathematical observations to cellular biologic function.

Toward the end of the nineteenth century, Galton recognized that twins could be useful for evaluating the nature-nurture argument that was raging at that time. Interest in the twin method for study of the relative importance of heredity and environment in humans has been increasing. One explanation for this interest is that many human traits are multifactorial (polygenic), are susceptible to environmental modification, and therefore are difficult to study by conventional methods. The twin method allows an approach to the study of such traits and is based on the principle that human twins are of two basic types: monozygotic (or identical) twins resulting from a single ovum fertilized by a single sperm, and dizygotic (or fraternal) twins resulting from fertilization of two ova by two sperm. It is axiomatic that monozygotic twins have identical genotypes, whereas dizygotic twins are no more closely related to each other than are any two siblings.[18] It also follows that differences between monozygotic twins result from environmental differences, whereas those between dizygotic twins result from differences in both heredity and environment.

To use the twin method, one must distinguish between the two types of zygosity. If both twins are identical for the trait in question (regardless of their zygosity), they are described as concordant. If they are unlike for the trait, they are discordant. Such intrapair differences are usually expressed in percentage figures for a group of twins being evaluated. For example, monozygous twins show a 33% concordance for CLP, whereas dizygous twins show only a 5% concordance.

Another method to estimate the heritability of a trait and to evaluate evidence of linkage of a phenotype with DNA polymorphisms is by sib-pair analysis. Heritability estimates can be generated from within- and between-sibship variance quantified by generalized linear models, with confounding factors controlled for where indicated. Polymorphic DNA markers may be tested for genetic linkage (proximity) to a gene influencing a particular phenotype by testing whether the magnitude of the phenotypic difference between two siblings is correlated with the alleles they share that are identical by descent (IBD). An allele is considered to be IBD if both members of a sibling pair inherited the same marker allele from the same parent. If a marker is linked to a gene contributing to the phenotype in question, then siblings with a similar (if quantitative) or the same (if discrete) phenotype would be expected to share more alleles IBD, whereas siblings with widely differing phenotypes would be expected to share few if any alleles IBD near any gene(s) influencing the phenotype.[19] In addition, another method of looking for DNA markers that are in linkage disequilibrium is to use the quantitative

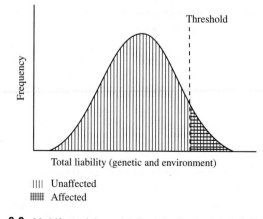

FIG. **6-9.** Multifactorial model for inheritance of cleft lip and palate.

transmission disequilibrium test. This analysis calculates the difference between the value of the quantitative trait in the offspring and the average value of the quantitative trait in all offspring in all families studied, while simultaneously considering the allele transmission from parent to offspring.[20] Thus, whereas the sib-pair linkage analysis involves two or more siblings, the quantitative transmission disequilibrium test involves trios of parents and one or more siblings.

Influence of Genetic Factors on Major Croniofacial, Oral, and, Dental Conditions

GENETICS AND DENTAL CARIES

It is clear from many dietary studies that variation in susceptibility to dental caries exists even under identical, controlled conditions.[21] This implies that, because of genetic differences, certain environmental factors are potentially more cariogenic for some people than for others. This is not to say that dental caries is an inherited disease; rather, genetic influences may modify the overt expression of this disease in the individual.

Fifty years ago, dental caries was presented to dental students as a disease that was so common that more than 99% of the general population was afflicted by it. Although it is still recognized as a common disease, the use of systemic and topical fluorides and persistence by organized dentistry to bring about changes in dietary habits and oral hygiene practices have contributed significantly to a remarkable decrease in the prevalence of this disorder, especially noted in children. Today, it is not unusual for a prepubertal-age child to be caries free.

Three essential interacting elements comprise the model system for dental caries that is most commonly used to discuss its etiology. These factors are microorganisms, substrate (fermentable carbohydrates), and host factors, such as tooth anatomy. It is in the last area of the host factors that genetics exerts a major influence on dental caries initiation.

Several investigators have studied the genetic aspects of dental caries in humans, using both the twin and the family pedigree approaches. Since dental caries is an age-dependent process, much of the reported data cannot be compared because of age differences in the various population groups studied. Nevertheless, the family observations by Klein and Palmer[22] and Klein[23] are worth noting. Their findings indicated that children have a caries experience remarkably similar to that of their parents when the susceptibility of both parents is the same (either high or low). When caries susceptibility of the two parents is dissimilar, however, the children's susceptibility tends to be more like that of the mother than that of the father. This finding was particularly evident in daughters.

Since dental caries is an infectious communicable disease, however, familial clustering may to some degree reflect familial environmental contact, with transmission of cariogenic bacteria to children at certain ages. Li and Caulfield found that mothers are the principle source of mutans streptococci to their infants, with a greater rate of transmission to female than male infants.[24]

The more common a genetic trait is, the more difficult it is to demonstrate its genetic character. Several authors have attempted to do this for dental caries by the study of twins. Book and Grahnen attempted to maximize differences in caries experience within families by selecting caries-free, 20-year-old men and comparing caries experience within their families.[25] Results showed that parents and siblings of caries-free propositi had significantly lower rates of decayed, missing, and filled teeth than the control families. The authors concluded that the observed differences are hereditary and probably polygenic in nature.

Studies of twins by Dahlberg and Dahlberg,[26] Mansbridge,[27] Horowitz, Osborne, and De George,[28] and Caldwell and Finn[29] indicated that genetic factors make a significant contribution to individual differences in caries susceptibility. However, most authors agree that this genetic component of dental caries is a minor one in comparison with the overall effect of environment. The conclusion from clinical twin and familial correlation studies and estimation of heritability studies regarding the degree of genetic influence on caries may be confounded by the already mentioned transmission of cariogenic bacteria within the family.

A review of inherited risks for susceptibility to caries found evidence of an association between altered dental enamel development in defined populations and an increased risk of caries, as well as a relationship between host immune complex genes and different levels of cariogenic bacteria and enamel defects.[30] Thus the individual's genotype may influence the likelihood of intraoral colonization of cariogenic bacteria, which further exemplifies the complexity of caries development. To further delineate the familial aspect of caries that is bacterial from host genetic factors, studies relating caries susceptibility to specific biochemical differences in individuals may be undertaken. For example, Goodman et al reported significant differences in salivary flow, pH, and salivary amylase activity between monozygotic and dizygotic twins.[31] In addition, genetic linkage studies on well-characterized populations with clearly defined caries experience will help define those host factors that have the greatest influence on the incidence of caries.[25]

Animal studies have been more productive. Hunt, Hoppert, and Rosen succeeded in establishing caries-resistant and caries-susceptible strains of rats using inbreeding techniques.[32] Although the resistant strain was challenged by oral inoculation of cariogenic bacteria, the resistant phenotype was maintained. These were the first studies to confirm the presence of important genetics elements influencing dental caries susceptibility.

From this information, it is clear that heredity plays an important but obscure role in the cause of dental caries. Studies in the 1970s and 1980s examined the influence of saliva proteins on dental plaque formation. These studies suggested a possible mechanism of action for genes regulating this multifactorial trait. A group of saliva proteins designated as the proline-rich proteins (PRPs) because of their high content of the amino acid proline have been linked to early plaque and pellicle formation.[33,34] PRPs closely resemble enamel matrix proteins in both composition and structure, which accounts for why they bond so tightly to hydroxylapatite crystals. Furthermore, the ability to produce these several types of PRPs is inherited as a group of autosomal codominant traits. At least eight different polymorphic PRPs are known, and all these proteins are coded for by a block of genes called the salivary protein complex, located on the short arm of human chromosome 12.[35,36] Only a few studies have attempted to associate these salivary protein phenotypes with oral disease states. Yu et al reported significant association between two specific PRPs phenotypes (Pa+ and Pr22) and an increase in dental caries scores in the permanent teeth of children 5 to 15 years of age.[37] This result suggested that persons with either or both of these two genotypes (Pa+ and/or Pr22) may be at significant risk for increased susceptibility to dental caries, whereas the allelic genes, Pa– and Pr11 or Pr12, appear to confer caries resistance. The mechanism of action could be related to the formation of a caries-susceptible plaque. Certainly, the most important result of an interaction between genetic and environmental factors is the production of dental plaque. It is through the plaque itself that dental caries is expressed as a disease process, and so plaque formation may be the critical element influenced by genetics in disease initiation.

In summary, susceptibility to human dental caries is influenced to a significant but minor degree by heredity. This genetic control is undoubtedly multifactorial in nature, and such a polygenic background strongly implies considerable environmental influence. Specific types of dental caries susceptibility representing the extremes of variation of this trait may ultimately prove to be monogenic traits, but at present the evidence is insufficient for a clear statement of such inheritance.

GENETICS AND PERIODONTAL DISEASE

The periodontal disease state is often described as a local inflammatory disease with possible underlying systemic factors. This disease is so widespread in human populations and has such widely varying clinicohistopathologic features that it seems certain that multiple diseases with multiple causes are being lumped together as a single entity. Periodontists suggest that there is evidence for the existence of several variant types of periodontal disease generally subclassified by the age of onset, severity of bone loss, oral hygiene status, and presence or absence of local factors. One might visualize a continuum of disease expression ranging from a localized gingivitis to a generalized periodontitis with severe bone and tooth loss. Such a complex disease shows both inflammatory and degenerative pathologic features.

It is easy to understand why genetic studies of this common problem have been neglected. As is true for dental caries, periodontal disease is common, occurs with a continuum of expressivity, and is greatly influenced by environmental conditions, such as diet, occlusion, and oral hygiene habits. All of these features fit the description of a multifactorial type of disease or at least of disease susceptibility.

Most periodontists believe that dental plaque formation is the critical first step in the initiation of chronic periodontal disease, and it is possible that the PRPs, which are influential in dental caries initiation through regulation of plaque formation, also play a role in the genetics of periodontal disease.

Most genetic studies of a trait make use of families with multiple affected individuals or twins. A carefully designed study of twins with periodontal disease by Ciancio, Hazen, and Curat was reported in 1969.[38] Using the Ramfjord index, which evaluates gingival inflammation, calculus formation, tooth mobility, and tooth loss in all four quadrants of the mouth, the authors examined 7 monozygotic and 12 dizygotic pairs of teenaged twins. They concluded that there was no evidence in these twins for significant heritability of any of these dental parameters.

Alternatively, Michalowicz et al published a large study of adult twins (mean age, 40 years) of which there were 63 monozygotic and 33 dizygotic pairs.[39] Using elements of the Ramfjord index as criteria for diagnosis, heritability estimates were calculated. The authors state that from 38% to 82% of the periodontal disease identified in these twins was attributable to genetic factors.

Investigation by Kornman et al into the association of different polymorphisms of inflammation-mediating genes and periodontal disease in adult nonsmokers indicate interleukin 1α and 1β (IL-1α and IL-1β) genotype may be a risk factor.[40] The IL-1β polymorphism was IL-1β+3953 and the IL-1α polymorphism was IL-1α-889. Nonsmokers aged 40 to 60 carrying the "2" allele (in either homozygous or heterozygous state) at both loci were observed to have nearly 19 times the risk of developing severe periodontitis of subjects homozygous for the "1" allele at either or both of these loci. However, in a review of subsequent studies, Greenstein and Hart[41] noted that the relationship of specific IL-1 genotypes and the level of crevicular fluid IL-1β is not clear, and that the ability of the genetic susceptibility test for severe chronic periodontitis based on the finding of Kornman et al[40] to forecast which patients will develop increased bleeding on probing, periodontitis, or loss of teeth or need for dental implants is ambiguous. It is evident that biochemical and molecular biologic techniques, in concert with clinical studies, will continue to be used in evaluating the heritable predisposing factors in periodontal disease.

Animal studies have not been a focus for examining the heredity of periodontal disease. Only the complex multifaceted periodontal disease of humans is available for study, and the variation in definitive diagnostic criteria that could be used to establish different types of periodontal disease increases the difficulty of studying this heterogeneous and complicated pathology. Early-onset periodontitis has been the subject of most family studies. Since several forms of early-onset periodontitis (e.g., localized prepubertal periodontitis, localized juvenile periodontitis [JP], and generalized JP) can be found in the same family, the expression of the underlying genetic defect appears to have the potential to be influenced by other genetic factors.[42]

Progress has been made in the study of rare genetic conditions or syndromes that can predispose to periodontal disease or have periodontal disease as a relatively consistent component of their pleiotropic effect. For example, leukocyte adhesion deficiency (LAD), type I and type II, are autosomal recessive (AR) disorders of the leukocyte adhesion cascade.[43] LAD type I has abnormalities in the integrin receptors of leukocytes resulting from mutations in the β2 integrin chain (ITGB2) gene leading to impaired adhesion and chemotaxis, which results in an increased susceptibility for severe infections and early-onset (prepubertal) periodontitis.[44,45] LAD type II is also an AR disorder secondary to mutation in the gene encoding guanosine 5'-diphosphate–fucose transporter 1 (FUCT1). The infectious episodes and the severity are much milder than those observed in LAD type I, and the only persistent clinical symptom is chronic severe periodontitis. The exact defect in the system is absence of the stalyl Lewis x (SleX) structure antigens, which are important ligands for the selectin on the leukocyte, which leads to a profound defect in leukocyte rolling, the first step in the adhesion cascade. This causes a marked decrease in chemotaxis accompanied by pronounced neutrophilia. Apart from the leukocyte defect, these patients suffer from severe growth and mental retardation and exhibit the rare Bombay blood group type.[43]

Ehlers-Danlos syndrome (EDS) is actually a collection of ten types distinguished on the basis of clinical symptoms and inheritance pattern. In addition to consistent early-onset periodontal disease, patients with EDS type VIII have variable hyperextensibility of the skin, ecchymotic pretibial lesions, minimal bruising, minimal to moderate joint hypermobility of the digits, and cigarette paper scars. Inheritance is AD. Early-onset periodontal disease may also be found in patients with EDS type IV. These individuals are usually characterized by type III collagen abnormalities with hyperextensibility of the skin, ecchymotic pretibial lesions, easy bruisability, cigarette paper scars, joint hypermobility of digits, pes planus, and, of greatest concern, arterial and intestinal ruptures. Like type VIII, type IV also has AD inheritance.[46] The presence or absence of type III collagen abnormalities has been taken to be a differentiating factor between the two types, with EDS type IV showing abnormal type III collagen. The considerable overlap in phenotype of these two types warrants careful family and clinical evaluation, and biochemical studies of collagen, when a patient with features of EDS and periodontal disease is evaluated.[47]

Chédiak-Higashi syndrome has frequently been linked with severe periodontitis.[45] This rare AR disorder is characterized by oculocutaneous hypopigmentation, severe immunologic deficiency with neutropenia and lack of natural killer cells, a bleeding tendency, and neurologic abnormalities. It is caused by mutations in the CHS1/LYST gene.[48]

Papillon-Lefèvre syndrome and Haim-Munk syndrome are two of the many different types of palmoplantar keratoderma, differing from the others by the occurrence of severe early-onset periodontitis with premature loss of the primary and permanent dentition. Haim-Munk syndrome is characterized in addition by arachnodactyly, acroosteolysis, and onychogryphosis.[49] Hart et al[50] have shown that both of these AR syndromes are due to different mutations in the cathepsin C (CTSC) gene.

EARLY-ONSET PERIODONTITIS

Early onset of periodontitis may occur in the primary dentition (prepubertal periodontitis), may develop during puberty (JP), or may be characterized by exceedingly rapid loss of alveolar bone (rapidly progressive periodontitis). Along with hypophosphatasia, prepubertal periodontitis appears to be the most commonly encountered cause of premature exfoliation of the primary teeth, especially in girls.[46]

JP has the following features:

1. An early onset of the breakdown of periodontal bone. This bone loss is of two types: chronic

periodontitis in a generalized form affecting any dental area, and a localized form in which the molar or incisor regions of bone are the most severely affected.

2. Bone destruction that is rapid and vertical, with specific microorganisms associated with the periodontal lesion.

3. Familial aggregation, especially in the molar and incisor types. It seems probable that the generalized and localized types represent two different aspects of the same disorder, so this discussion will consider them as a complex entity that goes by the name familial JP.

At least three different modes of inheritance have been proposed for JP. The early reports of Benjamin and Baer, and later that of Melnick et al, offered support for an XLD trait.[51,52] This conclusion was based on the observation that twice as many females were observed to be affected as males (see preceding criteria for XLD inheritance). However, Hart et al have shown that females are twice as likely as males to seek out treatment.[53] When this biased ascertainment is allowed for, the male/female ratio is essentially unity. Saxen demonstrated that a clinical phenotype found in Finland closely resembling JP (if not actually JP) showed an AR mode of inheritance.[54] This disorder may be peculiar to Finland. Boughman et al reported linkage of a gene in a single large family for an AD form of JP on chromosome 4 to another dental trait (dentinogenesis imperfecta, Shields type III).[55] Hart et al, in a study of 19 unrelated families, strongly excluded linkage between an early-onset periodontitis susceptibility gene and chromosome region 4q12-q13 assuming locus homogeneity.[56] They concluded that the previous report of linkage was a false positive, or that there are two or more unlinked forms of JP, with the form located in 4q12-q13 being less common. Dominant inheritance is probable for the type most prevalent in this country (Fig. 6-10).

Evaluation of the same IL-1α and IL-1β polymorphisms found by Kornman et al[40] to be associated with periodontitis in adult nonsmokers was performed in black and white families with two or more members affected with early-onset periodontitis by Diehl et al.[57] Interestingly, they found the IL-1 alleles associated with high risk of early-onset periodontitis to be the ones suggested previously to be correlated with low risk for severe adult periodontitis. They concluded that early-onset periodontitis is a complex, oligogenic disorder (i.e., involving a small number of genes), with IL-1 genetic variation having an important but not exclusive influence on disease risk.

GENETICS OF MALOCCLUSION

The study of occlusion pertains to relationships between teeth in the same dental arch, as well as between the two dental arches when the teeth come together. Many factors are involved in the definition of normal occlusion, and it is not possible in this chapter to discuss all of them. Some of the most important orofacial parameters of occlusion are airway function, soft tissue anatomy and function, size of the maxilla, size of the mandible (both rami and body), arch form, anatomy of teeth (including malformation), congenitally missing teeth, and rotation of teeth. All of these important elements must be included in the concept of occlusion.

Malocclusion is perhaps somewhat easier to define. One may simply say that malocclusion is a significant deviation from normal occlusion. However, this description is useful only if one considers the multiple aspects implicit in such a definition. Normal occlusion and malocclusion are dynamic concepts that involve the interrelationships of many factors, not a few of which have been shown to be influenced by genetic factors. For example, in a study of the association of the Pro561Thr (P56IT) variant in the growth hormone receptor (GHR) gene with craniofacial measurements on lateral cephalometrics radiographs by Yamaguchi et al, those who did not have the GHR P56IT allele had a significantly greater mandibular ramus length (condylion-gonion) than did those with the GHR P56IT allele in a normal Japanese sample of 50 men and 50 women.[58] The average mandibular ramus height in those with the GHR P56IT allele was 4.65 mm shorter than the average for those without the GHR P56IT allele. This significant correlation between the GHR P56IT allele and shorter mandibular ramus height was confirmed in an additional 80 women.

Theoretically, there are two general ways in which predisposing or causative factors for malocclusion could be due to heritable characteristics.[59] One would be inheritance of a disproportion between the size of the

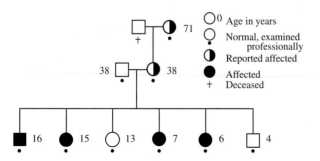

FIG. **6-10.** Pedigree of family with juvenile periodontitis, a dominant trait.

teeth and the jaws resulting in crowding or spacing, whereas the other would be inheritance of a disproportion in the position, size, or shape of the mandible and maxilla. As will be seen, genetic influences on each of these traits are rarely due to a single gene, which would be necessary for malocclusion to be due to the simple inheritance of discrete skeletal and dental characteristics. Instead they are often polygenic with the potential for environmental influence. Part of the practice of orthodontics is to use environmental (i.e., nongenetic) influences for the correction of malocclusion.

Dental anthropologists tell us that malocclusion is uncommon in pure racial populations. However, it has been debated whether this is due to the lack of procreation with other populations or the less refined diet often eaten by these typically isolated groups.

The experiments of Stockard et al in dogs have been cited as evidence that crossbreeding among inbred strains increases the incidence of malocclusion.[60] However, the anomalies they produced may have been due in part to the influence of a major gene or genes that have been bred to be part of specific breeds. It seems improbable that racial crossbreeding in humans could resemble the condition of these experiments and thereby result in a synergistic increase of orofacial malrelations. An exception on an individual basis may be when an individual with a dominant trait or syndrome that results in a malocclusion has a child. Depending on whether it is autosomal or X-linked, the dominant gene, if transmitted to an offspring, may also affect the offspring's occlusal development in a similar fashion as in the affected parent.

Studies of occlusion in twins have also been made. Lundstrom performed an intensive analysis of specific dentofacial attributes in twins and concluded that heredity played a significant role in determining the following characteristics: tooth size, width and length of the dental arch, height of the palate, crowding and spacing of teeth, and degree of overbite.[61] Kraus, Wise, and Frei made a cephalometric study of triplets in an attempt to assign an inherited basis to specific craniofacial morphologic features.[62] The authors looked at the lateral profile of the head and cranial vault, the outline of the calvaria, the cranial base, and the facial complex, which included both the upper and lower face and the maxillomandibular relationship. In addition, they selected 17 individual measurements of single portions of a given bone (e.g., posterior border of ramus). They concluded that morphology of an individual bone is under strong genetic control but that the environment plays a major role in determining how various bony elements are combined to achieve a harmonious or disharmonious craniofacial skeleton. This observation at least partly explains the remarkable differences sometimes seen in the facial patterns of identical twins and emphasizes the important role of environment in their development.

Litton et al reported class III malocclusion to be a heritable trait that is probably polygenic in nature.[63] Harris has shown that the craniofacial skeletal patterns of children with class II malocclusions are heritable and that there is a high resemblance to the skeletal patterns in their siblings with normal occlusion.[64] From this he concluded that the genetic basis for this resemblance is probably polygenic. Interestingly, Harris used the family skeletal patterns as predictors for treatment prognosis of the child with a class II malocclusion.[64]

King et al noted that many studies which estimate heritability of craniofacial structures may have a bias because they have generally involved subjects who had not undergone orthodontic treatment, and that often subjects judged to have an extreme malocclusion were excluded.[65] They found that, in contrast to the relatively high heritability of cephalometric variables and low heritability of occlusal variables in subjects with naturally occurring good occlusion, the heritability estimates for craniofacial skeletal variables in subjects with overt malocclusions were significantly lower and the heritability estimates for occlusal variations were significantly higher. This observation supports the idea that everyone does not react to specific environmental factors in the same manner, although those who are related are more likely to react in a similar fashion. To quote King et al, "We propose that the substantive measures of intersib similarity for occlusal traits reflect similar responses to environmental factors common to both siblings. That is, given genetically influenced facial types and growth patterns, siblings are likely to respond to environmental factors (e.g., reduced masticatory stress, chronic mouth breathing) in similar fashions. Malocclusions appear to be acquired, but the fundamental genetic control of craniofacial form often diverts siblings into comparable physiologic responses leading to development of similar malocclusions."[65]

Although we have some information about genetic influence on specific traits (e.g., missing teeth, occlusal patterns, tooth morphology, and even mandibular prognathism), these cases are exceptions, and we do not have sufficient information to make accurate predictions about the development of occlusion simply by studying the frequency of its occurrence in parents or even siblings. Admittedly, family patterns of resemblance are frequently obvious, but predictions must be made cautiously because of the genetic and environmental variables and their interaction, which are unknown and difficult to evaluate.

Unfortunately, at this time the results of studies on the genetic and environmental factors that influence the development of malocclusion are representative of the samples studied, not necessarily of any particular individual. In addition, the extent that a particular trait is influenced by genetic factors may have little if any effect on the success of environmental (treatment) intervention. Still, it may be that genetic factors that influenced a trait will also influence the response to intervention to alter that trait, or other genetic factors may be involved in the response. Therefore, the possibility of altering the environment to gain a more favorable occlusion theoretically exists even in individuals in whom the malocclusion does have a relatively high genetic influence. However, the question of how environmental and genetic factors interact is most relevant to clinical practice, because it may explain why a particular alteration of the environment (treatment) may be successful in one compliant patient and not in another.[66]

EXTERNAL APICAL ROOT RESORPTION

Basic descriptors of root resorption are based on the anatomical region of occurrence; that is, designations are internal root resorption and external root resorption (cervical root resorption and external apical root resorption [EARR]). EARR is a frequent iatrogenic outcome associated with orthodontic treatment and may also occur in the absence of orthodontic treatment.[67,68] Although orthodontic treatment is associated with some maxillary central incisor EARR in most patients, and more than one third of those treated experience greater than 3 mm of loss, severe EARR (more than 5 mm) occurs in 2% to 5%.[69,70]

Currently, there are no reliable markers to predict which patients will develop EARR nor how severe EARR will be following orthodontic tooth movement,[71] although the shape of the root does appear to be associated with the likelihood of EARR and is best examined on periapical rather than panoramic radiographs.[72] Even when duration of treatment is a factor, it along with several significant dentofacial structural measurements (such as overjet) do not account for enough of the observed variability to be useful as predictors of EARR by themselves.[69]

The degree and severity of EARR associated with orthodontic treatment is multifactorial, involving host and environmental factors, with genetic factors accounting for at least 50% of the variation. A polymorphism in the IL-1β (IL-1B) gene in orthodontically treated individuals accounts for 15% of the variation in maxillary central incisor EARR. Individuals homozygous for the IL-1B allele 1 have a 5.6-fold (95% confidence interval, 1.9 to 21.2) increased risk of EARR greater than 2 mm compared with individuals who are not homozygous for the IL-1B allele 1.[73] Although this is the

first genetic marker suggested to be associated with EARR, it accounts for too small an amount of the total variation to be predictive. Additional genetic studies such as the one that found genetic linkage for EARR with a marker on chromosome 18 near the RANK gene are needed to determine what other genes influence EARR.[74] Future estimation of susceptibility to EARR will likely require the analysis of a number of genes, root morphology, dental and facial measurement values, and the amount of tooth movement planned for treatment.

GENETICS OF CLEFT LIP AND PALATE

Studies of the CLP phenotype in twins indicate that monozygous twins have a 35% concordance rate, whereas dizygous twins show less than 5% concordance.[75] Information from two sources (families and twins) then establishes a genetic basis for CLP, but despite many extensive investigations, no simple pattern of inheritance has been demonstrated. This has led to proposal of a variety of genetic modes of inheritance for CLP, including dominance, recessiveness, and sex linkage, and has led ultimately to the documentation of modifying conditions that may be present, such as incomplete penetrance and variable gene expressivity.[76] There are three important reasons for the failure to resolve the question of a hereditary basis for clefts: (1) some clefts are of a nongenetic origin and should not be included in a genetic analysis; unfortunately, such cases are seldom recognized and are difficult to prove; (2) individuals who have increased genetic liability for having a child with CLP often fail to be recognized, but because they do not have CLP themselves they cannot be identified with certainty; this latter situation defines the problem of nonpenetrance for genes that control CLP[77]; and (3) CLP, although sometimes appearing to be relatively simple in origin, is undoubtedly a complex of diseases with different etiologies lumped together because of clinical disease resemblance (they all show clefting).

There are two clearly recognized groups of etiologically different clefts—cleft lip either with or without cleft palate (CL[P]) and isolated cleft palate (CP). These two entities, CL(P) and CP, occur as single cases in a family and as multiple cases in a family. In the former they are called sporadic, and in the latter they are called familial or multiplex. Some researchers refer to multiplex cases as those individuals with findings in addition to an oral cleft, even if a specific syndrome is not recognized. It should also be noted that the isolated CP that occurs without a cleft of the lip is different from the palatal cleft that occurs as a part of CLP. The embryology and developmental timing are both different, and isolated CP is more commonly

| TABLE **6-2** | Potential Etiologic Groups Within Cleft Lip with or without Cleft Palate (CL[P]) and Cleft Palate (CP) |

	SPORADIC CASES	FAMILIAL CASES	CLEFT SYNDROMES
CL(P)	74%	25%	1%
Recurrence risk	Less than 1%	16%	Risk varies from 0.1% to 50%
Isolated CP	80%	12%	8%
Recurrence risk	Less than 1%	16%	Risk varies from 0.1% to 50%

the result of an environmental teratogen than is CLP. When all potential study groups for CL(P) and CP are considered, the minimum number is six: three subgroups for CL(P) and three for CP. These three for each type of cleft are the sporadic and the familial groups and a small group of syndromes that feature CL(P) and/or CP. Although there are many such recognizable syndromes, they are relatively rare in occurrence and may not provide much information about the nonsyndromic clefting process. Thus, if these syndromic cases are omitted, the four groups that remain may yield useful information concerning possible genetic origin.

Table 6-2 gives a breakdown of the numbers to be found in these four groups. It can be seen that sporadic cases of both CL(P) and CP are in a large majority, comprising about three fourths of all cases. On the other hand, the familial cases, although not as common, still

make up 12% to 20% of cleft cases. As noted earlier, it is probable that minor and subtle facial changes are more likely to produce the best-correlated phenotype needed to pinpoint the cleft genotype. Part of the reason for this view is the suspicion that certain facial shapes are more predisposed to developing CLP than others.[78] Although this approach seems best for producing an accurately generated clefting phenotype, as yet there are few data to substantiate it. This also means that we must go a lot farther in our study of the developmental anatomy of the head and face.

Recurrence risks for CL(P) and CP have been reported in which penetrance was not considered. These data are frequently cited by genetic counselors as illustrating the lesser risk associated with a multifactorial than with a monogenic trait. The reader will note that these data consider CL(P) and CP without regard to the three groups discussed previously. These data, therefore, are average risk figures (Table 6-3).

The published data on nonsyndromic cleft populations comes from around the world (Japan, China, Hawaii, Denmark, Sweden, Great Britain, and North America). These studies make it clear that both CL(P) and CP are heterogeneous diseases. That is, there are multiple causes for the single phenotypes, CL(P), and CP. To summarize the generally accepted hereditary basis for CL(P) and CP: Single, nonsyndromic cases of CL(P) and CP, or sporadic clefts, are believed to be the result of a complex interaction between multiple genetic and environmental factors. Hence, their etiology is multifactorial in the true sense of the word, and the chance that these multiple factors would interact to produce a cleft phenotype in relatives is small, probably less than 1%.

| TABLE **6-3** | Recurrence Risks for Cleft Lip with or without Cleft Palate (CL[P]) and Isolated Cleft Palate (CP) |

	□—○ → ■, ?	MATING TYPE ■—○ → ?	□—● → ●, ?
Fogh-Andersen[76]	4%	2%	14%
CL(P)	12%	7%	17%
CP*			
Curtis and Walker[79]	4%	4%	19%
CL(P)	2%	6%	14%
CP*			
Curtis, Fraser, and Warburton[80]	4%	—	17%
CL(P)	7%	—	15%
CP*			

*Isolated cleft palate data were obtained from familes with cleft individuals, in addition to the immediate family unit.

The other nonsyndromic group consists of multiple cases of clefts that occur in a single family. These are called familial (or multiplex) and have been viewed by researchers as the "true" genetic cases. Familial occurrences of CL(P) and CP seem most likely to be accounted for by the action of a single major gene, but the influence of multifactorial trait factors is difficult to rule out. Thus we are left with the idea that both multifactorial and single major gene elements may have a role in producing sporadic and familial cases of CL(P) and CP.

REFERENCES

1. Chakravarti A: To a future of genetic medicine, *Nature* 409:822-823, 2001.
2. Everett ET, Hartsfield JK Jr: Mouse models for craniofacial anomalies. In *Biological mechanisms of tooth movement and craniofacial adaptation,* Boston, 2000, Harvard Society for the Advancement of Orthodontics.
3. Cobourne MT: Construction for the modern head: current concepts in craniofacial development, *J Orthod* 27:307-314, 2000.
4. Lejeune J, Turpin R, Gautier J: Le mongolisme: premier exemple d'aberration et autosomique humaine, *Ann Genet* 1:41-49, 1959.
5. Goodenough U: *Genetics,* ed 3, Philadelphia, 1984, WB Saunders.
6. Hopper JL: *Heritability in biostatistical genetics and genetic epidemiology,* New York, 2002, Wiley.
7. LaBuda MC, Gottesman II, Pauls DL: Usefulness of twin studies for exploring the etiology of childhood and adolescent psychiatric disorders, *Am J Med Genet* 48:47-59, 1993.
8. Croissant R, Guenther H, Slavkin H: How are embryonic pre-ameloblasts instructed by odontoblasts to synthesize enamel. In Slavkin HC, Greulich RC, editors: *Extracellular matrix influences on gene expression,* New York, 1975, Academic Press.
9. Sharpe PT: Neural crest and tooth morphogenesis, *Adv Dent Res* 15:4-7, 2001.
10. Thesleff I: Genetic basis of tooth development and dental defects. *Acta Odontol Scand* 58:191-194, 2000.
11. Witkop CJ, Sauk JJ: Defects of enamel. In Stewart R, Prescott G, editors: *Oral facial genetics,* St Louis, 1976, Mosby.
12. Dean JA et al: Dentin dysplasia, type II linkage to chromosome 4q, *J Craniofac Genet Dev Biol* 17:172-177, 1997.
13. Schulze C, Lenz F: Uber Zahnschmelzhypoplasie von unvollstandig dominatem geschlechtgebundenen Erbgang, *Z Mensch Vererb Konstitutionsl* 31:14-114, 1952.
14. Mulvihill JJ: Craniofacial syndromes: no such thing as a single gene disease, *Nat Genet* 9:101-103, 1995.
15. Park WJ, Bellus GA, Jabs EW: Mutations in fibroblast growth factor receptors: phenotypic consequences during eukaryotic development, *Am J Hum Genet* 57:748-754, 1995.
16. Escobar V, Bixler D: On the classification of the acrocephalosyndactyly syndromes, *Clin Genet* 12:169-178, 1977.
17. Everett ET et al: A novel FGFR2 gene mutation in Crouzon syndrome associated with apparent nonpenetrance, *Cleft Palate Craniofac J* 36:533-541, 1999.
18. Smith SM, Penrose LS: Monozygotic dizygotic twin diagnosis, *Ann Hum Genet* 19:289-293, 1955.
19. Kruglyak L, Lander ES: Complete multipoint sib-pair analysis of qualitative and quantitative traits, *Am J Hum Genet* 57:439-454, 1995.
20. Abecasis GR, Cardon LR, Cookson WO: A general test of association for quantitative trait in nuclear families, *Am J Hum Genet* 66:279-292, 2000.
21. Gustafsson BE et al: Vipeholm dental caries study: the effect of different levels of carbohydrate intake on caries activity in 436 individuals observed for 5 years, *Acta Odontol Scand* 11:232, 1954.
22. Klein H, Palmer CE: Studies of dental caries. V. Familial resemblance in caries experience in siblings, *Public Health Rep* 53:1353-1364, 1938.
23. Klein H: The family and dental disease. IV. Dental disease (DMF) experience in parents and offspring, *J Am Dent Assoc* 33:735-743, 1946.
24. Li Y, Caufield PW: The fidelity of initial acquisition of mutans streptococci by infants from their mothers, *J Dent Res* 74:681-685, 1995.
25. Book JA, Grahnen H: Clinical and genetical studies of dental caries. II. Parents and sibs of adult highly resistant (caries-free) proposition, *Odontol Rev* 4:1-53, 1953.
26. Dahlberg G, Dahlberg B: Uber Karies und andere Zahnveranderungen bei Zwillingen, *Uppsala Lakerf Forh* 47:395-416, 1942.
27. Mansbridge JN: Heredity and dental caries, *J Dent Res* 38:337-347, 1959.
28. Horowitz SL, Osborne RH, De George FV: Caries experience in twins, *Science* 128:300-301, 1958.
29. Caldwell RC, Finn SB: Comparisons of the caries experience between identical and fraternal twins and unrelated children, *J Dent Res* 39:693-694, 1960.
30. Shuler CF: Inherited risks for susceptibility to dental caries, *J Dent Educ* 65:1038-1045, 2001.
31. Goodman HO et al: Heritability in dental caries, certain oral microflora and salivary components, *Am J Hum Genet* 11:263-273, 1959.
32. Hunt HR, Hoppert CA, Rosen S: Genetic factors in experimental rat caries. In Sognnaes RF, editor: *Advances in experimental caries research,* Washington, DC, 1955, American Associates for the Advancement of Science.
33. Mayhall CW: Concerning the composition and source of the acquired enamel pellicle of human teeth, *Arch Oral Biol* 15:1327-1341, 1970.
34. Bennick A et al: The role of human salivary acidic proline-rich proteins in the formation of acquired dental pellicle in vivo and their fate after absorption to the human enamel surface, *Arch Oral Biol* 28:19-27, 1983.
35. Goodman PA et al: The human salivary protein complex (SPC): a large block of related genes, *Am J Hum Genet* 37:785-797, 1985.
36. Mamula PW et al: Localization of the human salivary protein complex (SPC) to chromosome band 12p13.2, *Cytogenet Cell Genet* 39:279-284, 1985.
37. Yu PL et al: Human parotid proline rich proteins: correlation of genetic polymorphisms to dental caries, *Genet Epidemiol* 3:147-152, 1986.

38. Ciancio SC, Hazen P, Curat JJ: Periodontal observations in twins, *J Periodontal Res* 4:42-45, 1969.

39. Michalowicz BS et al: Periodontal findings in adult twins, *J Periodontol* 62:293-299, 1991.

40. Kornman KS et al: The interleukin-1 genotype as a severity factor in adult periodontal disease, *J Clin Periodontol* 24: 72-77, 1997.

41. Greenstein G, Hart TC: Clinical utility of a genetic susceptibility test for severe chronic periodontitis: a critical evaluation, *J Am Dent Assoc* 133:452-459, 2002.

42. Schenkein HA: Inheritance as a determinant of susceptibility for periodontitis, *J Dent Educ* 62:840-851, 1998.

43. Etzioni A, Tonetti M: Leukocyte adhesion deficiency II—from A to almost Z, *Immunol Rev* 178:138-147, 2000.

44. Arnaout MA et al: Point mutations impairing cell surface expression of the common beta subunit (CD18) in a patient with leukocyte adhesion molecule (Leu-CAM) deficiency, *J Clin Invest* 85:977-981, 1990.

45. Meyle J, Gonzáles JR. Influences of systemic diseases on periodontitis in children and adolescents, *Periodontol 2000* 26:92-112, 2001.

46. Hartsfield JK Jr: Premature exfoliation of teeth in childhood and adolescence, *Adv Pediatr* 41:453-470, 1994.

47. Hartsfield JK Jr, Kousseff BG: Phenotypic overlap of Ehlers-Danlos syndrome types IV and VIII, *Am J Med Genet* 37: 465-470, 1990.

48. Nagle DL et al: Identification and mutation analysis of the complete gene for Chédiak-Higashi syndrome, *Nat Genet* 14:307-311, 1996.

49. Hart TC et al: Genetic studies of syndromes with severe periodontitis and palmoplantar hyperkeratosis, *J Periodontal Res* 32:81-89, 1997.

50. Hart TC et al: Haim-Munk syndrome and Papillon-Lefèvre syndrome are allelic mutations in cathepsin C, *J Med Genet* 37:88-94, 2000.

51. Benjamin SD, Baer PM: Familial patterns of advanced alveolar bone loss in adolescence (periodontosis), *J Am Soc Psychosom Dent Med* 5:82-88, 1967.

52. Melnick M, Shields ED, Bixler D: Periodontosis: a phenotypic and genetic analysis, *Oral Surg* 42:32-41, 1976.

53. Hart TC et al: Re-interpretation of the evidence for X-linked dominant inheritance of juvenile periodontitis, *J Periodontol* 63:169-172, 1992.

54. Saxen L: Heredity of juvenile periodontitis, *J Clin Periodontol* 7:276-288, 1989.

55. Boughman JA et al: An autosomal-dominant form of juvenile periodontitis: its localization to chromosome 4 and linkage to dentinogenesis imperfecta and GC, *J Craniofac Genet Dev Biol* 6:341-350, 1986.

56. Hart TC et al: Reevaluation of the chromosome 4q candidate region for early onset periodontitis, *Hum Genet* 91:416-422, 1993.

57. Diehl SR et al: Linkage disequilibrium of interleukin-1 genetic polymorphisms with early-onset periodontitis, *J Periodontol* 70:418-430, 1999.

58. Yamaguchi T, Maki K, Shibasaki Y: Growth hormone receptor gene variant and mandibular height in the normal Japanese population, *Am J Orthod Dentofacial Orthop* 119:650-653, 2001.

59. Proffit WR: *Contemporary orthodontics*, ed 3, St Louis, 1999, Mosby.

60. Stockard CR et al: The genetic and endocrine basis for differences in form and behavior, *Am Anat Memoirs* 19, 1941.

61. Lundstrom A: *Tooth size and occlusion in twins*, Stockholm, 1948, AB Fahlcrantz Boktryckeri.

62. Kraus BS, Wise WJ, Frei RA: Heredity and the craniofacial complex, *Am J Orthod* 45:172-217, 1959.

63. Litton SF et al: A genetic study of Class III malocclusion, *Am J Orthod* 58:565-577, 1970.

64. Harris JE: Genetic factors in the growth of the head: inheritance of the craniofacial complex and malocclusion, *Dent Clin North Am* 19(1):151-160, 1975.

65. King L, Harris EF, Tolley EA: Heritability of cephalometric and occlusal variables as assessed from siblings with overt malocclusions, *Am J Orthod Dentofacial Orthop* 104: 121-131, 1993.

66. Hartsfield JK Jr: Development of the vertical dimension: nature and nurture, *Semin Orthod* 8:113-119, 2002.

67. Harris EF, Butler ML: Patterns of incisor root resorption before and after orthodontic correction in cases with anterior open bites, *Am J Orthod Dentofacial Orthop* 101:112-119, 1992.

68. Harris EF, Robinson QC, Woods MA: An analysis of causes of apical root resorption in patients not treated orthodontically, *Quintessence Int* 24:417-428, 1993.

69. Taithongchai R, Sookkorn K, Killiany DM: Facial and dentoalveolar structure and the prediction of apical root shortening, *Am J Orthod Dentofacial Orthop* 110:296-302, 1996.

70. Killiany DM: Root resorption caused by orthodontic treatment: an evidence-based review of literature, *Semin Orthod* 5:128-133, 1999.

71. Vlaskalic V, Boyd RL, Baumrind S: Etiology and sequelae of root resorption, *Semin Orthod* 4:124-131, 1998.

72. Sameshima GT, Asgarifar KO: Assessment of root resorption and root shape: periapical vs. panoramic films, *Angle Orthod* 71:185-189, 2001.

73. Al-Qawasmi RA et al: Genetic predisposition to external apical root resorption in orthodontic patients: linkage and association of the interleukin 1B gene, *Am J Orthod Dentofacial Orthop* 123:242-252, 2003.

74. Al-Qawasmi RA et al: Genetic predisposition to external apical root resorption in orthodontic patients: linkage of chromosome-18 marker, *J Dent Res* 82:356-360, 2003.

75. Shields ED, Bixler D, Fogh-Andersen P: Facial clefts in Danish twins, *Cleft Palate J* 16:1-6, 1979.

76. Fogh-Andersen P: *Incidence of harelip and cleft palate*, Copenhagen, 1942, Nyt Nordisk Forlag.

77. Metrakos JD, Metrakos K, Baxter H: Clefts of the lip and palate in twins, including a discordant pair whose monozygosity was confirmed by skin transplants, *Plast Reconstr Surg* 22:109-122, 1958.

78. Ward RE, Moore ES, Hartsfield JK Jr: Morphometric characteristics of subjects with oral facial clefts and their relatives. In Wyszynski DF, editor: *Cleft lip and palate from origin to treatment*, New York, 2002, Oxford University Press.

79. Curtis EJ, Walker NF: *Etiological study of cleft lip and cleft palate*, Toronto, 1961, The Research Institute of the Hospital for Sick Children, University of Toronto.

80. Curtis EJ, Fraser FC, Warburton D: Congenital cleft lip and palate, *Am J Dis Child* 102:853-857, 1961.

COMMON DISTURBANCES IN CHILDREN
ALVEOLAR ABSCESS
CELLULITIS
DEVELOPMENTAL ANOMALIES OF THE TEETH
Odontoma
Fusion of the Teeth
Germination
Dens in Dente (Dens Invaginatus)
EARLY EXFOLIATION OF TEETH
Hypophosphatasia
Cherubism (Familial Fibrous Dysplasia)
Acrodynia
Hypophosphatemia (Familial or X-linked
Hypophosphatemic Rickets or Vitamin
D–Resistant Rickets)
Cyclic Neutropenia (Cyclic Hematopoiesis)
Other Disorders
ENAMEL HYPOPLASIA
Hypoplasia Resulting from Nutritional Deficiencies
Hypoplasia Related to Brain Injury and Neurologic
Defects
Hypoplasia Associated with Nephrotic Syndrome
Hypoplasia Associated with Allergies
Hypoplasia Associated with Lead Poisoning
(Plumbism)
Hypoplasia Caused by Local Infection and Trauma
Hypoplasia Associated with Cleft Lip and Palate
Hypoplasia Caused by X-Radiation and
Chemotherapy
Hypoplasia Resulting from Rubella Embryopathy
Treatment of Hypoplastic Teeth
Hypoplasia Caused by Fluoride (Dental Fluorosis)
Enamel Microabrasion to Remove Superficial
Enamel Discolorations
PREERUPTIVE "CARIES" (PREERUPTIVE CORONAL
RESORPTION OR PREERUPTIVE INTRACORONAL
RADIOLUCENCY)

TAURODONTISM
INHERITED DENTIN DEFECTS
Dentinogenesis Imperfecta (Hereditary Opalescent
Dentin)
Dentin Dysplasia
AMELOGENESIS IMPERFECTA
ENAMEL AND DENTIN APLASIA
AGENESIS OF TEETH
Anodontia
Hypodontia (Oligodontia)
Ectodermal Dysplasias
INTRINSIC DISCOLORATION OF TEETH
(PIGMENTATION OF TEETH)
Discoloration in Hyperbilirubinemia
Discoloration in Porphyria
Discoloration in Cystic Fibrosis
Discoloration in Tetracycline Therapy
Bleaching of Intrinsic Tooth Discoloration
MICROGNATHIA
ANOMALIES OF THE TONGUE
Macroglossia
Ankyloglossia (Tongue-Tie)
Fissured Tongue and Geographic Tongue (Benign
Migratory Glossitis)
Coated Tongue
White Strawberry Tongue
Black Hairy Tongue
Indentation of the Tongue Margin (Crenation)
Median Rhomboid Glossitis (Central Papillary
Atrophy of the Tongue)
Trauma to the Tongue with Emphasis on Tongue
Piercing
ABNORMAL LABIAL FRENUM
Frenectomy

COMMON DISTURBANCES IN CHILDREN

Dental care services have become more readily available to children, and caries prevention programs have become more effective. There has been a steady decline in the incidence and prevalence of dental caries in permanent teeth among U.S. children (see Chapter 10). However, according to the first-ever Surgeon General's report on oral health in America published in May 2000, dental caries is the single most common chronic childhood disease.[1] Periodontal disturbances are also common. Although severe forms of periodontal disease are rare in children, all experience at least mild gingivitis on occasion. Both caries and periodontal disease are, for the most part, acquired and preventable disturbances of the teeth and jaws. Other chapters of this book are devoted to a more in-depth discussion of the cause, prevention, and management of dental caries (see Chapters 10, 17, 18, and 19) and periodontal disturbances (see Chapters 11 and 20). Injuries to the teeth and supporting tissues represent another large category of acquired disturbances (see Chapter 21).

Many children have orthodontic conditions that justify corrective treatment, and for some of them the condition is serious enough to be categorized as deforming or crippling. Approximately 1 in 1000 children in the United States is born with a cleft lip or palate. These conditions are primarily developmental disturbances and are discussed in greater detail in Chapters 6 and 25 to 28.

ALVEOLAR ABSCESS

During the examination procedure the dentist may observe evidence of an acute or chronic alveolar abscess. An alveolar abscess associated with the pulpless permanent tooth is usually a specific lesion localized by a fibrous capsule produced by fibroblasts that differentiate from the periodontal membrane. The primary tooth abscess is usually evident as a more diffuse infection, and the surrounding tissue is less able to wall off the process. The virulence of the microorganisms and the ability of the tissues to react to the infection probably determine whether the infection will be acute or chronic.

In the early stages the acute alveolar abscess can be diagnosed based on radiographic evidence of a thickened periodontal membrane. The tooth is sensitive to percussion and movement, and the patient may have a slight fever. The acute symptoms of an alveolar abscess can be relieved by using antibiotic therapy. Relief of the symptoms is more efficient if drainage is also established (Fig. 7-1). Drainage may be established through the pulp chamber of the tooth and/or the associated gingiva or by extraction of the tooth. If extraction is

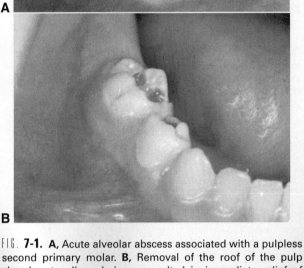

FIG. 7-1. A, Acute alveolar abscess associated with a pulpless second primary molar. **B,** Removal of the roof of the pulp chamber to allow drainage resulted in immediate relief of pain. After the swelling has been reduced, one can decide whether the tooth is to be treated or extracted.

selected as the best choice of treatment at the emergency appointment and the patient has an unremarkable medical history, concomitant antibiotic therapy is not always necessary. During this acute infection phase, however, it may be impossible to establish effective pain control for the extraction procedure with conventional out-patient techniques.

If establishing drainage through the pulp chamber is selected as part of the emergency treatment, a large opening should be made into the pulp chamber to permit drainage of the exudate. After initial débridement and rinsing, the opening to the chamber may be closed unless drainage persists to ooze indefinitely. Should pain occur during the excavation of tooth structure to establish drainage, the discomfort can be lessened if the tooth is stabilized by the dentist's fingers.

Warm saline mouth rinses often aid in localizing the infection and maintaining adequate drainage before endodontic treatment or extraction.

Chronic alveolar abscess, characterized by less soreness, is often a better-defined radiographic lesion. The patient will likely have some lymphadenopathy as well.

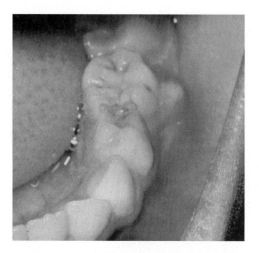

FIG. **7-2.** Chronic alveolar abscess associated with a pulpless second primary molar that is also a candidate for incision and drainage, in addition to removal of the roof of the pulp chamber to initiate root canal therapy if the tooth is to be saved.

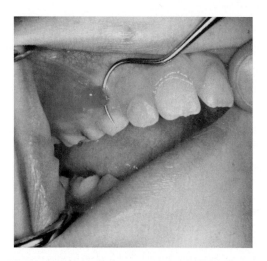

FIG. **7-3.** A pedunculated granulomatous lesion overlying the canine but associated with a chronic draining alveolar abscess of the maxillary right first primary molar.

Draining fistulas are also frequently associated with chronic alveolar abscesses. Usually, antibiotic therapy is unnecessary except in patients with an overriding systemic problem (e.g., patients susceptible to subacute bacterial endocarditis, patients with organ transplants, or those who are immunodeficient). Again, drainage and sterilization of the infected local area are necessary through root canal therapy for the involved tooth or through extraction. If the lesion has only recently passed the acute stage, there may be a pointing soft tissue abscess. In this situation, incising and draining the soft tissue may be indicated in addition to opening the tooth, especially if the tooth is to be treated endodontically (Fig. 7-2). If the lesion is in an advanced

chronic stage, drainage may already be established as a natural reaction (Fig. 7-3).

CELLULITIS

Cellulitis is a diffuse type of infection of the soft tissues that may be caused by a pulpless primary or permanent tooth. It often causes considerable swelling of the face or neck, and the tissue appears discolored.

Cellulitis is a very serious infection. It can be life-threatening and is a potential complication of all acute dental infections. It is usually a result of severe untreated caries in patients who do not receive regular dental care or who may have had dental care only for treatment of dental emergencies. It is not unusual for the parents to take the child with dental cellulitis to the hospital emergency department. The child appears acutely ill and may have an alarmingly high temperature with malaise and lethargy.

If a maxillary tooth is the problem, the swelling and redness may involve the eye (Fig. 7-4, *A*). If cellulitis is treated too late, serious complications, such as involvement of the central nervous system or a cavernous sinus thrombosis, could occur. If cellulitis results from an infected mandibular tooth, the diffuse swelling and infection will spread to the floor of the mouth along fascial planes, nerves, and vessels. If the infection involves the submandibular, sublingual, and submental spaces, it is called *Ludwig angina*. In this condition the tongue and floor of the mouth become elevated to the extent that the patient's airway is obstructed and swallowing is impossible.

The establishment of drainage, if possible, by opening the pulp chamber of the affected tooth is helpful in reducing the acute symptoms of cellulitis. However, the child may have difficulty opening the mouth to permit the procedure. Incision of soft tissue to establish drainage is not indicated in the early stages of cellulitis because of the diffuse, nonlocalized nature of the infection.

The offending organisms in cellulitis from dental infections are usually capable of producing hyaluronidase and fibrinolysins. These agents break down the intercellular cementing substance (hyaluronic acid) and fibrin, which permits the rapid spread of the infection. One of the broad-spectrum antibiotics should be prescribed early to reduce the possibility of the infection localizing and draining on the outer surface of the face (Fig. 7-4, *B*). It should be emphasized to the parents or patient that antibiotics will not heal the condition completely and that follow-up treatment of the tooth is essential.

If the infection is already severe when the parent or patient seeks treatment, a blood culture or a culture of exudate may be performed to identify the infecting organisms. Then, if the infection does not respond to the initial antibiotic therapy, a second, more appropriate

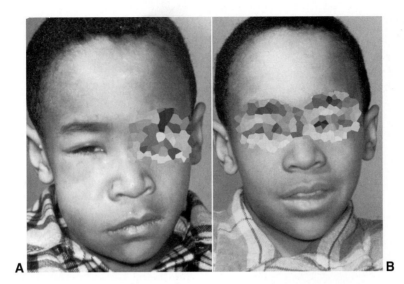

FIG. **7-4. A**, Patient appears to be acutely ill because of an infected permanent molar and resultant cellulitis. **B**, Use of broad-spectrum antibiotics reduced the acute symptoms of the disease and prevented extraoral drainage.

antibiotic may be selected after the causative organisms have been identified. Molinari has emphasized the continuing emergence of antibiotic-resistant bacterial strains that renders many common antimicrobial agents ineffective.[2]

The child with cellulitis should be hospitalized if the clinical signs or symptoms warrant very close monitoring or if there is any question as to whether the parents or patient will follow through with the prescribed treatment. Hospitalization is recommended especially in the case of Ludwig angina, since maintenance of a patent airway may require the assistance of medical personnel. In these severe cases, parenteral administration of antibiotics is also recommended, at least initially.

DEVELOPMENTAL ANOMALIES OF THE TEETH

ODONTOMA

The abnormal proliferation of cells of the enamel organ may result in an odontogenic tumor, commonly referred to as an *odontoma*. An odontoma may form as a result of continued budding of the primary or permanent tooth germ or as a result of an abnormal proliferation of the cells of the tooth germ, in which case an odontoma replaces the normal tooth (Figs. 7-5 and 7-6). The anomaly is discussed in detail in Chapter 8. An odontoma should be surgically removed before it can interfere with eruption of teeth in the area. The presence of an odontoma should alert the practitioner to inquire about the concurrent presence of dysphagia or a family history of dysphagia that is perhaps due to hypertrophy of the smooth muscles of the esophagus as a part of the rare autosomal dominant odontoma-dysphagia syndrome.[3]

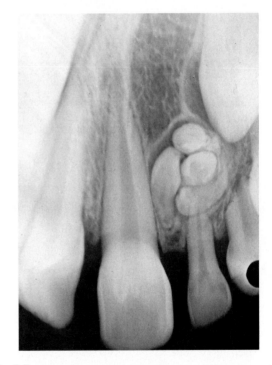

FIG. **7-5.** Compound composite odontoma. The anomalous structure consists of small structures resembling teeth.

FUSION OF THE TEETH

Fusion represents the union of two independently developing primary or permanent teeth. The condition is almost always limited to the anterior teeth and, like gemination (see the following discussion), may show a familial tendency.

The radiograph may show that the fusion is limited to the crowns and roots. Fused teeth will have separate

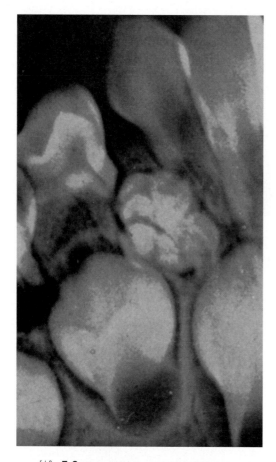

FIG. **7-6.** Complex composite odontoma.

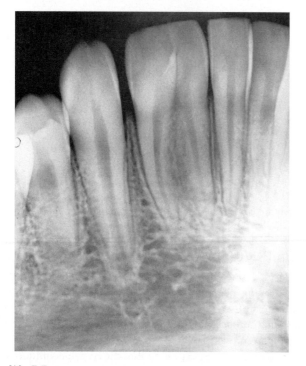

FIG. **7-7.** Fusion of a permanent central and lateral incisor.

pulp chambers and separate pulp canals (Fig. 7-7). Dental caries may develop in the line of fusion of the crowns, necessitating the placement of a restoration. A frequent finding in fusion of primary teeth is the congenital absence of one of the corresponding permanent teeth.

Delaney and Goldblatt reported an interesting case that illustrates the multidisciplinary approach that may be indicated in the clinical management of certain problems associated with fused teeth.[4] The disciplines of pediatric dentistry, endodontics, surgery, restorative dentistry, and orthodontics were represented in the initial management of the case, and a post and core and a crown restoration were anticipated for the future. Yet excellent results were obtained in only 6 months with an organized approach to a complex problem that involved the fusion of a supernumerary tooth to a maxillary central incisor, severe crowding, and a palatally displaced lateral incisor. One root of the fused teeth was treated endodontically. The fused teeth were then hemisectioned, and the endodontically treated tooth was restored while the separated tooth was sacrificed. Orthodontic repositioning of the palatally displaced lateral incisor and alignment of the anterior segment concluded the management of the problem. A case of bilateral fusion of primary incisors has also been reported by Eidelman.[5]

The presence of a single primary and permanent maxillary central incisor may at first appear to be a product of fusion. However, if the single tooth is in the midline, and symmetric with normal crown and root shape and size, then it may be an isolated finding or may be part of the solitary median maxillary central incisor syndrome. This is a heterogeneous condition that may include other midline developmental abnormalities of the brain and other structures that can be due to mutation in the sonic hedgehog (*SHH*) gene, *SIX3* gene, or other genetic abnormality.[6] The development of only one maxillary central incisor is an indication for further evaluation for other anomalies.

GEMINATION

A geminated tooth represents an attempted division of a single tooth germ by invagination occurring during the proliferation stage of the growth cycle of the tooth. The geminated tooth appears clinically as a bifid crown on a single root (Fig. 7-8). The crown is usually wider than normal, with a shallow groove extending from the incisal edge to the cervical region. The anomaly, which may follow a hereditary pattern of occurrence, is seen in both primary and permanent teeth, though it probably appears more frequently in primary teeth.

The treatment of a permanent anterior geminated tooth may involve reduction of the mesiodistal width of

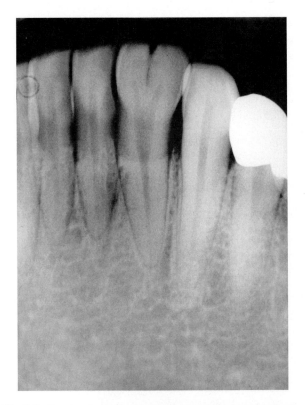

FIG. **7-8.** Gemination of a mandibular lateral incisor. The crown has a groove on the labial surface and is wider than normal.

the tooth to allow normal development of the occlusion. Periodic disking of the tooth is recommended when the crown is not excessively large, as is eventual preparation of the tooth for restoration if dentin is exposed. Secondary dentin formation and pulpal recession will follow judicial periodic reduction of crown size. Devitalization of the tooth and root canal therapy followed by the construction of a postcrown may be needed when the geminated tooth is large and malformed.

DENS IN DENTE (DENS INVAGINATUS)

The diagnosis of dens in dente (tooth within a tooth) can be verified by a radiograph. The developmental anomaly has been described as a lingual invagination of the enamel. This condition can occur in primary and permanent teeth. Unusual cases of dens invaginatus have been reported in a mandibular primary canine,[7] a maxillary primary central incisor,[8] and a mandibular second primary molar.[9] Dens in dente is most often seen in the permanent maxillary lateral incisors. The condition should be suspected whenever deep lingual pits are observed in maxillary permanent lateral incisors. Grahnen, Lindahl, and Omnell found in a study of 58 families that a similar anomaly was present in more than one third of the parents of children with dens in dente.[10] Within the same family some had dens in dente

and others had deep lingual pits, which indicates that the condition may be inherited as an autosomal dominant trait with variable expressivity and possibly incomplete penetrance (see Chapter 6 for definitions).

Anterior teeth with dens in dente are usually of normal shape and size. In other areas of the mouth, however, the tooth can have an anomalous appearance. A dens in dente is characterized by an invagination lined with enamel and the presence of a foramen cecum with the probability of a communication between the cavity of the invagination and the pulp chamber (Fig. 7-9).

Application of sealant or a restoration in the opening of the invagination is the recommended treatment to prevent pulpal involvement. If the condition is detected before complete eruption of the tooth, the removal of gingival tissue to facilitate cavity preparation and restoration may be indicated.

The advisability of performing endodontic procedures on such a tooth with pulpal degeneration depends on its pulp morphology and the restorability of the crown (Fig. 7-10).

EARLY EXFOLIATION OF TEETH

Variations in the time of eruption of the primary teeth and in the time of exfoliation are frequently observed in pediatric patients. A variation of as much as 18 months in the exfoliation time of primary teeth may be considered normal. However, this pattern must be consistent with other aspects of the dental development. Exfoliation of teeth in the absence of trauma in children younger than 5 years of age merits special attention because it can be related to pathologic conditions of local and systemic origin.

The early exfoliation of primary teeth resulting from periodontitis has been observed occasionally in young children, and this is discussed in Chapters 6 and 20. Along with hypophosphatasia, prepubertal periodontitis appears to be the most common cause of premature exfoliation of the primary teeth, especially in girls.

HYPOPHOSPHATASIA

The clinical dental finding diagnostic of hypophosphatasia in children is premature exfoliation of the anterior primary teeth associated with deficient cementum. The loss of teeth in the young child may be spontaneous or may result from a slight trauma. Severe gingival inflammation will be absent. The loss of alveolar bone may be limited to the anterior region. The disease is characterized by improper mineralization of bone caused by deficient alkaline phosphatase activity in serum, liver, bone, and kidney (tissue nonspecific). Increased levels of urinary phosphoethanolamine are also seen.

Ongoing study into the etiology of hypophosphatasia indicates that the usually lethal autosomal recessive

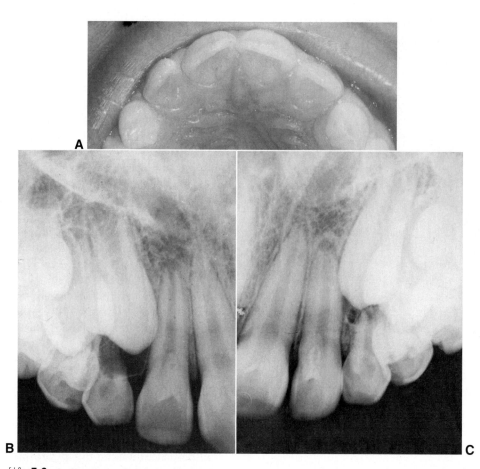

FIG. **7-9. A,** Small, "nonsticky" pits on the lingual surfaces of the maxillary lateral incisors are the only clues to the dens in dente condition of the teeth revealed radiographically in **B** and **C.**

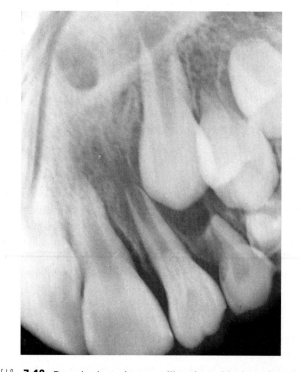

FIG. **7-10.** Dens in dente in a maxillary lateral incisor. A communication between the invagination and the pulp chamber apparently caused necrosis of the pulp.

infantile type (I), as well as the usually autosomal recessive milder juvenile type (II) and the autosomal dominant adult type (III), are due to different mutations and heterozygosity versus homozygosity in the tissue-nonspecific alkaline phosphatase *(TNSALP* or *ALPL)* gene. Hu et al state that, as a general rule, the earlier the appearance of the disease the greater the severity.[11] Early exfoliation of the primary teeth is usually associated with the juvenile type (II), although such a history may also be present in the adult type (III).[11] Diagnostic tests should include the determination of serum alkaline phosphatase levels for parents and siblings.

Pseudohypophosphatasia, first described by Scriver and Cameron, is a rare disorder in which the child has the phenotype of juvenile hypophosphatasia and elevated levels of urinary phosphoethanolamine but plasma alkaline phosphatase activity is normal.[12] However, the clinical findings are similar to those of juvenile hypophosphatasia.

CHERUBISM (FAMILIAL FIBROUS DYSPLASIA)

Cherubism is a rare childhood disease affecting jaw development. Cherubism is usually inherited as an autosomal dominant trait with somewhat reduced penetrance in females. The expression may be so variable that a clinically normal-appearing parent may have a history of prominent facial swellings or radiographic evidence of abnormal bone pattern in the mandible. Although disease progression is expected to stabilize or even regress after puberty, a few very aggressive cases, sometimes producing morbid results, have been reported.[13-16] At least four cases of nonfamilial cherubism have been reported, which suggests occasional sporadic occurrences from spontaneous mutations.[17-19]

Two independent groups of investigators[20,21] have demonstrated that the gene for cherubism maps to chromosome 4p16. Follow-up work by Ueki et al found that mutations in the gene encoding c-Abl–binding protein SH3BP2 on chromosome 4p16.3 causes cherubism.[22] They found several different *SH3BP2* gene mutations in patients with cherubism, which probably resulted in a gain of function or dominant-negative effect, although some other gene(s) may also cause cherubism in other patients. They postulated that the onset of cherubism and its anatomically circumscribed characteristics may be related to dental developmental processes in children, when signals unique to the mandible and maxilla are transmitted through the extracellular matrix, triggered by the eruption of secondary teeth.

A symmetric or asymmetric enlargement of the jaws may be noted at an early age. Numerous sharp, well-defined multilocular areas of bone destruction and thinning of the cortical plate are evident in the radiograph (Fig. 7-11). Teeth in the involved area are frequently exfoliated prematurely as a result of the loss of support or root resorption or, in permanent teeth, as a result of an interference in the development of roots. Spontaneous loss of the teeth may occur, or the child may pick the teeth out of the soft tissue.

McDonald and Shafer reported a case in which the mandible and maxilla of a 5-year-old girl were symmetrically enlarged.[23] Radiographs showed multilocular cystic involvement of both mandible and maxilla. A complete skeletal survey failed to reveal similar lesions in other bones. Microscopic examination of a segment of bone showed a large number of multinucleated giant cells scattered diffusely throughout a cellular stroma. The giant cells were large and irregular in shape and contained 30 to 40 nuclei. During a 10-year observation period the bony lesions had not progressed appreciably.

The patient illustrated in Fig. 7-11 was followed into adulthood, and her mouth was restored in a very satisfactory manner. A comparison of the full-face photographs in Fig. 7-11 (*A* and *I*) illustrates that, as the face increases in height, the "cherubic" appearance caused by the bilateral bulging of the bone of the mandible is less apparent. Seven permanent teeth in the upper and lower arches were retained and prepared for Baker

attachments. Complete dentures were constructed to restore function and improve appearance.

Pierce et al have reported their dental management of a mother and two daughters with inherited craniofacial fibrous dysplasia over a 15-year period.[24] The daughters exhibited clinical and radiographic appearances similar to that of the patient just described, but the authors consider fibrous dysplasia and cherubism to be separate entities. Their treatment of the daughters, though more aggressive, resulted in nearly complete dentitions. Treatment included surgical autotransplantation of several teeth and bony recontouring. Orthodontic therapy was also provided for one child. Orthodontics was recommended for the other child but was declined; her dental alignment was acceptable 3 years after surgery.

Peters has reported a study of 20 cases of cherubism in one family that confirmed an autosomal dominant pattern of inheritance.[25] The author preferred a conservative approach in managing the giant cell lesions, because they tend to resolve with maturity. Von Wowern has published an extensive review of the literature and a 36-year follow-up of families with cherubism.[26]

ACRODYNIA

The exposure of young children to minute amounts of mercury is responsible for a condition referred to as *acrodynia* or *pink disease*. Ointments and medications are the usual sources of the mercury. Weinstein and Bernstein recently reported on 20-month-old twin girls who presented to a hospital with the classic signs and symptoms of acrodynia.[27] Further investigation revealed that the girls had been receiving once- or twice-weekly doses of a mercury-containing teething powder during the preceding 4 months. Apparently such preparations are still available in some countries. Horowitz et al report on two young brothers diagnosed with acrodynia after playing repeatedly with a broken sphygmomanometer.[28] Dental amalgam restorations do not cause acrodynia.

The clinical features of the disease include fever, anorexia, desquamation of the soles and palms (causing them to be pink), sweating, tachycardia, gastrointestinal disturbance, and hypotonia. The oral findings include inflammation and ulceration of the mucous membrane, excessive salivation, loss of alveolar bone, and premature exfoliation of teeth.

HYPOPHOSPHATEMIA (FAMILIAL OR X-LINKED HYPOPHOSPHATEMIC RICKETS OR VITAMIN D–RESISTANT RICKETS)

As reported by Hartsfield, hypophosphatemia is the most common inherited abnormality of renal tubular transport.[29] Clinical features become evident in the second year of life. They include short stature and

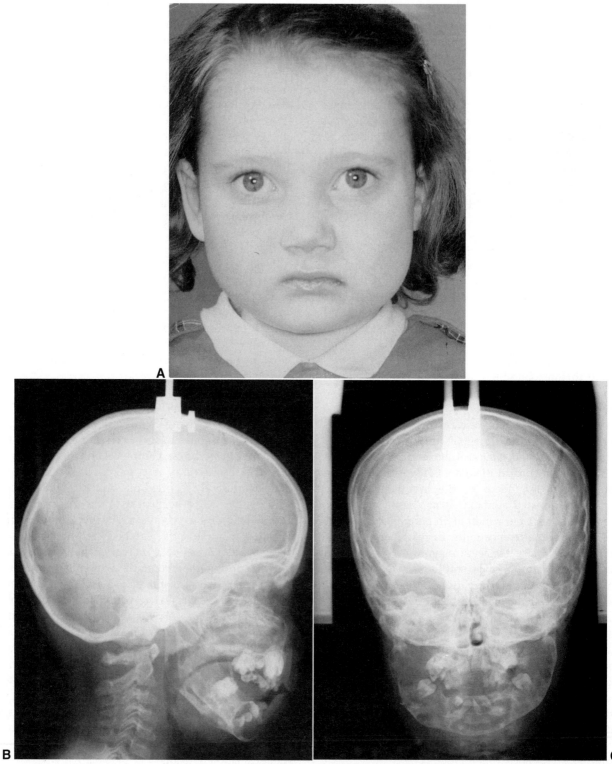

FIG. **7-11.** **A,** Enlargement of the cheeks caused by bilateral bulging of the bone of the mandible. **B** and **C,** lateral and anteroposterior cephalometric radiographs. Notice the displacement of the mandibular anterior teeth in a large area of bone destruction, the locular cystic involvement of the mandible and maxillae, and the number of missing teeth.

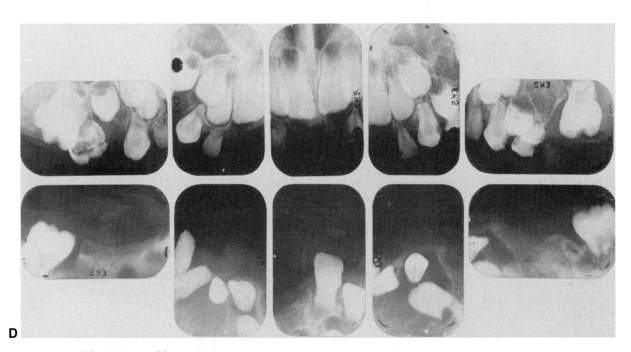

D

FIG. **7-11, cont'd D,** Full-mouth radiographs demonstrating large areas of bone destruction and several missing teeth.
Continued

bowing of the lower extremities in affected boys. Premature tooth exfoliation is sometimes also a feature. The inheritance pattern of the disease is usually X-linked dominant, and the disorder is twice as common in females as in males. The HYP Consortium of investigators found mutations in the *PHEX* (also called *PEX*) gene on the X chromosome in patients with this condition.[30]

Other dental manifestations often include apical radiolucencies, abscesses, and fistulas associated with pulp exposures in the primary and permanent teeth. The pulp exposures relate to the pulp horns extending to the dentinoenamel junction or even to the external surface of the tooth. The thin, hypomineralized enamel is abraded easily, which exposes the pulp. Dental radiographs show rickety bone trabeculations and absent or abnormal lamina dura.

McWhorter and Seale found that 25% of their patients diagnosed with vitamin D–resistant rickets (VDRR) were affected with abscesses in primary teeth.[31] The results of their study indicated that the presence of one abscess is a predictor of future abscesses in the same patient. The authors suggested that early prophylactic treatment of all posterior primary teeth with pulpotomies and crown placement may be the most conservative therapy for a VDRR patient who develops a spontaneous abscess. However, a follow-up retrospective study by Shroff, McWhorter, and Seale found the success rate for prophylactic pulpotomies in these patients to be only 44%.[32] They concluded that prophylactic pulpotomy therapy cannot be recommended for patients with VDRR based on the currently available data. They also suggested that a more aggressive approach using prophylactic pulpectomy as previously advocated by Rakocz, Keating, and Johnson may be indicated in these patients and encouraged further investigation in this area.[33]

CYCLIC NEUTROPENIA (CYCLIC HEMATOPOIESIS)

Cyclic neutropenia is an autosomal dominant condition in which affected individuals are at risk for opportunistic infection during intervals of neutropenia that occur in a 21-day cycle concomitant with oscillation in bone marrow blood cell production. Levels of monocytes, platelets, lymphocytes, and reticulocytes also cycle with the same frequency. Horwitz et al found several different single-base substitutions in the *ELA2* gene encoding neutrophil elastase (also known as leukocyte elastase, elastase 2, and medullasin) in affected individuals, and hypothesized that a perturbed interaction between neutrophil elastase and serpins or other substrates may regulate mechanisms governing the clocklike timing of hematopoiesis.[34]

The condition occurs at any age. Numerous cases in children have been reported. The patients manifest a fever, malaise, sore throat, stomatitis, and regional lymphadenopathy, as well as headache, cutaneous infection, and conjunctivitis. Children exhibit a severe gingivitis with ulceration. With a return of the neutrophil count to normal, the gingiva may return to a nearly normal clinical appearance. Children experiencing repeated insults from the condition have a

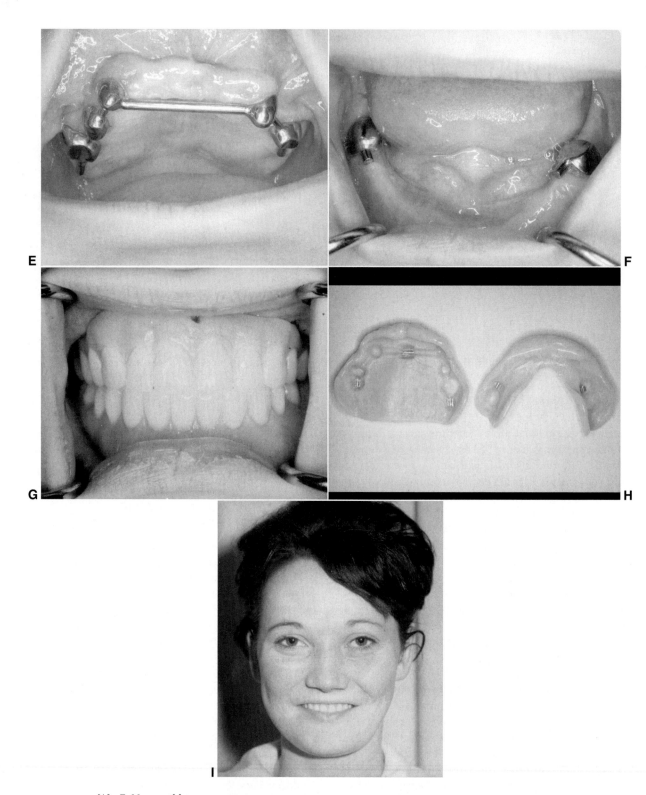

FIG. **7-11, cont'd E,** to **H,** When the patient was 18 years of age, the permanent teeth that had good support were prepared for Baker attachments, and complete dentures were constructed. **I,** The restored mouth and improved appearance of the adult. *(E to H courtesy Dr. Donald Cunningham.)*

considerable loss of supporting bone around the teeth. A case report by da Fonseca and Fontes describes a young woman who had suffered from poor oral health throughout her lifetime, and as she approached 21 years of age, all her remaining permanent teeth were finally removed.[35] Soon after the extractions the patient's blood counts improved to a level not previously seen by her hematologist.

OTHER DISORDERS

Premature exfoliation or marked mobility of teeth in childhood or adolescence has been associated in some cases with other systemic disorders, including acatalasia, Chédiak-Higashi syndrome, Coffin-Lowry syndrome, Down syndrome, Ehlers-Danlos syndrome types IV and VIII, Hajdu-Cheney syndrome, hyperpituitarism, hyperthyroidism, juvenile diabetes, Papillon-Lefèvre syndrome, progeria, Singleton-Merten syndrome, and some malignant diseases such as the histiocytosis X groups (see Chapter 8) and the leukemias (see Chapter 24).

ENAMEL HYPOPLASIA

Amelogenesis occurs in two stages. In the first stage, the enamel matrix forms, and in the second stage, the matrix undergoes calcification. Local or systemic factors that interfere with normal matrix formation cause enamel surface defects and irregularities called *enamel hypoplasia*. Factors that interfere with calcification and maturation of the enamel produce a condition termed *enamel hypocalcification*.

Enamel hypoplasia may be mild and may result in a pitting of the enamel surface or in the development of a horizontal line across the enamel of the crown. If ameloblastic activity has been disrupted for a long period, gross areas of irregular or imperfect enamel formation occur. Enamel hypoplasia is often seen as one component of many different syndromes.

Postnatal hypoplasia of the primary teeth is probably as common as hypoplasia of the permanent teeth, although the former usually does not occur in as severe a form. Hypoplasia of the primary enamel that forms before birth is rare, however (Fig. 7-12). In its mildest form, a prenatal disturbance is reflected as an accentuated neonatal ring in the primary tooth. In the severe type of neonatal disturbance, enamel formation is sometimes arrested at birth or during the neonatal period (Fig. 7-13). Postnatal amelogenesis is confined to the portion of the crown located cervically from the enamel area present at birth (Fig. 7-14).

Seow et al have observed that enamel hypoplasia of the primary teeth is common in prematurely born, very-low-birth-weight children; its pathogenesis is not understood clearly.[36] One likely mechanism is related to mineral deficiency, which may be diagnosed

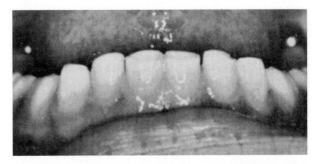

FIG. **7-12.** Prenatal enamel hypoplasia. The medical history revealed that the patient suffered from cerebral palsy as a result of premature birth (gestation, 6 months; birth weight, 2 lb, 5 oz). *(Courtesy Dr. Stanley C. Herman.)*

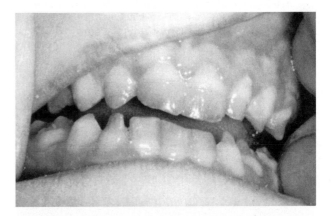

FIG. **7-13.** Neonatal enamel hypoplasia. Only the most cervical parts of the intrinsically stained areas are hypoplastic. The child experienced severe nutritional deficiency during the first month of extrauterine life. *(Courtesy Dr. Stanley C. Herman.)*

radiologically as demineralization of long bones. These authors believe that both local and systemic factors are involved. An important local factor is trauma from laryngoscopy and endotracheal intubation, which usually results in localized enamel hypoplasia involving only the left maxillary anterior teeth. Slayton et al examined 698 well-nourished and healthy children 4 to 5 years of age and found that 6% had at least one primary tooth with enamel hypoplasia.[37]

HYPOPLASIA RESULTING FROM NUTRITIONAL DEFICIENCIES

Many clinical investigations have been undertaken to determine the relationship between hypoplastic defects of enamel and systemic disabilities. Relatively little importance has been placed on exanthematous fevers, but deficiency states, particularly those related to deficiencies in vitamins A, C, and D, calcium, and phosphorus, can often be related to the occurrence of enamel hypoplasia.

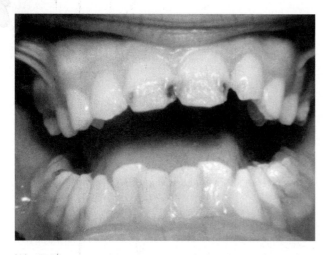

FIG. **7-14.** Enamel hypoplasia that occurred during infancy. A wide band of pitted enamel is evident on the maxillary and mandibular permanent incisors and first permanent molars. The child was severely affected with pneumonia at 6 months of age. *(Courtesy Dr. Stanley C. Herman.)*

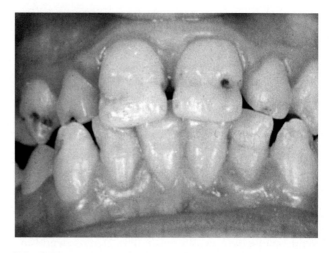

FIG. **7-16.** Enamel hypoplasia occurred during early childhood. Enamel formation on the incisal third of the lower incisors and the maxillary central incisors is normal.

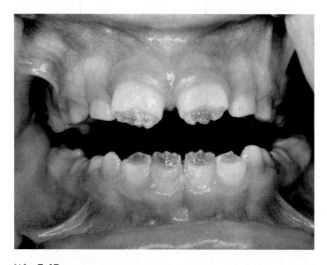

FIG. **7-15.** Enamel hypoplasia that developed as the result of a nutritional deficiency during infancy. The first permanent molars, maxillary central incisors, and mandibular incisors show hypoplastic enamel and dentin.

Sarnat and Schour observed that, in a group of 60 children who had adequate medical histories, two thirds of the hypoplastic disturbances occurred during infancy (birth to the end of the first year)[38] (Fig. 7-15). Approximately one third of enamel hypoplasia was found in the portion of teeth formed during early childhood (13 to 34 months) (Fig. 7-16). Less than 2% of enamel defects found originated in late childhood (35 to 80 months).

Sheldon, Bibby, and Bales sought to determine whether defects in enamel were related to the occurrence of systemic ailments.[39] They examined ground sections of 95 teeth from 34 patients for whom detailed medical histories were available. In more than 70% of the individuals a positive correlation was established between the time of formation of a band of defective enamel and the existence of some systemic disability. However, defects in enamel occurred in 23% of patients who had no history of systemic conditions that might have produced enamel defects. No enamel changes occurred in 6% of patients who had histories of disabilities that had produced enamel changes in other patients. Deficiencies of vitamins A, C, and D, calcium, and phosphorus were the most common causes of defective enamel formation.

Purvis et al, in a study of 112 infants with neonatal tetany in Edinburgh, observed that 63 (56%) later showed severe enamel hypoplasia of the primary teeth.[40] Histologic examinations revealed a prolonged disturbance of enamel formation in the 3 months before birth. An inverse relationship was demonstrated between the mean daily hours of bright sunshine in each calendar month and the incidence of neonatal tetany 3 months later. This observation suggested that enamel hypoplasia and neonatal tetany can be manifestations of vitamin D deficiency during pregnancy and are most likely the result of secondary hyperparathyroidism in the mother. A significantly higher mean maternal age and a preponderance of lower social class was also seen in the mothers of those in the tetany group. Another study in Edinburgh indicated that only 1% of pregnant mothers took vitamin D supplements.

Apparently in some children a mild deficiency state or systemic condition without clinical symptoms can interfere with ameloblastic activity and can produce a permanent defect in the developing enamel.

HYPOPLASIA RELATED TO BRAIN INJURY AND NEUROLOGIC DEFECTS

Herman and McDonald studied 120 children with cerebral palsy between 2½ and 10½ years of age (for whom complete medical records were available) to determine the prevalence of dental hypoplasia.[41] The researchers compared them with 117 healthy children in the same age group and observed enamel hypoplasia in 36% of the group with cerebral palsy and in 6% of the group without the disorder. A definite relationship between the time of occurrence of the possible factors that could have caused brain damage and the apparent time of origination of the enamel defect (based on its location in the enamel on the crown of the tooth) was established for 70% of the affected teeth of children with cerebral palsy (see Fig. 7-12). Evidence of enamel hypoplasia is an aid to the clinician and the research worker in determining when brain injury occurred in patients in whom the cause is not clearly defined.

Cohen and Diner observed that enamel defects occurred with greatest frequency in children with low intelligence quotients and a high incidence of neurologic defects.[42] They found that chronologically distributed enamel defects were a valuable aid in neurologic diagnosis, because they occur commonly in brain-damaged children. In addition, the defects indicate the time of insult to the developing fetus or infant even when the history is reportedly negative. Martinez et al examined 170 children between 4 and 17 years of age (mean age, 12.03 years) with mental retardation and no history of dental trauma.[43] They found that 37% of these children had dental enamel defects.

HYPOPLASIA ASSOCIATED WITH NEPHROTIC SYNDROME

Oliver and Owings observed enamel hypoplasia in permanent teeth in a high percentage of children with nephrotic syndrome and found a correlation between the time of severe renal disease and the estimated time at which the defective enamel formation occurred.[44] Similarly, Koch et al found a high incidence of enamel defects in the primary teeth of children who were diagnosed with chronic renal failure early in infancy.[45]

HYPOPLASIA ASSOCIATED WITH ALLERGIES

Rattner and Myers discovered a correlation between enamel defects of the primary dentition and the presence of severe allergic reactions.[46] Enamel defects were present in 26 of 45 children with congenital allergies. The enamel lesions were localized in the occlusal third of the primary canines and first molars.

HYPOPLASIA ASSOCIATED WITH LEAD POISONING (PLUMBISM)

Lawson and Stout observed that in areas of Charleston, South Carolina, containing very old frame buildings the incidence of pitting hypoplasia was approximately 100% greater than published standards or the incidence in their control group of children.[47] They suggest that dentists treating children with unexplained pitting hypoplasia should consider previous exposure to lead as a part of their health evaluation, particularly if the child is from a family in a low economic stratum.

Pearl and Roland have pointed out that the fetus of a lead-poisoned mother can be affected because lead readily crosses the placenta during pregnancy.[48] They observed significant delays in development and eruption of the primary teeth in the child of a lead-poisoned mother. They also listed pica (ingestion of unusual objects to satisfy an abnormal craving) as a common sign of plumbism in children 1 to 6 years old, as well as in their mothers. One mother admitted eating plaster from her apartment walls during several months of pregnancy.

HYPOPLASIA CAUSED BY LOCAL INFECTION AND TRAUMA

Enamel hypoplasia resulting from a deficiency state or a systemic condition will be evident on all the teeth that were undergoing matrix formation and calcification at the time of the insult. The hypoplasia will follow a definite pattern. Individual permanent teeth often have hypoplastic or hypocalcified areas on the crown that result from infection or trauma (Figs. 7-17 and 7-18).

Turner first described this localized type of hypoplasia.[49] He noted defects in the enamel of two premolars and traced the defects to apical infection of the nearest primary molar. Enamel hypoplasia resulting from local infection is called *Turner tooth*.

Bauer concluded from a study of autopsy material that the periapical inflammatory processes of primary teeth extend toward the buds of the pertinent permanent teeth and affect them during their prefunctional stage of eruption.[50] The infection fails to stimulate the development of a fibrous wall that would localize the lesion. Instead, the infection spreads diffusely through the bone around the buds of the successors and thereby affects the important protective layer of the young enamel, the united enamel epithelium.

Bauer found that in some cases the united enamel epithelium was destroyed and the enamel was exposed to inflammatory edema and to granulation tissue.[50] The granulation tissue later eroded the enamel and deposited a well-calcified, metaplastic, cementum-like substance on the surface of the deep excavation.

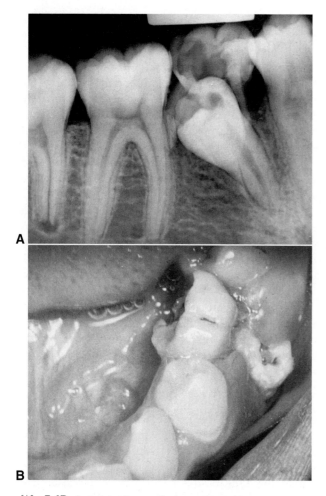

FIG. **7-17. A,** Infected mandibular second primary molar has caused hypoplasia of the second premolar and delayed eruption of the tooth. **B,** Hypoplasia is evident in the occlusal third of the second premolar.

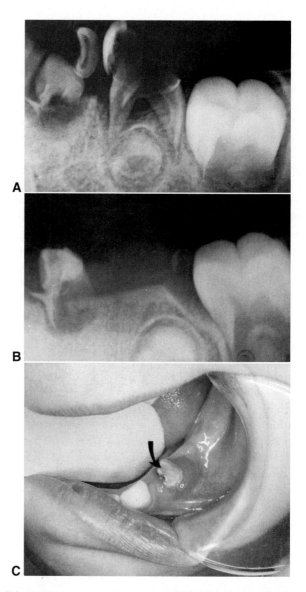

FIG. **7-18. A,** Only a root fragment remains as evidence of a pulpless first primary molar. The infection has affected the development of the first premolar. **B,** The second primary molar has been exfoliated prematurely. The first premolar is malformed as a result of the infection in the area. **C,** The malformed calcified mass *(arrow)* is surrounded by inflamed tissue.

A traumatic blow to an anterior primary tooth that causes its displacement apically can interfere with matrix formation or calcification of the underlying permanent tooth. The trauma or subsequent periapical infection frequently produces defects on the labial surface of the permanent incisor (Fig. 7-19). The retention of infected primary teeth, even if they are asymptomatic, is unjustifiable. The development of hypoplastic defects on the permanent tooth, its deflection from the normal path of eruption, and even death of the developing tooth may result.

HYPOPLASIA ASSOCIATED WITH CLEFT LIP AND PALATE

Mink studied the incidence of enamel hypoplasia of the maxillary anterior teeth in 98 patients with repaired bilateral and unilateral complete cleft lip and palate; the individuals ranged in age from 1½ to 18 years.[51] Among patients in the repaired unilateral and bilateral complete cleft lip and palate group, 66% of those with maxillary anterior primary teeth had one or more primary teeth affected with enamel hypoplasia; 92% of those with erupted maxillary anterior permanent teeth had one or more permanent teeth affected with enamel hypoplasia. Mink concluded that the permanent teeth are in earlier stages of development at the time of the surgical procedure and are more subject to damage.[51] Dixon also attributed many of the defects of tooth structure and formation observed in patients with cleft palate to the reparative surgery.[52] Vichi and Franchi, however, have suggested

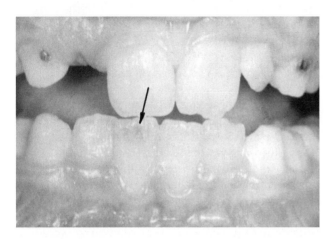

FIG. **7-19.** Hypoplastic defect on the labial surface of a mandibular permanent central incisor *(arrow)*. There was a history of trauma to the primary tooth.

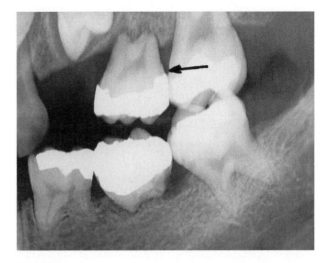

FIG. **7-20.** X-radiation caused hypoplastic defect on the crown of the first permanent molar *(arrow)* and stunting of root development.

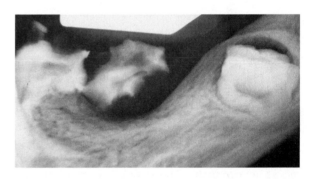

FIG. **7-21.** Absence of developing premolars and the malformed second permanent molar were caused by excessive x-radiation.

that dental anomalies, including hypoplasia, probably result from multiple causes.[53] They emphasize the difficulty in understanding the role played by genetic factors, postnatal environment, nutrition, and surgical influences in the development of the dental anomalies.

HYPOPLASIA CAUSED BY X-RADIATION AND CHEMOTHERAPY

Numerous dental abnormalities may result in surviving children who receive high-dose radiotherapy and chemotherapy during the time their teeth are forming. Kaste et al reviewed clinical and radiographic records of 423 survivors of acute lymphoblastic leukemia.[54] Among these patients they observed root stunting in 24.4%, microdontia in 18.9%, hypodontia in 8.5%, taurodontia in 5.9%, and overretention of primary teeth in 4%. The patients who were younger than 8 years old at diagnosis or who received cranial irradiation (in addition to chemotherapy) developed more dental abnormalities than those older than 8 years at diagnosis and those who did not receive cranial irradiation. They also noted that the resulting dental defects may affect the survivors' quality of life.

Maguire and Welbury point out that, as survival rates for children with cancer improve, the emphasis in therapy has moved from saving children at all costs to saving children at the least cost to the child, and therapy protocols are continually reviewed with this goal in mind.[55]

Children who receive high-dose x-radiation in the treatment of a malignancy are at risk for developing rampant caries in the irradiated area. The cause is generally believed to be associated with changes in salivary gland function and is discussed in Chapter 10.

Ameloblasts are somewhat resistant to x-radiation. However, a line of hypoplastic enamel that corresponds to the stage of development at the time of therapy may be seen (Fig. 7-20). Radiotherapy will have a more severe effect on the development of the dentin, and root formation will be stunted. Occasionally, development of the permanent teeth will be arrested (Fig. 7-21).

HYPOPLASIA RESULTING FROM RUBELLA EMBRYOPATHY

Musselman examined 50 children (average age, 2½ years) with congenital anomalies attributed to in utero infection with rubella.[56] Enamel hypoplasia was found in 90% of the affected children, compared with only 13% of unaffected children in a control group. Tapered teeth also occurred in 78% of the children with a history of rubella (Fig. 7-22). Nine of the children in the study group had notched teeth, but this defect was not present in any of the children in the control group.

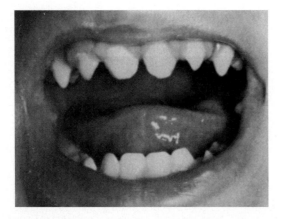

FIG. **7-22.** The mother of this child had rubella in the eighth week of pregnancy. The primary teeth were tapered and presented a rough hypoplastic surface. The child had a patent ductus arteriosus, pulmonary stenosis, and a cognitive disability. There was also a history of difficult feeding and dehydration at 2 months of age. *(Courtesy Dr. Robert Musselman.)*

TREATMENT OF HYPOPLASTIC TEETH

The contention that hypoplastic teeth are more susceptible to dental caries than normal teeth has little evidence to support it. Carious lesions do develop, however, in the enamel defects and in areas of the clinical crown where dentin is exposed. Small carious and precarious areas can be restored with resin or glass ionomer. The restoration is usually confined to the area of involvement. The occlusal third of the first permanent molar often shows gross evidence of hypoplasia, and treatment is necessary before the tooth fully erupts.

Hypoplastic primary and permanent teeth with large areas of defective enamel and exposed dentin may be sensitive as soon as they erupt. Satisfactory restoration may not be practical at this time. The topical application of fluoride has been found to decrease the sensitivity of the tooth. The application should be repeated as often as necessary to reduce sensitivity to thermal change and acid foods.

HYPOPLASIA CAUSED BY FLUORIDE (DENTAL FLUOROSIS)

Excess ingestion of fluoride can affect the ameloblasts during the tooth formation stage and can cause the clinical entity called *dental fluorosis* or *mottled enamel.* The appearance of enamel that is affected in its formation by excessive fluoride varies considerably. Although the more severe cases of dental fluorosis are associated with a high level of fluoride consumption, there is apparently a great deal of individual variation. The affected enamel is often limited superficially to the most outer surface and presents a white or brown opaque and/or pitted appearance.

Dental fluorosis is most often seen in permanent teeth, but it has also been observed in primary teeth. Levy et al observed fluorosis of primary teeth in 12.1% of 504 children.[57] It was observed most often on second primary molars. The middle of the first year of life seemed to be the most important time with regard to the development of fluorosis in the primary dentition based on their estimates of fluoride ingestion prenatally and during the first year of life in these children.

The existence of a genetic influence on the development of fluorosis is supported by the finding that some inbred strains of mice are much more susceptible to fluorosis than other strains who receive the same fluoride dosage under identical conditions. Studies of these differing mouse strains should identify candidate genes for study in human cases of dental and skeletal fluorosis.[58]

ENAMEL MICROABRASION TO REMOVE SUPERFICIAL ENAMEL DISCOLORATIONS

For many years some dentists have advocated the application of hydrochloric acid as an effective method for destaining mottled enamel. McClosky described a technique, originally advocated by Kane, that used 18% hydrochloric acid on the affected enamel surfaces.[59] Croll and Cavanaugh advocated a modified procedure that they called *enamel color modification by controlled hydrochloric acid–pumice abrasion.*[60,61] In their method, after the tooth or teeth are carefully isolated with a rubber dam and proper preparations have been made for safe use of the caustic agent, a slurry of fine pumice and 18% hydrochloric acid is applied under pressure and abrasion with a wooden stick. The slurry is rinsed away after each 5-second application until the desired color change has occurred. After a final rinsing with water, 1.1% neutral sodium fluoride gel is applied for 3 minutes. Next a fine fluoridated prophylactic paste is applied with a rotating rubber cup. Finally the enamel is polished with an aluminum oxide disk.

Dalzell, Howes, and Hubler investigated the effects of the three variables of time, number of applications, and pressure on enamel loss when applying a slurry of 18% hydrochloric acid and pumice.[62] They found that enamel loss increased as the level of each variable increased and that a greater amount of enamel loss occurred when levels of two or three variables increased simultaneously. The combination of ten 10-second applications or fifteen 5-second applications with 20 g of pressure resulted in enamel loss of slightly less than 250 µm.

Croll proposed a modified procedure called *enamel microabrasion* in which a specially prepared abrasive

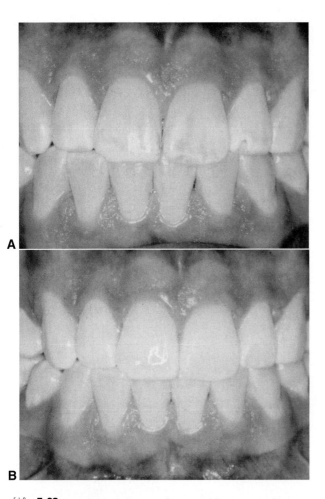

A

B

FIG. **7-23. A,** Mottled enamel. Because the brown pigmentation and white splotchy areas were objectionable, the teeth were treated by enamel microabrasion. **B,** Much of the pigment has been removed by the process.

compound (Prema*) is applied to the discolored enamel areas, similarly to prophylaxis paste, using a synthetic rubber applicator in a 10:1 gear-reduction handpiece.[63] Frequent water rinsings and reevaluation of the tooth for color correction are required. The instrumentation is continued until the undesirable coloration is removed or until a noticeable amount of enamel is being removed when the tooth is viewed from the incisal. Finally the abraded teeth are polished with a fine fluoridated prophylactic paste and given a 4-minute fluoride treatment (Fig. 7-23).

More recently Croll and Helpin have introduced a new delivery system for the microabrasion procedure.[64] A viscous, water-soluble abrasion slurry containing hydrochloric acid and silicon carbide microparticles (Opalustre†) is conveniently applied to the tooth surface

by a syringe. Vital tooth bleaching may be used in combination with enamel microabrasion to help remove deeper intrinsic discolorations. Bleaching is discussed later in this chapter.

PREERUPTIVE "CARIES" (PREERUPTIVE CORONAL RESORPTION OR PREERUPTIVE INTRACORONAL RADIOLUCENCY)

Occasionally, defects on the crowns of developing permanent teeth are evident radiographically, even though no infection of the primary tooth or surrounding area is apparent (Fig. 7-24). Muhler referred to this condition as *preeruptive "caries."*[65] Such a lesion often does resemble caries when it is observed clinically, and the destructive lesion progresses if it is not restored. As soon as the lesion is reasonably accessible, the tooth should be uncovered by removal of the overlying primary tooth or by surgical exposure. The carieslike dentin is then excavated, and the tooth is restored with a durable temporary or permanent restorative material. In some cases the lesion may be so extensive that indirect pulp therapy is justified (Fig. 7-25).

Mueller et al reported carieslike resorption bilaterally in mandibular permanent second molars of a 12-year-old patient.[66] Both lesions were successfully treated in a fashion similar to the treatment illustrated in Fig. 7-25. Holan, Eidelman, and Mass reported three cases in which similar successful management of preeruptive tooth defects was performed.[67] Their experience and a review of other reported cases suggest that impacted teeth or teeth delayed in eruption may be at higher risk for developing the lesions. Savage, Gentner, and Symons also published an informative literature review and case report relevant to this topic.[68]

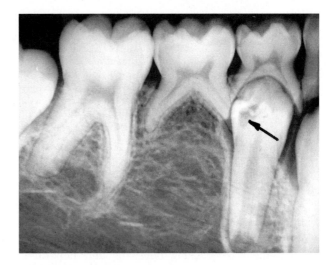

FIG. **7-24.** Preeruptive "caries" on the crown of an unerupted first premolar *(arrow).*

*Premier Dental Products, King of Prussia, Pa.
†Ultradent Products, South Jordan, Utah.

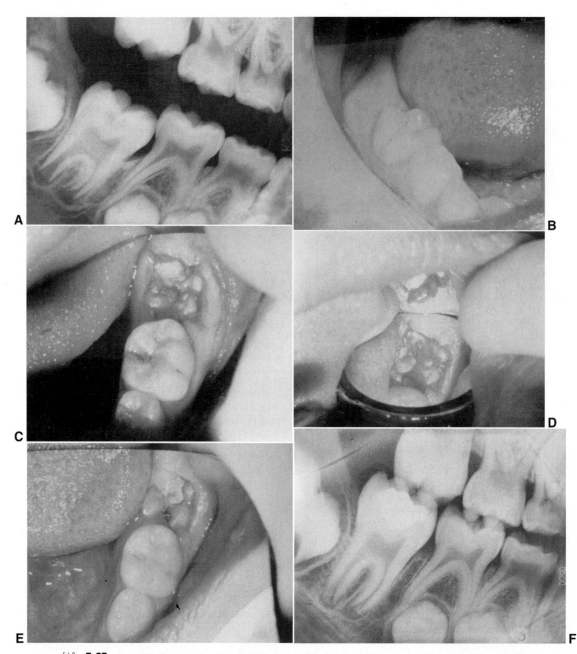

FIG. **7-25.** **A** and **B,** Preeruptive "caries" in a mandibular right first permanent molar that is still unerupted. **C,** Mirror view of the lesion on the occlusal surface of the unerupted tooth. **D,** Mirror view of excavated cavity after gross caries removal. **E,** Mirror view of temporary restoration 1 week postoperatively (dark spot on mesial marginal ridge area is an artifact). **F,** Nine months postoperatively, patient had continued normal root development and eruption of the tooth. The temporary restoration remained 3 months before the tooth was reentered and restored with amalgam. *(Courtesy Drs. George E. Krull and James R. Roche.)*

Seow, Wan, and McAllan[69] and Seow, Lu, and McAllan[70] have published retrospective studies to determine the prevalence of preeruptive dentin radiolucencies in permanent teeth using bite-wing and panoramic radiographs, respectively. In the study using bite-wing radiographs, the authors examined a set of films from 1959 subjects and observed 9919 unerupted permanent teeth. They found 126 subjects (6%) with 163 teeth (2%) exhibiting preeruptive dentin radiolucencies. In the study using panoramic radiographs, the investigators examined 1281 films of individual patients with 11,767 unerupted permanent teeth (incisors excluded). This

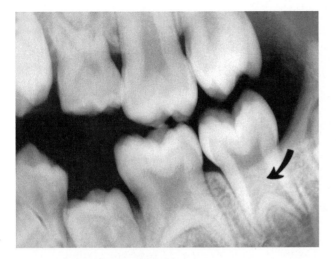

FIG. **7-26.** Taurodontism. Notice the elongated pulp chamber and short root canals *(arrow)*.

study identified 42 subjects (3%) with 57 teeth (0.5%) exhibiting preeruptive dentin defects. The authors emphasize the importance of carefully studying radiographic images of unerupted teeth so that early detection and treatment are possible.

TAURODONTISM

Lysell credits Keith with giving the name to the phenomenon known as *taurodontism.*[71] This anomaly is characterized by a tendency for the body of the tooth to enlarge at the expense of the roots. The pulp chamber is elongated and extends deeply into the region of the roots (Fig. 7-26). A similar condition is seen in the teeth of cud-chewing animals such as the bull (Latin, *taurus*).

Jaspers and Witkop noted that taurodontism is found in about 2.5% of adult whites as an isolated trait, as well as in individuals with syndromes such as tricho-dento-osseous syndrome, otodental dysplasia, and X-chromosome aneuploidies.[72] Mena observed a mother and seven children, four of whom showed evidence of taurodontism in the permanent or primary teeth, or both.[73] This was probably the first report of taurodontism of the primary dentition as a definite family trait in black children. Gedik and Çimen reported taurodontism of six primary molars of a 7-year-old boy who had no syndromes or systemic disease.[74] Other pedigrees have been consistent with autosomal dominant or autosomal recessive inheritance. The inheritance may also be polygenic.

The clinical significance of the condition becomes apparent if vital pulp therapy or root canal therapy is necessary.

INHERITED DENTIN DEFECTS

Two broad categories of heritable dentin defects, dentinogenesis imperfecta and dentin dysplasia, are identifiable, each with distinct subtypes.

DENTINOGENESIS IMPERFECTA (HEREDITARY OPALESCENT DENTIN)

Dentinogenesis imperfecta is inherited as an isolated autosomal dominant trait ("isolated" in this usage means that it occurs without other anomalies). Bixler, Conneally, and Christen observed this pattern in a six-generation family in which 34 members were studied.[75] There was 100% penetrance and consistent gene expression within a sibship. In a survey of 96,000 Michigan children, Witkop reported a prevalence of 1 in 8000 with the trait.[76] The anomaly may be seen with osteogenesis imperfecta (Fig. 7-27). A decade later, Witkop suggested that there are two distinct diseases.[77] He recommended that the term *hereditary opalescent dentin* be used for the disease that occurs as an isolated trait and the term *dentinogenesis imperfecta* be used for that which occurs in conjunction with osteogenesis imperfecta. Shields, Bixler, and El-Kafrawy recognized the difference and proposed a new classification: the dentin defect that occurs in association with osteogenesis imperfecta is termed *(Shields) type I dentinogenesis imperfecta* and that which occurs as an isolated trait is termed *(Shields) type II dentinogenesis imperfecta.*[78] In addition, the dentin defects seen in the isolated Brandywine triracial population in southern Maryland was termed *(Shields) type III dentinogenesis imperfecta.* These latter defects consisted of variable expression of the features of (Shields) type I (without osteogenesis imperfecta) and type II, shell-like teeth, and multiple pulp exposures (Fig. 7-28). In this condition normal dentin formation is confined to a thin layer next to the enamel and cementum, followed by a layer of disorderly dentin containing a few tubules. The roots of shell teeth are short, and the primary teeth may be exfoliated prematurely.

Mutations in the *DSPP* gene, which codes for the two major noncollagenous dentin matrix proteins, dentin sialoprotein (DSP) and dentin phosphoprotein (also known as phosphophorin), have been found in patients with (Shields) type II dentinogenesis imperfecta by Zhang et al[79] and by Xiao et al.[80] Sreenath et al noted in the *DSPP* knockout mouse that the teeth have a widened predentin zone and develop defective dentin mineralization similar in phenotype to that in human (Shields) type III dentinogenesis imperfecta; these findings imply that this gene may also be involved in the latter condition.[81]

The clinical picture of dentinogenesis imperfecta is one in which the primary and permanent teeth are a characteristic reddish brown to gray opalescent color. Soon after the primary dentition is complete, enamel often breaks away from the incisal edge of the anterior teeth and the occlusal surface of the posterior teeth. The exposed soft dentin abrades rapidly, occasionally to the

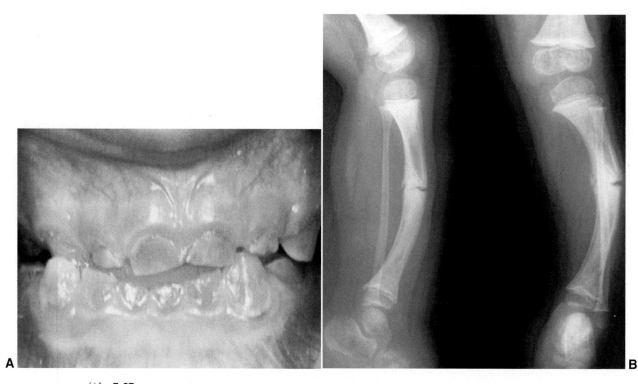

FIG. **7-27. A,** Five-year-old girl with dentinogenesis imperfecta and osteogenesis imperfecta. The child had sustained numerous fractures of the long bones. **B,** A fracture of the tibia is evident in the radiograph.

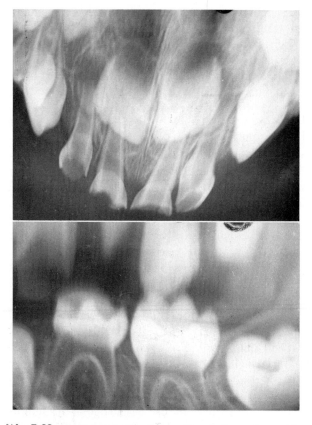

FIG. **7-28.** Shell teeth. The large size of the pulp cavities indicates the nonexistence of secondary dentin.

extent that the smooth, polished dentin surface is continuous with the gingival tissue (Fig. 7-29). Radiographs show slender roots and bulbous crowns. The pulp chamber is small or entirely absent, and the pulp canals are small and ribbonlike (Fig. 7-30). Periapical rarefaction in the primary dentition is occasionally observed. However, no satisfactory explanation has been offered, because the condition apparently is not related to pulp exposures and pulpal necrosis. Multiple root fractures are often seen, particularly in older patients. Crowns of the permanent teeth often seem to be of better quality and have less destruction. Occasionally they appear essentially normal clinically (Fig. 7-31).

The treatment of dentinogenesis imperfecta is difficult in both the primary and permanent dentitions. The placement of stainless steel crowns on the primary posterior teeth may be considered as a means of preventing gross abrasion of the tooth structure. Full-coverage restorations may be placed on the permanent teeth if the crowns need protection in late adolescence or young adulthood. Bonded veneer restorations on anterior teeth have also been used successfully for esthetic improvement in patients with dentinogenesis imperfecta when full-coverage restorations are unnecessary.

Teeth that have periapical rarefaction and root fracture should be removed. Extraction of the affected teeth is difficult because of the brittleness of the dentin.

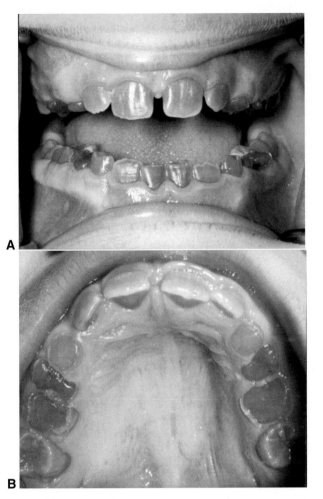

FIG. **7-29.** Dentinogenesis imperfecta. The primary teeth are severely abraded. Enamel is breaking away from the incisal edge of the lower permanent central incisors.

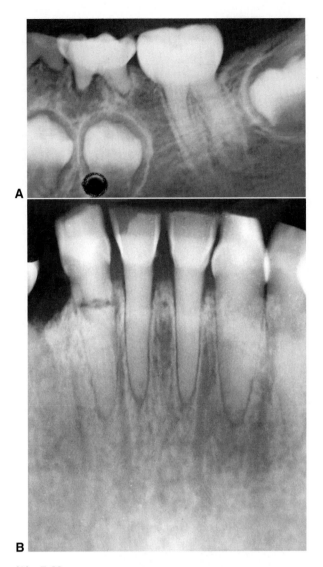

FIG. **7-30. A,** Slender roots with ribbonlike pulp canals and bulbous crowns are characteristic of dentinogenesis imperfecta. The primary molars show periapical rarefaction. **B,** Root fractures are common in older patients.

DENTIN DYSPLASIA

Dentin dysplasia is a rare disturbance of dentin formation that Shields, Bixler, and El-Kafrawy have categorized into two types: radicular dentin dysplasia (type I) and coronal dentin dysplasia (type II).[78] Both primary and secondary dentitions are affected in dentin dysplasia type I, which is inherited as an autosomal dominant trait. Radiographically the roots are short and may be more pointed than normal. Usually the root canals and pulp chambers are absent except for a chevron-shaped remnant in the crown. The color and general morphology of the crowns of the teeth are usually normal, although they may be slightly opalescent and blue or brown. Periapical radiolucencies may be present at the apices of affected teeth.

Dentin dysplasia type II is inherited as an autosomal dominant trait in which the primary dentition appears opalescent and on radiographs has obliterated pulp chambers, similar to the appearance in dentinogenesis imperfecta. Unlike in dentinogenesis imperfecta, however, in dentin dysplasia type II the permanent dentition has normal color and radiographically exhibits a thistle tube pulp configuration with pulp stones.

Dean et al, noting the phenotypic similarity of dentinogenesis imperfecta, Shields type II, to that in the primary dentition in dentin dysplasia type II, hypothesized that these conditions may be due to different alleles of the same gene.[82] Investigation of a family with 10 of 24 members affected in three generations showed that the candidate region for the dentin dysplasia type II gene overlaps the likely location of the gene for Shields type II dentinogenesis imperfecta. They suggested that a candidate gene for dentinogenesis imperfecta Shields type II and/or III should also be a candidate gene for dentin dysplasia type II. Subsequently Rajpar et al

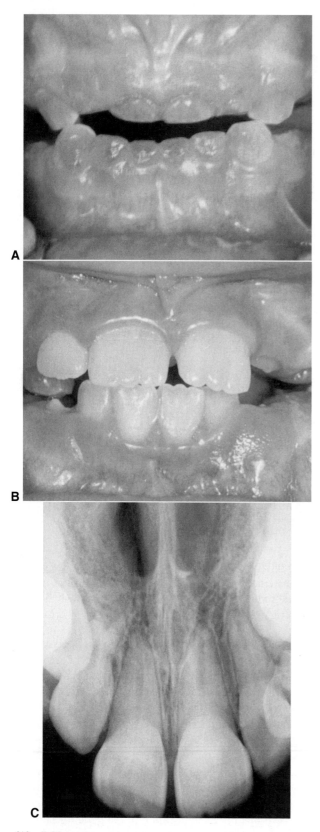

FIG. **7-31. A,** Four-year-old child with dentinogenesis imperfecta. **B,** The permanent teeth, in contrast to the primary teeth, are normal in color. **C,** The radiograph shows the typical picture of dentinogenesis imperfecta.

showed that a *DSPP* missense mutation was present in a family with dentin dysplasia type II, thereby confirming the hypothesis of Dean et al.[82,83]

AMELOGENESIS IMPERFECTA

As noted in Chapter 6, amelogenesis imperfecta is a developmental defect of the enamel with a heterogeneous etiology that affects the enamel of both the primary and permanent dentition. The anomaly occurs in the general population with an incidence of 1 in 14,000 to 1 in 16,000. Amelogenesis imperfecta has a wide range of clinical appearances with three broad categories observed: the hypocalcified type, the hypomaturation type, and the hypoplastic type. Although amelogenesis imperfecta can occur as a part of several syndromes, Cartwright, Kula, and Wright confirmed that the trait itself could also be associated with a skeletal anterior open bite.[84]

Some progress has been made in unraveling the molecular basis of the myriad clinical forms of amelogenesis imperfecta. Aldred and Crawford discussed the limitations of the existing classification systems and proposed an alternative classification based on the molecular defect, biochemical result, mode of inheritance, and phenotype.[85] Hart et al recommended a standardized nomenclature for describing amelogenesis imperfecta that causes alterations at the genomic, complementary DNA, and protein levels.[86,87] In addition, two clinically distinct forms of autosomal dominant amelogenesis imperfecta—smooth hypoplastic amelogenesis imperfecta and local hypoplastic amelogenesis imperfecta—are associated with mutations in the enamelin (*ENAM*) gene located at 4q21. An X-linked form (AIH1) has been found to be associated with as many as 12 mutations in the amelogenin (*AMELX*) gene, located at Xp21. However, at least one family has had the trait linked to another location on the chromosome, Xq22-q28.[88]

The defective tooth structure is limited to the enamel. On radiographic examination the pulpal outline appears to be normal, and the root morphology is not unlike that of normal teeth. The difference in the appearance and quality of the enamel is thought to be attributable to the state of enamel development at the time the defect occurs. In the hypoplastic type the enamel matrix appears to be imperfectly formed; although calcification subsequently occurs in the matrix and the enamel is hard, it is defective in amount and has a roughened, pitted surface (Fig. 7-32). In the hypocalcified type, matrix formation appears to be of normal thickness, but calcification is deficient and the enamel is soft (Fig. 7-33). In both of these more common types of the defect, the enamel becomes stained because of the roughness of the surface and the increased permeability.

In still another variant of amelogenesis imperfecta a thin, smooth covering of brownish yellow enamel is

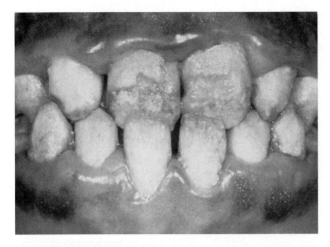

FIG. **7-32.** Both the primary and permanent teeth are affected by the hereditary anomaly amelogenesis imperfecta. The enamel is pitted but hard.

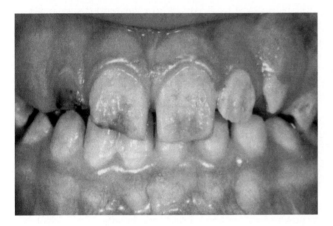

FIG. **7-33.** Hypocalcification type of amelogenesis imperfecta. The primary teeth were similarly affected. The enamel surface is soft.

present. In this type the enamel does not seem excessively susceptible to abrasion or caries (Figs. 7-34 and 7-35).

Congleton and Burkes reported three cases of amelogenesis imperfecta in which the patients also demonstrated taurodontism.[89] Others have identified cases with the clinical appearance of amelogenesis imperfecta and taurodontism along with strikingly curly hair and increased bone density (especially of the skull), and this has been identified as *tricho-dento-osseous syndrome*. Seow has suggested that some cases reported as amelogenesis imperfecta with taurodontism were actually cases of tricho-dento-osseous syndrome.[90] Price et al found that this autosomal dominant condition is caused by a mutation in the distal-less homeobox gene *DLX3*.[91] Even though the taurodontism and amelogenesis imperfecta traits in this condition are fully penetrant

in affected individuals, the osseous and hair features are variably expressed even when the same deletion is present in a family—findings which indicate that the variable expression is influenced by other genes and/or environmental factors. Further studies by Price et al have confirmed that tricho-dento-osseous syndrome and amelogenesis imperfecta of the hypomaturation-hypoplastic type with taurodontism are two genetically distinct conditions.[92]

The treatment of teeth with amelogenesis imperfecta–like defects depends on its severity and the demands of aesthetic improvement. When indicated, the teeth can be prepared for full-coverage restorations. For some cases of the hypomaturation and hypoplastic types, bonded veneer restorations may offer a more conservative alternative for management of the aesthetic problem of the anterior teeth. Patel et al have reported successful treatment with porcelain laminate veneer restorations.[93]

ENAMEL AND DENTIN APLASIA

Teeth that have some characteristics of both dentinogenesis imperfecta and amelogenesis imperfecta have been described in the literature. Chaudhry et al reported such a case and called the condition *odontogenesis imperfecta*.[94]

Schimmelpfennig and McDonald observed a similar dentition and termed it *enamel and dentin aplasia*.[95] The primary teeth were essentially devoid of enamel, and the smooth, severely abraded dentin was reddish brown. Radiographs showed normal alveolar bone around the roots of the teeth. Two teeth had pulp exposure and pulpal degeneration (Fig. 7-36). Radiolucent areas were present at the apices of the two primary teeth, with exposed and degenerated pulps. The pulp chambers and canals in all the primary teeth were extremely large, with no evidence that they were becoming obliterated. In ground sections of the primary teeth the dentinal tubules showed little evidence of a normal growth pattern. They were few and irregular, with a tendency toward branching. The cementum appeared normal and was acellular. No evidence of secondary dentin formation was found. A few fragments of enamel adhering to the dentin appeared thinner than normal, and few normal morphologic characteristics were present. The dentinoenamel junction was atypical in that it lacked the characteristic scalloping.

The permanent teeth, when they erupted, were partially covered with a thin, gray, poorly coalesced coating of enamel. Brown dentin could be seen on the labial aspect of the central incisors and at the base of the fissures of the first permanent molars. Stainless steel crown restorations were placed even before complete eruption to protect the teeth from continued abrasion.

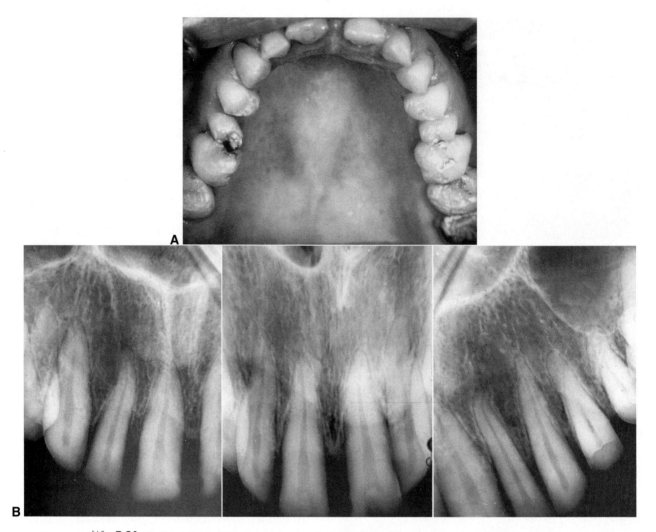

FIG. **7-34. A,** Case diagnosed as amelogenesis imperfecta. The permanent teeth have a thin covering of pigmented enamel. **B,** The radiographs show essentially normal root morphology. The crowns have a thin covering of enamel.

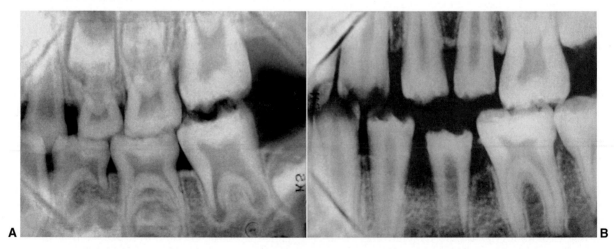

FIG. **7-35. A** and **B,** Left bite-wing radiographs of a patient with amelogenesis imperfecta. Radiograph in **B** was made 6 years after radiograph in **A** and demonstrates the maintenance of a caries-free dentition despite the thin enamel.

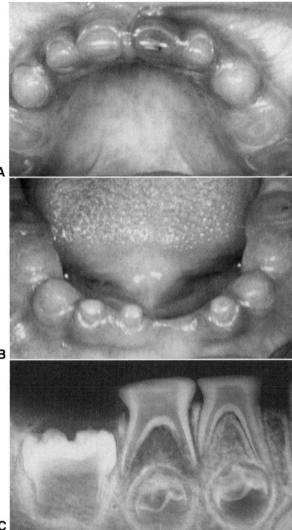

FIG. **7-36.** **A** and **B,** Severely abraded teeth are almost entirely devoid of enamel. The outline of a large pulp chamber can be seen through a thin covering of dentin. The mandibular second primary molars have pulp exposure. **C,** Radiograph shows large pulp canals and large pulp chambers. Apical rarefaction is associated with pulp exposure of the second primary molar.

AGENESIS OF TEETH

ANODONTIA

Anodontia, which implies complete failure of the teeth to develop, is a rare condition. Although agenesis of permanent teeth is often referred to as *congenital absence,* they would not, of course, be expected in the oral cavity at birth anyway. Gorlin, Herman, and Moss noted that, when agenesis occurs as an isolated trait, the primary dentition is not affected, and the inheritance is autosomal recessive.[96] Swallow reported on an 11-year-old boy who had a complete primary dentition but no permanent dentition.[97] Schneider also observed a 7-year-old white female with primary teeth but missing permanent teeth.[98] As is usually the case with presumed autosomal recessive inheritance, the hereditary background included no known consanguinity in the family or history of anodontia or ectodermal dysplasia in either the maternal or paternal lineages. Although consanguinity increases the likelihood that recessive traits or conditions will be expressed, most affected individuals do not have a family history of inbreeding. An overlay denture was constructed for the patient, which is often the treatment of choice. A comparable situation is shown in Fig. 7-37. Laird reported a similar patient in whom a complete primary dentition was present, but the only permanent teeth were maxillary first permanent molars.[99] Witkop studied two families in which both parents had peg or missing maxillary lateral incisors, which is an autosomal dominant trait with incomplete penetrance and variable expressivity, and concluded that agenesis of the permanent teeth can be an expression of the homozygous state of that gene.[100]

HYPODONTIA (OLIGODONTIA)

Agenesis of some teeth is referred to as *hypodontia,* which is preferable to the term *partial anodontia. Oligodontia* is sometimes used when only a few teeth develop. Hypodontia may occur without a family history of hypodontia, although it is often familial. It may also be found as a part of a syndrome, especially in an ectodermal dysplasia, although it usually occurs alone (isolated). Note that *isolated* in this usage means not occurring as part of a syndrome. It may still be familial.

Any one of the 32 permanent teeth may be missing. However, those most frequently missing in children are the mandibular second premolars, maxillary lateral incisors, and maxillary second premolars. This order of frequency has been confirmed in studies by Glenn[101] and by Grahnen.[102] The absence of teeth may be unilateral or bilateral. Glenn observed during an examination of 1702 children that 5% had a missing permanent tooth other than a third molar.[101] In 97% of the children the formation of the second premolar could be detected radiographically at 5.5 years of age and that of the lateral incisor at 3.5 years of age.

In addition to the already mentioned autosomal dominant hypoplasia or agenesis of the maxillary lateral incisors, Vastardis et al found absence of second premolars in one family showing an autosomal dominant pattern of inheritance to be caused by a mutation in the *MSX1* gene located at 4p16.1.[103] In contrast, evidence for the genetic heterogeneity of hypodontia is provided by the finding of a frameshift mutation (resulting in premature termination of translation and a shortened protein) in the human *PAX9* gene in a large

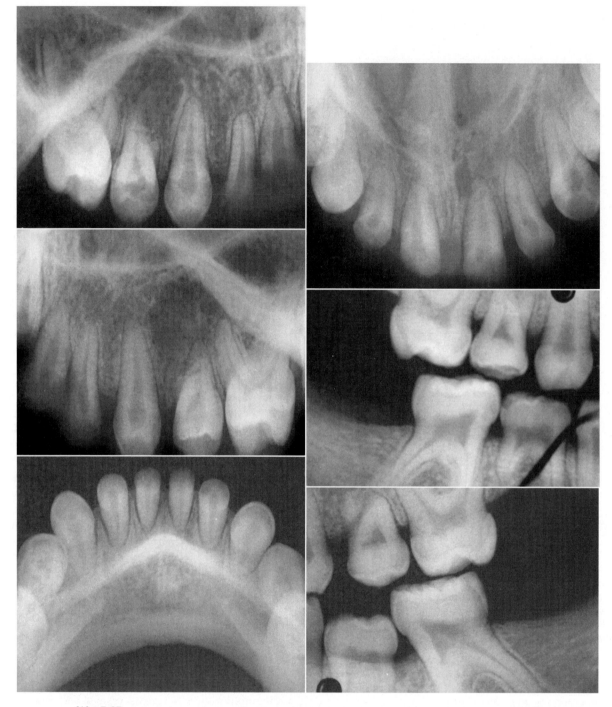

FIG. **7-37.** A complete primary dentition without evidence of permanent teeth in a 14-year-old girl.

family with autosomal dominant oligodontia.[104] X-linked inheritance of oligodontia or hypodontia through four generations of a family was described by Erpenstein and Pfeiffer.[105] Not only was there no male-to-male transmission, but males had oligodontia while females had hypodontia. Ahmad et al demonstrated

that hypodontia inherited in an autosomal recessive mode and associated with malformation of teeth, enamel hypoplasia, and failure of eruption could be linked to 16q12.1.[106]

Bennett and Ronk reported an unusual case of a 4-year-old boy with three missing primary teeth.[107] The mother related that the two missing mandibular central incisors erupted a few days after birth (neonatal teeth) and were removed because of a lack of root formation. The maxillary left first primary molar was congenitally missing as well. A panoramic radiograph of the patient also revealed the absence of multiple permanent tooth buds. The child did not exhibit any other signs or symptoms; he appeared normal in every other way, and there was no known familial history of missing teeth. A rare finding of nine congenitally missing primary teeth in a 3-year-old boy has been reported by Shashikiran, Karthik, and Subbareddy.[108] The boy's mother gave a history of consanguineous marriage. There was no known family history of missing teeth even among the patient's siblings. The primary teeth that were present appeared normal clinically and radiographically. The boy also exhibited ankyloglossia, and the frenum attachments were high in both arches. He did not show any evidence of other ectodermal disorders and otherwise appeared to be a normal young child.

Fleming, Nelson, and Gorlin have reported that a missing maxillary central incisor may occur as an isolated dental finding.[109] This anomaly has also been reported to occur in association with growth retardation with or without growth hormone deficiency, in association with autosomal dominant holoprosencephaly, and occasionally in association with other midline developmental defects. As already stated in the discussion of fusion of teeth, children with this dental anomaly should be referred for medical follow-up unless a comprehensive evaluation for a diagnosis has already been performed. Growth hormone therapy or some other form of treatment may be indicated.

ECTODERMAL DYSPLASIAS

The congenital absence of primary teeth is relatively rare. When a number of the primary teeth fail to develop, other ectodermal deficiencies are usually evident. There are more than 100 types of ectodermal dysplasia with varying anomalies of ectodermal derivatives, including both the primary and permanent teeth, hair, nails, and skin. Children with a number of missing primary and permanent teeth may have some or all of the signs of a type of ectodermal dysplasia and should undergo further evaluation.

One of the more common types of ectodermal dysplasia is X-linked recessive hypohidrotic ectodermal dysplasia (XLHED), also called *anhidrotic ectodermal dysplasia* and *Christ-Siemens-Touraine syndrome*. A rare autosomal recessive form also occurs that is clinically indistinguishable from XLHED. Hypodontia and dental hypoplasia, as well as hypotrichosis, hypohydrosis/ anhidrosis, and asteatosis are characteristic of XLHED. Secondary characteristics include a deficiency in salivary flow, protuberant lips, and a saddle-nose appearance.

The skin is often dry and scaly, and there is fissuring at the corners of the mouth. Mutations in the *EDA1* gene have been found in most patients with XLHED.[110]

Because the absence of teeth predisposes the child to a lack of alveolar process growth, the construction of dentures is complicated. However, as might be expected in at least most types of ectodermal dysplasia, skeletal structures are normal. Serial lateral cephalograms taken during childhood and adolescence have shown that the sagittal development of the jaw occurs in an essentially normal manner. A deficiency in sweat glands causes a predisposition to increased body temperature, and children with hypohidrosis/anhidrosis are extremely uncomfortable during hot weather. Many of them must reside in cool climates. Children with an ectodermal dysplasia usually have normal mentality and a normal life expectancy. Consanguinity increases the likelihood of expression of a trait or condition that is inherited in a recessive manner (Fig. 7-38), and may be one way a female with a normal karyotype can be affected.

The primary teeth that are present may be normal or reduced in size. The anterior teeth are often conical, which is characteristic of oligodontia associated with many types of ectodermal dysplasia. The primary molars without permanent successors have a tendency to become ankylosed.

The many types of ectodermal dysplasia with different modes of inheritance can be emphasized by describing a "tooth and nail" type of autosomal dominant ectodermal dysplasia, also called Witkop syndrome, reported by Giansanti, Long, and Rankin.[111] This ectodermal dysplasia is characterized by hypoplastic nails and hypodontia. A different mutation in the *MSX1* gene than that found when only hypodontia is present has been reported in a family with tooth and nail syndrome by Jumlongras et al.[112] In contrast to most nonsyndromic hypodontias, in which (excluding third molars) premolars and maxillary lateral incisors are most often missing, the mandibular incisors, second molars, and maxillary canines are most frequently absent. Overall, the teeth are generally not affected to the extent seen in XLHED, and there can be little involvement of the hair and sweat glands.[113]

For children with a large number of missing primary teeth, partial dentures can be constructed at an early age. Two-year-old and 3-year-old children have worn partial dentures successfully. Their ability to masticate food increases, and their nutritional status may improve. A partial denture can be adjusted or remade at intervals to allow for the eruption of permanent teeth. Denture construction at an early age may also reduce the psychologic problem of the child's feeling "different" (Fig. 7-39).

If the permanent teeth erupt in good position and in favorable relationship to each other, partial dentures

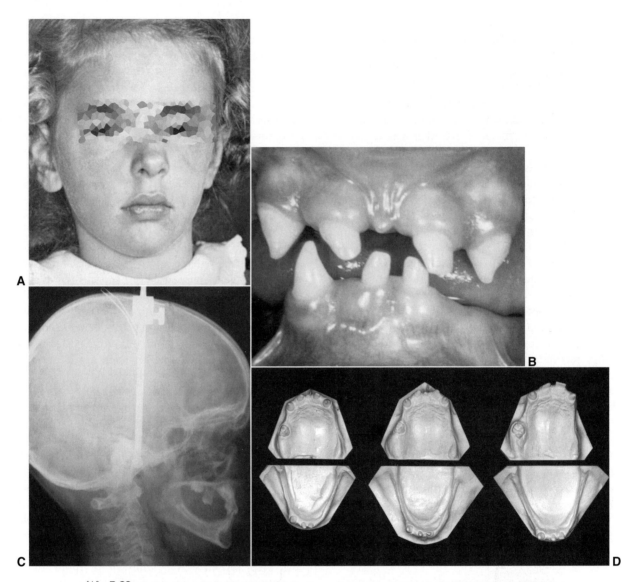

FIG. **7-38. A,** Four-year-old girl with many features of ectodermal dysplasia. There was a history of consanguinity. **B,** The anterior teeth were small and conical in shape. The lack of development of the alveolar process is evident in the photograph. **C,** The facial pattern was good even though many primary and permanent teeth were missing. **D,** Partial dentures were constructed, modified, and remade as additional teeth erupted. The models show how growth has occurred in the mandible and maxilla.

may serve until the child is old enough for implants or fixed bridgework as described in Chapter 22. Orthodontic and surgical procedures may be necessary before the prosthodontic treatment.

Bonding techniques have improved the ability to provide aesthetic interim restorations and greater function for patients with conical teeth with or without oligodontia or hypodontia. Nunn et al published a series of five papers (monthly, beginning in the March 2003 of the *British Dental Journal*) that outline the management of patients with hypodontia by a coordinated interdisciplinary team of dentists and demonstrate

the advantages of this approach.[114] Several dental specialties are represented on the team. Ideally, the initial responsibility for oversight and coordination of the patient's care begins in infancy with the services of a pediatric dentist. As the patient grows and develops through puberty, a general family practitioner may assume the oversight and coordination responsibilities.

When maxillary lateral incisors are missing, the occlusion and arches must be analyzed carefully to determine whether there is sufficient room within the arch to maintain space and to provide fixed bridgework. If space for a normal-sized lateral incisor replacement is

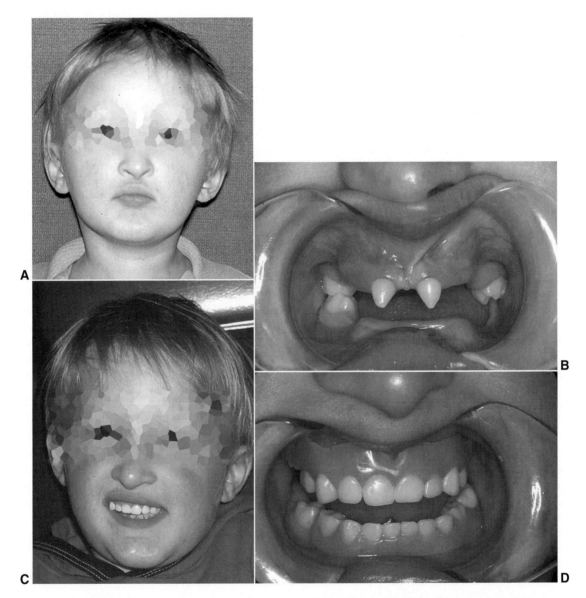

FIG. **7-39.** **A,** Four-year-old boy with characteristics of ectodermal dysplasia. Many primary and permanent teeth are congenitally missing. The skin is dry, and the hair is sparse. **B,** The anterior primary teeth are typically conical. **C** and **D,** A full maxillary overdenture and partial mandibular denture were constructed.

insufficient, the clinician may sometimes choose to move the canine forward into the lateral position and reshape it to make it appear more like a permanent lateral incisor.

INTRINSIC DISCOLORATION OF TEETH (PIGMENTATION OF TEETH)

The primary teeth occasionally have unusual pigmentation. Certain conditions arising from the pulp can cause the whole tooth to appear discolored. Factors causing these conditions include bloodborne pigment, blood decomposition within the pulp, and drugs used in procedures such as root canal therapy. Color changes in relation to trauma are discussed in Chapter 21.

DISCOLORATION IN HYPERBILIRUBINEMIA

Excess levels of bilirubin are released into the blood in a number of conditions.[115] If teeth are developing during periods of hyperbilirubinemia they may become intrinsically stained. The two most common disorders that cause this intrinsic staining are *erythroblastosis fetalis* and *biliary atresia*. Other less common causes are premature birth, ABO incompatibility, neonatal respiratory distress, significant internal hemorrhage, congenital hypothyroidism, biliary hypoplasia, tyrosinemia, α_1-antitrypsin deficiency, and neonatal hepatitis.

Erythroblastosis fetalis results from the transplacental passage of maternal antibody active against red blood cell antigens of the infant, which leads to an increased rate of red blood cell destruction.[116] It is a significant cause of anemia and jaundice in newborn infants despite the development of a method of prevention of maternal isoimmunization by Rh antigens; however, an infant from an Rh-negative mother's first pregnancy rarely contracts this hemolytic disease.

If an infant has had severe, persistent jaundice during the neonatal period, the primary teeth may have a characteristic blue-green color, although in a few instances brown teeth have been observed. The color of the pigmented tooth is gradually reduced. The fading in color is particularly noticeable in the anterior teeth.

Cullen has reported the occurrence of erythroblastosis fetalis produced by Kell immunization.[117] In utero, the maternal antibodies coat the fetal red blood cells and cause hemolysis. The fetus develops anemia with a resultant increase in the bilirubin content of the amniotic fluid. The newborn appears pale and anemic. Shortly after birth, jaundice occurs as a result of the high bilirubin levels.

DISCOLORATION IN PORPHYRIA

The porphyrias are inherited and acquired disorders in which the activities of the enzymes of the heme biosynthetic pathway are partially or almost completely deficient.[118] As a result, abnormally elevated levels of porphyrins and/or their precursors are produced, accumulate in tissues, and are excreted. Congenital erythropoietic porphyria (Günther disease) is a rare autosomal recessive form of the disease.

Children with congenital erythropoietic porphyria have red-colored urine, are hypersensitive to light, and develop subepidermal bullous lesions when their skin is exposed to sunlight. Their primary teeth are purplish brown as a result of the deposition of porphyrin in the developing structures. The permanent teeth also show evidence of intrinsic staining but to a lesser degree.

DISCOLORATION IN CYSTIC FIBROSIS

Cystic fibrosis is an inherited, chronic, multisystem, life-shortening disorder characterized primarily by obstruction and infection of the airways and poor digestion. It is autosomal recessive and is caused by mutations in both copies of the cystic fibrosis transmembrane regulator gene (CFTR). Zegarelli et al have suggested that tooth discoloration in persons with cystic fibrosis is a result of the disease alone; of therapeutic agents, especially tetracyclines; or of a combination of the two factors.[119] The possibility that there is at least in part an intrinsic developmental enamel abnormality secondary to the disease is supported by the investigations of Wright, Hall, and Grubb, who found abnormal enamel in the incisors of homozygous CFTR knockout mice.[120] Further studies by Arquitt, Boyd, and Wright also

strongly suggest that CFTR plays an important role in enamel formation.[121]

It is interesting to note that no papers attributing tooth discoloration in patients with cystic fibrosis to tetracycline therapy have been published in the major scientific journals in more than 10 years. Although many patients with cystic fibrosis who lived during the latter half of the twentieth century endured unsightly discolorations of their teeth because they received tetracycline therapy during a period when their tooth crowns were forming, physicians nowadays rarely, if ever, prescribe tetracyclines for any patients during their tooth-forming years. During the era when tetracycline therapy for children was common, Primosch reported on tetracycline tooth discolorations, enamel defects, and dental caries in 86 young patients with cystic fibrosis.[122] The incidence of dental caries in these patients was compared to that in control subjects matched for sex, race, exposure to optimally fluoridated water, chronologic age, and dental age. The findings indicated a high prevalence of tooth discolorations and enamel defects but a significantly reduced caries experience in the patients with cystic fibrosis who had received the tetracycline drugs.

DISCOLORATION IN TETRACYCLINE THERAPY

Dentists and physicians have observed that children who have received tetracycline therapy during the period of calcification of the primary or permanent teeth show a degree of pigmentation of the clinical crowns of the teeth. As Van der Bijl and Pitigoi-Aron pointed out, because the tetracyclines chelate calcium salts, the drugs are incorporated into bones and teeth during calcification.[123] The crowns of affected teeth are discolored, ranging from yellow to brown and from gray to black (Fig. 7-40). Currently most, if not all, infections in

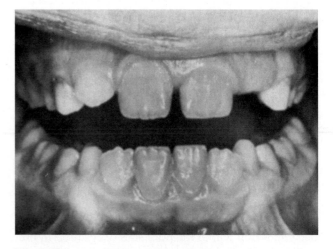

FIG. **7-40.** Pigmentation in tetracycline therapy. The permanent incisors that have erupted show a yellowish brown color.

children can be treated effectively with antibiotics that do not cause tooth discoloration. Consequently this previously common problem is now rarely encountered.

Tetracycline is deposited in the dentin and to a lesser extent in the enamel of teeth that are calcifying during the time the drug is administered. The location of the pigment in the tooth can be correlated with the stage of development of the tooth and the time and duration of drug administration. The tetracyclines, which are yellow, fluoresce under ultraviolet light. When tetracyclines in the dental structures darken from yellow to brown, the fluorescence diminishes because of the destruction of the fluorophore.

The exposure of the teeth to light results in slow oxidation, with a change in color of the pigment from yellow to brown. The larger the dose of drug relative to body weight, the deeper the pigmentation. The duration of exposure to the drug may be less important than the total dose relative to body weight.

Because tetracyclines can be transferred through the placenta, the crowns of the primary teeth may also show noticeable discoloration if tetracyclines are administered during pregnancy. Moffitt et al have observed that the critical period for tetracycline-related discoloration in the primary dentition is 4 months in utero to 3 months postpartum for maxillary and mandibular incisors and 5 months in utero to 9 months postpartum for maxillary and mandibular canines.[124] The sensitive period for tetracycline-induced discoloration in the permanent maxillary and mandibular incisors and canines is 3 to 5 months postpartum to about the seventh year of the child's life. The maxillary lateral incisors are an exception because they begin to calcify at 10 to 12 months postpartum.

BLEACHING OF INTRINSIC TOOTH DISCOLORATION

Vital bleaching of intrinsically discolored teeth became a very popular dental cosmetic procedure during the late twentieth century (Fig. 7-41). Several safe techniques are available to achieve tooth bleaching. The accepted procedures incorporate the use of a peroxide compound placed on the tooth surface that bleaches the intrinsic tooth pigments to a lighter hue. Adding energy to the peroxide compound, as in the form of heat, light, or laser radiation, may accelerate this process.

Although many dilute tooth-bleaching products are available over the counter, the most efficient and effective systems are provided or prescribed by a dentist. To be safe, bleaching procedures must be carefully performed and monitored. Although these procedures are usually performed on permanent teeth, Brantley, Barnes, and Haywood have reported successfully bleaching discolored primary teeth in a 4-year-old girl.[125]

It is beyond the scope of this textbook to describe the various bleaching techniques in detail. The reader is referred to current textbooks on endodontics or cosmetic dentistry for more information. Another valuable resource with considerable detailed information is the Special Supplement of the *Journal of the American Dental Association*, volume 128, April 1997. This supplement provides reports by numerous recognized bleaching experts presented during an international symposium on the subject of nonrestorative treatment of discolored teeth.

If the tooth discoloration is severe and bleaching does not adequately improve the condition, the dentist may consider masking the visible surfaces with bonded veneer restorations similar to those discussed in

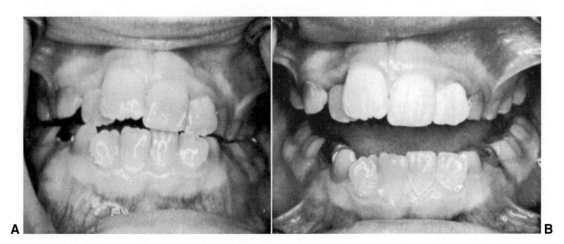

FIG. **7-41. A,** Tetracycline-pigmented teeth. **B,** The maxillary incisors have been bleached; the lower mandibular incisors are untreated.

Chapter 18. Bleaching and enamel microabrasion may be used in combination for certain types of discoloration, and these procedures may also be used as adjunctive steps before placement of veneer restorations.

MICROGNATHIA

Micrognathia is usually considered a congenital anomaly; however, the condition may be acquired in later life. The mandible is most often affected (Fig. 7-42). The etiology of congenital micrognathia appears to be heterogeneous. Deficient nutrition of the mother and intrauterine injury resulting from pressure or trauma have been suggested as possible causes. In addition, micrognathia may be part of the Robin sequence, which also includes cleft palate (especially in the posterior with a rounded distal edge) and glossoptosis. Although this developmental sequence may be sporadic, it is often the pleiotropic expression of a gene for a condition such as Stickler syndrome or velocardiofacial syndrome and warrants a clinical genetic evaluation.[126]

Infants with mandibular micrognathia have difficulty breathing and experience episodes of cyanosis, and must be kept in a ventral position as much as possible. The anterior portion of the mandible is positioned so that the tongue has little if any support and can fall backward, causing an obstruction.

Based on longitudinal growth studies Pruzansky and Richmond reported that, in most instances of congenital micrognathia, the increment in mandibular growth as related to total facial growth during infancy and early childhood is sufficient to overcome the extreme recessiveness of the chin at birth.[127] This is often referred to as "catch-up growth." Daskalogiannakis, Ross, and Tompson performed 29 cephalometric measurements, taken at three different ages, on 96 patients with Robin sequence and compared them to similar measurements in 50 patients with isolated clefting of the palate (control group).[128] They found that patients with Robin sequence had significantly smaller mandibles than the control group from approximately 5.5 years of age to 17 years of age. This finding suggests that the mandibles of patients with Robin sequence do not really grow proportionately more than those in others not affected by the disorder.

The nursing bottle may be used in the treatment of congenital micrognathia to help promote adequate function of the mandible. Because the infant should be made to reach for the nipple of the nursing bottle, the bottle should never be allowed to rest against the mandible. The parent is instructed to sit the infant on his or her lap in an upright position and place gentle forward pressure on the child's ramus with the thumb and fingers while offering the bottle. Thus the infant must extend the mandible to feed. Mandibular advancement by orthopedic force is sometimes recommended by Strohecker and Lahey.[129] Surgical mandibular

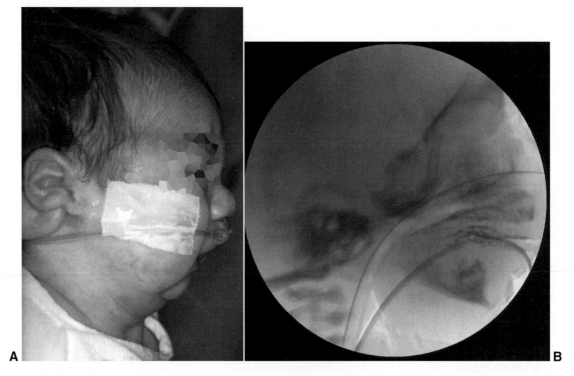

A   **B**

FIG. **7-42. A,** Micrognathia in a girl 1 month of age. The chin was noticeably recessive. **B,** The radiograph shows the extent of the development of the dentition at birth. When the patient was 1 year of age, the micrognathia was less noticeable.

reconstruction in some cases is another option proposed by James and Ma.[130]

Hotz and Gnoinsky have described the use of a special palatal obturator appliance to help infants born with Robin sequence.[131] In addition to providing coverage to seal the cleft palate, the appliance includes a posterior extension to simulate the missing soft palate structures including the uvula. The appliance seems to stimulate the infant to maintain a more normal tongue position. The improved tongue position significantly reduces the tendency for the infant to experience life-threatening apneic episodes. Dean et al also reported successful use of similar appliances in infants with Robin sequence.[132] Their study included 22 infants with severe airway obstruction. Their results supported the use of the obturator, but they also concluded that further study of treatment with these appliances was needed.

Acquired micrognathia may develop gradually and may not be evident until 4 to 6 years of age. This anomaly in growth is usually related to heredity. Ankylosis of the jaw caused by a birth injury or trauma in later life may result in an acquired type of micrognathia. Infection in the temporomandibular joint area can also cause arrested growth at the head of the condyle and lead to development of the acquired pattern of micrognathia. In cases of true ankylosis of the mandible, arthroplasty should be recommended.

ANOMALIES OF THE TONGUE

Pediatric patients with unremarkable medical histories rarely complain of symptomatic tongue lesions. However, the tongue should be inspected carefully during the examination procedure. Several benign conditions may be evident that should be brought to the attention of the parents.

Burket described four main types of papillae of the tongue.[133] Large circumvallate papillae, 10 to 15 in number, may be found on the posterior border of the dorsum. These papillae have a blood supply and are the site of numerous taste buds. Fungiform (mushroom-shaped) papillae may be distributed over the entire dorsum of the tongue; however, they are present in greater numbers at the tip and toward the lateral margins of the tongue. Inflammatory and atrophic changes occurring on the dorsum of the tongue may involve the vascularized fungiform papillae. The most numerous papillae of the tongue are the filiform papillae, which are thin and hairlike and evenly distributed over the dorsal surface. The filiform papillae are without a vascular core, and their continuous growth is slight. The foliate papillae represent a fourth type and are arranged in folds along the lateral margins of the tongue; the taste sensation is associated with these papillae.

MACROGLOSSIA

Macroglossia refers to a larger than normal size of the tongue. This condition may be either congenital or acquired. Congenital macroglossia, which is caused by an overdevelopment of the lingual musculature or vascular tissues, becomes increasingly apparent as the child develops.

An abnormally large tongue is characteristic of hypothyroidism, in which case the tongue is fissured and may extend from the mouth. Macroglossia is also commonly observed with type 2 glycogen-storage disease, neurofibromatosis type 1, and Beckwith-Wiedemann syndrome. It can be an isolated and sporadic (nonfamilial) trait or a familial (autosomal dominant) trait as studied by Reynoso et al.[134] Macroglossia has also been cited as a characteristic of Down syndrome. Occasionally an allergic reaction will cause a transitory enlargement of the tongue (angioneurotic edema). Both allergic reaction and injury can cause such severe enlargement of the tongue that a tracheotomy is necessary to maintain a patent airway.

A disproportionately large tongue may cause both an abnormal growth pattern of the jaw and malocclusion. Flaring of the lower anterior teeth and an Angle class III malocclusion are occasionally the result of macroglossia.

The treatment of macroglossia depends on its cause and severity. Surgical reduction of a portion of the tongue is occasionally necessary.

ANKYLOGLOSSIA (TONGUE-TIE)

In ankyloglossia a short lingual frenum extending from the tip of the tongue to the floor of the mouth and onto the lingual gingival tissue limits movements of the tongue and causes speech difficulties (Fig. 7-43). Stripping of the lingual tissues may occur if the tongue-tie is not corrected. Surgical reduction of the abnormal lingual frenum is indicated if it interferes with the infant's nursing (lingual frenectomy, frenotomy, or frenuloplasty). In the older child a reduction of the frenum should be recommended only if local conditions or speech problems warrant the treatment.

Ayers and Hilton reported a case of ankyloglossia in a 7-year-old boy who had been evaluated at his school for a speech problem.[135] The patient previously had routine dental examinations, but no treatment had been suggested by the dentist. Tongue mobility and speech patterns improved greatly after the frenum attachment was released surgically. The patient and parents reported very little postoperative discomfort. This history and the results are similar to those of the 6-year-old girl with ankyloglossia illustrated in Fig. 7-44. Messner and Lalakea, after studying 30 children aged 1 to 12 years with ankyloglossia, concluded that tongue mobility and speech improve significantly after frenuloplasty.[136]

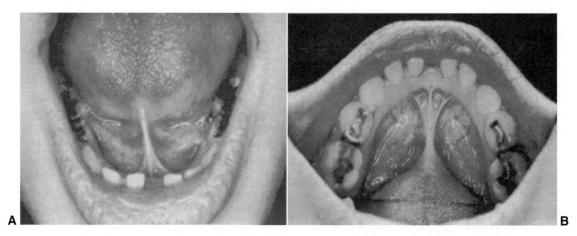

FIG. **7-43. A,** Ankyloglossia (tongue-tie). A short, heavy lingual frenum extends from the top of the tongue to the floor of the mouth and onto the lingual tissue. **B,** A mirror view of the abnormal frenum.

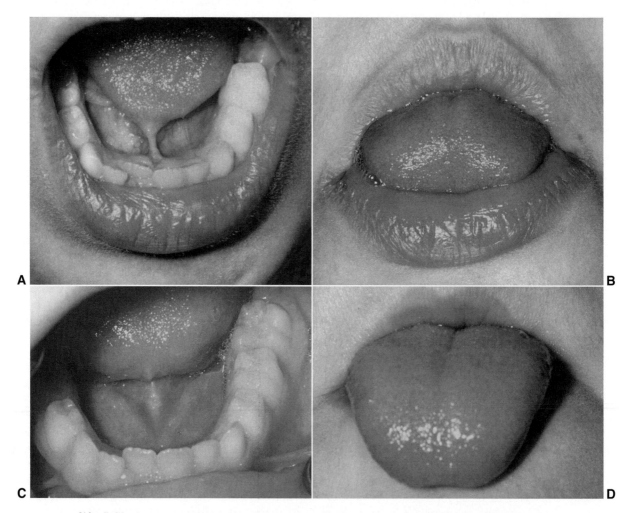

FIG. **7-44. A,** Ankyloglossia in a 6-year-old girl. **B,** Patient had limited tongue mobility and speech problems. **C,** Two weeks after surgical release. **D,** Tongue mobility and speech improved spontaneously.

FISSURED TONGUE AND GEOGRAPHIC TONGUE (BENIGN MIGRATORY GLOSSITIS)

A fissured tongue is seen in a small number of children and may be of no clinical significance, although it is sometimes associated with hypothyroidism and Down syndrome. The fissures on the dorsum of the tongue usually have a symmetric pattern and may be longitudinal or at right angles to the margin of the tongue. Vitamin B–complex deficiency may be associated with the fissuring. Treatment of the fissured tongue is generally unnecessary unless a mild inflammation develops at the base of the fissures from an accumulation of food debris. Brushing of the tongue and improved oral hygiene aid in reducing the inflammation and soreness.

A wandering type of lesion and probably the most common tongue anomaly is known as *geographic tongue.* Rahamimoff and Muhsam observed a 14% prevalence of migratory glossitis in 5000 children 2 years old and younger.[137] Kleinman, Swango, and Pindborg reported a prevalence of geographic tongue of 0.6% in 39,206 children aged 5 to 17 years.[138] Meskin, Redman, and Gorlin have observed the incidence of geographic tongue among college students to be 1.1%.[139]

Kullaa-Mikkonen studied the inheritance of fissured tongue in 31 families and concluded that fissured tongue with smooth-surfaced papillae is transmitted as an autosomal dominant trait with incomplete penetrance and is preceded by geographic tongue.[140] The severity of fissured tongue increased with age. Tongue fissuring with normal-appearing filiform papillae was found not to be familial and was not associated with geographic tongue.

Geographic tongue is often detected during routine dental examination of pediatric patients who are unaware of the condition. Red, smooth areas devoid of filiform papillae appear on the dorsum of the tongue. The margins of the lesions are well developed and slightly raised. The involved areas enlarge and migrate by extension of the desquamation of the papillae at one margin of the lesion and regeneration at the other (Fig. 7-45). Every few days a change can be noted in the pattern of the lesions. The condition is self-limited, however, and no treatment is necessary.

Bánóczy, Szabó, and Csiba have indicated that gastrointestinal disturbances associated with anemia may be related to migratory glossitis.[141] In addition, a psychosomatic disorder should be considered as a

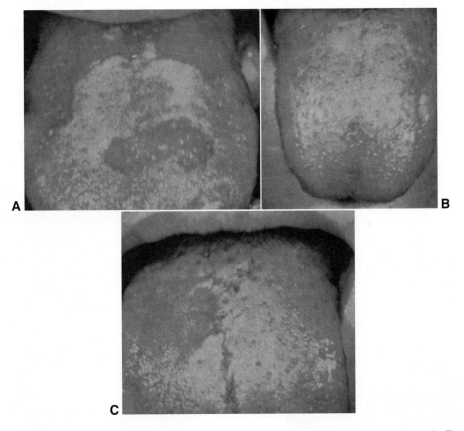

FIG. **7-45. A,** Geographic tongue. The smooth areas are devoid of filiform papillae. **B,** The pattern observed at the initial visit is indistinguishable 4 weeks later. **C,** In 1 year a new pattern is developing on the dorsum of the tongue.

possible etiologic factor. Histologically the process appears to be superficial, with desquamation of the keratin layers of papillae and inflammation of the corium.

COATED TONGUE

A white coating of the tongue is usually associated with local factors. The amount of coating on the tongue varies with the time of day and is related to oral hygiene and the character of the diet. The coating consists of food debris, microorganisms, and keratinized epithelium found on and around the filiform papillae (Fig. 7-46).

Children who have a congenital or acquired deficiency in salivary flow may have a coated tongue, occasionally to the extent that a dry crust appears on the dorsum of the tongue. Frequent rinsings with artificial saliva will palliate the condition. Systemic disease with associated fever and dehydration may also cause a coating, which is usually white but may become stained with foods or drugs. Increased ingestion of liquid is appropriate to alleviate this situation. Brushing the tongue with a toothbrush and dentifrice will reduce the coating.

WHITE STRAWBERRY TONGUE

An enlargement of the fungiform papillae extending above the level of the white desquamating filiform papillae gives the appearance of an unripe strawberry. The condition has been observed in cases of scarlet fever and Kawasaki disease in young children. During the course of scarlet fever and other acute febrile conditions the coating disappears, and the enlarged red papillae extend above a smooth denuded surface, which gives the appearance of a red strawberry or raspberry. The tongue will return to normal after recovery from the systemic condition.

BLACK HAIRY TONGUE

Black hairy tongue is rarely seen in children but occurs in young adults and has been related to the oral and systemic intake of antibiotics, smoking, and excessive ingestion of dark drinks such as coffee and tea (Fig. 7-47). Accumulations of keratin on the filiform papillae in the middle third of the tongue become elongated into hairlike processes, sometimes as long as 2.5 cm (1 inch). Neville et al note that the cause is uncertain but that an apparent increase in keratin production or a decrease in normal keratin desquamation results.[115] It is a benign condition with no serious sequelae. Rigorous hygienic procedures such as brushing and scraping the tongue may help control it. When the condition appears during antibiotic therapy, it usually disappears again without specific treatment after the antibiotics have been discontinued.

INDENTATION OF THE TONGUE MARGIN (CRENATION)

During the examination of the pediatric patient the dentist may notice a scalloping or crenation along the lingual periphery. Careful examination will reveal the markings to be caused by the tongue's lying against the lingual surfaces of the mandibular teeth. Although usually no significance can be attached to these crenations, they have been related to pressure habits, macroglossia, vitamin B–complex deficiency, and systemic disease that causes a reduction of muscle tone.

MEDIAN RHOMBOID GLOSSITIS (CENTRAL PAPILLARY ATROPHY OF THE TONGUE)

Median rhomboid glossitis is an oval, rhomboid, or diamond-shaped reddish patch on the dorsal surface of the tongue immediately anterior to the circumvallate papillae. Flat, slightly raised, or nodular, it stands out distinctly from the rest of the tongue because it has no filiform papillae. This atrophic area is usually

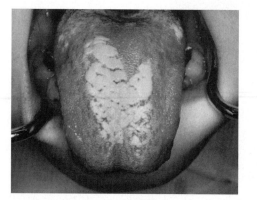

FIG. **7-46.** White coating of the tongue is usually associated with local factors.

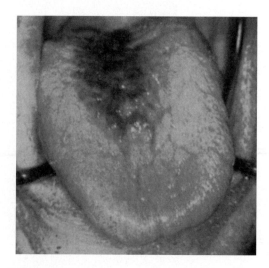

FIG. **7-47.** Black hairy tongue. This condition usually has no clinical significance.

asymptomatic. Long believed to be a developmental anomaly, the condition is now recognized almost exclusively to represent a chronic, localized, and mild candidal infection, as proposed by Cooke.[142]

Although median rhomboid glossitis occurs more often in adults, it is sometimes seen in teenagers and even occurs infrequently in younger children. It has been observed with high prevalence in HIV-positive children by Barasch et al.[143] Treatment with topical antifungal agents is appropriate.

TRAUMA TO THE TONGUE WITH EMPHASIS ON TONGUE PIERCING

A child may bite his or her tongue as a result of a traumatic blow or fall. The dentist may inadvertently traumatize the tongue with a cutting instrument during operative procedures. Deep laceration of the tongue requires suturing to minimize the scarring and to aid in hemorrhage control. In cases of severe injury the tongue should be examined carefully to detect any enlargement that might interfere with the maintenance of an open airway.

Tongue piercing, a deliberate trauma, is one of the popular types of body piercing occurring in all parts of the world today, especially among teenagers and young adults (Fig. 7-48). Tongue piercing is of particular interest in dentistry because it carries a high risk of adverse intraoral sequellae and can have significant systemic effects as well. The scientific literature has exploded with documented cases of complications following piercing procedures. Fractured teeth, dental abrasion, and gingival recession are reported to be common sequelae.[144-146] Other observed complications with life-threatening potential include brain abscess,[147] cephalic tetanus,[148] endocarditis,[149] Ludwig angina,[150] and upper airway compromise.[151] Whenever appropriate, dentists should counsel their patients and other members of the community about the serious risks associated with this form of body art. If patients insist on wearing tongue ornaments and other such body jewelry, they should be advised at least to remove them during athletic activities in which the risk of injury is very high.[152]

ABNORMAL LABIAL FRENUM

A maxillary midline diastema is frequently seen in preschool children and in those in the mixed dentition stage. It is important to determine whether the diastema is normal for that particular time of development or is related to an abnormal maxillary labial frenum.

A midline diastema may be considered normal for many children during the time of eruption of the permanent maxillary central incisors. When the incisors first erupt, they may be separated by bone, and the crowns incline distally because of the crowding of the roots. With the eruption of the lateral incisors and the permanent canines, the midline diastema will be reduced, and in most cases normal contact between the central incisors will develop (see Fig. 27-55).

Insufficient tooth mass in the maxillary anterior region, the presence of peg lateral incisors, or the congenital absence of lateral incisors may cause a diastema. Other factors and anomalies, including a midline supernumerary tooth, an oral habit, macroglossia, and abnormally large mandibular anterior teeth, should be considered as possible causes (in addition to an abnormal labial frenum) of the midline diastema.

The labial frenum is composed of two layers of epithelium enclosing a loose vascular connective tissue. Muscle fibers, if present, are derived from the orbicularis oris muscle.

The origin of the maxillary frenum is at the midline on the inner surface of the lip. The origin is often wide, but the tissue of the frenum itself narrows in width and is inserted in the midline into the outer layer of periosteum and into the connective tissue of the internal maxillary suture and the alveolar process. The exact attachment site is variable. It can be several millimeters above the crest of the ridge or on the ridge, or the fibers may pass between the central incisors and attach to the palatine papilla.

Many dentists delay considering an abnormal labial frenum as the cause of a diastema until all the maxillary permanent anterior teeth, including the canines, have erupted. This approach may be considered generally correct. However, other diagnostic points should be kept in mind.

One can carry out a simple diagnostic test for an abnormal frenum during mid to late mixed dentition by observing the location of the alveolar attachment when intermittent pressure is exerted on the frenum. If a

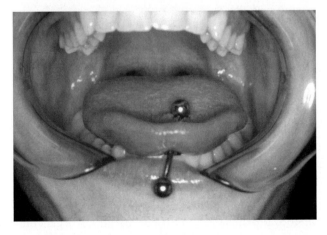

FIG. **7-48.** An example of a tongue ornament very popular among teenagers and young adults.

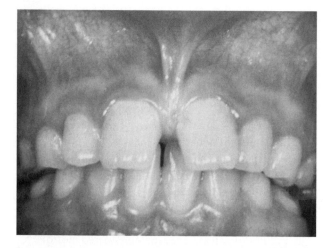

FIG. **7-49.** Abnormal labial frenum. There is blanching of the free marginal tissue between the central incisors and also of the palatine papilla. A frenectomy is indicated.

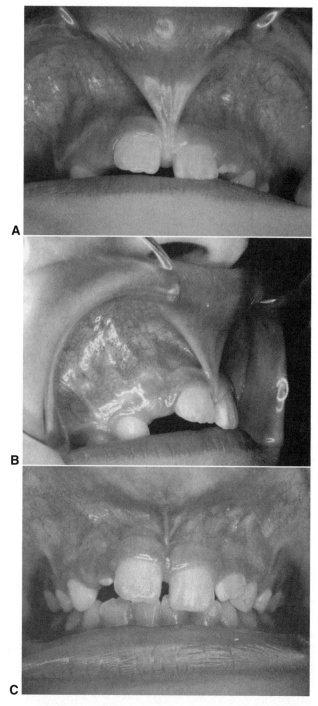

FIG. **7-50. A,** Abnormal labial frenum in an 8-year-old child. The heavy, fan-shaped band of tissue interfered with speech and presented an undesirable appearance. **B,** An oblique view of the abnormal frenum. **C,** A much more desirable appearance is observed 6 months after the frenectomy.

heavy band of tissue with a broad, fanlike base is attached to the palatine papilla and produces blanching of the papilla, it is safe to predict that the frenum will unfavorably influence the development of the anterior occlusion (Fig. 7-49).

The abnormal labial frenum, in addition to causing a midline diastema, can produce other undesirable clinical conditions. The heavy band of tissue and low attachment can interfere with toothbrushing by making it difficult to place the brush at the proper level in the vestibule to brush in the conventional manner. If fibers of the frenum attach into the free marginal tissue, stretching of the lip during mastication and speech may cause stripping of the tissue from the neck of the tooth. Such attachment may also cause the accumulation of food particles and eventual pocket formation. The abnormal frenum may restrict movements of the lip, may interfere with speech, and may produce an undesirable cosmetic result (Fig. 7-50).

FRENECTOMY

The decision regarding treatment of the labial frenum should be made only after a careful evaluation to determine whether the result will be undesirable if the condition is allowed to remain.

In the surgical technique, a wedge-shaped section of tissue is removed, including the tissue between the central incisors and the tissue extending palatally to the nasal palatine papilla (Figs. 7-50 and 7-51). Lateral incisions are made on either side of the frenum to the depth of the underlying bone. The free marginal tissue on the mesial side of the central incisors should not be disturbed. The wedge of tissue can be picked up with tissue forceps and excised with tissue shears at an area close enough to the origin of the frenum to provide a desirable cosmetic effect. Sutures are placed inside the lip to approximate the free tissue margins. It is generally unnecessary to suture or pack the tissue between the incisors.

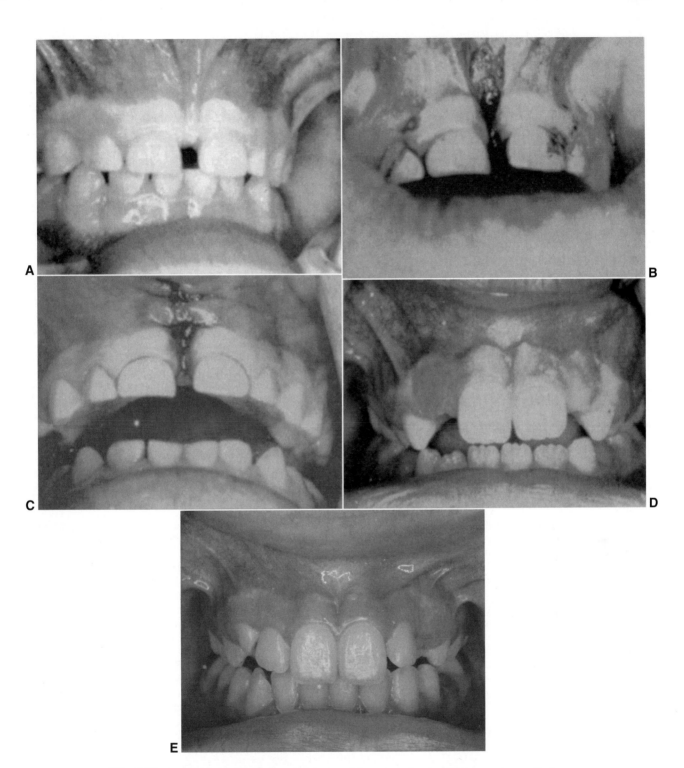

FIG. **7-51. A,** Abnormal labial frenum observed in a preschool child is causing a diastema between the primary central incisors and is interfering with normal movement of the upper lip. **B,** A wedge-shaped section of tissue including the frenum has been removed. **C,** Two sutures have been placed to approximate the tissue margins. **D,** The permanent incisors have erupted. No reattachment of the frenum fibers has occurred. **E,** A desirable result of the frenectomy is evident 5 years after the surgical procedure.

REFERENCES

1. US Department of Health and Human Services: Oral health in America: a report of the Surgeon General, Rockville, Md, 2000, US Department of Health and Human Services, National Institute of Dental and Craniofacial Research, National Institutes of Health.
2. Molinari JM: Microbial disease trends and acquired antibiotic resistance. Part I. *Compendium* 18:106-108, 1997.
3. Bader G: Odontomatosis (multiple odontomas), *Oral Surg Oral Med Oral Pathol* 23:770-773, 1967.
4. Delaney GM, Goldblatt LI: Fused teeth: a multidisciplinary approach to treatment, *J Am Dent Assoc* 103:732-734, 1981.
5. Eidelman E: Fusion of maxillary primary central and lateral incisors bilaterally, *Pediatr Dent* 3:346-347, 1981.
6. Nanni L et al: SSH mutation is associated with solitary median maxillary central incisor: a study of 13 patients and review of the literature, *Am J Med Genet* 102:1-10, 2001.
7. Holan G: Dens invaginatus in a primary canine: a case report, *Int J Paediatr Dent* 8:61-64, 1998.
8. Kupietzky A: Detection of dens invaginatus in a one-year-old infant, *Pediatr Dent* 22:148-150, 2000.
9. Eden EK, Koca H, Sen BH: Dens invaginatus in a primary molar: report of a case, *J Dent Child* 69:49-53, 2002.
10. Grahnen H, Lindahl B, Omnell KA: Dens invaginatus. I. A clinical, roentgenological and genetical study of permanent upper lateral incisors, *Odont Rev* 10:115-137, 1959.
11. Hu CC et al: A clinical and research protocol for characterizing patients with hypophosphatasia, *Pediatr Dent* 18:17-23, 1996.
12. Scriver CR, Cameron D: Pseudohypophosphatasia, *N Engl J Med* 281:604-606, 1969.
13. Ayoub AF, el-Mofty SS: Cherubism: report of an aggressive case and review of the literature, *J Oral Maxillofac Surg* 51:702-705, 1993.
14. Kalentar Motamedi MH: Treatment of cherubism with locally aggressive behavior presenting in adulthood: report of four cases and a proposed new grading system, *J Oral Maxillofac Surg* 56:1336-1342, 1998.
15. Silva EC et al: An extreme case of cherubism, *Br J Oral Maxillofac Surg* 40:45-48, 2002.
16. Timosca GC et al: Aggressive form of cherubism: report of a case, *J Oral Maxillofac Surg* 58:336-344, 2000.
17. Grunebaum M, Tiqva P: Nonfamilial cherubism: report of two cases, *J Oral Surg* 31:632-635, 1973.
18. DeTomasi DC, Hann JR, Stewart HM Jr: Cherubism: report of a nonfamilial case, *J Am Dent Assoc* 111:455-457, 1985.
19. Rattan V et al: Non-familial cherubism—a case report, *J Indian Soc Pedod Prev Dent* 15:118-120, 1997.
20. Mangion J et al: The gene for cherubism maps to chromosome 4p16.3, *Am J Hum Genet* 65:151-157, 1999.
21. Tiziani V et al: The gene for cherubism maps to chromosome 4p16, *Am J Hum Genet* 65:158-166, 1999.
22. Ueki Y et al: Mutations in the gene encoding c-Abl-binding protein SH3BP2 cause cherubism, *Nat Genet* 28:125-126, 2001.
23. McDonald RE, Shafer WG: Disseminated juvenile fibrous dysplasia of the jaws, *Am J Dis Child* 89:354-358, 1955.
24. Pierce AM et al: Fifteen-year follow-up of a family with inherited craniofacial fibrous dysplasia, *J Oral Maxillofac Surg* 54:780-788, 1996.
25. Peters WJN: Cherubism: a study of twenty cases from one family, *Oral Surg* 47:307-311, 1979.
26. Von Wowern N: Cherubism: a 36-year long-term follow-up of two generations in different families and review of the literature, *Oral Surg Oral Med Oral Pathol Oral Radiol Endod* 90:765-772, 2000.
27. Weinstein M, Bernstein S: Pink ladies: mercury poisoning in twin girls, *CMAJ* 168:201-203, 2003.
28. Horowitz Y et al: Acrodynia: a case report of two siblings, *Arch Dis Child* 86:453-455, 2002.
29. Hartsfield JK Jr: Premature exfoliation of teeth in childhood and adolescence, *Adv Pediatr* 41:453-470, 1994.
30. HYP Consortium: A gene (HYP) with homologies to endopeptidases is mutated in patients with X-linked hypophosphatemic rickets, *Nat Genet* 11:130-136, 1995.
31. McWhorter AG, Seale NS: Prevalence of dental abscess in a population of children with vitamin D–resistant rickets, *Pediatr Dent* 13:91-96, 1991.
32. Shroff DV, McWhorter AG, Seale NS: Evaluation of aggressive pulp therapy in a population of vitamin D–resistant rickets patients: a follow-up of 4 cases, *Pediatr Dent* 24:347-349, 2002.
33. Rakocz M, Keating J 3rd, Johnson R: Management of the primary dentition in vitamin D–resistant rickets, *Oral Surg Oral Med Oral Pathol* 54:166-171, 1982.
34. Horwitz M et al: Mutations in ELA2, encoding neutrophil elastase, define a 21-day biological clock in cyclic haematopoiesis, *Nat Genet* 23:433-436, 1999.
35. da Fonseca MA, Fontes F: Early tooth loss due to cyclic neutropenia: long-term follow-up of one patient, *Spec Care Dentist* 20:187-190, 2000.
36. Seow WK et al: Mineral deficiency in the pathogenesis of enamel hypoplasia in prematurely born, very low birthweight children, *Pediatr Dent* 11:297-302, 1989.
37. Slayton RL et al: Prevalence of enamel hypoplasia and isolated opacities in the primary dentition, *Pediatr Dent* 32:32-36, 2001.
38. Sarnat BG, Schour I: Enamel hypoplasia (chronologic enamel aplasia) in relation to systemic disease: a chronologic, morphologic, and etiologic classification, *J Am Dent Assoc* 28:1989-2000, 1941; 29:67-75, 1942.
39. Sheldon M, Bibby BG, Bales MS: Relationship between microscopic enamel defects and infantile disabilities, *J Dent Res* 24:109-116, 1945.
40. Purvis RJ et al: Enamel hypoplasia of the teeth associated with neonatal tetany: a manifestation of maternal vitamin D deficiency, *Lancet* 2:811-814, 1973.
41. Herman SC, McDonald RE: Enamel hypoplasia in cerebral palsied children, *J Dent Child* 30:46-49, 1963.
42. Cohen HJ, Diner H: The significance of developmental dental enamel defects in neurological diagnosis, *Pediatrics* 46:737-747, 1970.
43. Martinez A et al: Prevalence of developmental enamel defects in mentally retarded children, *J Dent Child* 69:151-155, 2002.
44. Oliver WJ, Owings CL: Hypoplastic enamel associated with the nephrotic syndrome, *Pediatrics* 32:399-406, 1963.
45. Koch MJ et al: Enamel hypoplasia of primary teeth in chronic renal failure, *Pediatr Nephrol* 13:68-72, 1999.
46. Rattner LJ, Myers HM: Occurrence of enamel hypoplasia in children with congenital allergies, *J Dent Res* 41:646-649, 1962.
47. Lawson BF, Stout FW: The incidence of enamel hypoplasia associated with chronic lead poisoning, *S C Dent J* 29:5-10, 1971.

48. Pearl M, Roland NM: Delayed primary dentition in a case of congenital lead poisoning, *J Dent Child* 47:269-271, 1980.

49. Turner JG: Two cases of hypoplasia of enamel, *Br J Dent Sci* 55:227-228, 1912.

50. Bauer WH: Effect of periapical processes of deciduous teeth on the buds of permanent teeth, *Am J Orthod* 32:232-241, 1946.

51. Mink JR: Relationship of enamel hypoplasia and trauma in repaired cleft lip and palate, thesis, Indianapolis, 1961, Indiana University School of Dentistry.

52. Dixon DA: Defects of structure and formation of the teeth in persons with cleft palate and the effect of reparative surgery on dental tissues, *Oral Surg Oral Med Oral Pathol* 25:435-446, 1968.

53. Vichi M, Franchi L: Abnormalities of the maxillary incisors in children with cleft lip and palate, *J Dent Child* 62:412-417, 1995.

54. Kaste SC et al: Dental abnormalities in children treated for acute lymphoblastic leukemia, *Leukemia* 11:792-796, 1997.

55. Maguire A, Welbury RR: Long-term effects of antineoplastic chemotherapy and radiotherapy on dental development, *Dent Update* 23(5):188-194, 1996.

56. Musselman RJ: Dental defects and rubella embryopathy: a clinical study of fifty children, thesis, Indianapolis, 1968, Indiana University School of Dentistry.

57. Levy SM et al: Primary tooth fluorosis and fluoride intake during the first year of life, *Community Dent Oral Epidemiol* 30:286-295, 2002.

58. Everett ET et al: Dental fluorosis: variability among different inbred mouse strains, *J Dent Res* 81:794-798, 2002.

59. McCloskey RJ: A technique for removal of fluorosis stains, *J Am Dent Assoc* 109:63-64, 1984.

60. Croll TP, Cavanaugh RR: Enamel color modification by controlled hydrochloric acid-pumice abrasion. I. Technique and examples, *Quintessence Int* 17:81-86, 1986.

61. Croll TP, Cavanaugh RR: Enamel color modification by controlled hydrochloric acid-pumice abrasion. II. Further examples, *Quintessence Int* 17:157-164, 1986.

62. Dalzell DP, Howes RI, Hubler PM: Microabrasion: effect of time, number of applications, and pressure on enamel loss, *Pediatr Dent* 17:207-211, 1995.

63. Croll TP: Enamel microabrasion: observations after 10 years, *J Am Dent Assoc* 128(suppl):45S-50S, 1997.

64. Croll TP, Helpin ML: Enamel microabrasion: a new approach, *J Esthet Dent* 12:64-71, 2000.

65. Muhler JC: Effect of apical inflammation of the primary teeth on dental caries in the permanent teeth, *J Dent Child* 24:209-210, 1957.

66. Mueller BH et al: "Caries-like" resorption of unerupted permanent teeth, *J Pedod* 4:166-172, 1980.

67. Holan G, Eidelman E, Mass E: Pre-eruptive coronal resorption of permanent teeth: report of three cases and their treatments, *Pediatr Dent* 16:373-377, 1994.

68. Savage NW, Gentner M, Symons AL: Preeruptive intra-coronal radiolucencies: review and report of case, *J Dent Child* 65:36-40, 1998.

69. Seow WK, Wan A, McAllan LH: The prevalence of pre-eruptive dentin radiolucencies in the permanent dentition, *Pediatr Dent* 26:26-33, 1999.

70. Seow WK, Lu PC, McAllan LH: Prevalence of pre-eruptive intracoronal dentin defects from panoramic radiographs, *Pediatr Dent* 26:332-339, 1999.

71. Lysell L: Taurodontism: a case report and a survey of the literature, *Odontol Rev* 13(2):158-174, 1962.

72. Jaspers MT, Witkop CJ Jr: Taurodontism: an isolated trait associated with syndromes and X-chromosomal aneuploidy, *Am J Hum Genet* 32:396-413, 1980.

73. Mena CA: Taurodontism, *Oral Surg* 32:812-823, 1971.

74. Gedik R, Çimen M: Multiple taurodontism: report of case, *J Dent Child* 67:216-217, 2000.

75. Bixler D, Conneally PM, Christen AG: Dentinogenesis imperfecta: genetic variations in a six-generation family, *J Dent Res* 69:1196-1199, 1969.

76. Witkop CJ Jr: *Genetics and dental health,* New York, 1961, McGraw-Hill.

77. Witkop CJ Jr: Manifestations of genetic diseases in the human pulp, *Oral Surg* 32:278-316, 1971.

78. Shields SD, Bixler D, El-Kafrawy AM: A proposal classification for heritable human dentin defects with a description of a new entity, *Arch Oral Biol* 18:543-554, 1973.

79. Zhang X et al: DSPP mutation in dentinogenesis imperfecta Shields type II, *Nat Genet* 27:151–152, 2001.

80. Xiao S et al: Dentinogenesis imperfecta 1 with or without progressive hearing loss is associated with distinct mutations in DSPP, *Nat Genet* 27:201–204, 2001.

81. Sreenath T et al: Dentin sialophosphoprotein knockout mouse teeth display widened predentin zone and develop defective dentin mineralization similar to human dentinogenesis imperfecta type III, *J Biol Chem* 278:24874-24880, 2003.

82. Dean JA et al: Dentin dysplasia, type II linkage to chromosome 4q, *J Craniofac Genet Dev Biol* 17:172-177, 1997.

83. Rajpar MH et al: Mutation of the signal peptide region of the bicistronic gene DSPP affects translocation to the endoplasmic reticulum and results in defective dentine biomineralization, *Hum Mol Genet* 11:2559-2565, 2002.

84. Cartwright AR, Kula K, Wright JT: Craniofacial features associated with amelogenesis imperfecta, *J Craniofac Genet Dev Biol* 19:148-156, 1999.

85. Aldred MJ, Crawford PJ: Amelogenesis imperfecta—towards a new classification, *Oral Dis* 1:2-5, 1995.

86. Hart PS et al: A nomenclature for X-linked amelogenesis imperfecta, *Arch Oral Biol* 47:255-260, 2002.

87. Hart PS et al: Identification of the enamelin (g.8344delG) mutation in a new kindred and presentation of a standardized ENAM nomenclature, *Arch Oral Biol* 48:589-596, 2003.

88. Aldred MJ et al: Genetic heterogeneity in X-linked amelogenesis imperfecta, *Genomics* 14:567-573, 1992.

89. Congleton J, Burkes EJ: Amelogenesis imperfecta with taurodontism, *Oral Surg* 48:540-544, 1979.

90. Seow WK: Taurodontism of the mandibular first permanent molar distinguishes between the tricho-dento-osseous (TDO) syndrome and amelogenesis imperfecta, *Clin Genet* 43:240-246, 1993.

91. Price JA et al: A common DLX3 gene mutation is responsible for tricho-dento-osseous syndrome in Virginia and North Carolina families, *J Med Genet* 35:825-828, 1998.

92. Price JA et al: Tricho-dento-osseous syndrome and amelogenesis imperfecta with taurodontism are genetically distinct conditions, *Clin Genet* 56:35-40, 1999.

93. Patel RA et al: X-linked (recessive) hypomaturation amelogenesis imperfecta: a prosthodontic, genetic, and histopathologic report, *J Prosthet Dent* 66:398-402, 1991.

94. Chaudhry AP et al: Odontogenesis imperfecta: report of a case, *Oral Surg* 14:1099-1103, 1961.

95. Schimmelpfennig CB, McDonald RE: Enamel and dentin aplasia: report of a case, *Oral Surg* 6:1444-1449, 1953.

96. Gorlin RJ, Herman NG, Moss SJ: Complete absence of the permanent dentition: an autosomal recessive disorder, *Am J Med Genet* 5:207-209, 1980 (letter).

97. Swallow JN: Complete anodontia of the permanent dentition, *Br Dent J* 107:143-145, 1959.

98. Schneider PE: Complete anodontia of the permanent dentition: case report, *Pediatr Dent* 12:112-114, 1990.

99. Laird GS: Congenital anodontia, *J Am Dent Assoc* 51:722, 1955.

100. Witkop CJ Jr: Agenesis of succedaneous teeth: an expression of the homozygous state of the gene for the pegged or missing maxillary lateral incisor trait, *Am J Med Genet* 26:431-436, 1987.

101. Glenn FB: A consecutive six-year study of the prevalence of congenitally missing teeth in private practice of two geographically separated areas, *J Dent Child* 31:269-270, 1964.

102. Grahnen H: Hypodontia in the permanent dentition, *Dent Abstr* 3:308-309, 1957.

103. Vastardis H et al: A human MSX1 homeodomain missense mutation causes selective tooth agenesis, *Nat Genet* 13: 417-421, 1996.

104. Stockton DW et al: Mutation of PAX9 is associated with oligodontia, *Nat Genet* 24:18-19, 2000.

105. Erpenstein H, Pfeiffer RA: Geschlechsgebunden-dominant erbliche zahnunterzahl, *Humangenetik* 4:280-293, 1967.

106. Ahmad W et al: A locus for autosomal recessive hypodontia with associated dental anomalies maps to chromosome 16q12.1, *Am J Hum Genet* 62:987-991, 1998 (letter).

107. Bennett CG, Ronk SL: Congenitally missing primary teeth: report of case, *J Dent Child* 47:346-348, 1980.

108. Shashikiran ND, Karthik V, Subbareddy VV: Multiple congenitally missing primary teeth: report of a case, *Pediatr Dent* 24:149-152, 2002.

109. Fleming P, Nelson J, Gorlin RJ: Single maxillary central incisor in association with mid-line anomalies, *Br Dent J* 168:476-479, 1990.

110. Monreal AW, Zonana J, Ferguson B: Identification of a new splice form of the EDA1 gene permits detection of nearly all X-linked hypohidrotic ectodermal dysplasia mutations, *Am J Hum Genet* 63:380-389, 1998.

111. Giansanti JS, Long SM, Rankin JL: The "tooth and nail" type of autosomal dominant ectodermal dysplasia, *Oral Surg* 37:576-582, 1974.

112. Jumlongras D et al: A nonsense mutation in MSX1 causes Witkop syndrome, *Am J Hum Genet* 69:67-74, 2001.

113. Hudson CD, Witkop CJ Jr: Autosomal dominant hypodontia with nail dysgenesis, *Oral Surg* 39:409-423, 1975.

114. Nunn JH et al: The interdisciplinary management of hypodontia: background and role of paediatric dentistry, *Br Dent J* 194:245-251, 2003.

115. Neville BW et al: *Oral and maxillofacial pathology*, ed 2, Philadelphia, 2002, WB Saunders.

116. Stoll BJ, Kliegman RM: Hemolytic disease of the newborn (erythroblastosis fetalis). In Behrman RE, Kliegman RM, Jenson HB, editors: *Nelson textbook of pediatrics*, ed 17, Philadelphia, 2004, WB Saunders, pp 601-606.

117. Cullen LP: Erythroblastosis fetalis produced by Kell immunization: dental findings, *Pediatr Dent* 12:393-395, 1990.

118. Sassa S: The Porphyrias. In Behrman RE, Kliegman RM, Jenson HB: *Nelson textbook of pediatrics*, ed 17, Philadelphia, 2004, WB Saunders, pp 495-504.

119. Zegarelli EV et al: Discoloration of teeth in a 24-year-old patient with cystic fibrosis of the pancreas not primarily associated with tetracycline therapy, *Oral Surg* 24:62-64, 1967.

120. Wright JT, Hall KI, Grubb BR: Enamel mineral composition of normal and cystic fibrosis transgenic mice, *Adv Dent Res* 10:270-274, 1996.

121. Arquitt CK, Boyd C, Wright JT: Cystic fibrosis transmembrane regulator gene (CFTR) is associated with abnormal enamel formation, *J Dent Res* 81:492-496, 2002.

122. Primosch RE: Tetracycline discoloration, enamel defects, and dental caries in patients with cystic fibrosis, *Oral Surg* 50:301-308, 1980.

123. Van der Bijl P, Pitigoi-Aron G: Tetracyclines and calcified tissues, *Ann Dent* 54:69-72, 1995.

124. Moffitt JM et al: Prediction of tetracycline-induced tooth discoloration, *J Am Dent Assoc* 88:547-552, 1974.

125. Brantley DH, Barnes KP, Haywood VB: Bleaching primary teeth with 10% carbamide peroxide, *Pediatr Dent* 23: 514-516, 2001.

126. Gorlin RJ, Cohen MM Jr, Hennekam RCM: *Syndromes of the head and neck*, ed 4, New York, 2001, Oxford University Press.

127. Pruzansky S, Richmond JB: Growth of mandible in infants with micrognathia: clinical implications, *Am J Dis Child* 88:29-42, 1954.

128. Daskalogiannakis J, Ross RB, Tompson BD: The mandibular catch-up growth controversy in Pierre Robin sequence, *Am J Orthod Dentofacial Orthop* 120:280-285, 2001.

129. Strohecker B, Lahey D: Mandibular elongation by bone distraction: treatment for mandibular hypoplasia with Robin sequence, *Plast Surg Nurs* 17:8-10, 15, 1997.

130. James D, Ma L: Mandibular reconstruction in children with obstructive sleep apnea due to micrognathia, *Plast Reconstr Surg* 100:1131-1137, 1997.

131. Hotz M, Gnoinski W: Clefts of the secondary palate associated with the "Pierre Robin syndrome." Management by early maxillary orthopaedics, *Swed Dent J Suppl* 15:89-98, 1982.

132. Dean J et al: Prevention of airway obstruction in Pierre Robin sequence via obturator use, *Pediatr Dent* 24:173-174, 2002 (abstract).

133. Burket LW: *Oral medicine: diagnosis and treatment*, ed 7, Philadelphia, 1977, JB Lippincott.

134. Reynoso MC et al: Autosomal dominant congenital macroglossia: further delineation of the syndrome, *Genet Couns* 5:151-154, 1994.

135. Ayers FJ, Hilton LM: Treatment of ankyloglossia: report of case, *J Dent Child* 44:237-239, 1977.

136. Messner AH and Lalakea ML: The effect of ankyloglossia on speech in children, *Otolaryngol Head Neck Surg* 127:539-545, 2002.

137. Rahamimoff P, Muhsam HV: Some observations on 1,246 cases of geographic tongue, *AMA J Dis Child* 93:519-525, 1957.

138. Kleinman DV, Swango PA, Pindborg JJ: Epidemiology of oral mucosal lesions in United States schoolchildren: 1986-87, *Community Dent Oral Epidemiol* 22:243-253, 1994.

139. Meskin LH, Redman RS, Gorlin RJ: Incidence of geographic tongue among 3,668 students at the University of Minnesota, *J Dent Res* 42:895, 1963.

140. Kullaa-Mikkonen A: Familial study of fissured tongue, *Scand J Dent Res* 96:366-375, 1988.

141. Bánóczy J, Szabó L, Csiba A: Migratory glossitis: a clinical-histologic review of seventy cases, *Oral Surg* 39:113-121, 1975.

142. Cooke BE: Median rhomboid glossitis. Candidiasis and not a developmental anomaly, *Br J Dermatol* 93:399-405, 1975.

143. Barasch A et al: Oral soft tissue manifestations in HIV-positive vs. HIV-negative children from an inner city population: a two-year observational study, *Pediatr Dent* 22:215-220, 2000.

144. Campbell A et al: Tongue piercing: impact of time and barbell stem length on lingual gingival recession and tooth chipping, *J Periodontol* 73:289-297, 2002.

145. De Moor RJ et al: Tongue piercing and associated oral and dental complications, *Endod Dent Traumotol* 16:232-237, 2000.

146. Ram D, Peretz B: Tongue piercing and insertion of metal studs: three cases of dental and oral consequences, *J Dent Child* 67:326-329, 2000.

147. Martinello RA, Cooney EL: Cerebellar brain abscess associated with tongue piercing, *Clin Infect Dis* 36:e32-34, 2003.

148. Dyce O et al: Tongue piercing. The new "rusty nail"? *Head Neck* 22:728-732, 2000.

149. Akhondi H, Rahimi AR: *Haemophilus aphrophilus* endocarditis after tongue piercing, *Emerg Infect Dis* 8:850-851, 2002.

150. Perkins CS, Meisner J, Harrison JM: A complication of tongue piercing, *Br Dent J* 182:147-148, 1997.

151. Keogh IJ, O'Leary G: Serious complication of tongue piercing, *J Laryngol Otol* 115:233-234, 2001.

152. McGeary SP, Studen-Pavlovich D, Ranalli DN: Oral piercing in athletes: implications for general dentists, *Gen Dent* 50:168-172, 2002.

8

Tumors of the Oral Soft Tissues and Cysts and Tumors of the Bone

JOHN S. McDONALD

Not only is it the responsibility of the dental practitioner to oversee the care and maintenance of the teeth and periodontium of each patient, but also it is at least as important to monitor and help maintain the overall health and well-being of that individual as manifested in the orofacial and head and neck structures that are so obviously within the purview of the dental profession. It is all too easy to focus strictly on the dental needs of the patient and remain oblivious to subtle or even not so subtle lumps, bumps, swellings, or changes in texture or color that may signify the presence of a reactive or a hamartomatous overgrowth of tissue or a benign or malignant disease. Oral tumors occur too often for the dentist to take the attitude that these lesions happen only in someone else's patients.

The purpose of this chapter is not to present a comprehensive treatise on oral tumors and cysts in children but to provide an overview of some of the more frequently encountered ones that may be found in the oral soft tissues and bone in the pediatric age group.

BENIGN TUMORS OF THE ORAL SOFT TISSUE

SQUAMOUS PAPILLOMA AND VERRUCA VULGARIS

The squamous papilloma is a relatively common, benign neoplasm that arises from the surface epithelium. It is typically an exophytic lesion whose surface may vary from cauliflower-like to fingerlike in appearance, and although it is generally a pedunculated lesion, it may arise from a sessile base. Although the average age of occurrence is in the fourth decade of life, nearly 20% of cases have been noted by Abbey, Page, and Sawyer and by Greer and Goldman to occur before 20 years of age.[1,2] The most common sites of occurrence appear to be the tongue and palatal complex, followed by the buccal mucosa, gingiva, and lips. This lesion is also seen with some frequency on the alveolar ridge, floor of the mouth, and retromolar pad regions.

Oral verruca vulgaris, or oral warts, are exophytic papillomatous lesions indistinguishable clinically from oral squamous cell papillomas. Like their skin counterpart, the common wart (verruca vulgaris), they are a viral disorder associated with the human papillomavirus (HPV) and may be spread to the oral cavity in children through autoinoculation by finger or thumb sucking (Fig. 8-1). According to Praetorius's review of HPV-associated diseases of oral mucosa, types 2 and 57 were most commonly found.[3] In addition, DNA types 6, 11, and 16 have been demonstrated in oral verrucae as reported by Naghashfar et al as well as by Zeuss, Miller, and White.[4,5]

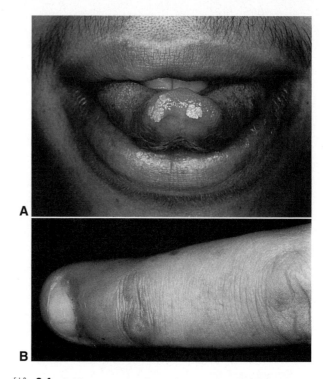

FIG. **8-1. A,** Verruca vulgaris on the anterior tip of the tongue. This is an example of autoinoculation from finger sucking. **B,** Notice the wart on this patient's finger from which he inoculated his tongue. *(Courtesy Dr. Mark L. Bernstein.)*

Although the histopathologic differences between squamous papilloma and verruca vulgaris are subtle, these lesions are distinguishable from one another, and HPV has been detected in some squamous papillomas. In one study by Jenson et al, HPV was found in two of five multiple papillomas, and in another study by Löning et al, it was reported that five of six clinically and morphologically defined papillomas tested positive for HPV-associated antigens.[6,7] Syrjänen, Syrjänen, and Lamburg used the in situ DNA hybridization technique and reported the presence of HPV antigens in 57% of squamous papillomas studied.[8] The types of HPV identified in the study of Syrjänen et al and in a subsequent report by Eversole and Laipis were HPV-6 and HPV-11.[9] Ward et al detected the presence of HPV DNA types 6 and 11 in 68% of clinically diagnosed and histologically confirmed oral squamous cell papillomas analyzed by the highly sensitive polymerase chain reaction technique followed by dot blot hybridization of the polymerase chain reaction product with digoxigenin-labeled, type-specific oligonucleotide probes for HPV DNA types 6, 11, 16, and 18.[10]

Histologically, the papilloma is seen as a proliferation of the spinous cell layer in a papillary pattern, often with hyperkeratosis, acanthosis, and basilar hyperplasia. Mitotic figures may be prominent. The supporting fibrous connective tissue stroma often contains prominent numbers of small blood vessels as well as an inflammatory cell infiltrate. The presence of a coarse keratohyalin granular cell layer and vacuolated cells with pyknotic nuclei (koilocytes) may be used to differentiate verruca vulgaris from a squamous papilloma. Treatment of either the oral squamous papilloma or verruca vulgaris is best accomplished by complete surgical excision of the lesion, including the base.

FIBROMA

The fibroma is the most common benign soft tissue tumor found in the oral cavity. It is characteristically a dome-shaped lesion with a sessile base and a smooth surface that is usually the color of the surrounding mucosa. It may vary from firm to flaccid in texture and most commonly occurs in sites predisposed to irritation or trauma, such as the buccal mucosa, lip, tongue, gingiva, and hard palate. It may occur at any age. Sometimes termed *focal fibrous hyperplasia,* a fibroma occurring in the oral cavity is reactive in nature, being basically either a reactive type of fibrous hyperplasia or in some cases a healed pyogenic granuloma that has undergone sclerosis.

Histologically the fibroma is a dome-shaped lesion composed of a fibrous connective tissue stroma that may vary from loose and delicate to quite dense in its appearance, with an overlying layer of stratified squamous epithelium. Treatment consists of simple surgical excision. There is little propensity for recurrence.

PYOGENIC GRANULOMA, PERIPHERAL OSSIFYING FIBROMA, AND PERIPHERAL GIANT CELL GRANULOMA

The pyogenic granuloma is a relatively common soft-tissue tumor that arises from the fibrous connective tissue of the skin or mucous membranes. Originally believed to be a botryomycotic infection, it is now known to be a reactive inflammatory process in which an exuberant fibrovascular proliferation of the connective tissue occurs secondary to some low-grade, chronic irritation.

Clinically the pyogenic granuloma is a raised lesion on either a sessile or a pedunculated base. Its surface may have a smooth, lobulated, or, occasionally, warty appearance that is erythematous and often ulcerated (Fig. 8-2). Depending on the age of the lesion, it will vary in texture from soft to firm and is suggestive of an ulcerated fibroma. Because of the pronounced vascularity of these lesions, they often bleed easily when probed. A review of pyogenic granulomas of the oral cavity by Angelopoulos revealed a 65% to 70% incidence of occurrence on the gingiva, most commonly the maxillary anterior labial gingiva, followed by the lips, tongue, buccal mucosa, palate, mucolabial or mucobuccal fold, and alveolar mucosa of edentulous areas.[11]

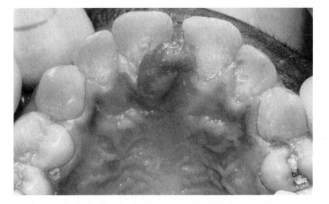

FIG. **8-2.** Pyogenic granuloma arising from the interdental papilla between the maxillary central incisors. The surface is lobulated with erythema and ulceration. There was poor oral hygiene with heavy accumulation of plaque on the lingual surfaces of the teeth.

Twenty-seven percent of cases in his series of 46 patients were in individuals younger than 20 years of age. Lawoyin, Arotiba, and Dosumu reviewed 38 cases from Ibadan, Nigeria, and reported an age range of 5 to 75 years (mean age, 33 years) with the main site of occurrence on the gingiva (74%), which closely approximates the findings of Angelopoulos.[11,12]

Histologically the pyogenic granuloma presents as a remarkable proliferation of plump fibroblasts and endothelial cells with the formation of prominent numbers of thin-walled, endothelium-lined vascular channels. A polymorphous inflammatory cell infiltrate is present, and the overlying surface epithelium is often ulcerated. Treatment consists of surgical excision, with care being taken to completely remove any local irritant that may still be present that would predispose to recurrence of the lesion.

In addition to an ulcerated fibroma, which in fact may itself be a nearly healed or sclerosed pyogenic granuloma, both the peripheral ossifying fibroma and peripheral giant cell granuloma must be considered in the differential diagnosis of pyogenic granuloma because these lesions are clinically indistinguishable from it. The peripheral ossifying fibroma, which has also been called the *peripheral odontogenic fibroma,* is a reactive lesion believed to be of periodontal ligament origin that occurs exclusively on the gingiva. In the largest series of cases, reported by Cundiff, 50% of the lesions were noted to occur in individuals between 5 and 25 years of age, with the peak incidence at 13 years.[13] The lesions were approximately equally divided between the maxilla and the mandible, with more than 80% of the lesions in both jaws occurring anterior to the molar area.

Over time, the terms *peripheral ossifying fibroma* and *peripheral odontogenic fibroma* have been used synonymously, which has introduced considerable confusion into the literature. In an attempt to clarify the confusion in nomenclature, Gardner proposed that the term *peripheral odontogenic fibroma* (World Health Organization [WHO] type) be used to denote the rare peripheral counterpart of the central odontogenic fibroma (WHO type) and that the term *peripheral ossifying fibroma* be retained and used to denote the relatively common reactive gingival lesion.[14] Clinically the peripheral odontogenic fibroma (WHO type) must be considered in the differential diagnosis of dome-shaped or nodular, usually nonulcerated, growths on the gingiva.

Histologically the peripheral ossifying fibroma demonstrates a proliferation of plump fibroblasts in a characteristic stroma of delicate, interlacing collagen fibrils. Osteoid and calcified material varying from dystrophic calcification to spicules of lamellar bone may be found in the lesion. The surface epithelium is often ulcerated. Although simple surgical excision is the treatment of choice, recurrences are not uncommon and were reported by Cundiff and by Eversole and Rovin in 16% and 20% of cases, respectively.[13,15]

The peripheral giant cell granuloma, like the peripheral ossifying fibroma, is a lesion unique to the oral cavity, occurring only on the gingiva or, in the case of the peripheral giant cell granuloma, also on the alveolar mucosa of edentulous areas. Like the pyogenic granuloma and peripheral ossifying fibroma, the peripheral giant cell granuloma may represent an unusual response to tissue injury. It is distinguishable from the pyogenic granuloma and peripheral ossifying fibroma only on the basis of its unique histomorphology, which is essentially identical to that of the central giant cell granuloma that is discussed later in this chapter. As reported by Giansanti and Waldron in their review of 720 cases, 33% were seen in patients under 20 years of age, which concurs with the findings of a study by Andersen, Fejerskov, and Philipsen, who reported 33 of 97 cases occurring in individuals between 5 and 15 years of age.[16,17] There is a nearly 2:1 predilection of females to males, with the mandible being involved more often than the maxilla. Nedir, Lombardi, and Samson point out that although it is quite rare, root resorption may be associated with peripheral giant cell granuloma.[18]

The peripheral giant cell granuloma is best treated by complete surgical excision, with care taken to excise it at its base. Little tendency for recurrence has been noted.

NEUROFIBROMA AND NEUROFIBROMATOSIS (VON RECKLINGHAUSEN'S DISEASE)

Neurofibroma is a benign neural neoplasm of Schwann cell origin of which several clinical forms are recognized. The solitary neurofibroma may present in the skin or oral mucous membranes as a soft tumor with a sessile or pedunculated base. Some neurofibromas are diffuse, presenting as a soft, nonspecific tissue mass or swelling. Although patients with neurofibromatosis may have either solitary or diffuse neurofibromas, the presence of either lesion does not in itself herald the diagnosis of this syndrome. The presence of a third form, the plexiform neurofibroma, is, however, considered to be diagnostic of neurofibromatosis. The plexiform neurofibroma differs from either the solitary or diffuse form in that it remains confined to the perineurium, presenting as a tortuous, fusiform enlargement of a nerve.

Neurofibromatosis type 1 (NF1), known as von Recklinghausen's disease, is a relatively common disease showing autosomal dominant inheritance with complete penetrance, variable clinical expressivity and pleiotropy, and age-dependent expression of clinical manifestations. It occurs in approximately 1 in 3000 live births with an equal sex predilection. It is carried on chromosome 17, and there is growing evidence that the tumor-suppressing properties of neurofibromin (the NF1 gene product) may be impaired or lost. It is said to be the most common single-gene disorder to affect the human nervous system. The criterion for diagnosis is the presence of two or more of the following features: six or more café-au-lait spots (1.5 cm or larger in postpubertal individuals, 0.5 cm or larger in prepubertal individuals), two or more neurofibromas of any type or one or more plexiform neurofibromas, freckling in the axillary or inguinal region, optic glioma, two or more pigmented iris hamartomas or Lisch nodules, dysplasia of the sphenoid bone or dysplasia or thinning of long bone cortex (pseudarthrosis), and a first-degree relative with NF1.

The NF1 gene is a tumor-suppressor gene, and thus patients with neurofibromatosis are at increased risk of developing benign and malignant tumors. In a study by Young, Hyman, and North, 5% of 495 adults and children diagnosed at their clinic had neoplasms, including both central nervous system and non–central nervous system neoplasms.[19] Poyhonen, Niemela, and Herva found the risk of malignancy in NF1 in Finland to be 8%, with the most common being malignant peripheral nerve sheath tumors.[20]

Intraorally, neurofibromas may present as nodular lesions on either a sessile or pedunculated base, often with a normal, pink mucosal color (Fig. 8-3); as a diffuse, ill-defined swelling with a firm to doughy consistency; or as a diffuse, noncompressible mass. They are most frequently found on the tongue and buccal mucosa but occasionally present as intraosseous lesions, which occur most commonly in the posterior mandible (Fig. 8-4).

The most common radiographic findings according to Lee, Yan, and Pharoah include an increase in bone

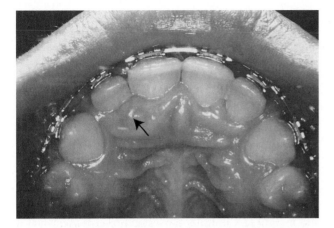

FIG. **8-3.** A 14-year-old boy undergoing orthodontic therapy was referred for evaluation of gingival hyperplasia on the lingual surfaces of the maxillary incisors and a firm swelling on the palatal side of tooth number 9 that was found after biopsy to be a neurofibroma *(arrow).*

density, enlarged mandibular foramen, lateral bowing of the mandibular ramus, increase in dimensions of the coronoid notch, and decrease in the mandibular angle.[21] In six cases for which computed tomographic scans were available, enlargement of the mandibular foramen and concavity of the medial surface of the ramus were seen.

A great deal of histomorphologic variability may be noted, from relatively circumscribed but nonencapsulated solitary neurofibromas to diffuse and plexiform neurofibromas. The diffuse neurofibroma is characterized by its infiltrative growth pattern along connective planes and its Wagner and Meissner tactile corpuscles. Plexiform neurofibromas are characterized by fascicles of neoplastic Schwann cells and collagen within a myxoid matrix that is confined to the perineurium. Mast cells are common findings within neurofibromas.

Solitary soft lesions are best treated by simple surgical excision and show little propensity for recurrence. Surgical excision of diffuse neurofibromas is difficult because of their diffuse, infiltrating nature. Plexiform neurofibromas are also difficult to treat as they have a tendency to grow along the course of a nerve, which results in frequent recurrences. According to Needle et al, children younger than 10 years of age; children with plexiform neurofibromas in the head, face, and neck; and those with tumors that cannot be almost completely removed are at particular risk for progression of their lesions.[22]

HEMANGIOMA

The hemangioma is a common, benign, vasoformative tumor that frequently occurs in the head and neck in children. It is generally believed to be hamartomatous rather than neoplastic in nature. Most hemangiomas are either present at birth or develop within the first year of life. It is believed that even those lesions that do not appear until adult life may have been present but not clinically evident until they began to enlarge. The classification of hemangiomas arising within the head and neck is confusing at best, and a discussion of it is not within the scope of this chapter.

Hemangiomas arising in the oral soft tissues most commonly affect the tongue, lips, and buccal mucosa. Clinically, they may be flat or raised and may vary from deep red to blue in color. Their histologic classification is based on the size of the vascular spaces. A capillary hemangioma is composed of many tiny capillaries with a pronounced endothelial cell proliferation. A cellular hemangioma consists principally of a proliferation of endothelial cells with only small numbers of discernible capillaries. A cavernous hemangioma is characterized by large, blood-filled sinusoidal spaces lined by endothelial cells and supported by a fibrous stroma. Hemangiomas may also occur centrally within either the mandible or maxilla.

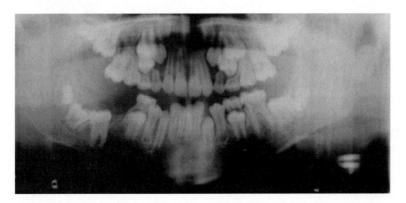

FIG. **8-4.** Neurofibroma involving the molar region and ramus of the right mandible in a child with neurofibromatosis. *(Courtesy Dr. Robin Cotton.)*

Central hemangiomas of bone may be asymptomatic, picked up only as incidental radiographic findings, or they may cause pain and swelling. They are typically well circumscribed, radiolucent lesions with no characteristic radiographic pattern to denote their underlying nature. Occasionally, loose or displaced teeth may be seen. The central hemangioma of bone bears a radiographic similarity to any number of other relatively well-circumscribed unilocular or multilocular radiolucent lesions in the jaws. Therefore it is advisable to aspirate such lesions with a needle before surgery or dental extraction to avoid the possibility of severe blood loss or exsanguination caused by the inability to control the resultant profuse bleeding.

The treatment for hemangiomas varies with the type, location, and size of the lesion involved. Many lesions spontaneously involute with age, especially those that are noted early and cease growing during the first year of life. Others require no treatment because of their small size and innocuous nature.

LYMPHANGIOMA

Lymphangiomas are thought to arise as a benign hamartomatous proliferation of sequestered lymphatic rests. Forming along tissue planes or penetrating adjacent tissue, they become canalized and, in the congenital absence of venous drainage, accumulate fluid. The majority becomes clinically evident early in life; however, a small number may not be manifest for a number of years. Lymphangiomas are classified on a histologic basis into three types: capillary lymphangiomas, cavernous lymphangiomas, and cystic hygroma. The capillary lymphangioma is typically composed of a proliferation of thin-walled, endothelium-lined channels primarily devoid of erythrocytes. The cavernous lymphangioma is characterized by the presence of dilated sinusoidal endothelium-lined vascular channels devoid of erythrocytes. The cystic hygroma is a macroscopic form of the cavernous lymphangioma, with large sinusoidal spaces lined with a single layer of endothelial cells that form multilocular cystic masses of varying sizes. Lymphangiomas of the oral soft tissues occur most commonly on the tongue, lips, and buccal mucosa. They are often elevated and nodular in appearance and may have the same color as the surrounding mucosa. Treatment is generally not indicated for small oral mucosal lymphangiomas; partial or complete spontaneous involution is occasionally noted.

Although cystic hygromas may be found in sites in the oral cavity, such as the tongue, they most frequently appear as a mass in the neck, occasionally extending into the mediastinum. Most commonly presenting as an asymptomatic soft tissue mass, they are usually slow growing; however, they may undergo sudden enlargement in the presence of trauma, inflammation, internal hemorrhage, or respiratory tract infection. Large cystic hygromas may encroach on the airway and esophagus, leading to difficulty in swallowing and even causing airway obstruction.

CONGENITAL EPULIS (GINGIVAL GRANULAR CELL TUMOR) OF THE NEWBORN

The congenital epulis of the newborn is a rare lesion of uncertain histogenesis that occurs exclusively in newborn infants, chiefly on the maxillary anterior alveolar ridge and less commonly on the mandibular anterior alveolar ridge. Although usually solitary lesions, they may be multiple, most often affecting both the maxilla and mandible. Clinically the lesion presents at birth as a pink, smooth to lobulated, pedunculated mass that may vary in size from a few millimeters to more than 7 cm in diameter. More than 90% of cases occur in girls (Fig. 8-5).

Ugras et al point out that, while typically considered a lesion of uncertain histogenesis, immunohistochemical studies have revealed strong and diffuse cytoplasmic staining for neuron-specific enolase and vimentin, which suggests that the congenital epulis may be derived from uncommitted nerve-related mesenchymal cells.[23]

Although histologic similarities to the granular cell myoblastoma have long been noted, the epithelium over the congenital epulis is generally thin without rete ridge formation, whereas the giant cell myoblastoma is characterized by pseudoepitheliomatous hyperplasia of

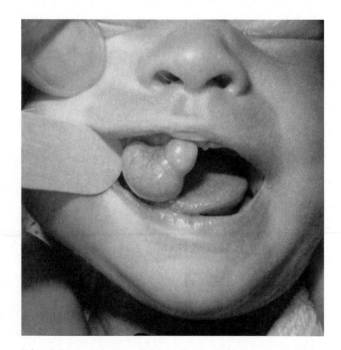

FIG. **8-5.** Congenital epulis of the newborn. *(Courtesy Dr. Robin Cotton.)*

the overlying epithelium; distinct differences are obvious on both ultrastructural and immunohistochemical evaluation.

Although the clinical presence of the congenital epulis may frighten parents, it ceases to grow following birth and is entirely benign, with some cases undergoing spontaneous involution. The usual treatment is simple surgical excision, with care taken not to interfere with the developing dentition. There is no propensity for recurrence, even in those cases in which the lesion is incompletely removed.

MUCOCELE

The mucocele, or *mucus retention phenomenon*, as it is often called, is a salivary gland lesion of traumatic origin that forms when the main duct of a minor salivary gland is torn with subsequent extravasation of mucus into the fibrous connective tissue so that a cystlike cavity is produced. The wall of this cavity is formed by compressed bundles of collagen fibrils, and its lumen contains inspissated mucin.

Mucoceles are noted to occur most commonly on the lower lip, with the floor of the mouth and buccal mucosa being the next most frequent sites of involvement. Mucoceles are only rarely seen on the upper lip, retromolar pad, or palate. Although they may occur at any age and have been reported to be present at birth, they tend to be noted most frequently in the second and third decades of life. No obvious sex predilection is noted.

A mucocele may be located either in the superficial mucosa, where it is typically seen as a fluid-filled vesicle or blister (Fig. 8-6), or deep within the connective tissue as a fluctuant nodule with the overlying mucosa normal in color. There may be spontaneous drainage of the

inspissated mucin with temporary resolution, especially in superficial lesions, and subsequent recurrence as the mucous saliva continues to drain into the connective tissue at the site of the torn duct. Fibrosis may be observed over the surface of long-standing lesions where chronic periodic drainage has taken place.

Treatment is by surgical excision, with removal of the involved accessory salivary gland. Marsupialization will only result in recurrence.

RANULA

Ranula is the clinical term for a mucocele occurring on the floor of the mouth after trauma to components of the sublingual glands. Two varieties of ranula exist: cystic (mucus retention cyst) and pseudocystic (mucus retention phenomenon or mucocele). In the cystic type, there is partial obstruction of the distal end of a sublingual gland duct that results in a small epithelial-lined cyst usually less than 1 cm in diameter. However, the most common variety of ranula (which is pseudocystic) forms as a result of extravasation of mucus into the fibrous connective tissue after a tear in a sublingual gland duct and, as in the case of a mucocele, arises as a result of the escape of mucus into the adjacent connective tissue. The clinical term *plunging ranula* is used when extravasated mucus dissects through the mylohyoid muscle and along the fascial planes of the neck, producing a swelling evident in the floor of the mouth.

Ranulas are typically slowly enlarging, fluctuant masses occurring to one side of the midline of the floor of the mouth and are so named because of their resemblance to the bloated underside of a frog's belly (Fig. 8-7). Lesions are usually treated by marsupialization, with occasional recurrence being noted. Chronic recurrence may require excision of the entire involved gland.

BENIGN TUMORS OF BONE
FIBRO-OSSEOUS LESIONS OF THE JAWS

The fibro-osseous lesions of the jaws include a diverse group of lesions sharing as a common denominator the replacement of normal bone architecture by a benign fibrous stroma containing varying amounts of mineralized material, including woven bone, lamellar bone, and curvilinear trabeculae or spherical calcifications. The mineralized material may histologically resemble bone and/or cementum. Because of the similar histomorphology of these lesions, diagnosis is best made on the basis of distinguishing clinical and radiographic as well as histologic features. This group of lesions includes fibrous dysplasia (considered a developmental process), reactive or dysplastic processes grouped under the collective term *cemento-osseous dysplasia,* and ossifying fibroma, which is a benign neoplasm. Because of the frequency of occurrence of fibrous dysplasia and

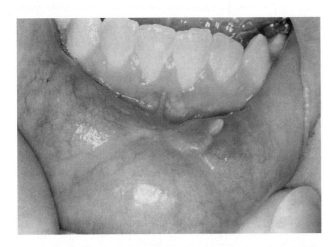

FIG. **8-6.** Mucocele on the lower lip. Notice the small white area of fibrosis where the mucocele has spontaneously drained with healing on the roof of the lesion, only to have the mucocele recur.

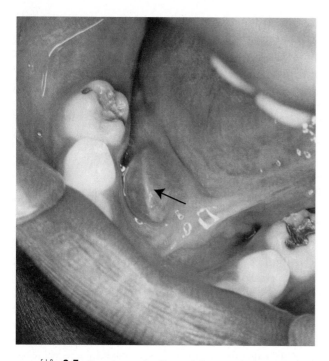

FIG. **8-7.** Ranula on the floor of the mouth *(arrow).*

ossifying fibroma of bone in the jaws of children, and the relative lack of occurrence of the cemento-osseous dysplasia group of lesions, only the former two are discussed here.

FIBROUS DYSPLASIA

Fibrous dysplasia of the jaws is a distinct clinicopathologic entity that is generally considered to be a nonneoplastic developmental lesion of bone. One of a variety of disease entities included in the spectrum of benign fibro-osseous lesions of the jaws, it is distinguished from the others by its clinical and radiographic features. In the child and adolescent, it has most often been confused with the ossifying and cementifying fibroma, which is a benign neoplasm believed to be of periodontal ligament origin. Fibrous dysplasia is caused by a somatic activating mutation of the alpha subunit of the G protein (Gsalpha) that ultimately results in abnormalities of osteoblast differentiation and therefore of bone matrix. Progression of the lesion results from an increase in osteoblastic bone resorption.

Two forms of fibrous dysplasia exist, the relatively rare polyostotic form of the disease and the considerably more common monostotic fibrous dysplasia. A severe form of polyostotic fibrous dysplasia called *McCune-Albright syndrome* is associated with café-au-lait macules on the skin and a variety of endocrine disorders, including Cushing's syndrome, hyperthyroidism, hyperparathyroidism, diabetes mellitus, and precocious puberty.

Monostotic fibrous dysplasia is seen with approximately equal frequency in males and females, with the maxilla being involved more frequently than the mandible. Maxillary involvement can be an especially serious form of the disease, frequently involving contiguous bones across suture lines, including the maxillary sinus, floor of the orbit, sphenoid bone, base of the skull, and occiput. This form of the disease has been called *craniofacial fibrous dysplasia* and is not truly monostotic in its nature.

Monostotic fibrous dysplasia tends to develop early in life. Of 22 cases reported in one study by Waldron and Giansanti, 9 patients were initially diagnosed as having fibrous dysplasia before 20 years of age, with a reliable clinical history of occurrence in the first or second decade of life in an additional 6 cases.[24] The most common clinical manifestation is a painless swelling of the jaws characterized by a smooth, uniform, fusiform expansion of the involved alveolar ridge. Obliteration of the mucobuccal or mucolabial fold is a common feature, with the overlying mucosa being normal in appearance. When the maxilla is involved, elevation of the eye may be noted.

Radiographically, maxillary lesions most often show a ground-glass appearance of the bone, whereas mandibular lesions usually show either a ground-glass or a mixed radiolucent-radiopaque appearance (Fig. 8-8). Their borders are typically poorly defined, except for the anterior portion of some maxillary lesions, which may appear to be well circumscribed. Divergence of roots may be noted, and in children in whom developing permanent teeth are present there may be displacement of teeth with noneruption (see Fig. 8-8). Other potential distinguishing radiographic findings as reported by Petrikowski et al include superior displacement of the mandibular canal and a fingerprint bone pattern as well as displacement of the maxillary sinus cortex, alteration of the lamina dura because of the abnormal bone pattern, and narrowing of the periodontal ligament space.[25]

Histologically there is a benign fibrous stroma with bony trabeculae varying from woven to lamellar in appearance, proportionate to the relative maturity of the lesion.

Monostotic fibrous dysplasia of the jaws is typically a slow-growing, painless, progressive enlargement of bone whose growth pattern often stabilizes with time as maturation in skeletal growth is reached. Because of the benign nature of this lesion, as well as the fact that surgically its margins are ill defined and blend into the surrounding normal bone, conservative therapy is indicated. Surgery, chiefly in the form of osseous recontouring, should be considered only in those cases in which there is functional or significant cosmetic deformity and then usually only after stabilization of the

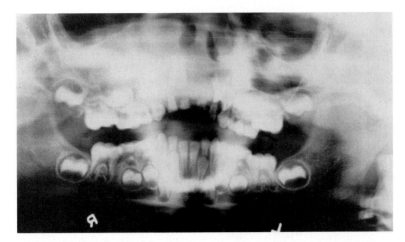

FIG. **8-8.** Panelipse radiograph for a child with fibrous dysplasia presenting as a uniformly radiodense lesion crossing the midline with poorly defined borders blending into the surrounding bone. Notice the displacement of the developing teeth.

disease process. Because this is a benign lesion of bone, radiation therapy is contraindicated because of the possibility of development of a postradiation sarcoma in the area.

OSSIFYING AND CEMENTIFYING FIBROMA

The ossifying fibroma is a benign neoplasm of bone grouped with fibrous dysplasia and other benign nonodontogenic tumors under the broad category of benign fibro-osseous lesions of the jaws. As with other benign fibro-osseous lesions, it is characterized histologically by a benign fibrous stroma, with formation of variable amounts of woven-appearing bone, lamellar bone, and spherical to annular to amorphous cementum-like calcifications. Although it was traditionally considered to be an odontogenic neoplasm of periodontal ligament origin affecting the tooth-bearing areas of the jaws, the occurrence of histologically identical neoplasms in the temporal, frontal, ethmoid, and sphenoid bones leaves this concept in doubt. When the predominant calcified component is bone, the term is *ossifying fibroma*. When cementum or cementum-like calcifications predominate, the term is *cementifying fibroma*. When both bone and cementum-like tissues are present, the lesions are termed *cemento-ossifying fibromas*. Although there is a predilection for occurrence in the third and fourth decades of life, the ossifying fibroma is found with some frequency in patients younger than 20 years of age. The mandible is involved more often than the maxilla, with the molar and premolar region of the mandible being the most common site of occurrence.

The ossifying fibroma may be entirely asymptomatic, being discovered on routine radiographic examination, or may present as a painless expansion of bone. Radiographically the ossifying fibroma is a well-circumscribed lesion, often with a well-demarcated sclerotic border (Fig. 8-9). Beyond this, the radiographic features are quite variable, as demonstrated by Eversole, Leider, and Nelson.[26] It most frequently presents as a unilocular radiolucency with or without radiopaque foci, which may be superimposed over teeth, may be interposed between contiguous teeth, or may reside in edentulous regions. Aggressively expansile lesions with or without radiopaque foci as well as multilocular expansile lesions may also be noted. Divergence of roots of teeth and/or root resorption may be noted with varying degrees of frequency. Eversole, Leider, and Nelson reported root

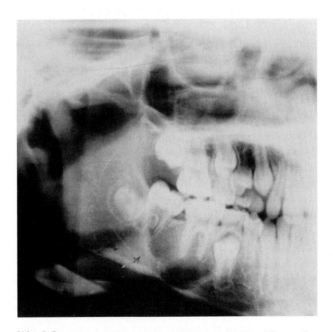

FIG. **8-9.** Ossifying fibroma in a 10-year-old boy. The radiograph shows a well-circumscribed, expansile, radiolucent lesion with thinning of the inferior cortical plate of bone. *(Courtesy Dr. Mark L. Bernstein.)*

divergence in 17% of their cases, whereas root resorption was encountered in 11%.[26] These rates are considerably lower than those observed by Sciubba and Younai, who noted tooth displacement or root divergence in 33% of cases and root resorption in 44%.[27] Cortical thinning and bony expansion with clinical deformity have been reported in as many as 91% of cases.

Studies by Eversole, Leider, and Nelson and by Sciubba and Younai have pointed out that the behavior of the ossifying fibroma is unpredictable when either radiographic or histologic criteria are employed.[26,27] Initial treatment is by enucleation or curettage where possible, with the frequency of recurrence varying from 0% as reported by Waldron to 28% in a series reported by Eversole, Leider, and Nelson.[26,28]

JUVENILE ACTIVE OSSIFYING FIBROMA

The term *juvenile active ossifying fibroma* (JOF) encompasses two distinct histopathologic variants of an aggressive form of ossifying fibroma involving the craniofacial bones: the psammomatoid juvenile ossifying fibroma (PsJOF) and trabecular juvenile ossifying fibroma (TrJOF). El-Mofty, in a review of the literature, reported six new cases of JOF, three of the psammomatoid type and three of the trabecular variant.[29] The PsJOF was noted to occur predominantly in the sinonasal and orbital bones in patients with a mean age range of 16 to 33 years (range, 3 months to 72 years), whereas the TrJOF primarily affected the jaws in patients with a mean age range of 8 1/2 to 12 years (range, 2 to 12 years). Aggressive growth was noted to occur in some, but not all, cases of both types. El-Mofty proposed that these histologic, demographic, and clinical differences between PsJOF and TrJOF warranted their classification as two distinct clinicopathologic entities.

CENTRAL GIANT CELL GRANULOMA

The central giant cell granuloma (CGCG) of the jaws is a relatively common lesion of bone that is generally thought to be nonneoplastic in nature. There is considerable discussion in the literature as to the relationship of CGCG of the jaws to giant cell tumor of bone. It has been suggested by Waldron and Shafer, as well as by Auclair et al, among others, that the CGCG and giant cell tumor of other bones represent a spectrum of a single disease process, with the differences in clinical behavior partially accounted for by differences in age distribution and by the site of occurrence, among other factors.[30,31] The CGCG of the jaws occurs most commonly during the first 30 years of life, with more than 60% of lesions noted before 20 years of age and nearly 50% occurring in patients younger than 16 years of age. The CGCG occurs more often in females than in males. It may be found in either jaw, but the mandible is involved twice as often as the maxilla. Although it is generally accepted that the majority of lesions occur in the anterior portion of the jaw, anterior to the first permanent molar, Kaffe et al, in a study of 80 cases of CGCG, found that nearly 50% of their cases occurred in the molar, ramus, and tuberosity regions.[32]

Although usually asymptomatic, CGCG may be an expansile lesion with or without divergence of teeth. Radiographically the CGCG may vary from a unilocular radiolucency to a multilocular expansile bone-destructive lesion with faint trabeculation and an ill-defined border (Fig. 8-10). Both displacement and noneruption of teeth may be noted. Histologically the CGCG is composed of a delicate, fibrous connective tissue stroma, interspersed with multinucleated giant cells, plump fibroblasts, and capillaries. Prominent numbers of extravasated red blood cells with associated hemosiderin pigment are often scattered throughout the fibrous connective tissue. Varying amounts of osteoid and trabeculae of bone are also noted.

Traditionally, treatment of CGCG has consisted of complete curettage or conservative surgical excision. Auclair et al, however, have pointed out that the recurrence rate may be higher than previously suggested in the literature.[31] In their series, 5 of the 25 patients for whom follow-up information was available developed recurrence. The average age of these five patients was 11 years compared with an average age of 29 years for patients without recurrence. All five of the patients with recurrence were under the age of 17 years, and these patients accounted for 45% of all those in this age group

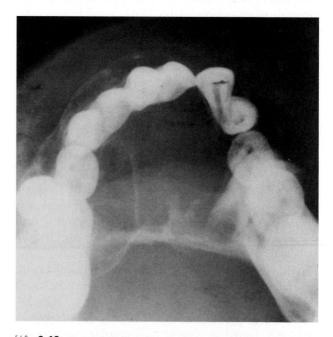

FIG. **8-10.** Central giant cell granuloma involving the anterior mandible presenting radiographically as a multilocular, radiolucent lesion with expansion and thinning of the cortical plates. Notice also the faint trabeculation within the lesion.

with follow-up. Minic and Stajcic studied 31 cases of CGCG of the jaws in 29 patients.[33] Seven lesions demonstrated cortical perforation and soft tissue extension. Lesions recurred in five cases, all of which showed microscopically confirmed cortical perforation at the time of first occurrence. Hence, despite the good prognosis for patients with this condition, close long-term follow-up would seem to be indicated, particularly in those cases in which cortical perforation is noted. In cases in which less radical nonsurgical treatment options are desirable, especially to avoid disfigurement, intralesional injections with triamcinolone acetonide have been used successfully to stop lesional growth, possibly effecting some regression in size and providing bony filling of the osteolytic lesion. Radiation therapy is contraindicated.

ODONTOGENIC CYSTS

PRIMORDIAL CYST

Traditionally the primordial cyst was considered to be a relatively uncommon type of odontogenic cyst formed by cystic degeneration of the enamel organ (primordium) before the formation of enamel or dentin. Primordial cysts are usually asymptomatic and are most likely to be found on routine radiographic examination. Because of this, although they begin to evolve when the enamel organ is developing before the formation of the enamel or dentin, they may not be noticed or become clinically evident for many years.

Radiographically, the primordial cyst may be a well-circumscribed, unilocular- or multilocular-appearing radiolucent lesion in a location where a permanent tooth failed to develop and where none has been extracted. Such cysts are more commonly found in the third molar region but may occur in any location where a permanent tooth would have formed.

Although more typically lined by nonkeratinizing, stratified squamous odontogenic cyst-lining epithelium with a fibrous connective tissue wall, the primordial cyst may present as a histologically distinct type of odontogenic cyst, the odontogenic keratocyst. In one large series of cases reported by Brannon, 60 of 135 (44.4%) of primordial cysts were histologically odontogenic keratocysts.[34] Some authors have concluded that all primordial cysts are odontogenic keratocysts and use the two terms synonymously. As shown by Brannon, however, this practice ignores the histologic evidence to the contrary.

Appropriate treatment for the primordial cyst is surgical removal unless an extremely large bone-destructive lesion is present, in which case cystotomy with placement of a polyethylene drain followed by cystectomy when the cyst has reached a manageable size is the treatment of choice. If the lesion is found histologically to be an odontogenic keratocyst, the chance for recurrence is high.

DENTIGEROUS CYST

The dentigerous cyst is a relatively common type of odontogenic cyst associated with the crown of an impacted, embedded, or otherwise unerupted tooth. Although these lesions are typically asymptomatic and are usually found on routine radiographic examination, they may be large, destructive, expansile lesions of bone. The radiographic appearance is that of a well-defined radiolucent lesion that may be unilocular or multilocular in its appearance. The lesion may vary in size from one in which the differentiation from an enlarged dental follicle is, at best, arbitrary to a large, bone-destructive lesion that may resorb the roots of primary teeth, cause the divergence of or completely displace permanent teeth, and produce large areas of bone destruction in either the mandible or the maxilla (Fig. 8-11).

In addition to its potential for bone destruction and because of the multipotential nature of this epithelium derived from the dental lamina, several entities may arise in or be associated with the wall of a dentigerous cyst. In a study by Brannon, 8.5% of clinical dentigerous cysts were found histologically to be odontogenic keratocysts.[34] Although ameloblastomas are relatively uncommon in children, McMillan and Smillie believe that the majority of ameloblastomas associated with dentigerous cysts arise in children or adolescents.[35] Studies by Leider, Eversole, and Barkin and by Gardner and Corio have shown that in 50% to 80% of cases cystic ameloblastoma appeared radiographically as dentigerous cysts.[36,37] Also, based on histopathologic features,

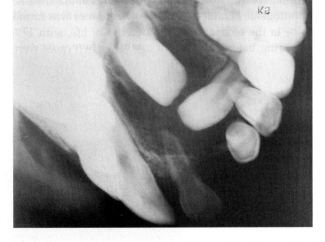

FIG. 8-11. A dentigerous cyst in an 8-year-old girl associated with the developing maxillary central incisor with bone destruction and expansion, as well as displacement of the lateral incisor.

of teeth. The average age of patients with ameloblastoma is said to be approximately 36 years, with more than 80% of the lesions occurring in the mandible and more than 70% occurring in the molar-ramus area.

At first glance, with the average age of occurrence of ameloblastomas in the fourth decade of life, the discussion of this entity in a pediatric context would not appear to be particularly relevant to this chapter. In 1977, however, Robinson and Martinez described the unicystic ameloblastoma, which they felt to be a prognostically distinct entity.[44] In the 20 patients they studied, the average age of occurrence was 21 years, and half of their patients were below the age of 20 years. Clinically and radiographically the lesions were described as having the features of a nonneoplastic cyst, with the majority mimicking dentigerous cysts.

Philipsen and Reichert presented a critical review of 193 cases of unicystic ameloblastoma in the literature.[45] They found that the mean age at the time of diagnosis of unicystic ameloblastoma was most closely related to one clinical feature: the presence of an impacted tooth. They termed cases associated with an impacted tooth the dentigerous type and those not associated with an impacted tooth the nondentigerous type. The mean age at diagnosis of the dentigerous variant was 16.5 years, whereas that of the nondentigerous type was 35.2 years.

Kahn published a clinicopathologic analysis of 38 cases of ameloblastoma (37 intraosseous, 1 peripheral) in individuals younger than 20 years of age.[46] In the 19 years and under age group, the average age at diagnosis was 10.4 years with no obvious sex predilection. All of the 37 intraosseous cases reported in this study occurred in the mandible, with 80% occurring in the molar-ramus area. The most common presenting symptom was swelling, noted in 54% of cases. Sixty-nine percent of cases for which information was available were found to be associated with impacted teeth. In 29% of cases, teeth were displaced. In cases available for review radiographically, 72% of lesions were unilocular with a well-demarcated border and 28% were multilocular in appearance. Of the 37 intraosseous cases reported in this study, 31 were unicystic (radiographically unilocular or multilocular) and 5 were conventional ameloblastomas, all of which were multilocular radiographically. In a series of 21 cases of unicystic ameloblastoma reported by Rosenstein et al, all lesions were also reported to be in the mandible.[47]

As alluded to previously, ameloblastomas may present as either unilocular or multilocular radiolucent lesions, with or without bony expansion. Cystic-appearing spaces may be compartmentalized by separate, distinct septa of bone. Unicystic ameloblastoma, which is considered a distinct prognostic entity, occurs almost exclusively in the mandible, predominantly in the posterior part. Although most commonly found in

association with the crowns of impacted teeth, unicystic ameloblastomas may be seen in interradicular, periapical, or edentulous regions.

Ameloblastomas are distinguished by their histologic resemblance to the enamel organ. Regardless of age or location, ameloblastomas demonstrate singly or in combination a variety of distinct histologic patterns. They are frequently characterized by discrete islands of neoplastic odontogenic epithelium with a peripheral layer of columnar to cuboidal epithelial cells that are palisaded in their appearance with polarization of the nuclei. The central portions of these islands of neoplastic odontogenic epithelium are composed of cells that resemble the stellate reticulum. In some lesions, these central areas may take on an acanthomatous or granular appearance. The plexiform pattern is most frequently encountered in the pediatric age group, with arrangement of tumor cells as a network of interconnecting strands of cells. An important histologic finding in the unicystic form, other than the observation of ameloblastic change in the cyst lining itself, is the presence of a significant luminal and/or mural component characterized by a proliferation of ameloblastic odontogenic epithelium into the lumen of the cyst, the fibrous cyst wall, or both. Mural invasion of the cyst wall portends a higher risk of recurrence for this lesion.

Therapy is by surgical removal, the method of which will vary according to the location and clinical and radiographic extent of the lesion. Although a recurrence rate of 55% to 90% has been found for ameloblastomas of all types that have been treated by curettage, the cystic form, which is the type found most commonly in children, was noted in a study by Gardner and Corio to recur only 11% of the time after the same treatment.[37] After a mean follow-up of 5.2 years, Kahn found recurrence in 7% of cases in which lesions were initially treated by enucleation and/or curettage (cauterized).[46] It has been recommended, however, that unicystic ameloblastomas with proliferation of epithelium into the fibrous wall of the cyst be treated as aggressively as conventional ameloblastomas.

ADENOMATOID ODONTOGENIC TUMOR

The adenomatoid odontogenic tumor (AOT) is a benign, probably hamartomatous, epithelial tumor that occurs in two intraosseous forms (follicular and extrafollicular) as well as a peripheral variant. It has also been known as adenoameloblastoma, which is extremely misleading because it behaves clinically in a distinctly different fashion than does ameloblastoma.

In 1998 Philipsen and Reichart presented an update on data collected since Philipsen et al reviewed the biologic profile of 499 cases of AOT in 1991, with approximately 250 more cases added since that time.[48,49] The AOT can be subclassified into three variants based on clinical and radiologic findings. Two of these are central or intraosseous variants. The first is the follicular (dentigerous) type in which the tumor is found in association with the crown of an impacted tooth, with the most likely provisional diagnosis being that of a dentigerous cyst. The second and less commonly reported intraosseous variant of the AOT is the extrafollicular type in which there is no association with the crown of an impacted tooth and with the most likely provisional diagnosis being that of a residual, radicular, globulomaxillary, or lateral periodontal cyst, depending upon its location. The third variant of AOT is the peripheral or extraosseous variant, which may appear clinically as a fibroma. Approximately 95% of AOTs are reported as being the intrabony or central type, with the follicular variant accounting for 71%. Although most often asymptomatic, the tumor frequently causes a painless swelling exhibiting slow but progressive growth.

AOTs occur most commonly in the second decade of life. Nearly 70% of patients are younger than 20 years of age and more than 50% of cases occur in the teenage years. Females are involved twice as often as males, and the intraosseous lesions have been noted to occur nearly twice as frequently in the maxilla as in the mandible, with a noticeable predilection for occurrence in the canine and incisor regions. The rare peripheral type is found almost entirely in the anterior maxillary region.

The most common radiographic finding is that of a unilocular radiolucent lesion, which as previously stated may appear radiographically as a dentigerous cyst (Fig. 8-14) or as a residual, radicular, globulomaxillary, or lateral periodontal cyst, depending on its location. Radiopacities of varying size and density are often present. Because these are space-occupying lesions, divergence of roots and displacement of teeth may be noted.

Histologically the AOT is composed of neoplastic odontogenic epithelium with a distinct histologic appearance: an encapsulated proliferation of swirling strands of spindle-shaped or polygonal epithelial cells within which are nodules of ductlike or rosettelike structures composed of a row of definite cuboidal to columnar epithelial cells; these may be empty or may contain variable amounts of an amorphous eosinophilic material, which may become calcified in some areas.

Because these lesions are in almost all cases well encapsulated and show an identical benign biologic behavior, conservative surgical enucleation and curettage is the treatment of choice. There is no propensity for recurrence.

ODONTOGENIC MYXOMA

The odontogenic myxoma is an uncommon benign mesodermal neoplasm of the jaws that is thought to arise from the mesenchymal portion of the odontogenic

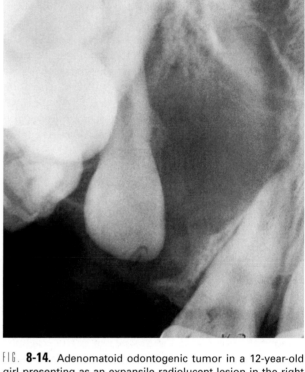

FIG. **8-14.** Adenomatoid odontogenic tumor in a 12-year-old girl presenting as an expansile radiolucent lesion in the right maxilla associated with the lateral incisor. The lesion was curetted, and the lateral incisor was allowed to erupt and was orthodontically moved into proper alignment. *(Courtesy Dr. Dan J. Crocker.)*

apparatus. Kaffe, Naor, and Buchner reviewed the English-language literature on odontogenic myxoma published between 1965 and 1995.[50] Their review included 162 cases from the literature and 2 new cases. Two thirds of the cases involved the mandible and one third of the cases involved the maxilla, with the molar and premolar region being the most common site of occurrence. Although the majority of cases were diagnosed in the second to fourth decades, 34% of the cases were in patients 20 years of age or younger.

Several cases have been reported as occurring in association with impacted or missing teeth; however, at least in the case of unerupted teeth, this is an uncommon finding. In addition, several cases have been noted to occur in non–tooth-bearing areas, such as the condyle and the condylar neck. Clinically, these are usually painless lesions that may show mobility and divergence of teeth.

Radiographically, odontogenic myxomas may be unilocular or multilocular lesions that may cause expansion and thinning and destruction of the cortical plates of bone, and displacement of teeth. Multilocular lesions often exhibit a mottled or honeycombed appearance. There is no universal agreement as to the relative frequency of presentation as a unilocular versus a multilocular radiographic appearance. In their analysis of 10 cases of odontogenic myxoma in childhood, Keszler, Dominguez, and Giannunzio found the most frequent image to be a unilocular lesion with cortical expansion.[51] In the review by Kaffe, Naor, and Buchner of cases from all age groups, a multilocular appearance was noted in 55% of cases, with a significant correlation between the size of the lesion and its locularity.[50] Perhaps the findings by Keszler, Dominguez, and Giannunzio can be accounted for based on a smaller lesional size in their pediatric cases.[51]

Histologically, the odontogenic myxoma is made up of stellate to spindle-shaped cells with delicate fibrillar interlacing processes, which produce a loose myxoid appearance. Occasional nests of inactive odontogenic epithelium may be noted, interspersed within this fibromyxoid stroma.

The appropriate treatment for the odontogenic myxoma is still a matter of debate and is certainly dependent on its size and location. The preferred treatment is complete surgical excision, which may prove difficult because of infiltration and expansion of the tumor into bone, and the absence of a true capsule. Treatment is complicated by the understandable reluctance to perform wide surgical excision of a benign lesion, especially in a child. Periodic follow-up to check for recurrence is important. In Keszler, Dominguez, and Giannunzio's series of 10 cases, two patients experienced recurrence within the first year after surgery.[51]

AMELOBLASTIC FIBROMA

The ameloblastic fibroma is a true mixed neoplasm of odontogenic origin characterized by the proliferation of both odontogenic epithelium and mesenchymal tissue without the formation of enamel or dentin. It is generally believed to be a less aggressive lesion than the ameloblastoma. The average age of occurrence is approximately 14 years with no obvious sex predilection noted. The lesion occurs in the mandible in approximately 70% of cases, primarily in the molar region. Its initial clinical presentation is most often swelling; however, it is not uncommonly asymptomatic, being found on routine radiographic examination. Radiographically, it may be a unilocular or multilocular radiolucent lesion, usually with well-defined, often sclerotic borders, and may be found in association with unerupted or displaced teeth.

The ameloblastic fibroma has a characteristic histologic appearance, with nests and strands of cuboidal to columnar epithelial cells proliferating along with a primitive-appearing mesenchymal component that resembles the developing dental papilla.

Treatment is by surgical removal that is complete but conservative compared with that advocated for the ameloblastoma. At one time, simple surgical excision was advocated, because there was believed to be little chance for recurrence. Recent evidence, however, indicates that the recurrence rate is higher than originally suspected, and somewhat more aggressive surgical therapy is indicated than was previously recommended.

AMELOBLASTIC FIBRO-ODONTOMA

As reviewed by Philipsen, Reichart, and Praetorius, the WHO defines this lesion as "a lesion similar to ameloblastic fibroma, but also showing inductive changes that lead to the formation of both dentine and enamel."[52] Philipsen, Reichart, and Praetorius updated the review by Slootweg, bringing the total number of cases in the literature to 86.[52,53] The average age of recurrence has been reported as 9 years. The majority of cases are found in the posterior mandible, and the ratio of lesions in this location to those in both the anterior and posterior maxilla is 2.4:1. Described as a painless, slow-growing, and expanding tumor, the lesion is associated with unerupted teeth in 83% of cases, which often leads to its diagnosis. Size may vary from lesions evident only microscopically to a large mass up to 6 cm or more in its greatest dimension.

Histologically the epithelial and mesenchymal components are those of an ameloblastic fibroma, with the formation of osteodentin or dentin-like material and enamel matrix.

Philipsen, Reichart, and Praetorius agreed with Slootweg that the ameloblastic fibro-odontoma is a hamartomatous lesion but also proposed that it is a stage preceding the development of a complex odontoma.[52, 53] In his review, Takeda argued that ameloblastic fibro-odontoma should not be considered a hamartoma because rare cases showing true neoplastic behavior exist and because the existence of a malignant variant has been reported.[54] Conservative surgical enucleation is considered to be the treatment of choice, and recurrence is unlikely.

ODONTOMA

Odontomas are mixed odontogenic tumors in which both the epithelial and mesenchymal components have undergone functional differentiation to the point that both enamel and dentin are formed. The most common of the odontogenic tumors, odontomas are believed to be hamartomatous rather than neoplastic in nature. The WHO has classified odontomas into two types depending on their degree of morphodifferentiation. The compound odontoma is a lesion in which all the dental tissues are represented in an orderly fashion so that there is at least superficial anatomic resemblance to teeth. In a complex odontoma, on the other hand, although all the dental tissues are represented, they are formed in such a rudimentary fashion that there is little or no morphologic similarity to normal tooth formation (Fig. 8-15).

Budnick, in a review of 65 cases from the literature and 84 from the Emory University School of Dentistry Pathology Department, reported that compound odontomas have a propensity for occurrence in the canine and incisor region, being found more often in the maxilla than in the mandible, whereas complex odontomas show a predilection for occurrence in the posterior jaws.[55] In a review, Philipsen, Reichart, and Praetorius also found the posterior mandible to be the most frequent site of occurrence followed by the anterior maxilla.[52] Compound odontomas have been reported by Slootweg as having a mean age of occurrence of 14.8 years compared to 20.3 years of age for complex odontomas, possibly because the odontogenic tissue in the anterior jaws where the compound odontoma predominantly occurs has finished its differentiation

earlier than tissues in the posterior part of the jaw.[53] Budnick and Kaugars, Miller, and Abbey did not differentiate between clinical types of odontomas; however, they noted a mean age of detection of 14.8 and 16 years of age, respectively.[55,56] Kaugars, Miller, and Abbey have argued that, because the radiographic and histologic distinction between the compound and complex odontomas is poorly defined and because no appreciable clinical difference separates them, differentiation of these two types of odontomas cannot be justified given the obliquity of the diagnostic criteria.[56] Philipsen, Reichart, and Praetorius take exception to this concept, holding the view that complex and compound odontomas are pathogenetically different.[52] They believe that complex odontomas are the terminal stage in the series of hamartomatous lesions that they termed the developing complex odontoma line and that includes the ameloblastic fibro-dentinoma, the ameloblastic fibro-odontoma, and what they call the hamartomatous type of ameloblastic fibroma (they argue that ameloblastic fibromas occurring after the age of 20 years represent a benign neoplasm, whereas those occurring during childhood [i.e., during the tooth-development age group] are likely to be nonneoplastic hamartomatous lesions). They feel that the compound odontoma represents a malformation with a high degree of histomorphologic differentiation similar to the process producing supernumerary teeth, "multiple schizodontia," or locally conditioned hyperactivity of the dental lamina.

Although odontomas are usually asymptomatic, they may be the cause of noneruption or impaction of teeth and retained primary teeth (see Fig. 8-15). In the series of cases by Kaugars, Miller, and Abbey, odontomas were found to be in association with an unerupted tooth in 48% of cases and in conjunction with a dentigerous cyst in 28% of cases.[56]

Odontomas are most commonly found on routine radiographic examination, presenting as an irregular radiopaque mass or as small, toothlike structures. The lesions are typically asymptomatic, and the most common presenting symptom is usually lack of eruption of a permanent tooth or bony expansion or swelling. The recommended treatment for an odontoma is conservative surgical excision, with care taken to remove the surrounding soft tissue. No propensity for recurrence has been noted.

MALIGNANT TUMORS

FIBROMATOSIS AND FIBROSARCOMA IN INFANCY AND CHILDHOOD

As reviewed by Fisher, these neoplasms are part of a large group of benign and malignant lesions that present as subcutaneous or deep tumor masses, often with alarmingly rapid growth.[57] The fibromatoses are

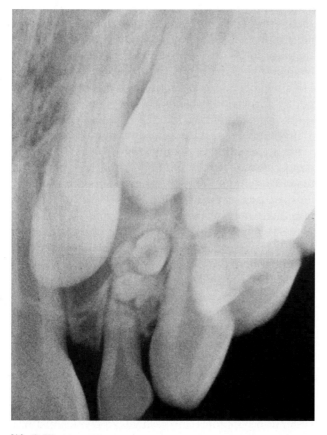

FIG. 8-15. Complex composite odontoma delaying eruption of the lateral incisor.

characterized by a proliferation of spindle-shaped or oval bland and uniform cells without pleomorphism or giant cells. They are marked by their propensity for local infiltration and recurrence. Although they may kill by local extension, technically they are benign, because they do not metastasize.

The common or desmoid type of infantile fibromatosis is found from birth to 5 years (usually before 2 years of age) in the shoulder and upper arm, thigh, or head and neck region.[57] The literature suggests that conservative surgery with the goal of achieving a wide lesion-free margin should be attempted as a primary means of control. Radiation therapy should be used only as a last step in the young patient because of the risk of disturbance of skeletal growth and potential for radiation-induced sarcoma. Chemotherapy may have a role in the treatment of children with inoperable disease.

Fibrosarcoma is a malignant neoplasm of fibroblastic and myofibroblastic differentiation. According to Fisher, congenital and infantile fibrosarcoma is a relatively rare tumor that usually is manifest in the first year of life, especially in the first 3 months, and almost always before 4 years of age.[57] It is distinguished from fibromatosis by cellular pleomorphism, increased mitotic activity, and its potential for metastasis. Less cellular examples may also occur in older children and resemble adult-type desmoids. Fibrosarcoma that occurs in children younger than 4 years of age is much less likely to metastasize than it is in adults and has more in common with infantile aggressive fibromatosis than it does with the adult form of the disease. Although recurrence is possible, metastases are rare, and the majority of cases are cured by wide local excision. Adjuvant radiation therapy and chemotherapy are reserved for inoperable, recurrent, or metastatic cases.

MALIGNANT LYMPHOMA

Malignant lymphomas are neoplasms of lymphoreticular origin that are divided into two main categories: non-Hodgkin's lymphoma (NHL) and Hodgkin's lymphoma (HL, or Hodgkin's disease). As a group, malignant lymphomas represent the most frequently encountered malignant tumors in the head and neck in children and are approximately equally divided in their frequency between HL and NHL.

Hodgkin's Lymphoma (Hodgkin's Disease). Hodgkin's lymphoma (HL) is a malignant neoplasm of lymphoreticular origin distinguished from NHL by diverse but distinctive morphologic features with one common denominator, the presence of Reed-Sternberg cells or their variants, which are widely accepted as the neoplastic cells in this disease. HL is characterized by a bimodal age distribution with the first peak incidence at approximately 25 years of age and the second peak at approximately 65 years of age. Although the first peak

incidence is noted in adolescence and young adulthood, HL may be found even in very young children. Males are affected more often than females.

The staging of Hodgkin's disease is anatomically based because of it's propensity to spread contiguously from one lymph node group to the next. The Ann Arbor staging classification was initially reported in 1971 by Carbone et al.[58] In 1989 the Ann Arbor staging was modified at a meeting in Cotswolds, England.[59] The Cotswolds modifications validated the use of computed tomographic scanning for the identification of intraabdominal disease, formally introduced bulk of disease into the staging system, and included the concept of unconfirmed complete remission. According to these modifications of the Ann Arbor staging system, stage I HL signifies disease involving one lymph node region or lymphoid structure (e.g., spleen, thymus, Waldeyer ring); stage II signifies involvement of two or more lymph node regions on the same side of the diaphragm, most often in the neck and mediastinum; stage III indicates disease on both sides of the diaphragm (III1 with or without involvement of splenic, hilar, celiac, or portal nodes [upper abdomen] and III2 with involvement of paraaortic, iliac, and mesenteric nodes [lower abdomen]); and stage IV indicates the presence of involvement of extralymphatic sites, most often the liver and/or lungs, bone marrow, or bone. Symptoms such as unexplained fever with oral temperatures higher than 38° C for 3 or more consecutive days, shaking chills, drenching night sweats, and unexplained weight loss of 10% or more of body weight over a 6-month period are considered "B" symptoms that impart a worse prognosis within each stage.

HL in the head and neck most commonly presents as a firm, rubbery, asymmetrically enlarged, nontender mass in the cervical lymph node chain. The lesion occurs primarily in lymph nodes, and involvement of the oral cavity or oropharynx, including the Waldeyer tonsillar ring, is uncommon. HL is classified into four histologic subtypes: lymphocyte predominant, nodular sclerosing, mixed cellularity, and lymphocyte depletion. The nodular lymphocyte–predominant form has been separated from the classic disease.

The most important prognostic variable in newly diagnosed cases of HL is the clinical stage, and the strongest predictive factor for patients with relapse after initial treatment is the duration of the initial response. Most treatment programs for limited-stage HL include chemotherapy and involved-field radiation therapy. With advances in therapy, current 5-year recurrence-free survival has been achieved by 95% or more of patients with stage I or II nonbulky disease and absence of systemic B symptoms (mediastinal lymphadenopathy is considered bulky). Five-year survival rates for patients with bulky disease, B symptoms, and/or advanced stage III or IV disease are between 80% and 94%. For patients who have experienced relapse after initial combined-modality therapy and those who experience multiple relapses, hematopoietic stem cell transplantation may offer hope of long-term remission.

Non-Hodgkin's Lymphomas. The NHLs are a heterogenous group of neoplasms of the lymphoid system that may arise in the head and neck in the lymph nodes (nodal), in extranodal lymphatic areas (the Waldeyer tonsillar ring), or in extranodal, extralymphatic tissue, such as the mandible, salivary glands, pharynx, deep fascial spaces, paranasal sinuses, the orbit, and other areas. As pointed out by Miller, Young, and Novakovic, Wright, McKeever, and Carter, and Skarin and Dorfman, the classification of NHL has changed substantially in the past 25 years.[60-62] Childhood NHL differs from adult NHL in that the majority of childhood cases are high grade, demonstrate a diffuse growth pattern, and commonly involve extranodal sites.

The majority of cases fall into one of three types: small, noncleaved cell lymphoma, Burkitt's type (some authors use the terms Burkitt's lymphoma and small, noncleaved lymphoma synonymously; some use Burkitt's lymphoma and non–Burkitt's lymphoma as subtypes of small, noncleaved cell lymphoma; and others speak of the two as "related" entities); lymphoblastic lymphoma; and anaplastic large cell lymphoma. The separation of each of these can be made on the basis of morphologic and immunohistochemical features. Unlike HL, which spreads to contiguous lymph node groups, NHL spreads in an unpredictable fashion, so that most patients present with stage III or IV disease.

Ribeiro et al studied 87 consecutively treated children with NHL arising in the head and neck region.[63] Thirty-one children had primary nodal NHL, whereas 56 had extranodal NHL. Their data indicate that, unlike adults, children whose primary head and neck NHLs were extranodal had a significantly worse treatment outcome than those whose primary tumors were nodal. Children whose tumors were extranodal and extralymphatic had an even worse outcome than the others. Owing to the anatomical sites of origin of NHL in childhood, the majority of patients do not present with peripheral lymphadenopathy. When lymphadenopathy is present, it may appear as a firm, nontender swelling.

The use of effective risk-adapted multiagent chemotherapy along with improvements in supportive care have resulted in marked improvements in cure rates for all stages and subtypes of NHL in children, with event-free survival ranging from 70% to 90% depending on the stage and subtype of disease. Stage of disease and tumor burden are now used to select the intensity and length of therapy rather than serving as a major indicator of outlook for survival.

RHABDOMYOSARCOMA

Rhabdomyosarcoma, a malignant neoplasm of skeletal muscle origin, is the most common soft tissue sarcoma in children, accounting for more than half of all such lesions occurring in childhood. There are two key age ranges for the occurrence of rhabdomyosarcoma in children: 2 to 6 years of age and adolescence. According to Miser and Pizzo, the early peak is due primarily to occurrences in the head and neck region and genitourinary tract.[64]

Three histologic subtypes are recognized: embryonal and its botryoid variant, alveolar, and pleomorphic. The embryonal subtype accounts for most rhabdomyosarcomas in infancy and childhood that occur within the deep soft tissues or along mucosal surfaces.

The most common clinical finding is a mass occurring in any region of the head and neck where striated muscle or its mesenchymal progenitor cells exist. There are three primary sites of involvement for rhabdomyosarcoma in the head and neck in children: the eyelid and orbit, parapharyngeal sites, and remaining head and neck sites. The parapharyngeal sites include the pterygopalatine and infratemporal fossa, nasal cavity, nasopharynx, paranasal sinuses, and middle ear and mastoid. Orally, the tonsil and soft palate, tongue, and cheek are most frequently involved. Typically a rapidly growing, often nonulcerated soft tissue mass, rhabdomyosarcoma typically metastasizes by hematogenous routes to lungs, bone, and brain but may also disseminate via the lymphatics or by direct extension.

As discussed by Kraus, Saenz, and Gallamudi, rhabdomyosarcomas arising in the head and neck region are characterized by a wide variation in survival rate depending on the site, with orbital lesions associated the highest survival rates of any site in the body and parapharyngeal tumors having a worse prognosis.[65] Age, sex, resectability, and tumor-node-metastasis (TNM) stage are also important prognostic variables. In their review, Simon et al pointed out that children 11 years of age or younger with a tumor 5 cm or smaller had the best survival, whereas patients older than 11 years with a tumor larger than 5 cm had the worst survival outcome.[66] A multimodality approach to therapy consisting of multiagent chemotherapy, surgery, and external-beam radiotherapy has improved survival. In the study by Kraus, Saenz, and Gallamudi, overall 5-year survival was 74%, with each variable contributing to the TNM stage being statistically significant in determining survival.[65]

OSTEOGENIC SARCOMA

Osteogenic sarcoma is an uncommon, highly malignant, primary neoplasm of bone with a soft tissue counterpart with a similar histomorphology. As pointed out by with nearly all patients having micrometastatic disease at the time of diagnosis. In the Intergroup Ewing's Sarcoma Study as reported by Siegal et al, the prognosis for head and neck Ewing's sarcoma was noted to be significantly better than that for Ewing's sarcoma over-all.[73] Of their patients who had been followed in the study for more than 3 years, 80% were alive and well without known progressive recurrent or metastatic disease. Of the 10 patients who had survived 5 years or longer, none had subsequently died, and of the 5 patients in their study who had died, none had gnathic involvement.

Therapy consists of systemic multiagent chemo-therapy along with local control, which may consist of surgery, radiation therapy, or a combination of the two, depending on the age of the patient, the location of the primary tumor, and the functional consequences of therapy. Because of the potential for postradiation sarcomas, particularly bone sarcoma in the field of radiation treatment, the importance of local control of the disease with surgery and safe local control with radiation is now emphasized. Patients with clinically detectable metastases at the time of diagnosis and those with relapse after initial therapy have a significantly poorer prognosis. As pointed out by Rodriguez-Galindo, Spunt, and Pappo in their overview, chemotherapy dose intensification and the use of megatherapy with auto-logous hematopoietic stem cell transplantation are routinely used at a number of treatment centers for these high-risk patients.[79]

LANGERHANS' CELL HISTIOCYTOSIS (HISTIOCYTOSIS X)

Langerhans' cell histiocytosis (LCH) is the current desig-nation replacing the term *histiocytosis X* introduced by Lichtenstein in 1953 as a unifying designation for several previous eponyms, including Letterer-Siwe disease, Hand-Schüller-Christian disease, and eosinophilic granuloma (LCH of bone).[80]

Although clinical forms of LCH were first described at least a century ago, the etiology and patho-genesis of Langerhans' cell histiocytosis remains obscure, with the one common denominator being the Langerhans' cell, a bone marrow–derived, antigen-presenting dendritic cell. Langerhans' cells reside in the skin, thymus, and mucosal epithelium, including the oropharynx and nasopharynx, esophagus, bronchi, and cervix and, as reviewed by Lam, are said to be the most potent antigen-presenting cells in the body.[81]

Histologically, LCH is characterized by the presence of uniform sheets of large round Langerhans' histio-cytes with a homogenous pink cytoplasm when stained with hematoxylin and eosin, interspersed with variable numbers of eosinophils, lymphocytes, plasma cells, and multinucleated giant cells, particularly in lesions of

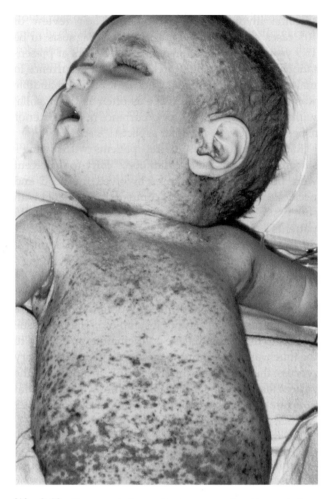

FIG. **8-18.** Characteristic erythematous scaly skin rash in a 5½-month-old infant with Letterer-Siwe disease.

bone. Langerhans' cells are characterized ultrastructurally by the presence of Langerhans' or Birbeck granules, rod-shaped organelles that may have a vesicular portion imparting the so-called tennis racquet appearance under the electron microscope.

The clinical manifestations of LCH are variable and historically were divided into distinct entities. The term *Letterer-Siwe disease* has been used as a moniker for an acute fulminating proliferative disorder involving Langerhans' histiocytes that chiefly affects infants and children under the age of 3. It is often characterized initially by the development of a scaly erythematous skin rash initially most prominent on the trunk but pro-gressing to involve the scalp and extremities (Fig. 8-18). This is accompanied by a persistent low-grade fever, anemia, thrombocytopenia, hepatosplenomegaly, and lymphadenopathy.

Bony involvement, indistinguishable from that found in Hand-Schüller-Christian disease, and eosinophilic granuloma of bone may be noted (Fig. 8-19). Oral lesions with pain, swelling, ulceration, gingival necrosis, and

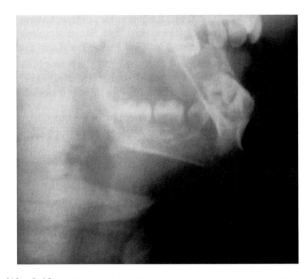

FIG. **8-19.** Diffuse destruction of maxillary and mandibular alveolar bone around the developing primary teeth in the same patient as in Fig. 8-18. Notice also destruction of the left angle and ramus of the mandible.

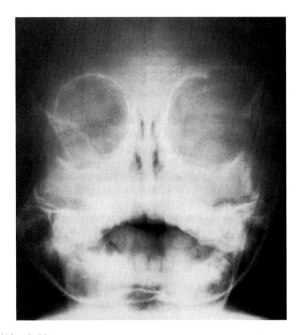

FIG. **8-20.** Radiograph for a 12-month-old girl with Hand-Schüller-Christian disease. There is an expansile, radiolucent lesion in the right body of the mandible as well as destruction of the greater wing of the sphenoid and supraorbital rim on the left.

destruction of alveolar bone with premature exfoliation of the teeth may be an early manifestation of Letterer-Siwe disease. Although multiagent chemotherapy may result in regression of the disease in some cases, patients with this form of the disease have a relatively poor prognosis.

The term *Hand-Schüller-Christian disease* has been used to describe the chronic, disseminated form of LCH, which is characterized by the development of multifocal eosinophilic granulomas of bone, lymphadenopathy, and visceral involvement, especially hepatosplenomegaly (Fig. 8-20). The classical clinical triad that has often been described for this disease is the occurrence of punched out–appearing radiolucent defects in membranous bones, exophthalmos, and diabetes insipidus. Chronic otitis media is also a frequent symptom. Although usually diagnosed early in the first decade of life, Hand-Schüller-Christian disease has been reported by McDonald et al to occur as late as the sixth decade.[82]

The treatment varies according to the extent of the disease, with surgical curettage or radiation therapy being used to treat focal disease. Multiagent chemotherapy has proved to be relatively successful in the long-term control of disseminated disease.

Eosinophilic granuloma is the most common and also least severe form of LCH. It is characterized by single or multiple usually well-defined radiolucent bony lesions, most often accompanied by pain and swelling. Older children and young adults most commonly display this form of the disease. In addition to the mandible and skull, the femur, humerus, ribs, and pelvis are also frequently involved. The maxilla is involved less frequently than the mandible, with the midposterior

mandible being the most common site of occurrence. Skin and visceral involvement such as that described for Hand-Schüller-Christian and Letterer-Siwe diseases are absent. A variety of options exist for patients with this form of the disease. After confirmation of the diagnosis by biopsy, the lesion may be left alone for observation, it may be surgically curetted or excised, intralesional injections of corticosteroids may be given, or low-dose radiotherapy may be used. As noted in the review by Ardekian et al, the recurrence rate of eosinophilic granuloma ranges from 1.6% to 25%.[83] Their study was the first to use a standardized treatment regimen of surgery and radiation therapy. A 7.3% recurrence rate was reported.

REFERENCES

1. Abbey LM, Page DG, Sawyer DR: The clinical and histopathologic features of a series of 464 oral squamous cell papillomas, *Oral Surg* 49:419-428, 1980.
2. Greer RO, Goldman HM: Oral papillomas: clinicopathologic evaluation and retrospective examination for dyskeratosis in 110 lesions, *Oral Surg* 38:435-440, 1974.
3. Praetorius F: HPV-associated diseases of oral mucosa, *Clin Dermatol* 15:399-413, 1997.
4. Naghashfar Z et al: Identification of genital tract papillomavirus HPV-6 and HPV-16 in warts of the oral cavity, *J Med Virol* 17:313-324, 1985.
5. Zeuss MS, Miller CS, White DK: In situ hybridization analysis of human papillomavirus DNA in oral mucosal lesions, *Oral Surg Oral Med Oral Pathol* 71:714-20, 1991.

9

Eruption of the Teeth: Local, Systemic, and Congenital Factors That Influence the Process

RALPH E. McDONALD

DAVID R. AVERY

JEFFREY A. DEAN

CHAPTER OUTLINE

CHRONOLOGIC DEVELOPMENT AND ERUPTION OF THE TEETH

A variety of developmental defects that are evident after eruption of the primary and permanent teeth can be related to systemic and local factors that influence matrix formation and the calcification process. Thus it is important that the dentist be able to explain to the parents the time factors related to the early stages of tooth calcification both in utero and during infancy.

Lunt and Law made a careful review of the literature on the calcification of the primary teeth.[1] They compared their findings with the values in Table 9-1 showing Logan and Kronfeld's chronology of human dentition, which has been an accepted standard for many years.[2] They offered a revised table that establishes earlier ages than those previously accepted for initial calcification (Table 9-2). A similar review was carried out for the ages at which the primary teeth erupt.[3]

Lunt and Law concluded after reviewing the work of Kraus and Jordan (1965) and of Nomata (1964) that Table 9-1 should be modified.[4,5] The sequence of calcification of the primary teeth should be changed to central incisor, first molar, lateral incisor, canine, and second molar. They determined that the times of initial calcification of the primary teeth are 2 to 6 weeks earlier than those given in Table 9-1. They also concluded that the maxillary teeth are generally ahead of the mandibular teeth in development. Exceptions are the second molars, which generally are advanced in the mandible, and the lateral incisors and canines, which at times may be ahead in the mandible.

Lunt and Law also believe that the lateral incisor, first molar, and canine tend to erupt earlier in the maxilla than in the mandible; the Logan and Kronfeld table suggests that eruption in the mandible is generally ahead of that in the maxilla. The ages at which primary teeth erupt are 2 months or more later than suggested in the Logan and Kronfeld table.

It should be remembered that the time of eruption of both primary and permanent teeth varies greatly. Variations of 6 months on either side of the usual eruption date may be considered normal for a given child. Interestingly, a study by Parner et al compared the well-known general acceleration of the physical development of children over the past century with their own observations of the emergence of permanent teeth.[6] They found that the emergence of permanent teeth has not been subject to a similar acceleration; in fact, the mean age of eruption has increased slightly, but only by a few days per year. They conclude that the age of eruption of the permanent teeth is a much more stable phenomenon than other aspects of physical development of children.

Numerous in vivo animal experiments and human radiographic studies have been done to better understand the process of tooth eruption. Although many theories have been advanced, the factors responsible for the eruption of the teeth are not fully understood. The factors that have been related to the eruption of teeth include elongation of the root, forces exerted by the vascular tissues around and beneath the root, growth of the alveolar bone, growth of dentin, growth and pull of the periodontal membrane, hormonal influences, presence of a viable dental follicle, pressure from the muscular action, and resorption of the alveolar crest.

A series of experiments by Cahill and Marks have established that a viable dental follicle is required for tooth eruption.[7] Further studies by Marks and Cahill resulted in the conclusion that "tooth eruption is a series of metabolic events in alveolar bone characterized by bone resorption and formation on opposite sides of the dental follicle and the tooth does not contribute to this process."[8]

Baume, Becks, and Evans reported evidence that tooth eruption is influenced by pituitary growth hormone and thyroid hormone.[9] Philbrick et al have demonstrated that parathyroid hormone–related protein is required for tooth eruption.[10]

Shumaker and El Hadary observed in a radiographic study that each tooth starts to move toward occlusion at approximately the time of crown completion.[11] The interval from crown completion and the beginning of eruption until the tooth is in full occlusion is approximately 5 years for permanent teeth.

Grøn observed in her study of 874 Boston children that tooth emergence appeared to be more closely associated with the stage of root formation than with the chronologic or skeletal age of the child.[12] By the time of clinical emergence approximately three fourths of root formation had occurred. Teeth reach occlusion before the root development is complete.

Demirjian and Levesque presented a large sample of 5437 radiographs from a homogeneous (French-Canadian) population.[13] They used this sample to investigate the sexual differences in the development of permanent mandibular teeth from the early stages of calcification to closure of the apex. The analysis of the developmental curves of individual teeth shows a common pattern, namely, the similarity in timing between the sexes for the early stages of development. For the first stages of crown formation, which they refer to as A, B, and C, there was no difference between boys and girls in the chronology of the dental calcification in the majority of teeth. For the fourth stage, D, which represents the completion of crown development, girls were more advanced than boys by an average of 0.35 year for four teeth. For the stages of root development the mean difference between the sexes for all teeth was 0.54 year; the largest difference was for the canine

| TABLE **9-1** | Chronology of the Human Dentition

TOOTH	HARD TISSUE FORMATION BEGINS	AMOUNT OF ENAMEL FORMED AT BIRTH	ENAMEL COMPLETED	ERUPTION	ROOT COMPLETED
DECIDUOUS DENTITION					
Maxillary					
Central incisor	4 mo in utero	Five sixths	1^1/$_2$ mo	7^1/$_2$ mo	1^1/$_2$ yr
Lateral incisor	4^1/$_2$ mo in utero	Two thirds	2^1/$_2$ mo	9 mo	2 yr
Cuspid	5 mo in utero	One third	9 mo	18 mo	3^1/$_4$ yr
First molar	5 mo in utero	Cusps united	6 mo	14 mo	2^1/$_2$ yr
Second molar	6 mo in utero	Cusp tips still isolated	11 mo	24 mo	3 yr
Mandibular					
Central incisor	4^1/$_2$ mo in utero	Three fifths	2^1/$_2$ mo	6 mo	1^1/$_2$ yr
Lateral incisor	4^1/$_2$ mo in utero	Three fifths	3 mo	7 mo	1^1/$_2$ yr
Cuspid	5 mo in utero	One third	9 mo	16 mo	3^1/$_4$ yr
First molar	5 mo in utero	Cusps united	5^1/$_2$ mo	12 mo	2^1/$_4$ yr
Second molar	6 mo in utero	Cusp tips still isolated	10 mo	20 mo	3 yr
PERMANENT DENTITION					
Maxillary					
Central incisor	3-4 mo		4-5 yr	7-8 yr	10 yr
Lateral incisor	10-12 mo		4-5 yr	8-9 yr	11 yr
Cuspid	4-5 mo		6-7 yr	11-12 yr	13-15 yr
First bicuspid	1^1/$_2$-1^3/$_4$ yr		5-6 yr	10-11 yr	12-13 yr
Second bicuspid	2-2^1/$_4$ yr		6-7 yr	10-12 yr	12-14 yr
First molar	At birth	Sometimes a trace	2^1/$_2$-3 yr	6-7 yr	9-10 yr
Second molar	2^1/$_2$-3 yr		7-8 yr	12-13 yr	14-16 yr
Third molar	7-9 yr		12-16 yr	17-21 yr	18-25 yr
Mandibular					
Central incisor	3-4 mo		4-5 yr	6-7 yr	9 yr
Lateral incisor	3-4 mo		4-5 yr	7-8 yr	10 yr
Cuspid	4-5 mo		6-7 yr	9-10 yr	12-14 yr
First bicuspid	1^3/$_4$-2 yr		5-6 yr	10-12 yr	12-13 yr
Second bicuspid	2^1/$_4$-2^1/$_2$ yr		6-7 yr	11-12 yr	13-14 yr
First molar	At birth	Sometimes a trace	2^1/$_2$-3 yr	6-7 yr	9-10 yr
Second molar	2^1/$_2$-3 yr		7-8 yr	11-13 yr	14-15 yr
Third molar	8-10 yr		12-16 yr	17-21 yr	18-25 yr

From Kronfeld R: *Bur* 35:18-25, 1935 (based on research by WHG Logan and R Kronfeld); adapted by Kronfeld R, Schour I: *J Am Dent Assoc* 26: 18-32, 1939; further adapted by McCall JO, Wald SS: *Clinical dental roentgenology: technic and interpretation including roentgen studies of the child and young adult,* Philadelphia, 1940, WB Saunders.

(0.90 year). The data from Demirjian and Levesque show the importance of sexual dimorphism during the period of root development rather than during the period of crown development.[13]

The tooth eruption process is clearly quite complex, and many different mechanisms are undoubtedly involved. Some of the leading scientists who are contributing to a better understanding of the tooth eruption process have written review articles to help consolidate the facts and theories associated with this process. A review article by Wise et al focuses on the molecular signals that initiate tooth eruption.[14] These researchers state that tooth eruption is a complex and tightly regulated process that involves cells of the tooth organ and the surrounding alveolus. Mononuclear cells (osteoclast precursors) must be recruited into the dental follicle prior to the onset of eruption. These cells, in turn, fuse to form osteoclasts that resorb alveolar bone, creating an eruption pathway for the tooth to exit its bony crypt. In recent years, knowledge of the biology of tooth eruption has greatly increased. What has emerged is the realization that interactions of osteoblasts, osteoclasts, and dental follicles involve a complex interplay of regulatory genes that encode various transcription

TABLE 9-2 Modification of the Table "Chronology of the Human Dentition" Suggested by Lunt and Law for the Calcification and Eruption of the Primary Dentition

TOOTH	HARD TISSUE FORMATION BEGINS	AMOUNT OF ENAMEL FORMED AT BIRTH	ENAMEL COMPLETED	ERUPTION (±1 SD)	ROOT COMPLETED
DECIDUOUS DENTITION					
Maxillary					
Central incisor	14 (13-16) wk in utero	Five sixths	1½ mo	10 (8-12) mo	1½ yr
Lateral incisor	16 (14²/₃-16½) wk in utero	Two thirds	2½ mo	11 (9-13) mo	2 yr
Canine	17 (15-18) wk in utero	One third	9 mo	19 (16-22) mo	3¼ yr
First molar	15½ (14½-17) wk in utero	Cusps united; occlusal completely calcified plus half to three fourths crown height	6 mo	16 (13-19) mo boys, 16 (14-18) mo girls	2½ yr
Second molar	19 (16-23½) wk in utero	Cusps united; occlusal incompletely calcified; calcified tissue covers one fifth to one fourth crown height	11 mo	29 (25-33) mo	3 yr
Mandibular					
Central incisor	14 (13-16) wk in utero	Three fifths	2½ mo	8 (6-10) mo	1½ yr
Lateral incisor	16 (14²/₃-) wk in utero	Three fifths	3 mo	13 (10-16) mo	1½ yr
Canine	17 (16-) wk in utero	One third	9 mo	20 (17-23) mo	3¼ yr
First molar	15½ (14½-17) wk in utero	Cusps united; occlusal completely calcified	5½ mo	16 (14-18) mo	2¼ yr
Second molar	18 (17-19½) wk in utero	Cusps united; occlusal incompletely calcified	10 mo	27 (23-31) mo boys, 27 (24-30) mo girls	3 yr

From Lunt RC, Law DB: *J Am Dent Assoc* 89:8720-879, 1974.
SD, Standard deviation.

factors, protooncogenes, and soluble factors. For the clinician faced with treating both simple and complex dental complications arising from abnormal tooth eruption, knowledge of the basic molecular mechanisms involved is essential (Fig. 9-1). A paper by Kardos reviews the evidence for a tooth-eruptive force as well as its direction and source.[15] Finally, an extensive review by Marks and Schroeder analyzes experimental data to identify the basic principles of tooth eruption and offers their guiding theories of the process.[16] Readers who wish to obtain more information about the details of the tooth eruption process are referred to these review articles.

INFLUENCE OF PREMATURE LOSS OF PRIMARY MOLARS ON ERUPTION TIME OF THEIR SUCCESSORS

Posen, after reviewing the records of children in the Burlington study who had undergone unilateral extraction of primary molars, came to the following conclusions: Eruption of the premolar teeth is delayed in children who lose primary molars at 4 or 5 years of age and before.[17] If extraction of the primary molars occurs after the age of 5 years, there is a decrease in the delay of premolar eruption. At 8, 9, and 10 years of age, premolar eruption resulting from premature loss of primary teeth is greatly accelerated. Hartsfield stated that premature loss of teeth associated with systemic disease usually results from some change in the immune system or connective tissue.[18] The most common of these conditions appears to be hypophosphatasia and early-onset periodontitis.

VARIATIONS IN THE SEQUENCE OF ERUPTION

The mandibular first permanent molars are often the first permanent teeth to erupt. They are quickly followed by the mandibular central incisors. Lo and Moyers found little or no clinical significance to the eruption of the incisors before the molars.[19]

After analyzing serial records of 16,000 children in Newburgh and Kingston, New York, Carlos and Gittelsohn concluded that the average eruption time of the lower central incisors was earlier than that of the first molars by about 1½ months in both boys and girls.[20] Of considerable interest was the gender difference in the

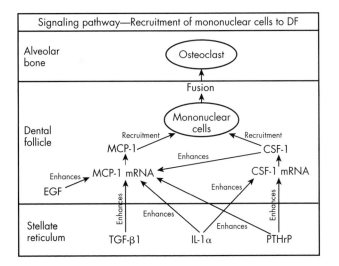

FIG. **9-1.** Paracrine signaling between the stellate reticulum and dental follicle (DF) results in the synthesis and secretion of chemotactic molecules, colony-stimulating factor 1 (CSF-1) and monocyte chemotactic protein 1 (MCP-1) for recruitment of mononuclear cells. *EGF,* Epidermal growth factor; *IL-1α,* interleukin 1α; *PTHrP,* parathyroid hormone–related peptide; *mRNA,* messenger RNA; *TGF-β1,* transforming growth factor β1. *(Reprinted with permission from Wise GE et al: Crit Rev Oral Biol Med 12[4]:323-335, 2002.)*

eruption sequence of permanent teeth. The mandibular canine erupted before the maxillary and mandibular first premolars in girls. In boys the eruption order was reversed—the maxillary and mandibular first premolars erupted before the mandibular canine.

Moyers stated that the most common sequence of eruption of permanent teeth in the mandible is first molar, central incisor, lateral incisor, canine, first premolar, second premolar, and second molar.[21] The most common sequence for the eruption of the maxillary permanent teeth is first molar, central incisor, lateral incisor, first premolar, second premolar, canine, and second molar (Fig. 9-2). He identified these common sequences in each arch to be favorable for maintaining the length of the arches during the transitional dentition.

It is desirable that the mandibular canine erupt before the first and second premolars. This sequence aids in maintaining adequate arch length and in preventing lingual tipping of the incisors. Lingual tipping of the incisors not only causes a loss of arch length but also

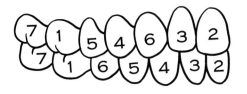

FIG. **9-2.** Desirable eruption sequence for the permanent teeth.

allows the development of an increased overbite. An abnormal lip musculature or an oral habit that causes a greater force on the lower incisors than can be compensated by the tongue allows a collapse of the anterior segment. For this reason use of a passive lingual arch appliance is often indicated when the primary canines have been lost prematurely or when the sequence of eruption is undesirable.

A deficiency in arch length can occur if the mandibular second permanent molar develops and erupts before the second premolar. Eruption of the second permanent molar first encourages mesial migration or tipping of the first permanent molar and encroachment on the space needed for the second premolar. The importance of maintaining the second primary molar until its replacement by the second premolar is discussed in Chapter 27.

In the maxillary arch the first premolar ideally should erupt before the second premolar, and they should be followed by the canine. The untimely loss of primary molars in the maxillary arch, which allows the first permanent molar to drift and tip mesially, results in the permanent canine's being blocked out of the arch, usually to the labial side.

The position of the developing second permanent molar in the maxillary arch and its relationship to the first permanent molar should be given special attention. Its eruption before the premolars and canine can cause a loss of arch length, just as in the mandibular arch.

The eruption of the maxillary canine is often delayed because of an abnormal position or devious eruption path. This delayed eruption should be considered along with its possible effect on the alignment of the maxillary teeth. The significance of the sequence of the eruption of permanent teeth is considered further in Chapter 27.

LINGUAL ERUPTION OF MANDIBULAR PERMANENT INCISORS

The eruption of mandibular permanent incisors lingual to retained primary incisors is often a source of concern for parents. The primary teeth may have undergone extensive root resorption and may be held only by soft tissues. In other instances the roots may not have undergone normal resorption and the teeth remain solidly in place. It is common for mandibular permanent incisors to erupt lingually, and this pattern should be considered essentially normal. It is seen both in patients with an obvious arch length inadequacy (Fig. 9-3) and in those with a desirable amount of spacing of the primary incisors (Fig. 9-4). In either case the tongue and continued alveolar growth seem to play an important role in influencing the permanent incisors into a more normal position with time. Although there may be insufficient room in the arch for the newly erupted permanent

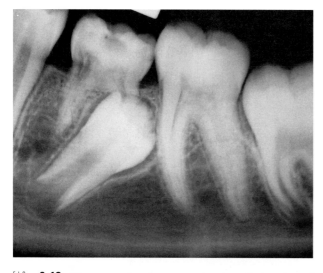

FIG. **9-12.** The second primary molar is ankylosed and below the normal plane of occlusion. There is evidence of root resorption and deposition of bone into the resorbed areas.

primary teeth had no permanent successors.[46] Brown also reported a higher prevalence of developmentally absent premolar teeth in patients with ankylosis.[47] It is often suggested that there is a relationship between congenital absence of permanent teeth and ankylosed primary teeth. Steigman, Koyoumdjisky-Kaye, and Matrai have discounted this relationship.[48] Based on observation and a careful review of the literature, they reported that there appears to be no causal relationship between ankylosed precursors and congenital absence of their successors.

Normal resorption of the primary molar begins on the inner surface or the lingual surface of the roots. The resorption process is not continuous but is interrupted by periods of inactivity or rest. A reparative process follows periods of resorption. In the course of this reparative phase a solid union often develops between the bone and the primary tooth. This intermittent resorption and repair may explain the varying degrees of firmness of the primary teeth before their exfoliation. Extensive bony ankylosis of the primary tooth may prevent normal exfoliation, as well as the eruption of the permanent successor.

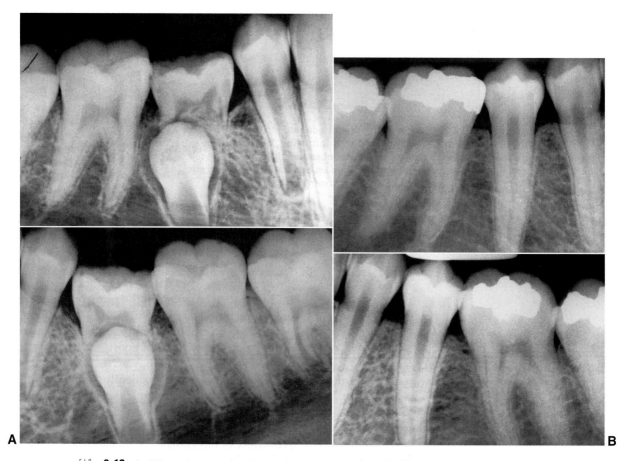

FIG. **9-13. A,** Bilateral ankylosis of second primary molars. **B,** The ankylosed molars were eventually shed, and the second premolars erupted into good occlusion. Frequently the ankylosed teeth must be removed surgically.

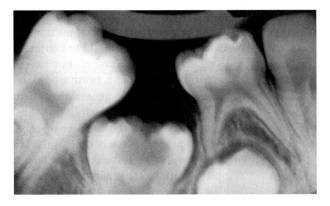

FIG. **9-14.** Ankylosed second primary molar with a carious lesion in the occlusal surface. This tooth probably became ankylosed soon after root resorption began.

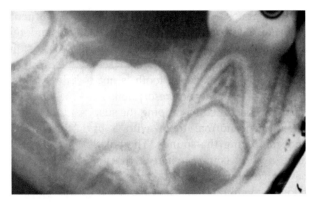

FIG. **9-15.** An ankylosed, deeply embedded second primary molar. Surgical removal of this tooth is indicated.

Ankylosis of the primary molar to the alveolar bone does not usually occur until after its root resorption begins. If ankylosis occurs early, eruption of adjacent teeth may progress enough that the ankylosed tooth is far below the normal plane of occlusion and may even be partially covered with soft tissue (Fig. 9-14). An epithelium-lined track will, however, extend from the oral cavity to the tooth. Ankylosis may occasionally occur even before the eruption and complete root formation of the primary tooth (Fig. 9-15). Tsukamoto and Braham reported a case of apparent early ankylosis of a mandibular second primary molar that was not diagnosed until the patient was 10 years of age; at that time the succedaneous second premolar was lying malposed but occlusal to the unerupted primary molar.[49] Ankylosis can also occur late in the resorption of the primary roots and even then can interfere with the eruption of the underlying permanent tooth (Fig. 9-16).

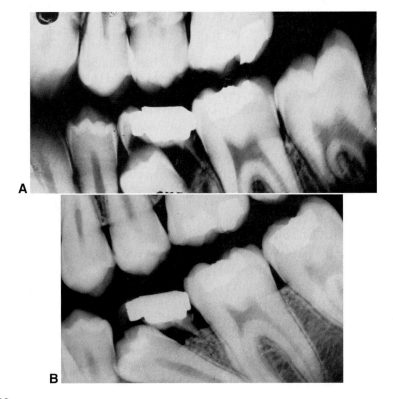

FIG. **9-16. A,** A small spicule of root of the primary tooth is ankylosed to the alveolar bone. This was overlooked at the time of the routine examination. **B,** One year later the second primary molar is still retained, and the second premolar has moved into a more unfavorable position.

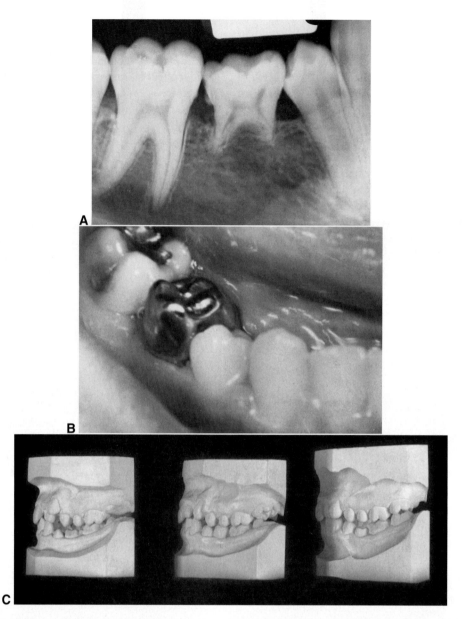

FIG. **9-18. A,** Ankylosed primary molar without a permanent successor. **B,** Mesiodistal width of the primary molar was reduced to allow the premolar to erupt, and an overlay was constructed to establish occlusion with the opposing teeth. **C,** Models at the left show the original condition. Center models show the occlusion at the time the overlay was placed on the ankylosed tooth. Models at the right show the continued eruption of the adjacent teeth that occurred in the subsequent 18-month period.

TRISOMY 21 SYNDROME (DOWN SYNDROME)

Trisomy 21 syndrome (Down syndrome [DS]) is one of the congenital anomalies in which delayed eruption of the teeth frequently occurs. The first primary teeth may not appear until 2 years of age, and the dentition may not be complete until 5 years of age. The eruption often follows an abnormal sequence, and some of the primary teeth may be retained until 15 years of age. A study of 127 males and 128 females with DS by Ondarza et al found that, on average, 6 primary teeth were delayed in

eruption in boys and 11 primary teeth were delayed in girls.[58] A similar study of 116 males and 124 females with DS by Jara et al showed delayed eruption of 13 permanent teeth in boys and 8 permanent teeth in girls.[59] These studies seem to confirm that delayed tooth eruption is common but sporadic in children with DS.

Earlier literature refers to DS as "mongolism," but the use of this term is inappropriate according to Schreiner and it may be insulting to the affected families.[60] DS occurs very early in embryonic development, possibly

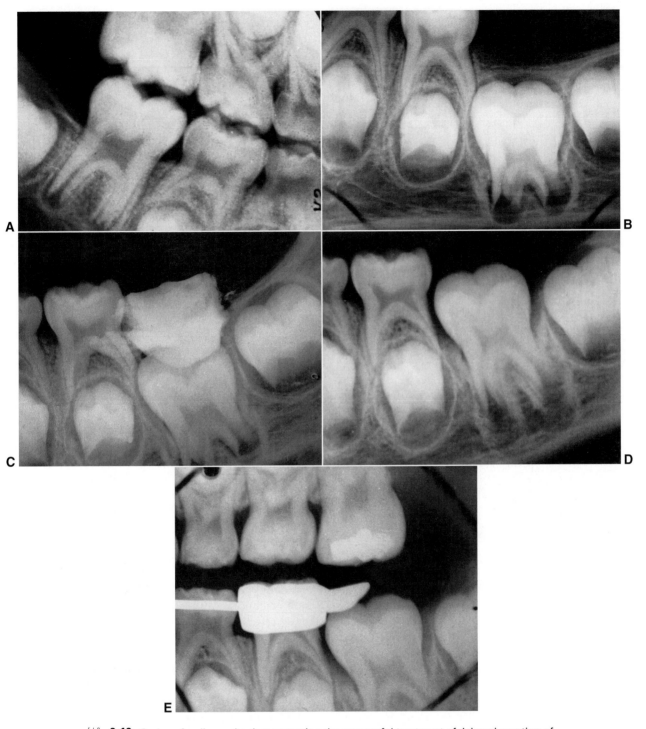

FIG. **9-19.** Series of radiographs demonstrating the successful treatment of delayed eruption of a first permanent molar. **A,** The first permanent molar has erupted on the right side. **B,** The left first permanent molar remains embedded in bone and is probably ankylosed. **C,** Soft tissue and bone have been removed, and surgical cement has been placed over the unerupted tooth. **D,** Within 3 months the first permanent molar has moved occlusally. **E,** The lingual arch and distal extension hold the surgical cement in position and prevent continued eruption of the opposing molar.

Continued

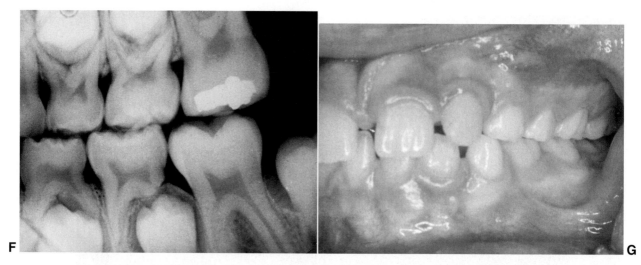

F   G

FIG. **9-19, cont'd** F and G, The first permanent molar has erupted, and the occlusion is good. Notice the progressive resorption of the distal root of the mandibular second primary molar.

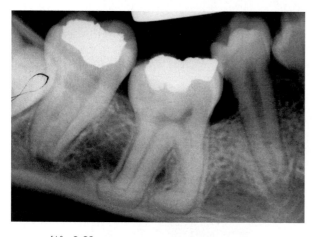

FIG. **9-20.** Ankylosed first permanent molar.

during the first cell divisions. Anomalies of the eye and external ear are seen, and congenital heart defects are often present. The occurrence of DS is frequently related to maternal age. Benda reported the frequency of DS to be approximately 1.5 per 1000 births for mothers in the 18- to 29-year-old age group.[61] The frequency increases for maternal ages of 30 years and higher, reaching 29 per 1000 in the 40-year-old and older age group and a high of 91 per 1000 in the 44-year-old age group.

The cause of DS is trisomy 21, that is, the presence of three number 21 chromosomes rather than the normal two (diploid). The diagnosis of DS in a child is not usually difficult to make because of the characteristic facial pattern (Fig. 9-22). The orbits are small, the eyes slope upward, and the bridge of the nose is more depressed than normal. Cohen, in a study of 194 children with DS, reported that 54% demonstrated anomalies in the formation of the external ear, characterized by outstanding

"lap" ear with flat or absent helix.[62] Mental retardation is another characteristic finding, with most children in the mild to moderate range of disability (see Table 3-3).

Landau made a cephalometric comparison of children with DS and their normal siblings.[63] Retardation in the growth of the maxillae and mandible was evident in those with DS. Both the maxillae and mandible were positioned anteriorly under the cranial base. The upper facial height was found to be significantly smaller. The midface was also found to be small in the vertical and horizontal dimensions. The smaller jaws contribute to a tendency for protrusion of the tongue and dental crowding, both of which may compromise good occlusion development. The tongue also tends to be larger than normal.

Many children with DS have chronic inflammation of the conjunctiva and a history of repeated respiratory tract infections. The use of antibiotics has reduced the incidence of chronic infection and has resulted in fewer deaths from infection.

Tannenbaum and also Baer and Benjamin observed that the prevalence and severity of periodontal disease in children with DS are much higher than the norm.[64,65] A high prevalence of necrotizing ulcerative gingivitis was also observed. After reviewing the available literature Cichon, Crawford, and Grimm concluded that individuals with DS have a higher prevalence of periodontal disease than otherwise normal, age-matched control groups and other mentally disabled patients of similar age distribution.[66] Furthermore the reports of exaggerated immunoinflammatory responses of the tissues in DS patients cannot be explained by poor oral hygiene alone and may be the result of impaired cell-mediated and humoral immunities and deficient

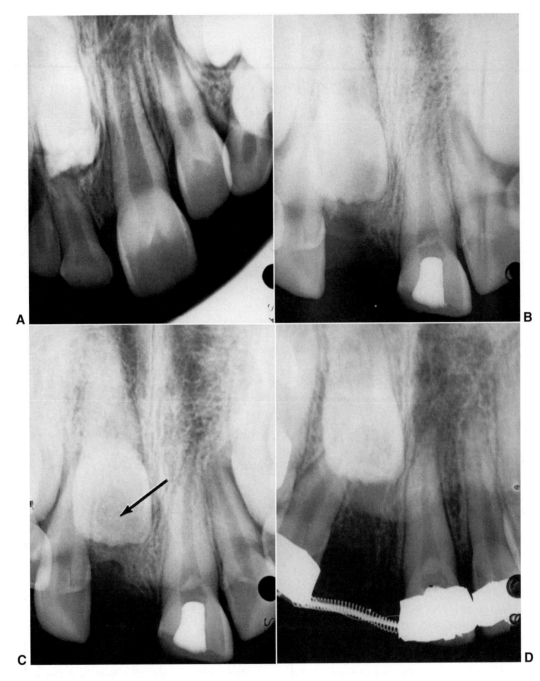

FIG. **9-21.** Ankylosis by inostosis. **A,** A mesiodens has delayed the eruption of the maxillary right permanent central incisor. **B,** The primary incisors and the mesiodens were removed. During the surgical removal of the mesiodens, there was apparently damage to the enamel epithelium. **C,** There is evidence of resorption of the enamel of the unerupted incisor and ankylosis of the tooth. **D,** The left central incisor crown sustained a fracture and pulp exposure. A calcium hydroxide pulpotomy was successfully performed, which resulted in continued root development.

phagocytic systems. Cichon et al's study of 10 DS patients aged 20 to 31 years demonstrated that the young age of onset, the severe destruction, and the pathogenesis of disease in the periodontal tissues were consistent with a juvenile periodontitis disease pattern.

Morinushi, Lopatin, and Van Poperin obtained blood samples and conducted gingival health assessments of 75 individuals with DS aged 2 to 18 years.[67] The extent of gingival inflammation and the antibody titers of the DS subjects suggested that colonization of certain pathogenic organisms for periodontal disease had occurred

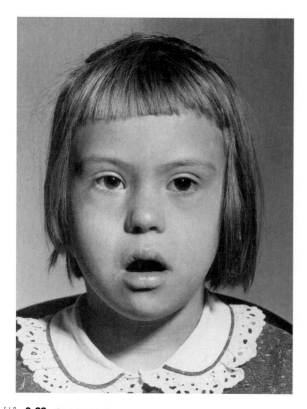

FIG. **9-22.** Child with Down syndrome, 8 years of age. *(Courtesy Dr. Mace Landau.)*

before 5 years of age. The prevalence and extent of gingivitis was significantly higher than in normal children. The antibody titers also suggested that colonization of additional pathogenic organisms increased with age. The authors believe that there are abnormalities in the systemic defenses that are responsible for the early onset of disease in the DS subjects. Similarly, Carlstedt et al have demonstrated significantly higher oral colonization with *Candida albicans* in DS children compared with an age- and sex-matched control group.[68] They believe that abnormalities of the immune response in DS children are responsible for their greater susceptibility to oral mucosal disease.

Dental caries susceptibility is usually low in those with DS. This finding has been reported by Johnson, Young, and Gallios, who noted a much lower dental caries incidence in both the primary and the permanent dentition.[69] Brown and Cunningham found in a study of DS children that 44% were caries free.[70] Shapira and Stabholz successfully demonstrated caries reduction and improved periodontal health during a 30-month period after initiating a comprehensive preventive oral health program for 20 children with DS.[71]

Although some children with low cognitive ability are unmanageable for dental procedures, most are pleasant, cheerful, affectionate, and well behaved.

They can often be managed in the dental office in a conventional manner. The possibility of reduced resistance to infection should be considered in the dental management of the child with DS.

CLEIDOCRANIAL DYSPLASIA

A rare congenital syndrome that has dental significance is cleidocranial dysplasia (CCD), which has also been referred to as *cleidocranial dysostosis, osteodentin dysplasia, mutational dysostosis,* and *Marie-Sainton syndrome.* Transmission of the condition is by either parent to a child of either sex, so that the disorder thus follows a true mendelian dominant pattern. CCD can also occur sporadically with no apparent hereditary influence and with no predilection for race. The diagnosis is based on the finding of an absence of clavicles, although there may be remnants of the clavicles, as evidenced by the presence of the sternal and acromial ends. The fontanels are large, and radiographs of the head show open sutures, even late in the child's life. The sinuses, particularly the frontal sinus, are usually small.

Richardson and Deussen performed cephalometric analyses of 17 patients with CCD.[72] They found that, on average, the patients exhibited mandibular prognathism caused by increased mandibular lengths and short cranial bases. The maxillae tended to be short vertically but not anteroposteriorly. Somewhat similar findings have been reported by Jensen and Kreiborg in their study of 22 children with CCD.[73]

The development of the dentition is delayed. Complete primary dentition at 15 years of age resulting from delayed resorption of the deciduous teeth and delayed eruption of the permanent teeth is not uncommon (Fig. 9-23). One of the important distinguishing characteristics is the presence of supernumerary teeth. Some children may have only a few supernumerary teeth in the anterior region of the mouth; others may have a large number of extra teeth throughout the mouth. Even with removal of the primary and

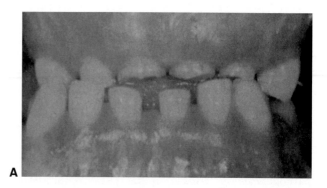

A

FIG. **9-23.** Cleidocranial dysplasia. **A,** A Primary dentition is still present at 15 years of age.   *Continued*

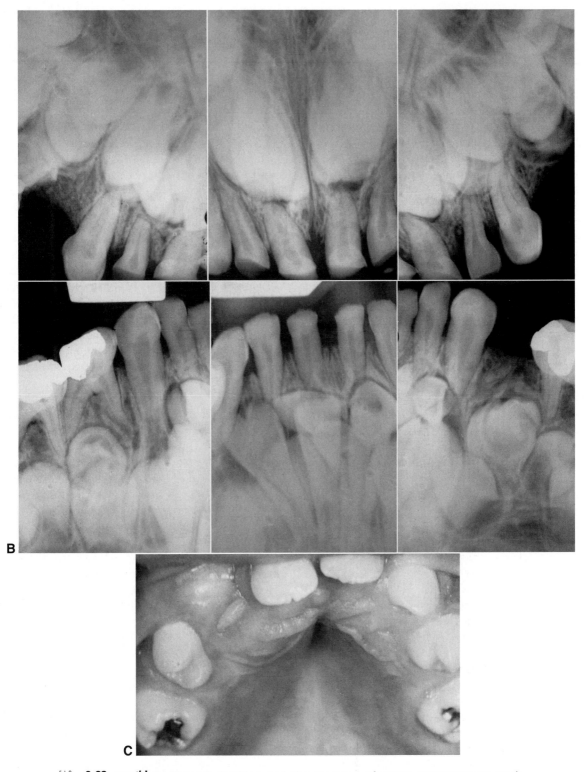

FIG. **9-23, cont'd B,** Delayed dentition and the presence of many supernumerary teeth. **C,** Removal of supernumerary teeth in the maxillary arch caused irregular and delayed eruption of some of the permanent teeth.

supernumerary teeth, eruption of the permanent dentition, without orthodontic intervention, is often delayed and irregular. Other reports by Jensen and Kreiborg, based on their experiences and longitudinal study of 19 patients with CCD, provide information to help clinicians predict the location and time of onset of formation of supernumerary teeth. This information should help the clinician optimally time the surgical treatment(s).[74,75]

Hutton, Bixler, and Garner have reported the successful dental management of a patient with CCD over a 15-year period.[76] The patient was first seen at 2 years of age. Treatment consisted of timed extractions of primary and supernumerary teeth and conservative uncovering of the permanent teeth. The surgical procedures were planned according to progressive radiographic evidence of the development of the permanent teeth. This management results in a nearly normal but slightly delayed eruption sequence. Orthodontic treatment was begun at 14 years of age, and by 16 years of age the patient displayed acceptable occlusion and normal vertical dimension, root development, and periodontal bone support.

Learning from their experiences with the long-term management of 16 patients with CCD, Becker et al advocate cooperative efforts by clinicians from the disciplines of pediatric dentistry, oral and maxillofacial surgery, and orthodontics and dentofacial orthopedics.[77] The pediatric dentist serves as the coordinator of overall oral health care and disease prevention during an extended treatment regimen that usually includes two surgical interventions and three stages of orthodontic surgery.

Delayed eruption has also been reported in other forms of osteopetroses.

HYPOTHYROIDISM

Hypothyroidism is another possible cause of delayed eruption. Patients in whom the function of the thyroid gland is extremely deficient have characteristic dental findings.

Congenital Hypothyroidism (Cretinism). Hypothyroidism occurring at birth and during the period of most rapid growth, if undetected and untreated, causes mental deficiency and dwarfism. This condition was referred to as *cretinism* in earlier medical and dental literatures. Congenital hypothyroidism is the result of an absence or underdevelopment of the thyroid gland and insufficient levels of thyroid hormone (Fig. 9-24). Today it is routinely diagnosed and corrected at birth because of mandatory blood screening of newborn infants. An inadequately treated child with congenital hypothyroidism is a small and disproportionate person, with abnormally short arms and legs. The head is disproportionately large, although the trunk

shows less deviation from the norm. Obesity is common.

Without adequate hormonal therapy the dentition of the child with congenital hypothyroidism is delayed in all stages, including eruption of the primary teeth, exfoliation of the primary teeth, and eruption of the permanent teeth. The teeth are normal in size but are crowded in jaws that are smaller than normal. The tongue is large and may protrude from the mouth. The abnormal size of the tongue and its position often cause an anterior open bite and flaring of the anterior teeth. The crowding of the teeth, malocclusion, and mouth breathing cause a chronic hyperplastic type of gingivitis.

Although untreated congenital hypothyroidism is rare, even in developing countries, Loevy, Aduss, and Rosenthal published a case report documenting the condition discovered in a 19-year-old boy.[78] The patient presented with a complete caries-free primary dentition and partially erupted maxillary first permanent molars. All primary teeth showed some abrasion. At a subsequent oral examination 1 year and 9 months after appropriate L-thyroxine therapy was initiated, several primary teeth had exfoliated, permanent incisors and first molars had erupted, and radiographs showed additional development of other permanent teeth.

Juvenile Hypothyroidism (Acquired Hypothyroidism). Juvenile hypothyroidism results from a malfunction of the thyroid gland, usually between 6 and 12 years of age. Because the deficiency occurs after the period of rapid growth, the unusual facial and body pattern characteristic of a person with congenital hypothyroidism is not present. However, obesity is evident to a lesser degree. In the untreated case of juvenile hypothyroidism, delayed exfoliation of the primary teeth and delayed eruption of the permanent teeth are characteristic. A child with a chronologic age of 14 years may have a dentition in a stage of development comparable with that of a child 9 or 10 years of age (Fig. 9-25).

HYPOPITUITARISM

A pronounced deceleration of the growth of the bones and soft tissues of the body will result from a deficiency in secretion of the growth hormone. Pituitary dwarfism is the result of an early hypofunction of the pituitary gland. Again, early diagnosis is routine because of the mandatory blood screening of newborn infants for congenital hypothyroidism.

An individual with pituitary dwarfism is well proportioned but resembles a child of considerably younger chronologic age (Fig. 9-26). The dentition is essentially normal in size.

Delayed eruption of the dentition is characteristic. In severe cases the primary teeth do not undergo

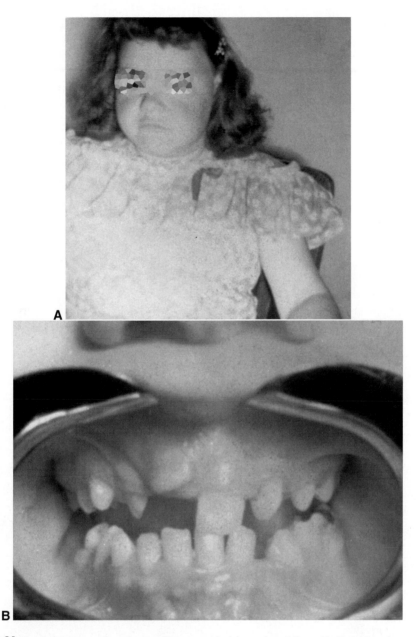

FIG. **9-24. A,** A 24-year-old patient with congenital hypothyroidism. **B,** Dentition is greatly delayed. With the administration of thyroxine, the eruption of the permanent teeth was accelerated. *(Courtesy Dr. David F. Mitchell.)*

resorption but instead may be retained throughout the life of the person. The underlying permanent teeth continue to develop but do not erupt. Extraction of the deciduous teeth is not indicated, since eruption of the permanent teeth cannot be assured. Some degree of cognitive disability often occurs.

ACHONDROPLASTIC DWARFISM

Achondroplastic dwarfism, also diagnosed at birth, demonstrates a few characteristic dental findings. Growth of the extremities is limited because of a lack of calcification in the cartilage of the long bones. Stature improvements have been reported with surgical lengthening of the limbs and also with growth hormone therapy. The head is disproportionately large, although the trunk is normal in size. The fingers may be of almost equal length, and the hands are plump. The fontanels are open at birth. The upper face is underdeveloped, and the bridge of the nose is depressed.

Although the etiology of achondroplastic dwarfism is unknown, it is clearly an autosomal dominant disorder although sporadic spontaneous mutations occur.

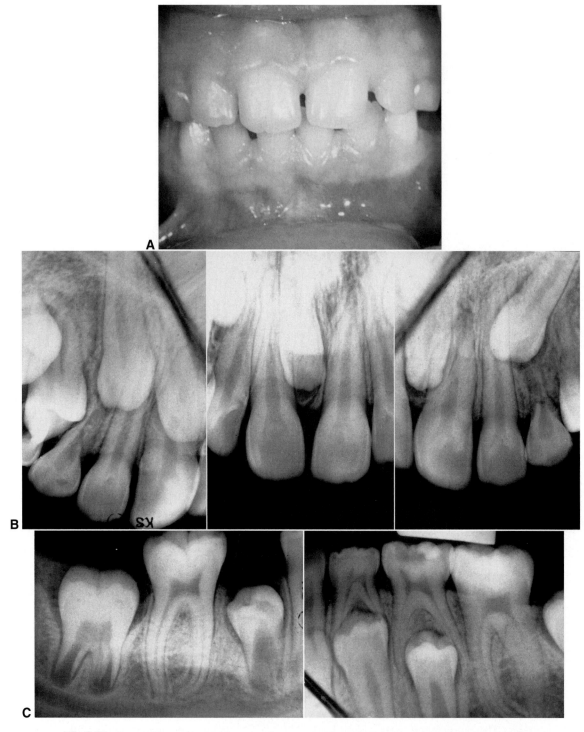

FIG. **9-25.** **A,** A 14-year-old girl who was diagnosed as having juvenile hypothyroidism. **B,** The occlusion was essentially normal but was delayed in its development. **C,** Delayed development of the teeth in juvenile hypothyroidism. The maxillary midline supernumerary tooth is a coincidental finding.

There is some evidence that the condition is more likely to occur when the ages of the parents differ significantly. In contrast to DS, the increased age of the father may be related to the occurrence of the condition.

Deficient growth in the cranial base is evident in many individuals with achondroplastic dwarfism. The maxilla may be small, with resultant crowding of the teeth and a tendency for open bite. A chronic

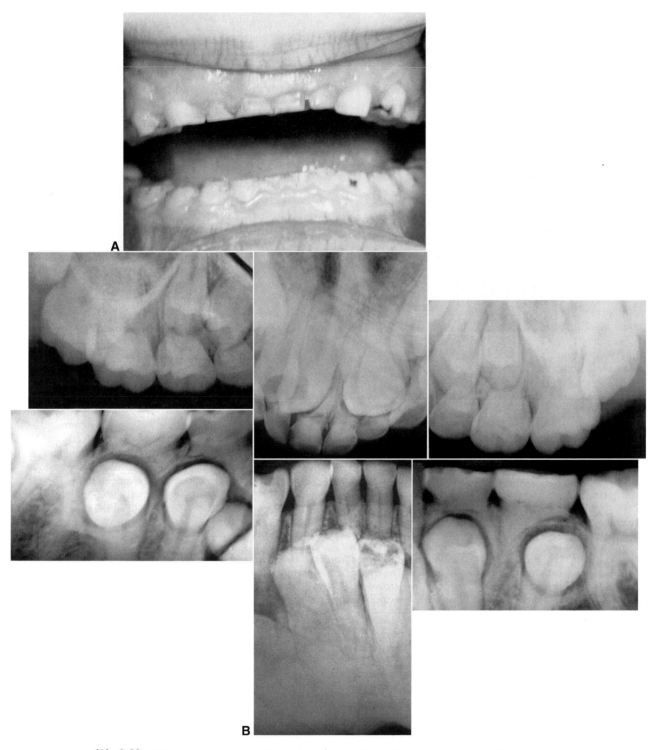

FIG. **9-26.** A 28-year-old woman diagnosed as having hypopituitary dwarfism. **A,** Complete primary dentition at 28 years of age. The first permanent molars have erupted. **B,** The roots of the primary teeth have not been resorbed to an appreciable degree, though some permanent teeth show complete development.

gingivitis is usually present. However, this condition may be related to the malocclusion and crowding of the teeth. In the patient shown in Fig. 9-27, the development of the dentition was slightly delayed.

OTHER CAUSES

Delayed eruption of the teeth has been linked to other disorders, including fibromatosis gingivae (see Chapter 20), Albright hereditary osteodystrophy,

We know that good oral health is an integral component of good general health. Although enjoying good oral health includes more than just having healthy teeth, many children have inadequate oral and general health because of active and uncontrolled dental caries. According to the first-ever United States Surgeon General's report on oral health in America published in May 2000, dental caries is the single most common chronic childhood disease.[1] Dental caries is five times more common than asthma and seven times more common than hay fever. Furthermore, as Edelstein and Douglass noted, dental caries is not self-limiting, like the common cold, nor amenable to treatment with a simple course of antibiotics, like an ear infection.[2] After analyzing the National Health Interview Survey data from 1993 through 1996, Newacheck et al concluded that dental care is the most prevalent unmet health need among American children.[3] Much other available data verify that we learned a great deal during the twentieth century about preventing dental caries, but other variables that contribute to the spread of the disease among many people in the world continue to thwart our efforts to eliminate this major health problem. Although effective methods are known for prevention and management of the disease, the unmet need for treatment, especially in children, does not seem to be diminishing. Gift has estimated that 51 million school hours per year are lost in the United States, because of dental-related illness.[4]

The National Institutes of Health sponsored a Consensus Development Conference on Diagnosis and Management of Dental Caries Throughout Life in March 2001.[5] Thirty-four papers were presented by recognized experts on dental caries. The October 2001 issue of the *Journal of Dental Education* published the entire proceedings of that conference. Only a few of the papers from the conference are specifically cited in the references for this chapter. However, the complete journal issue provides many good updates on the diagnosis and management of dental caries.

ETIOLOGY OF DENTAL CARIES

For as long as the science of dentistry has existed, there has been theorizing about the cause of dental caries. Today, all experts on dental caries generally agree that it is an infectious and communicable disease and that multiple factors influence the initiation and progression of the disease. The disease is recognized to require a host (tooth in the oral environment), a dietary substrate, and aciduric bacteria.[6] The saliva (also considered a host component), the substrate, and the bacteria form a biofilm (plaque) that adheres to the tooth surface. Over time the presence of the substrate serves as a nutrient for the bacteria, and the bacteria produce acids that can demineralize the tooth. The flow, dilution, buffering, and remineralizing capacity of saliva are also recognized to be critical factors that affect, and in some ways regulate, the progression and regression of the disease. If the oral environment is balanced and favorable, saliva can contribute to strengthening of the tooth by supplying the components known to help build strong apatite structure. If the oral environment is unfavorable (too much acid is produced too often), an adequate flow of saliva can help dilute and buffer the acid, and thus slow the rate of damage to the tooth or even repair it. The critical pH for dissolution of enamel has been shown to be about 5.5. Once the process reaches dentin, dissolution can occur at a considerably higher pH. In addition, we know of many anatomic, behavioral, dietary, genetic, social (and cultural), socioeconomic, and therapeutic variables that can significantly influence the level of caries activity favorably or unfavorably.

We recognize dental caries as a preventable disease. Furthermore we know that the disease typically begins in enamel and progresses slowly in the early stages of the process. Rampant caries is an exception to the typical course and is discussed later. Cavitation of the tooth structure is quite a late stage of the disease. Prior to cavitation, the progress of the disease may be arrested and/or reversed if a favorable oral environment can be achieved. Even after cavitation occurs, if the pulp is not yet involved and if the cavitated area is open enough to be self-cleansing ("plaque-free"), the caries process can halt and become an "arrested lesion." Arrested lesions typically exhibit much coronal destruction, but the remaining exposed dentin is hard and usually very dark, there is no evidence of pulpal damage, and the patient has no pain. We also must emphasize that treating a carious tooth by providing a restoration does not cure the disease. If the unfavorable oral environment that caused the cavity persists, so will the disease, and more restorations will be required in time. Treating the oral infection by reducing the number of cariogenic microorganisms and establishing a favorable oral environment to promote predominantly remineralization of tooth structure over time will stop the caries process and cure the disease. Curing the disease currently requires modifications by the patient and/or caretaker and relies on their compliance in making the necessary modifications. Research efforts are ongoing to find a feasible method of achieving caries immunity that would be far less dependent on patient compliance.

Studies by Orland[7] and by Fitzgerald, Jordan, and Achard[8] demonstrated that dental caries will not occur in the absence of microorganisms. Animals maintained in a germ-free environment did not develop caries even when fed a high-carbohydrate diet. However, dental caries did develop in these animals when they were inoculated with microorganisms from caries-active animals and then fed cariogenic diets.

A number of microorganisms can produce enough acid to decalcify tooth structure, particularly aciduric streptococci, lactobacilli, diphtheroids, yeasts, staphylococci, and certain strains of sarcinae. *Streptococcus mutans* has been implicated as one of the major and most virulent of the caries-producing organisms. Consequently *S. mutans* has been targeted in a large share of research. Loesche conducted an extensive review of the literature regarding the etiology of caries. He concluded that the evidence suggests that *S. mutans*, possibly *Streptococcus sobrinus*, and lactobacilli are human odontopathogens. He stated that aciduricity appears to be the most consistent attribute of *S. mutans* and is associated with its cariogenicity. He also observed that other aciduric species such as *S. sobrinus* may be more important in smooth-surface decay and are perhaps associated with rampant caries. Loesche concluded the review with the suggestion that treatment strategies that interfere with the colonization of *S. mutans* may have a profound effect on the incidence of caries in humans.[9] As caries research proceeds, there seems to be increasing evidence that disease may result from a group of microbial species in the tooth-adhering biofilm. Currently, which combinations of organisms are most blameworthy is not clear.

Wan et al have published a series of three papers that report on 111 infants whom they observed to 2 years of age. They found *S. mutans* colonization in infants as young as 3 months, and over 50% of the predentate infants were infected by 6 months of age. By 24 months of age, 84% of the children harbored the bacteria.[10-12] Investigations by Davey and Rogers[13] and by Berkowitz and Jones[14] have confirmed that *S. mutans* is transmitted orally from mother to infant, whereas Brown, Junner, and Liew[15] have demonstrated a relationship between the numbers of *S. mutans* present in mothers and infants. Research by Kohler, Andreen, and Jonsson demonstrated that reducing the numbers of oral *S. mutans* in mothers delayed the colonization of the organisms in the mouths of their children.[16] Their findings also showed that 52% of the children who carried *S. mutans* at 3 years of age had caries, whereas only 3% of the children without demonstrable *S. mutans* had caries at the same age. In 1988, these same investigators reported that, the earlier the colonization of *S. mutans* in the mouths of children, the higher the caries prevalence at 4 years of age.[17] Caufield, Cutter, and Dasanayake suggested the possibility of a "window of infectivity" between 19 and 33 months of age during which most children acquire the cariogenic organisms.[18] The mother was the most common source of transmission of the bacteria to the child. In a group of 122 children 6 to 24 months of age, Mohan et al found

oral mutans streptococci colonization in 20% of the children under 14 months of age.[19] In addition, logistic regression models that controlled for both age and number of teeth indicated that children who consumed sweetened beverages in their baby bottle were four times more likely to have mutans streptococci than children who only consumed milk. Although investigations to elucidate how and when mutans streptococci are transmitted to children are continuing, essentially all experts agree that the earlier transmission occurs, the higher the caries risk.

The acids that initially decalcify the enamel have a pH of 5.5 to 5.2 or less and are formed in the plaque material, which has been described as an organic nitrogenous mass of microorganisms firmly attached to the tooth structure. This film, which exists primarily in the susceptible areas of the teeth, has received a great deal of attention. Considerable emphasis is currently being given to plaque and its relationship to oral disease. Methods of chemical plaque control are being investigated. The method that has received the most attention during the past decade is the use of antimicrobial agents whose action is selective against certain types of microorganisms, including *S. mutans*. Chlorhexidine and other agents are available in antimicrobial oral rinse solutions. Another approach involves the use of monomolecular layers on the tooth surface that prevent the adherence of microorganisms. Perhaps we will learn how to make enamel resistant to bacterial colonization (plaque formation) and consequently reduce both caries and gingival disease.

The acids involved in the initiation of the caries process are normal metabolic by-products of the microorganisms and are generated by the metabolism of carbohydrates. Because the outer surface of enamel is far more resistant to demineralization by acid than is the deeper portion of enamel, the greatest amount of demineralization occurs 10 to 15 μm beneath the enamel surface (Fig. 10-1). The continuation of this process results in the formation of an incipient subsurface enamel lesion that is first observed clinically as a so-called white spot. Unless the demineralization is arrested or reversed (remineralization) the subsurface lesion will continue to enlarge, with the eventual collapse of the thin surface layer and the formation of a cavitated lesion.

Remineralization of incipient subsurface lesions may occur as long as the surface layer of the enamel remains intact. Saliva, which is supersaturated with calcium and phosphate and has acid-buffering capability, diffuses into plaque, where it neutralizes the microbial acids and repairs the damaged enamel. The time required for remineralization to replace the hydroxyapatite lost during demineralization is determined by the age of the plaque, the nature of the carbohydrate consumed, and the presence or absence of fluoride. For example, it has

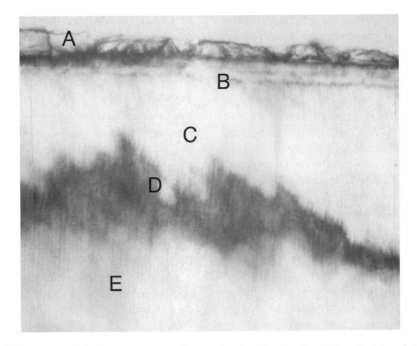

FIG. **10-1.** Polarized light appearance of natural subsurface caries lesion that has imbibed quinoline (100×). **A,** Calculus, **B,** Intact surface area (surface zone IV). **C,** Demineralized area (body of lesion III). **D,** Remineralized area (dark zone II). **E,** Advancing front (translucent zone I).

been suggested that, in the presence of dental plaque that has developed for 12 hours or less, the enamel demineralization resulting from a single exposure to sucrose will be remineralized by saliva within about 10 minutes. In contrast, a period of at least 4 hours is required for saliva to repair the damage to enamel resulting from a similar exposure to sucrose in the presence of dental plaque that is 48 or more hours old. As is noted later in this chapter, the presence of fluoride has a profound effect on the remineralization process; not only does fluoride greatly enhance the rate of remineralization of enamel by saliva but it also results in the formation of a fluorhydroxyapatite during the process, which increases the resistance of the remineralized enamel to future attack by acids. Fluoride also has antimicrobial effects.

Thus the development of dental caries may be considered as a continuous dynamic process involving repeating periods of demineralization by organic acids of microbial origin and subsequent remineralization by salivary components (or therapeutic agents), but in which the overall oral environment is imbalanced toward demineralization. Several factors influence the degree of vulnerability of the tooth.

CARIES PREVALENCE IN PRESCHOOL CHILDREN

Weddell and Klein examined 441 children who ranged in age from 6 to 36 months and resided in a community with water fluoridation.[20] They found dental caries in 4.2% of the children 12 to 17 months of age, 19.8% of those 24 to 29 months of age, and 36.4% of those 30 to 36 months of age. Children in the middle and middle-low socioeconomic groups showed a trend toward higher caries frequencies. Edelstein and Tinanoff found that 30.5% of 200 preschool children had caries detectable by visual or radiographic examination.[21] These children were recruited from a private pediatric dental office and ranged in age from 5 months to 5 years 11 months (mean, 3 years 8 months).

Douglass et al determined the caries prevalence of 3- to 4-year-old children from a fluoridated community in Connecticut who were enrolled in the same Head Start program.[22] They compared the caries prevalence in 517 children enrolled in 1999 with that in 311 children enrolled in 1991. They found a caries prevalence of 38% in the children enrolled in 1999 and 49% in those enrolled in 1991. They noted, however, that the children enrolled in 1999 had a greater severity of maxillary anterior caries. Tang et al performed dental caries examinations on 5171 preschool children recruited from public health assistance programs in Arizona.[23] They found caries in 6.4% of 1-year-olds, nearly 20% of 2-year-olds, 35% of 3-year-olds, and 49% of 4-year-old children in the study.

In general, other reports of caries prevalence among children in various parts of the world show rates that seem to be comparable to those cited here. Another common element of caries prevalence in the United

States and throughout the world is that children from families in low socioeconomic groups consistently have greater caries prevalences than their peers from families at a higher socioeconomic level. Vargas, Crall, and Schneider reported that 27.4% of a sample of 3889 children 2 to 5 years of age had at least one decayed or filled primary tooth.[24] These children were part of a larger sample of individuals included in the third National Health and Nutrition Examination Survey (NHANES III, 1988-1994). This sample of children was 51.4% male and 48.6% female, with an ethnic distribution of 64.1% non-Hispanic white, 16.0% black, 9.5% Mexican American, and 10.4% other ethnicity. The family incomes for these children were distributed into four groups categorized from low to high, and these groups comprised 27.9%, 25.5%, 21.6%, and 24.9% of the sample, respectively.

In a longitudinal evaluation of caries patterns in 317 children followed an average of 7.8 years in private dental practices, Greenwell et al made several noteworthy discoveries.[25] They found that 84% of the children who were caries free in the primary dentition remained caries free in the mixed dentition. Children with pit and fissure caries in the primary dentition were more likely to develop smooth-surface caries of primary teeth than the caries-free children. Fifty-seven percent of the children with proximal lesions in primary molars in the primary dentition developed additional primary molar proximal lesions in the mixed dentition. Children with faciolingual decay (nursing caries) were at the highest risk of any group for developing additional carious lesions. These investigators also discovered levels of caries susceptibility in children that can be characterized as caries free, pit and fissure caries, and proximal molar caries patterns.

CARIES PREVALENCE IN SCHOOLCHILDREN

The report by Vargas, Crall, and Schneider provides additional representative data for schoolchildren as well.[24] Their report revealed that 61.0% of the sample of children 6 to 12 years of age had at least one decayed or filled primary tooth. Furthermore, in the sample of 4116 children 6 to 14 years of age, 40.0% had at least one decayed or filled permanent tooth. Of the 1383 children 15 to 18 years of age, 89.8% had at least one decayed or filled permanent tooth. The ethnic and family income distributions for children in these different age groups were comparable to those outlined in detail for the preschool children. This information, along with that in many other published reports, clearly indicates that managing the disease of dental caries among children remains a formidable task despite the advances we have made in our various preventive programs. Edelstein and Douglass have noted, "The popular statement that

half of U.S. schoolchildren have never experienced tooth decay fails profoundly to reflect the extremity and severity of this still highly prevalent condition of childhood."[2]

RAMPANT DENTAL CARIES

There is no complete agreement on the definition of rampant caries or on the clinical picture of this condition. It has been generally accepted, however, that the disease referred to as rampant caries is, in terms of human history, relatively new. Rampant caries has been defined by Massler as a "suddenly appearing, widespread, rapidly burrowing type of caries, resulting in early involvement of the pulp and affecting those teeth usually regarded as immune to ordinary decay."[26]

There is no evidence that the mechanism of the decay process is different in rampant caries or that it occurs only in teeth that are malformed or inferior in composition. On the contrary, rampant caries can occur suddenly in teeth that were previously sound for many years. The sudden onset of the disease suggests that an overwhelming imbalance of the oral environment has occurred, and some factor(s) in the caries process seems to accelerate it so that it becomes uncontrollable; it is then referred to as *rampant caries.*

When a patient has what is considered an excessive amount of tooth decay, one must determine whether that person actually has a high susceptibility and truly rampant caries of sudden onset or whether the oral condition represents years of neglect and inadequate dental care. Young teenagers seem to be particularly susceptible to rampant caries, though it has been observed in both children and adults of all ages (Figs. 10-2 and 10-3).

There is considerable evidence that emotional disturbances may be a causative factor in some cases of rampant caries. Repressed emotions and fears, dissatisfaction with achievement, rebellion against a home situation, a feeling of inferiority, a traumatic school experience, and continuous general tension and anxiety have been observed in children and adults who have rampant dental caries. Because adolescence is often considered to be a time of difficult adjustment, the increased incidence of rampant caries in this age group lends support to this theory. An emotional disturbance may initiate an unusual craving for sweets or the habit of snacking, which in turn might influence the incidence of dental caries. On the other hand, a noticeable salivary deficiency is not an uncommon finding in tense, nervous, or disturbed persons. Indeed, various forms of stress in both children and adults, as well as various medications (such as tranquilizers and sedatives) commonly taken to help persons cope with stress, are associated with decreased salivary flow and decreased caries resistance

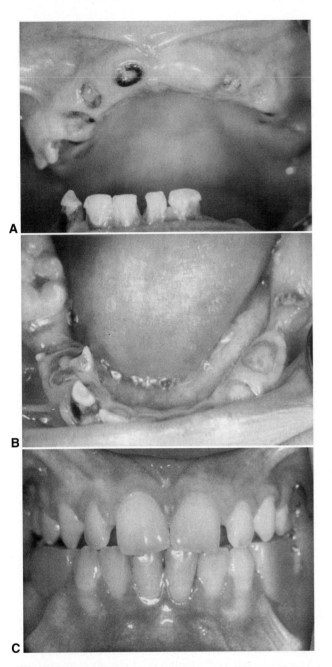

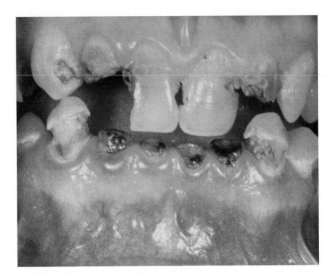

FIG. **10-3.** Teenaged patient with rampant caries. Occasionally a full-mouth extraction must be recommended if there is gross destruction with pulpal involvement.

FIG. **10-2. A,** Rampant dental caries and evidence of dental neglect in preschool child. There has been gross destruction of the clinical crowns of the primary teeth. **B,** Recently erupted first permanent molar with an extensive carious lesion. The destruction process evident in the primary teeth at an early age would be expected to continue in the permanent teeth. **C,** Same patient at 10 years of age. A preventive and corrective program has maintained the permanent teeth.

caused by impaired remineralization. It is well known that radiation therapy to the head and neck often results in significantly diminished salivary function and may place patients at high risk for severe caries development.

EARLY CHILDHOOD CARIES, SEVERE EARLY CHILDHOOD CARIES, NURSING CARIES, BABY BOTTLE TOOTH DECAY

The American Academy of Pediatric Dentistry (AAPD) defines early childhood caries (ECC) as the presence of one or more decayed (noncavitated or cavitated), missing (due to caries), or filled tooth surfaces in any primary tooth in a child 71 months of age or younger. The Academy also specifies that, in children younger than 3 years of age, any sign of smooth-surface caries is indicative of severe early childhood caries (S-ECC).[27]

For many years it has been recognized that, after eruption of the primary teeth begins, excessively frequent bottle feedings and/or prolonged bottle or breast feedings is often associated with early and rampant caries. The clinical appearance of the teeth in S-ECC in a child 2, 3, or 4 years of age is typical and follows a definite pattern.[28] There is early carious involvement of the maxillary anterior teeth, the maxillary and mandibular first primary molars, and sometimes the mandibular canines (Fig. 10-4). The mandibular incisors are usually unaffected. A discussion with the parents often reveals an inappropriate feeding pattern: the child has been put to bed at afternoon naptime and/or at night with a nursing bottle holding milk or a sugar-containing beverage. The child falls asleep, and the liquid becomes pooled around the teeth (the lower anterior teeth tend to be protected by the tongue). It would seem that the carbohydrate-containing liquid provides an excellent culture medium for acidogenic microorganisms. Salivary flow is also decreased during sleep, and clearance of the liquid from the oral cavity is slowed.

Gardner, Norwood, and Eisenson reported four case histories in which the same pattern of caries was observed, and in each child the condition was attributed to a specific breast-feeding habit.[29] In each case the mother explained that human milk was the main source of nutrition. The investigators recommend that from birth the infant should be held while feeding. The child who falls asleep while nursing should be burped and then placed in bed. In addition, the parent should start brushing the child's teeth as soon as they erupt and should discontinue nursing as soon as the child can drink from a cup—at approximately 12 months of age.

The AAPD endorses the policy statement of the American Academy of Pediatrics (AAP) on breast-feeding and the use of human milk.[30] The AAP statement includes the acknowledgment that "breast-feeding ensures the best possible health as well as the best development and psychosocial outcomes for the infant." However, both organizations discourage extended or excessive frequency of feeding times (from the breast or bottle) and encourage appropriate oral hygiene measures for infants and toddlers.

Dilley, Dilley, and Machen observed a large number of children with prolonged nursing habit caries and concluded that there was no association between the nursing habit and family background, except that the families were predominantly from lower socioeconomic groups.[31] All subjects demonstrated prolonged breast-feeding or bottle feeding, with milk reported to be the liquid most often used in the bottle. Parents indicated that they did not know when weaning should occur and when oral hygiene should be instituted. The authors also observed nearly symmetric caries patterns.

Hallonsten et al screened 3000 children 18 months of age for dental caries and ongoing breast-feeding.[32] Twelve (19.7%) of the 61 children still being breast-fed had caries, while 51 (1.7%) of the 2939 children not being breast-fed had caries. The authors found that children who experience prolonged breast-feeding tend to develop unsuitable dietary habits that put them at risk for caries at an early age.

There is considerable scientific evidence from experiments in vitro and in animal models to suggest that some dairy products such as bovine milk and cheese as well as human breast milk are not cariogenic and may actually be protective to tooth structure and promote remineralization under certain conditions. Similar experiments show that many infant formulas, with refined food additives, do promote caries. These issues are discussed in more detail later. Suffice it to say here that we have much yet to learn about caries progression in both the more typical disease and this rampant form. It is prudent to counsel parents to practice good oral

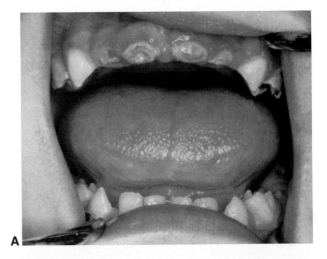

FIG. **10-4. A,** Severe early childhood caries in a 20-month-old child. There is extensive carious involvement of the maxillary primary incisors and first molars.

hygiene measures for the child and to avoid inappropriate feeding habits that are associated with S-ECC.

S-ECC may be prevented by early counseling of the parents. This is one reason for suggesting that children receive their first dental examination between 6 and 12 months of age, when S-ECC is not likely to have developed. In a comprehensive report prepared for the Oral Health Subcommittee of the Healthy Mothers–Healthy Babies Coalition, Ripa states, "Priority needs to be given to a major national educational program directed toward educating the public about nursing caries."[33] The educational program must involve direct contact with pregnant women, parents, and other caregivers in population subgroups with a high prevalence of nursing caries.

ADDITIONAL FACTORS KNOWN TO INFLUENCE DENTAL CARIES

SALIVA

Although saliva was identified in the etiology section earlier as part of the host component and thus a primary part of the caries process, the role of saliva overall is so unique and special that further discussion is warranted here regarding its influence on several aspects of the caries process that may help produce favorable environments to combat the process. Any patient with a salivary deficiency, from any cause, is at higher risk for caries activity.

It is generally accepted that the dental caries process is controlled to a large extent by a natural protective mechanism inherent within the saliva. Many properties of saliva have been investigated to learn their possible role in the caries process. Considerable importance has been placed on the salivary pH, the acid-neutralizing

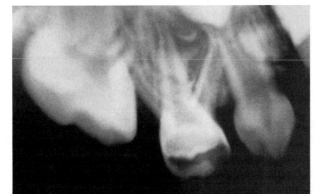

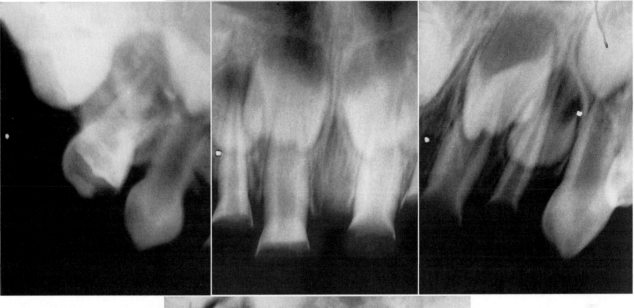

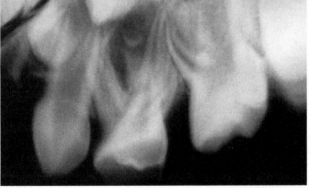

FIG. **10-4, cont'd. B,** Radiographs of the maxillary arch. Maxillary incisors are indicated for extraction. Notice the deep caries in the first primary molars. The primary second molars have not erupted.

power, and the calcium, fluoride, and phosphorus content. It has long been suggested that in addition to these properties the rate of flow and the viscosity of saliva may influence the development of caries. The normal salivary flow aids in the solution of food debris on which microorganisms thrive. In addition, the saliva manifests a variety of antibacterial and other antiinfectious properties. All known characteristics of saliva seem somehow relevant to the process of dental caries.

Saliva is secreted by three paired masses of cells—the submaxillary, sublingual, and parotid glands. Small accessory glands are also scattered over the oral mucous membranes. Each of these has its own duct.

The salivary glands are under the control of the autonomic (involuntary) nervous system, receiving fibers from both its parasympathetic and sympathetic divisions. Stimulation of either the parasympathetic (chorda tympani) fibers or the sympathetic fibers to the submaxillary or sublingual gland causes a secretion of saliva. The secretion resulting from parasympathetic stimulation is profuse and watery in most animals. Sympathetic stimulation, however, causes a scanty secretion of a thick, mucinous juice. Stimulation of the parasympathetic fibers to the parotid gland causes a profuse, watery secretion, but stimulation of the sympathetic fibers causes no secretion.

Salivary Deficiency. One of the first descriptions of a severe salivary deficiency with its deleterious effect on the dentition was reported by Hutchinson in 1888.[34] Since that time many reports have emphasized the importance of a normal flow of saliva in preventing a breakdown of the dentition. A reduction in the salivary flow may be temporary or permanent. When the quantity is only moderately reduced, the oral structures may appear normal. A pronounced reduction or complete absence of saliva, however, will result in a septic mouth with rampant caries (Fig. 10-5). In addition to the rapid destruction of the teeth, there may be dryness and cracking of the lips, with fissuring at the corners of the mouth, burning and soreness of the mucous membranes, crusting of the tongue and palate, and sometimes paresthesia of the tongue or mucous membrane.

There are many reasons for a reduction in salivary flow. Acquired salivary dysfunction may be the result of a psychologic or emotional disturbance and, again, may be either temporary or permanent. During the acute stages, mumps may cause a temporary reduction in salivary flow. Immune disorders, such as Sjögren syndrome, and genetic conditions, such as hypohidrotic

ectodermal dysplasia, often exhibit chronic xerostomia. Many oncology patients receive head and neck or total-body irradiation that also results in salivary gland dysfunction. An interruption in the central pathways of the secretory nerves has been suggested as a cause of salivary failure, but this is usually overshadowed by definite neurologic signs and symptoms. Similarly, a deficiency of vitamin B complex has been reported as a cause of salivary gland dysfunction.

One study indicated that the minimum effective dose of many of the antihistaminic drugs can reduce salivary flow by as much as 50%.[35] Dryness of the mouth may occur after the use of a variety of tranquilizers and antihistamines. It has likewise been observed that dry mouth and rampant caries may accompany a systemic condition, such as myasthenia gravis. In this disease the acetylcholine that is necessary for the proper transmission of nerve impulses is destroyed; as a result the salivary glands do not receive adequate stimulation.

Previous work has shown a great deal of individual variation in the amount of saliva produced by stimulation of the glands. The range is from less than a measurable amount in patients with acquired or congenital dysfunction of the salivary glands to 65 ml during a 15-minute period of stimulation and collection. Patients with deficient salivary flow often have excessive or rampant caries. In contrast, patients with greater than average salivary flow are usually relatively free from dental caries.

Determination of Salivary Flow. If a patient has no known existing conditions that may cause hyposalivation and if the clinician notices a small pool of saliva in the floor of the mouth during oral examination, it is not unreasonable to assume that the patient has adequate salivary quantity and flow. Little information is available about salivary flow rates in children, but Crossner reports that in children 5 to 15 years of age the rate of mixed whole stimulated saliva increases with age, and boys have consistently higher rates than girls.[36] If inadequate salivary flow is known to exist or is suspected, measurement of salivary flow can provide a baseline useful for comparing with later measurements after implementation of adjunctive therapy.

To evaluate the adequacy of salivary flow, Zunt recommends establishing the unstimulated salivary flow (USF) rate.[37] The USF rate is measured after a period of 1 hour without eating, drinking, chewing gum, or brushing the teeth. Sitting in the "coachman" position, on the edge of the dental chair, the patient passively drools into a funnel inserted into a graduated cylinder for 5 minutes. The eyes should remain open except for blinking during the 5-minute collection period. The head and neck should be bent, and the arms should rest comfortably on the thighs or knees.

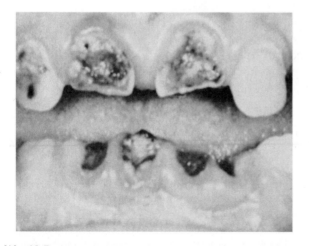

FIG. **10-5.** Rampant dental caries in a 9-year-old boy. There was a septic dry mouth caused by the congenital absence of salivary glands.

The volume of saliva collected in the cylinder after 5 minutes is divided by 5 to determine the USF. A USF rate of less than 0.1 ml per minute is diagnostic of salivary gland hypofunction. If the USF rate is less than 0.1 ml per minute, the next step is to measure the stimulated salivary flow (SSF). The patient should chew unflavored paraffin for 45 chews or 1 minute and expectorate into a funnel inserted into a graduated cylinder. The SSF rate should be 1 to 2 ml per minute; less than 0.5 ml per minute is scored as an abnormal rate. A convenient alternative method for measuring USF is the modified Schirmer technique, which uses a calibrated paper test strip to collect saliva in the floor of the mouth.

In patients who are known or suspected to have salivary deficiency, it is not unusual to find a salivary flow ranging from slightly below normal to practically a dry mouth. If there is a deficiency of saliva or a dry mouth, the cause should be sought. Sometimes the cause is readily determinable; sometimes it is obscure. An emotional disturbance should not be overlooked as a cause in a patient of any age. Psychotherapy may be helpful in these cases. If the cause cannot readily be determined, perhaps it should be assumed that the sparse flow is related to inadequacies in the diet, particularly a vitamin deficiency or excessive sugar consumption to the exclusion of needed foods. Monthly quantitative analyses of the saliva should be performed to determine whether dietary improvement is accompanied by an increased flow.

If the salivary glands have not undergone degenerative or metaplastic change and if the nerve pathways between the central nervous system and the salivary glands are still intact, salivary stimulants may be recommended. If dryness of the mouth is attributable to dehydration, increased fluid intake should be recommended. The use of gustatory stimulants (sugar-free candy) or masticatory stimulants (xylitol gum) has been suggested as an adjunct to encourage salivation. Prescription sialagogue medications, also known as secretagogues, such as pilocarpine and cevimeline may be of benefit in improving the salivary flow rate in patients with Sjögren syndrome or with radiation damage to salivary glands. The use of sialagogue medications has not been studied in pediatric populations, but these agents are considered very safe for most adult patients and have been used successfully in older children. The use of salivary substitutes has been suggested by Shannon, McCrary, and Starcke as helpful in preventing soft tissue problems associated with dry mouth.[38] Saliva substitutes, as well as fluoride and chlorhexidine rinses, are also reported to enhance remineralization and promote resistance to demineralization of tooth surfaces, and may help prevent radiation-induced caries.

Viscosity of Saliva. It has long been suggested that the viscosity of saliva is related to the rate of dental decay. Both thick, ropy saliva and thin, watery saliva have been blamed for rampant dental caries. Previous work conducted at Indiana University has shown a statistically significant direct relationship between the viscosity of saliva and the number of decayed, missing, and filled teeth.[39] This relationship held true for all members of the observation group, regardless of age. Patients with thick, ropy saliva invariably had poor oral hygiene. The teeth were covered with stain or plaque, and the rate of dental caries ranged from greater than average to rampant.

No evidence exists that viscosity changes with age under normal conditions. This property of the saliva is governed not only by the particular set of glands stimulated but also by the type of nervous stimulation and the amount of mucin (glycoprotein) present.

We have observed that children who consume excessive amounts of carbohydrates often have not only a sparse flow but also a viscous saliva. Even minimal doses of some antihistaminic drugs will result in a greatly increased viscosity of saliva in some persons.[35]

There are apparently only a limited number of ways to alter the viscosity of saliva. Reduction of refined sugar intake may be effective in some patients.

Although relatively little information specific to salivary function, flow, and viscosity in children is available, an excellent review article by Leone and Oppenheim provides much additional information regarding the relationship between saliva and dental caries for the interested reader.[40]

SOCIOECONOMIC STATUS

The Surgeon General's report of 2000 indicated that one in four American children is born into poverty.[1] It noted that children and adolescents living in poverty suffer twice as much tooth decay as their more affluent peers and that their disease is more likely to go untreated. The report also mentioned that, although continuing reductions of dental caries in permanent teeth have been achieved, caries prevalence in primary teeth has stabilized or possibly increased in some population groups. A Census Bureau report published in March 2003 showed that the poverty rate for children in the United States rose in 2002, whereas it dropped for people 65 years and older.[41] Nearly half of the 35 million people living in poverty were children. These are alarming data calling attention to a huge unmet oral health care need in our country.

Following the report of the Surgeon General, Edelstein pointed out that, paradoxically, children living in poverty also have the highest rates of dental insurance coverage, largely through the Medicaid program and the State Children's Health Insurance

Program.[42] Yet Medicaid-eligible children who have cavities have twice the number of carious teeth and twice the number of visits for pain relief but fewer total dental visits than children in families with higher incomes. He also notes that these disparities continue into adolescence and young adulthood but to a lesser degree. Because practitioners have the opportunity to assess the oral health of poor children individually, they will identify some patients at low risk for dental caries. However, the available data confirm that, from a demographic perspective, economically poor children are at high risk for dental caries.

ANATOMIC CHARACTERISTICS OF THE TEETH

Certain teeth of many patients, particularly permanent teeth, seem vulnerable to dental caries as they emerge and, in caries-active mouths, they may show evidence of the attack almost coincident with their eruption into the oral cavity. Because enamel calcification is incomplete at the time of eruption of the teeth and an additional period of about 2 years is required for the calcification process to be completed by exposure to saliva, the teeth are especially susceptible to caries formation during the first 2 years after eruption. Permanent molars often have incompletely coalesced pits and fissures that allow the dental plaque material to be retained at the base of the defect, sometimes in contact with exposed dentin. These defects or anatomic characteristics can readily be seen if the tooth is dried and the debris and plaque removed. In addition to occlusal surfaces, lingual pits on the maxillary permanent molars, buccal pits on the mandibular permanent molars, and lingual pits on the maxillary permanent lateral incisors are vulnerable areas in which the process of dental caries can proceed rapidly.

ARRANGEMENT OF THE TEETH IN THE ARCH

Crowded and irregular teeth are not readily cleansed during the natural masticatory process. It is likewise difficult for the patient to clean the mouth properly with a toothbrush and floss if the teeth are crowded or overlapped. This condition therefore may contribute to the problem of dental caries.

PRESENCE OF DENTAL APPLIANCES AND RESTORATIONS

Partial dentures, space maintainers, and orthodontic appliances often encourage the retention of food debris and plaque material and have been shown to result in an increase in the bacterial population. Few patients keep their mouths meticulously clean, and even those who make an attempt may be hampered by the presence of dental appliances that retain plaque material between brushings. Patients who have had moderate dental caries activity in the past might be expected to have increased caries activity after the placement of appliances in the mouth unless they practice unusually good oral hygiene.

Rosenbloom and Tinanoff evaluated the S. mutans level of patients before, during, and after orthodontic treatment.[43] S. mutans levels were significantly elevated during active treatment. When samples were taken 6 to 15 weeks into the retention phase of treatment, however, the microbial levels were found to have decreased significantly to levels comparable to those of untreated children.

Dentists have known for many years that the tooth structure at the interface with restorative material is especially vulnerable to recurrent caries. Clinical studies suggest that dentists and their patients should not expect successful restorative treatment to reduce a patient's risk for future development of carious lesions. Tinanoff, Siegrist, and Lang found higher numbers of salivary S. mutans in patients after they received restorative treatment.[44] Wright et al observed significant reductions in the number of mutans streptococci and lactobacilli immediately after restoration; however, mutans streptococci returned to prerestoration levels in many of their subjects.[45] Gregory, El-Rahman, and Avery observed that postoperative counts of salivary streptococci essentially equaled the preoperative counts after all restorative work had been completed in their patients.[46] Effective prevention programs are required to protect the patient from additional caries and to better justify the investment in restorative care.

HEREDITARY FACTORS

Although parents of children with excessive or rampant caries tend to blame the condition on hereditary factors or tendencies, and some scientific evidence as reviewed in Chapter 6 acknowledges certain genetic influences on the caries process, most authors agree that genetic influences on dental caries are relatively minor in comparison with the overall effect of environmental factors. The fact that children acquire their dietary habits, oral hygiene habits, and oral microflora from their parents makes dental caries more an environmental than a hereditary disease. Although several hereditary factors identified in Chapter 6 may be influential in promoting or preventing dental caries activity, available effective preventive therapies along with proper dietary and plaque control measures can override the hereditary factors that contribute to caries development.

EARLY DETECTION OF DISEASE ACTIVITY

Traditionally, dentists have relied upon a visual-tactile-radiographic procedure for the detection of dental caries. This procedure involves the visual identification of demineralized areas (typically white spots) or suspicious pits or fissures and the use of the dental explorer to determine the presence of a loss of continuity or breaks in the enamel and assess the softness or resilience of the enamel. Carious lesions located on interproximal tooth surfaces have generally been detected with the use of bitewing radiographs. These procedures have been used routinely in virtually every dental office in the United States for the past 50 years.

Because the reversal of the caries process depends on an intact surface layer of the lesion and the typical use of the dental explorer to probe the suspicious areas often results in the rupture of the surface layer covering early lesions, the use of the dental explorer to probe enamel is no longer recommended. The recommended use of the dental explorer is to judiciously remove plaque and debris to permit visual inspection of pits and fissures.

This understanding of the nature of the caries process also emphasizes the need for alternative methods for the early detection of dental caries. Lesions detected on radiographs have generally progressed to the initial involvement of dentin. Thus, the increased desire of dental professionals and patients for more conservative restorative procedures as well as the implementation of measures to control and reverse the caries process led to significant efforts to develop technologies for the early detection of dental caries. Although a variety of new technologies are being explored for this purpose, only three of these technologies are currently available for clinical dental practice.[47]

INFRARED LASER FLUORESCENCE (DIAGNOdent)

An instrument designed to facilitate the detection of dental caries, DIAGNOdent,* has recently become available in several countries. This instrument was developed for the detection and quantification of dental caries of occlusal and smooth surfaces. It uses a diode laser light source and a fiber-optic cable that transmits the light to a hand-held probe with a fiber-optic eye in the tip. The light is absorbed and induces infrared fluorescence by organic and inorganic materials. The emitted fluorescence is collected at the probe tip, transmitted through ascending fibers, and processed and presented on a display window as an integer between 0 and 99. Increased fluorescence reflects carious tooth substance, particularly for numerical values higher than about 20. What material is responsible for the fluorescence is still under investigation, but it appears to be bacterial metabolites, particularly the porphyrins.

An appreciable number of in vitro studies and a few in vivo (clinical) studies of the performance of this instrument have been reported in the past 5 years.

The results of the various in vitro studies have indicated that the DIAGNOdent instrument is capable of detecting relatively advanced carious lesions, and DIAGNOdent readings show a very good correlation with histologic evidence of caries but not with the depth of the lesions into dentin. These studies have also demonstrated the instrument to exhibit excellent reproducibility and good to excellent sensitivity. However, the results of the in vitro studies have also indicated that the readings are influenced by several variables, including the degree of dehydration of the lesion, the presence of dental plaque, and the presence of various types of stain in occlusal fissures.

The results of clinical investigations have shown significant differences in readings between different DIAGNOdent instruments with regard to occlusal caries, which raises questions regarding the selection of a value of 20 or 25 to indicate the presence of caries. For a given instrument, intraoperator reliability was generally very good and interoperator reliability typically ranged from good to very good. Further, DIAGNOdent readings increased linearly with clinical histologic measurements, and therefore the instrument was reported to be able to distinguish with good sensitivity between sound tooth structure or shallow enamel caries and deeper carious lesions in enamel or lesions extending into dentin. Recent studies, however, have not been able to confirm the narrow range of values related to lesion extent reported previously. The instrument is very good at indicating the presence of deeper lesions in enamel or into dentin that may not be apparent yet on radiographs but is unable to reliably indicate the depth of a dentinal lesion.

The DIAGNOdent instrument appears to be particularly useful for confirming the presence of occlusal caries. Especially with the judicious use of the dental explorer to remove oral debris from occlusal pits and fissures, the DIAGNOdent is capable of confirming the presence or absence of caries in otherwise suspicious areas. Instrument readings higher than 20 or 25 reflect the likely presence of caries, and higher readings generally reflect more extensive lesion progression, although there does not appear to be a linear relation between the readings and the extent of the lesions. Prudent use of the instrument can identify early lesions that should be considered for preventive rather than restorative treatment.

DIGITAL IMAGING FIBER-OPTIC TRANS-ILLUMINATION (DIFOTI)

Conventional clinical caries examinations routinely use transillumination to identify lesions located on the interproximal surfaces of the anterior teeth. For at least 30 years a fiber-optic transillumination (FOTI) instrument has been available for clinical use. It provides an

*Kaltenbach & Voigt GmbH & Co., Bismarckring 39.

TABLE **10-1** American Academy of Pediatrics Dentistry Caries-Risk Assessment Tool

CARIES RISK INDICATORS	LOW RISK	MODERATE RISK	HIGH RISK
CLINICAL CONDITIONS	• No carious teeth in past 24 months	• Carious teeth in the past 24 months	• Carious teeth in the past 12 months
	• No enamel demineralization (enamel caries "white spot lesions")	• One area of enamel demineralization (enamel caries "white spot lesions")	• More than one area of enamel demineralization (enamel caries "white spot lesions")
			• Radiographic enamel caries
	• No visible plaque; no gingivitis	• Gingivitis[a]	• Visible plaque on anterior (front) teeth
			• High titers of mutans streptococci
			• Wearing dental of Orthodontic appliances[b]
			• Enamel hypoplasia[c]
ENVIRONMENTAL CHARACTERSTICS	• Optimal systemic and topical fluoride exposure[d]	• Suboptimal systemic fluoride exposure with optimal topical exposure[d]	• Suboptimal topical fluoride expsure[d]
	• Consumption of simple sugars or foods strongly associated with caries initiation[e] primarily at mealtimes	• Occasional (e.g., one or two) between-meal exposures to simple sugars or foods strongly associated with caries	• Frequent (e.g., three or more) between-meal exposures to simple sugars or foods strongly associated with caries
	• High caregiver socioeconimic status[f]	• Midlevel caregiver socioeconomic status (e.g., eligible for school lunch program or SCHIP)	• Low-level caregiver socioeconomic status (e.g., eligible for Mediacid)
	• Regular use of dental care in an established dental home	• Irregular use of dental services	• No usual source of dental care
GENERAL HEALTH CONDITIONS			• Active caries present in the mother
			• Children with special health care needs[g]
			• Conditions impairing saliva composition/flow[h]

Adapted from American Academy of Pediatric Dentistry: Policy on the use of a caries-risk assessment tool (CAT) for infants, children and adolescents, *Pediatr Dent* 24(7 suppl):17, 2002 (special issue: Reference manual 2002-2003).

SCHIP, State Children's Health Insurance Program.

[a]Although microbial organisms responsible for gingivitis may be different from those primarily implicated in dental caries, the presence of gingivitis is an indicator of poor infrequent oral hygiene practices and has been associated with caries progression.

[b]Orthodontic appliances include both fixed and removable appliances, space maintainers, and other devices that remain in the mouth continuously or for prolonged time intervals and which may trap food and plaque, prevent oral hygiene, compromise access of tooth surfaces to fluoride, or otherwise create an environment supporting dental caries initiation.

[c]Tooth anatomy and hypoplastic defects such as poorly formed enamel, developmental pits, and deep pits may predispose a child to develop dental caries.

[d]Optimal systemic and topical fluoride exposure is based on the American Dental Association/American Academy of Pediatrics guidelines for exposure from fluoride drinking water and/or supplementation and use of a fluoride dentifrice.

[e]Examples of sources of simple sugars include carbonated beverages, cookies, cake, candy, cereal, potato chips, French fries, corn chips, pretzels, breads, juices, and fruits. Clinicians using caries-risk assessment should investigate individual exposures to sugars known to be involved in caries initiation.

[f]National surveys have demonstrated that children from low-income and moderate-income households are more likely to have dental caries and more decayed or filled primary teeth than children from more affluent households. Also, within income levels, minority children are more likely to have caries. Thus, sociodemographic status should be viewed as an initial indicator of risk that may be offset by the absence of other risk indicators.

[g]Children with special health care needs are those who have or are at increased risk for a chronic physical, developmental, behavioral, or emotional condition and who also require health and related services of a type or amount beyond that required by children generally (Source: Newacheck PW et al: New estimates of children with special health care needs and implications for the State Children's Health Insurance Program. Maternal and Child Health Policy Research Center Fact Sheet, No. 4, March, 1998).

[h]Alteration in salivary flow can be the result of congenital or acquired conditions, surgery, radiation, medication of age related changes in salivary function. Any condition, treatment, or process known or reported to alter saliva flow should be considered an indication of risk unless proven otherwise.

- No combination of risk indicators was consistently considered a good predictor when applied to different populations, across different age groups. In general, however, the best indicators of caries risk were easily obtained from dental charts and did not require additional testing.
- Previous caries experience was an important predictor for primary, permanent, and root surface caries in most models tested.
- Most of the research in this area has been done in children, for both primary and permanent teeth.

It is also obvious from their report that the caries-risk assessment process is very much a work in progress at this time. Further refinements will continue for some time in the future.

Of course, accurate caries-risk assessments of patients can guide clinicians and health care facilities toward better allocation of their time and resources for their high-risk patients. As our accuracy and efficiency in identifying patients with active disease or high potential to develop disease improves and as parents and patients (and, it is hoped, health care insurance plans) accept this newer approach to care, the standard "6-month recall visit" for children may change to a more customized plan for individual patients or groups of patients. Children who are at low risk for caries and do not present with other oral conditions that need frequent monitoring may not require oral health care visits as often as those at high risk (with or without active disease), whereas compliant high-risk patients may, at times, require frequent visits and multiple forms of caries control therapies in addition to their voluntary modification of caries-promoting dietary and behavioral habits.

CONTROL OF DENTAL CARIES

Many practical measures for the control of dental caries are applicable to private practice. Most practitioners have tried control measures with varying degrees of success. One cannot emphasize too strongly, however, that no single measure for the control of dental caries will be entirely satisfactory. At the present time all possible preventive measures and approaches must be considered in the hope of successfully controlling and preventing the caries process.

Pediatric dentists who see patients on a referral basis may hear a parent remark, "My child has so many cavities that my dentist doesn't know where to start." Although it is true that the problem may at first seem overwhelming, a systematic, understanding approach will often result in a gratifying response. An outline of procedures for the control of active and/or rampant caries in cooperative and communicative patients follows. With this approach and with patient cooperation, the problem can usually be explained and brought

under control. The successful management of active dental caries, however, depends on the parents' and/or patient's interest in maintaining the patient's teeth and their cooperation in a customized and specific caries control program.

CONTROL OF ALL ACTIVE CARIOUS LESIONS

When rampant caries occurs, the first steps are to initiate treatment of all carious lesions to stop or at least slow the progression of the disease and to identify the most important causes of the existing condition. Next, and even simultaneously, if possible, the practitioner begins working with the parents and/or the patient to achieve the appropriate behavioral modifications required to prevent recurrence. The problem may then be approached in a systematic manner. Invariably modifications in oral hygiene procedures and dietary habits will be necessary. Often, achieving patient compliance with the recommended modifications is the greatest challenge of all.

If the initial restorative treatment is to be done in one appointment under general anesthesia or in one or two appointments with sedation, control of the existing lesions will be definitive at that time. If the restorative care is to be performed over several visits in the outpatient setting, gross caries excavation as an initial approach in the control of rampant dental caries has several advantages. The removal of the superficial caries and the filling of the cavity with a glass ionomer material or zinc oxide–eugenol cement (IRM*) will at least temporarily arrest the caries process and prevent its rapid progression to the dental pulp. Gross caries removal can usually be accomplished easily in one appointment. If there are many extensive carious lesions, however, a second appointment may be necessary.

An alternative approach for some compliant children (with compliant parents) old enough to rinse and expectorate and for compliant adolescents is to initiate intensive and multiple antimicrobial and topical fluoride therapies in conjunction with the necessary behavioral life-style modifications, and then to proceed systematically with restorations and other indicated therapies.

REDUCTION IN THE INTAKE OF FREELY FERMENTABLE CARBOHYDRATES

Some excellent studies have been reported that show a relationship between diet and dental caries. As a result of these studies, considerable emphasis has been given to this phase of the caries control program. There is also much evidence to confirm that between-meal snacking and the frequency of eating and drinking are related to dental caries incidence.

---

*Intermediate Restorative Material, LD Caulk Co., Milford, DE, 19963.

Gustafsson et al conducted a well-controlled study of dental caries, now considered a classic, and observed that a group of patients whose diet was high in fat, low in carbohydrates, and practically free of sugar had low caries activity.[50] When refined sugar was added to the diet in the form of a mealtime supplement, there was still little or no caries activity. However, when caramels were given between meals, a statistically significant increase in the number of new carious lesions occurred. It was concluded from these studies that dental caries activity could be increased by the consumption of sugar if the sugar were in a form easily retained on the tooth surface. The more frequently this form of sugar was consumed between meals, the greater was the tendency for an increase in dental caries.

Weiss and Trithart reported additional evidence for the relationship between the incidence of dental caries and between-meal eating habits.[51] In a group of preschool children it was found that most between-meal snacks were of high sugar content or were high in adhesiveness. The children who did not eat between meals had 3.3 decayed, extracted, or filled primary teeth (deft), whereas those who ate four or more items between meals had a deft rate of 9.8.

As mentioned earlier, sweetened liquids provided to young children in nursing bottles can have enormous cariogenic potential. Likewise, the carbonated soft drinks and other sweetened drinks so popular with older children and adolescents are readily available today. Frequent ingestion of these drinks is another form of snacking that can promote and accelerate caries progression.

In view of the results of these and many other subsequent well-controlled studies, another consideration in the clinical control of dental caries could be a determination of eating habits by having the patient keep a 7-day record of all food eaten at mealtime and between meals. The record should then be evaluated to determine the adequacy of the diet and the amount of freely fermentable carbohydrates. The number of servings of food in each of the basic five food groups should be determined and compared with the recommended number of servings outlined in Figs. 10-6 and 10-7, and Table 10-2. The basic diet analysis form (Box 10-1) has been found to be helpful in evaluating the adequacy of the diet.

Figs. 10-6 and 10-7 and Table 10-2 provide appropriate guidelines to assist in assessing the adequacy of the patient's diet. Fig. 10-6 illustrates the Food Guide Pyramid, which presents the recommendations of the National Academy of Sciences and the U.S. Department of Agriculture. Fig. 10-7 shows the Guide to Good Eating, which presents the recommendations of the National Dairy Council (NDC). These two guides are designed for individuals who are school-aged and older. The NDC has also proposed guidelines for preschool children. The NDC guidelines for children are summarized in Table 10-2.

An evaluation of 500 consecutive records of children coming to the Indiana University Clinic has demonstrated that only a small percentage has adequate diets. The majority of children have noteworthy deficiencies in one or more of the basic five food groups.

Investigations by Schachtele and Jensen[52] as well as by Park, Ashmore, and Stookey[53] have indicated that the acidity of plaque located in interproximal areas, which generally have less exposure to saliva, may remain below the critical pH for periods in excess of 2 hours after carbohydrate ingestion. Because foods containing sugars in solution as well as retentive sugars are included in the diet analysis, 20 minutes may be considered as the minimal time each exposure permits acid concentrations to be available in the bacterial plaque (Fig. 10-8).

The following can be used in explaining the dental caries process to a parent or child:

Fermentable carbohydrate + Oral bacteria within plaque → Acid within plaque

Acid + Susceptible tooth → Tooth decay

Foods in the five basic groups should not be included in the fermentable carbohydrate calculation (with some exceptions) unless free sugar is added during their preparation. One exception is dry cereal, because it is considered a refined food. Cereals may be retained on the teeth for long periods of time; in addition, many of them are sugar coated and some are high in sucrose content. Although the cariogenicity of a food may be related to its sucrose content, its consistency, the time of consumption, and the conditions under which it is eaten, dietary counseling should involve particular consideration of sucrose consumption between meals.

Dried fruits, including raisins, prunes, peaches, apricots, and dates, have a high sugar content; therefore their sugar equivalents should also be included in the diet analysis. These are foods commonly eaten by children between meals, and there is no reason to believe that they are any less cariogenic than refined foods. Although honey is considered a natural food, its sugar equivalent should be considered, in addition to that of syrups and other spreads for bread.

Rather than insist that the patient follow a strict dietary routine severely restricted in carbohydrates, the dentist should suggest a basic diet. The purpose of limiting a diet to the basic five food groups is twofold. An adequate diet is fundamental to general good health and is, of course, essential during the period of tooth formation to help ensure the development of normal

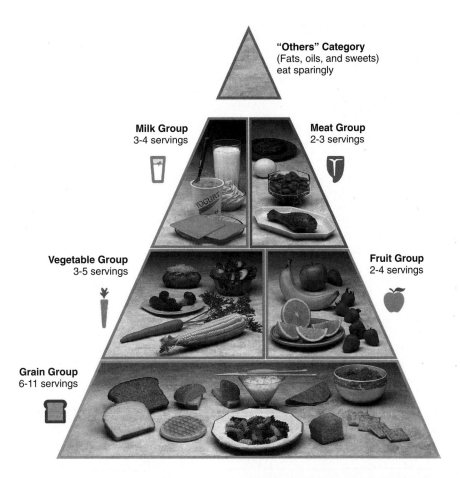

"Others" Category
(Fats, oils, and sweets)
eat sparingly

Milk Group
3-4 servings

Meat Group
2-3 servings

Vegetable Group
3-5 servings

Fruit Group
2-4 servings

Grain Group
6-11 servings

How many servings are right for me?

The pyramid shows a range of servings for each food group. The number of servings that are right for you depends on how many calories you need, which in turn depends on your age, sex, size, and activity level. Almost everyone should have at least the lowest number of servings in the ranges. The following calorie level suggestions are based on recommendations of the National Academy of Sciences and on calorie intakes reported by people in national food consumption surveys.

For adults and teens

1600 calories is about right for many sedentary women and some older adults.

2200 calories is about right for most children, teenage girls, active women, and many sedentary men. Women who are pregnant or breastfeeding may need somewhat more.

2800 calories is about right for teenage boys, many active men, and some very active women.

Sample Diets for a Day at Three Calorie Levels			
	Lower about **1600**	Moderate about **2200**	Higher about **2800**
Bread group servings	6	9	11
Vegetable group servings	3	4	5
Fruit group servings	2	3	4
Milk group servings	2-3[1]	2-3[1]	2-3[1]
Meat group (ounces)	5	6	7
Total fat (grams)	53	73	93

[1] Women who are pregnant or breastfeeding, teenagers, and young adults to age 24 need 3 servings.

FIG. **10-6.** Food Guide Pyramid. *(From US Department of Agriculture, 1992.)*

tooth structure. In addition, however, it is a well-established fact that if children and adults closely follow the recommended basic diet and consume a diet containing adequate amounts of protein, fresh fruit, and vegetables, the appetite for snacks between meals will be decreased.

REDUCTION OF DENTAL PLAQUE (AND MICROORGANISMS) WITH GOOD ORAL HYGIENE PROCEDURES

The next chapter of this text discusses the importance of good oral hygiene in more detail, but it must be mentioned here as a critically important component of

GUIDE TO GOOD EATING

Anyone can eat for good health. Just follow these 2 simple steps:

1. *Eat foods from all Five Food Groups every day.* Each food group provides you with different nutrients.

2. *Eat different foods from each food group every day.* Some foods in a food group are better sources of a nutrient than others. By eating several foods from each food group, you increase your chance of getting all the nutrients you need.

Every day eat: *Suggested Serving Sizes*

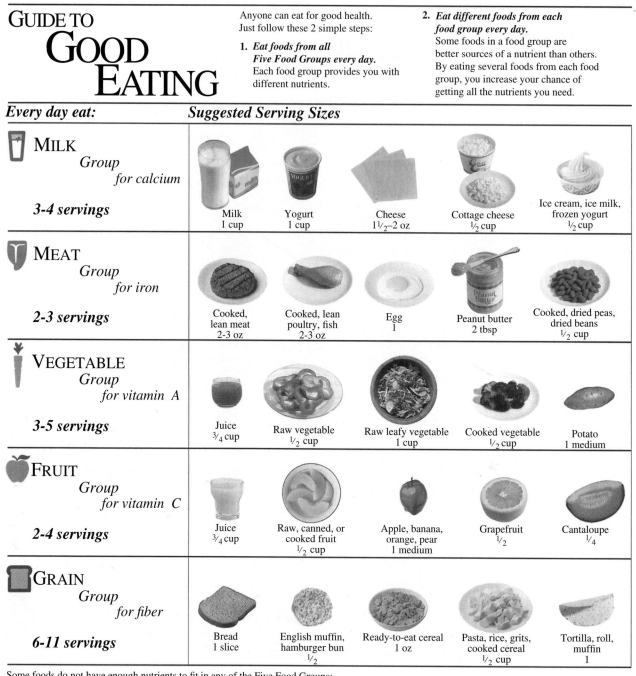

MILK *Group for calcium*
3-4 servings

Milk 1 cup | Yogurt 1 cup | Cheese 1½–2 oz | Cottage cheese ½ cup | Ice cream, ice milk, frozen yogurt ½ cup

MEAT *Group for iron*
2-3 servings

Cooked, lean meat 2-3 oz | Cooked, lean poultry, fish 2-3 oz | Egg 1 | Peanut butter 2 tbsp | Cooked, dried peas, dried beans ½ cup

VEGETABLE *Group for vitamin A*
3-5 servings

Juice ¾ cup | Raw vegetable ½ cup | Raw leafy vegetable 1 cup | Cooked vegetable ½ cup | Potato 1 medium

FRUIT *Group for vitamin C*
2-4 servings

Juice ¾ cup | Raw, canned, or cooked fruit ½ cup | Apple, banana, orange, pear 1 medium | Grapefruit ½ | Cantaloupe ¼

GRAIN *Group for fiber*
6-11 servings

Bread 1 slice | English muffin, hamburger bun ½ | Ready-to-eat cereal 1 oz | Pasta, rice, grits, cooked cereal ½ cup | Tortilla, roll, muffin 1

Some foods do not have enough nutrients to fit in any of the Five Food Groups; these foods are called "Others". These foods are okay to eat in moderation. They should not replace foods from the Five Food Groups.

"OTHERS" *category*

Fats and oils, sweets, salty snacks, alcohol, other beverages, and condiments

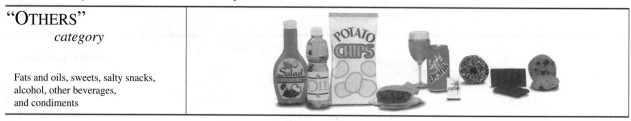

FIG. **10-7.** Guide to Good Eating. *(Reprinted by permission of the National Dairy Council, Rosemont, Ill.)*

TABLE 10-2 Recommended Food Servings for Children

FOOD GROUP	PRESCHOOL	6-12 YEARS	TEEN GIRLS	TEEN BOYS
Milk	3	3-4	4	4
Meat	2	2-3	2-3	2-3
Vegetables	3	3-4	3-4	4-5
Fruit	2	2-3	2-3	3-4
Grain	4	6-9	6-9	9-11

Adapted from the Guide to Good Eating, ed 6, and Food Models Teacher/Leader Guide for Early Childhood Educators, Rosemont, Ill, National Dairy Council.

any caries control program. Berenie, Ripa, and Leske studied the relationship between frequency of toothbrushing, oral hygiene, gingival health, and caries in 384 children, 9 to 13 years of age, who resided in a fluoride-deficient western New York community.[54] Of the children studied, 37% brushed their teeth once a day, 37% brushed twice a day, and 13% brushed less than once a day. The remaining children in the group, approximately 13%, brushed their teeth three or more times each day. A trend toward decreased scores for decayed, missing, or filled permanent teeth (DMFT) and decayed, missing, or filled permanent tooth surfaces (DMFS) accompanied increased daily brushing. The increased frequency of daily toothbrushing had its most significant positive effect on the level of oral hygiene.

Beal et al studied the caries incidence and gingival health of children who were 11 to 12 years old at the start of the study.[55] The children's dental cleanliness was evaluated at yearly examinations for a 3-year period. The children whose dental cleanliness was consistently good had lower caries increments than those whose dental cleanliness was consistently bad. Horowitz et al have demonstrated the benefits of a school-based plaque removal program in a 3-year study of children in grades 5 to 8.[56] At the end of the study the adjusted mean DMFS scores were 13% lower in the supervised plaque removal group than in the control group.

The difference between groups was accounted for entirely by a 26% difference in affected mesial and distal surfaces, a figure that approached statistical significance ($p = 0.07$). Similarly, Tsamtsouris, White, and Clark have demonstrated that supervised toothbrushing with instruction produces significantly and consistently lower plaque scores, even in preschool children, than were achieved through a control test of the same children when they were neither supervised nor instructed.[57] The investigators concluded that constant reinforcement is necessary to maintain effective plaque control in preschool children.

Wright, Banting, and Feasby conducted a clinical study to evaluate the effect of frequent interdental flossing on the incidence of proximal dental caries.[58] Schoolchildren from a fluoride-deficient area were studied after clinical and radiographic examinations were performed. Based on the observations of this study, the authors concluded that frequent interdental flossing resulted in a 50% reduction in the incidence of proximal caries in primary teeth during a 20-month period. The longer the period of interdental flossing, the greater the benefit; however, there was little residual effect after flossing was discontinued.

USE OF FLUORIDES AND TOPICAL ANTIMICROBIAL AGENTS

Without doubt the repeated use of fluorides is of critical importance for the control and prevention of dental caries in both children and adults. Numerous controlled clinical investigations have consistently demonstrated the cariostatic properties of fluoride provided in a variety of manners. These studies have also shown that the maximal benefit from fluoride is achieved only through the use of multiple delivery systems.

Existing evidence indicates that the cariostatic activity of fluoride involves several different mechanisms. The ingestion of fluoride results in its incorporation into the dentin and enamel of unerupted teeth; this makes the teeth more resistant to acid attack after eruption into the oral cavity. In addition, ingested fluoride is secreted into saliva. Although it is present in low concentrations, the

BOX 10-1 Basic Diet Analysis Form

WEEKLY REQUIREMENT	TOTAL SERVINGS CONSUMED	ACTUAL DEFICIENCY	PERCENT OF TOTAL
Bread, cereal, rice, and pasta group			
Vegetable group			
Fruit group			
Milk, yogurt, and cheese group			
Meat, poultry, fish, dry beans, eggs, and nuts group			

Fermentable carbohydrate exposures											
Form	Day of week										Total number of exposures
Sugar in solution	During meal										
	End of meal										
	Between meals										
Solid and retentive sugar-containing foods	During meal										
	End of meal										
	Between meals										

Grand total: _____

Total exposures × 20 min. = _____

Which specific food items are the offenders?   Suggested substitutes:

1. _____   1. _____

2. _____   2. _____

3. _____   3. _____

4. _____   4. _____

FIG. **10-8.** Form for analysis of ingested fermentable carbohydrates.

fluoride is accumulated in plaque, where it decreases microbial acid production and enhances the remineralization of the underlying enamel. Fluoride from saliva is also incorporated into the enamel of newly erupted teeth, thereby enhancing enamel calcification (frequently called *enamel maturation*), which decreases caries susceptibility. As a topically applied therapeutic agent, fluoride is effective in preventing future lesion development, in arresting or at least slowing the progression of active cavitated lesions, and in remineralizing active incipient lesions. Topical fluoride also has some antimicrobial properties.

The exposure of the teeth to fluoride through professional application of fluoride solutions, gels, foams, and varnishes plus exposure from dentifrices and other fluoride preparations used at home engages almost all of the foregoing mechanisms except the preeruptive incorporation into enamel. Although it is difficult to separate the benefits of the different mechanisms of action of fluoride, research has suggested that the predominant mechanism is the impact of fluoride on the remineralization of demineralized enamel. Numerous studies have shown that the presence of fluoride greatly enhances the rate of remineralization of demineralized enamel and dentin. Moreover, tooth structure remineralized in the presence of fluoride contains increased concentrations of fluorhydroxyapatite, which makes the remineralized tissue more resistant to future attack by acids than was the original structure. In view of fluoride's multiple mechanisms of action, it is not surprising that treatment with fluoride through multiple delivery systems has additive benefits. This supports the recommendation that frequent exposure to fluoride is beneficial for maximal caries prevention and control.

Communal Water Fluoridation. Research studies and observations in private practice continue to support the contention that fluoridation of the communal water supply is the most effective method of reducing the dental caries problem in the general population.

In 1998, Stookey noted that approximately half of the population of the United States enjoys the benefits of fluoridated communal water supplies.[59]

Cohen has cited observations in Philadelphia, the first city with a population over 1 million to fluoridate its water supply.[60] The reduction in DMFT has averaged 75% at 6 years of age, 54.5% at 8 years, 42.6% at 12 years, and 46.7% at 14 years. A 50% reduction in the decay rate has been noted in the primary teeth.

Murray and Rugg-Gunn reviewed 94 studies, conducted in 20 countries, to help clarify varying reports on the benefits to primary teeth of communal water fluoridation.[61] A thorough review of the data clearly showed that water fluoridation provides protection for primary teeth against dental caries but to a somewhat lesser degree than for permanent teeth. The caries reduction benefits to primary teeth ranged between 40% and 50%, whereas the range for permanent teeth was between 50% and 60%.

Carmichael et al[62] and Rock, Gordon, and Bradnock[63] have reported data in separate studies comparing the caries incidence in children living in two fluoridated communities with that in children living in two nonfluoridated communities in England. The role of fluoridation in reducing dental caries is obvious in both studies. The study by Carmichael et al also demonstrated that children in lower social classes gain an even greater caries prevention benefit than children in higher social classes. The reason is that, as a group, the children in the lower social classes have a higher prevalence of proximal carious lesions, and proximal tooth surfaces derive the greatest benefit from fluoridation.

The protection afforded by the ingestion of fluoridated water persists throughout the lifetime of the person. Investigations by Russell and Elvolve[64] and by Englander, Reuss, and Kesel,[65] as well as other studies, have shown that the continuous ingestion of fluoridated water during adulthood decreases the prevalence of dental caries by about the same magnitude observed in children. In addition, Stamm and Banting have reported a 56% decrease in the prevalence of root-surface caries in adults who lived continuously in a fluoridated community.[66]

The posteruptive benefits associated with the ingestion of fluoridated water also have been demonstrated. Arnold et al[67] as well as Hayes, Littleton, and White[68] have reported that the posteruptive ingestion of fluoridated water can result in decreases in caries prevalence as great as 30%. Similarly, Hardwick, Teasdale, and Bloodworth have reported a 27% reduction in caries prevalence after 4 years of ingestion of fluoridated water by teenagers who were 12 years of age when fluoridation was initiated.[69] These observations are consistent with the multiple mechanisms of action of fluoride cited earlier and support the significant contribution of the exposure of the teeth to fluoride even in the very low concentrations present in fluoridated drinking water.

More recent studies concerning the reduced prevalence of dental caries associated with the presence of fluoride in communal water supplies have demonstrated appreciably lesser benefits, typically ranging between 18% and 30%.[70-72] This decrease in attributable benefit is due to the so-called halo effect associated with the preparation of numerous foods and beverages in fluoridated communities and their consumption in nonfluoridated communities. Recent reports have attempted to quantify this halo effect by measuring the fluoride intake of children residing in communities that do not have a fluoridated communal water supply and have shown that fluoride ingestion is nearly 70% that of residents of optimally fluoridated communities.[73-75] Thus it is not surprising that only modest differences in caries prevalence rates are noted between children residing in fluoridated and nonfluoridated communities.

When fluoridation is discontinued in a community, an increase in the dental caries incidence will follow. Way has reported that, after a 2-year lapse of drinking fluoride-free water in Galesburg, Illinois, children experienced as much as a 38% increase in tooth decay.[76] Lemke, Doherty, and Arra have reported that in Antigo, Wisconsin, a city of 9600, tooth decay rose 92% among kindergarten children, 183% among second-graders, and 100% among fourth-graders when fluoridation was discontinued.[77]

Attwood and Blinkhorn reported on the dental health of schoolchildren in Stranraer, Scotland, 5 years after fluoridation of their water supply had ended.[78] They found that, among 5-year-old children, the dmft score had increased to 3.08 compared with 2.48 among the same age group 5 years earlier. After 5 years of no fluoridation, the scores for decayed, missing, or filled primary teeth (dmft) and DMFT were quite similar to the scores of children from another city in the same region (Annan, Scotland) that had never had fluoridated water. Most of the 44% difference in dmft scores and the 50% difference in DMFT scores that previously favored the Stranraer children was lost 5 years after the fluoride had been removed from their water. The authors point out that, although there is a general decline in dental caries because of the almost universal use of fluoride toothpaste (the Annan children also had lower dmft and DMFT scores at the end of the study), fluoridation of water has a significantly beneficial added effect.

Eichenbaum, Dunn, and Tinanoff reported interesting information related to the long-term impact of communal fluoridation on the private practice of pediatric dentistry.[79] A survey conducted from 1948 to 1950 showed that 86% of the pediatric patients in a private pediatric dental practice needed restorative treatment, and nearly half of these children required pulp therapy. The results of this survey encouraged the city health officials to implement dental health education and preventive programs that included communal water fluoridation. A survey of the same practice almost 30 years later (1977 to 1979) revealed a dramatic change in the restorative needs of the children. The majority of children needed no restorations, and the number of teeth with pulp involvement was negligible.

In 1986, Smith estimated that the average annual cost of fluoridating communal water supplies is approximately 25 cents per person.[80] Gish pointed out in 1979 that the annual cost varies with the size of the community and may range from approximately $1.50 per person in very small communities to as low as 10 cents per person in larger metropolitan areas.[81] These estimates are still valid, with just upward adjustment for inflation. Communal water fluoridation remains by far the most cost-effective caries prevention measure available.

Horowitz, Heifetz, and Law have reported findings that have relevance for the millions of Americans who are deprived of the benefits of community water fluoridation because they live in areas not served by central water supplies.[82] The water supply of a rural school was fluoridated for 12 years at a level of 5 ppm, which is 4.5 times the optimum level for community fluoridation in the area. In the final survey, children who had

attended the school continuously during the study had 39% fewer DMFT than did their counterparts who had not attended the school continuously. Late-erupting teeth (canines, premolars, and second molars) demonstrated twice as much caries protection as early-erupting teeth (incisors and first molars). In both categories of teeth the greatest benefits were observed on proximal surfaces, with as much as 69% less caries for late-erupting teeth.

Considerable research related to the effect of school water fluoridation on dental caries has been conducted using even higher concentrations of fluoride. Heifetz, Horowitz, and Brunelle completed another 12-year study in Seagrove, North Carolina, where school water is fluoridated at the level of 6.3 ppm, or approximately seven times the optimum recommended for community water fluoridation.[83] Observations after 12 years show only a slight improvement in DMFS reduction compared with the earlier 12-year study using 5 ppm (or 4.5 times the optimum). The researchers concluded that there is little justification for recommending the higher fluoride level for school water fluoridation programs.

When these investigations were conducted, it was thought that school water fluoridation would provide a mechanism for children in rural, nonfluoridated areas to receive the public health benefits of fluoride. At its peak, school water fluoridation programs were in operation in 13 states, serving about 170,000 children in 470 schools. However, numerous problems associated with equipment maintenance and monitoring coupled with the recently recognized impact of increased amounts of fluoride in the food chain (i.e., the halo effect) has led the Centers for Disease Control and Prevention (CDC) to discontinue promoting these programs in the United States. In 2001 the Task Force on Community Preventive Services of the CDC strongly recommended community water fluoridation and school-based or school-linked pit and fissure sealant delivery programs for prevention and control of dental caries.[84] However, the Task Force found insufficient evidence of effectiveness for the remaining interventions reviewed, including school water fluoridation.

Fluoride-Containing Dentifrices. Extensive research initiated in the early 1950s ultimately resulted in the identification of the first fluoride-containing dentifrice* capable of decreasing the incidence of dental caries. This dentifrice contained stannous fluoride (SnF_2) in combination with calcium pyrophosphate as the cleaning and polishing system and in 1964 was accepted as the first therapeutic dentifrice by the Council on Dental Therapeutics of the American Dental Association (ADA) based on more than 20 clinical trials. The significance of this original development has been profound;

---

*Crest, Procter & Gamble, Cincinnati, Ohio.

in fact, a review by Jenkins concluded that the general decline in caries prevalence in Britain and other developed countries appears to be attributable in large part to the widespread use of effective fluoride-containing dentifrices.[85] Caretakers should be counseled so they know that no more than a small, pea-sized amount of fluoridated toothpaste should be used when they brush the teeth of infants and other very young children.

For nearly three decades after the completion of the first successful clinical trial in 1954, this stannous fluoride dentifrice served as a standard of reference for the development of additional fluoride dentifrices as well as for efforts to identify even more effective compositions. An extensive review of the literature by Stookey in 1985 indicated that more than 140 clinical trials of fluoride dentifrices had been reported.[86] These investigations identified several fluoride dentifrice systems with demonstrated cariostatic activity and verified the commercial availability of many such systems. In the United States at the present time, 49 dentifrice formulations from 15 manufacturers have received the Seal of Approval of the ADA. These ADA-accepted dentifrices now comprise approximately 90% of all dentifrices sold in the United States. Fluoride dentifrices similarly represent 85% to 90% of the dentifrice sales in Britain as well as several in other countries.

Before 1981, attempts to identify a fluoride dentifrice system significantly more effective than the original stannous fluoride formulation were unsuccessful. However, in 1981 the results of two clinical studies demonstrated the superiority of a sodium fluoride composition.[87,88] A clinical study of 3 years' duration was conducted by Beiswanger, Gish, and Mallatt[87] to determine the effect of a sodium fluoride–silica abrasive dentifrice on dental caries. The dentifrice, containing 0.243% sodium fluoride, was compared with stannous fluoride in a study group of 1824 schoolchildren 6 to 14 years of age in Indiana cities where water supplies were fluoride deficient (containing less than 0.35 ppm fluoride). After 3 years the group brushing with the sodium fluoride dentifrice had significantly lower DMFT and DMFS increments than the group brushing with the stannous fluoride dentifrice. Two independent examiners found that the reductions were 14.8% and 10.5% for DMFT and 16.4% and 13.1% for DMFS. These results are consistent with those reported by Zacherl in which the sodium fluoride dentifrice resulted in a 40.7% decrease in DMFS compared with a 23.4% decrease observed with the stannous fluoride dentifrice.[88] Similarly, studies conducted by Gerdin[89] and by Edlund and Koch[90] indicated that the use of sodium fluoride dentifrices by children resulted in significantly fewer caries than the use of dentifrices containing sodium monofluorophosphate. The results of these studies and several similar reports led Stookey to conclude in 1985 that the use of

sodium fluoride in a highly compatible formulation resulted in greater cariostatic activity than the use of other fluoride dentifrice systems available at that time.[86]

Topical Fluorides in the Dental Office. The periodic professional topical application of more concentrated fluoride solutions, gels, foams, or varnishes has been repeatedly demonstrated to result in a significant reduction in the incidence of dental caries in both children and adults as well as the arrestment of incipient lesions. As a result, professional topical fluoride applications are routinely recommended for all children and adolescents. Even in the absence of dental caries activity, topical fluoride applications to children are recommended as a means of raising the fluoride content of the enamel of newly erupted teeth and thereby increasing the resistance of these teeth to caries formation.

Historically the periodic topical application of fluoride was first demonstrated to be effective for the prevention of dental caries in the early 1940s. Since that time, many hundreds of publications have provided additional data to confirm the efficacy of professionally applied topical fluoride treatments for caries prevention.

A 4-minute treatment time has been typically recommended for professionally applied topical fluoride solutions, gels, or foams. Recently some manufacturers recommend only a 1-minute application. It is known that most of the fluoride uptake in the enamel occurs during the first minute after application. However, measurable benefits do continue to accrue for approximately 4 minutes if the topical preparation remains in contact with the teeth. We continue to recommend the 4-minute application whenever possible. If gel or foam is applied with a tray technique, use of an ample amount will force the substance into the proximal areas. The trays should be about one third to one half full for gel and full (level with the edge) for foam. Usually both upper and lower trays are inserted at once to complete the topical fluoride treatment in one 4-minute application. Some trays are supplied as a connected double set (Fig. 10-9). The patient sits in an upright position with head tipped slightly forward to allow excess saliva and fluoride to flow toward the lips. Patients who follow instructions well may be provided with the high-velocity evacuator tip to help control the drooling themselves, or they may be given a plastic "drool bag" that enables them to tip the head forward even more and catch the drooled liquid in the bag, which is later discarded. The dentist or appropriate office staff should supervise the treatment and provide assistance as needed. If necessary the auxiliary may manipulate the evacuator tip or help hold the patient's head forward and the trays in place over the drool bag. Patients requiring assistance also often need positive reinforcement during the procedure. Extra caution and special application techniques are required when topical solutions, gels, or foams are

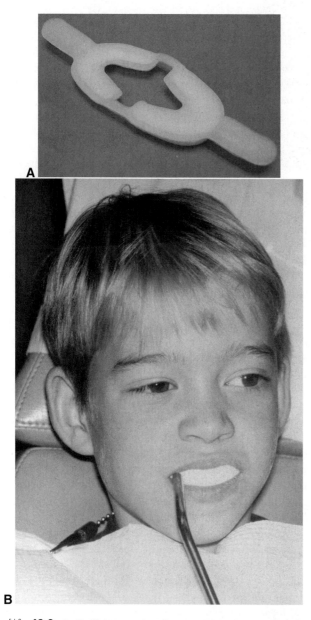

FIG. 10-9. **A,** Sufficient topical fluoride foam is placed in the upper and lower trays so that each tray is filled approximately level with the edge of the tray. **B,** The teeth are dried and the trays are inserted in the patient's mouth to provide a complete-mouth topical fluoride treatment in a single 4-minute application. The evacuator tip is positioned to remove the excess saliva and foam as the liquids flow toward the lips.

placed in the mouths of young children (around 4 years old and younger). The agent is usually brushed on to the teeth in small amounts and the excess is wiped away with gauze.

The results of independent clinical trials have seriously questioned the need for dental prophylaxis before the topical application of acidulated phosphate fluoride (APF). Ripa et al compared the caries incidence during a 3-year period in children given semiannual topical

applications of APF after different cleaning procedures.[91] Before each fluoride treatment the children either received conventional prophylaxis using a non-fluoride prophylactic paste, performed supervised toothbrushing and flossing, or rinsed their mouths with water. Caries increments after 3 years were essentially identical in all the treatment groups, a finding which indicates that the manner of cleaning the teeth before the APF treatment may not influence the cariostatic activity of the fluoride applications. Similarly designed clinical trials were conducted by Houpt, Koenigsberg, and Shey[92] and by Katz et al[93]; in both instances the results were comparable to those observed by Ripa et al.[91] An additional study by Bijella et al likewise demonstrated that the presence or absence of a prophylactic procedure did not alter the efficacy of a topical APF application.[94] Collectively these studies indicate that prophylaxis before an APF topical application may be an optional procedure with regard to caries reduction.

Beginning with reports by Ekstrand et al[95] and by LeCompte and Whitford,[96] several investigators have expressed concern regarding the amount of fluoride swallowed by children during a topical fluoride application. These reports indicated that, depending on the manner of application, 15 to 31 mg of fluoride may be swallowed during the treatment. Stookey et al explored the feasibility of permitting patients to rinse after a topical fluoride application as a means of reducing fluoride ingestion.[97] However, they observed that rinsing with water after a topical fluoride application significantly decreased fluoride deposition in incipient carious lesions. A report by LeCompte and Doyle indicated that one could drastically reduce the amount of fluoride ingested during topical fluoride application to about 1.6 mg by using only the necessary amount of fluoride gel, having the patient seated in an upright position, using high-velocity saliva evacuation during the treatment, and asking the patient to expectorate thoroughly for 1 minute after completion of the treatment.[98] Thus the latter procedures are recommended to minimize fluoride ingestion during the application, particularly in younger children, and the patient should be encouraged not to eat, drink, or rinse for 30 minutes after the treatment to maximize fluoride uptake in enamel.

Fluoride-containing varnishes have been widely used in Europe and other parts of the world for approximately 40 years but were not available in the United States until 1994. The first fluoride varnish was introduced in Europe in 1964 and contained 5.0% sodium fluoride (or 2.26% fluoride). A second product was introduced in Europe in 1975 and contained 0.9% silane fluoride (or 0.1% fluoride). Much more research has been conducted using the sodium fluoride system, and it is the most widely accepted.

Petersson,[99] Horowitz and Ismail,[100] and Petersson et al[101] have reviewed the numerous controlled clinical trials of fluoride varnishes and concluded that these materials are equally as effective as professional topical fluoride applications for the prevention of dental caries in children. Seppa et al investigated the effect of the sodium fluoride varnish in children with a high past caries experience and found that this measure resulted in numerically fewer new caries lesions than was achieved with semiannual applications of an APF gel during a 3-year study period.[102] These investigators also noted that the data for use of this varnish satisfied the criteria of the ADA for the claim of being "at least as good as" professionally applied topical fluoride gels. Helfenstein and Steiner performed a statistical meta-analysis of the data from a number of clinical trials and found that use of the sodium fluoride varnish resulted in an overall reduction in caries of 38% in the permanent teeth.[103] In general, slightly lower average benefits of about 30% have been observed in studies of varnish use on primary teeth.

The sodium fluoride varnish is particularly recommended for use in preschool-aged children because of its ease of application and equal efficacy to APF systems.[59] Before application of the varnish, the teeth receive prophylaxis or are brushed with a dentifrice to remove plaque and oral debris. The varnish is then applied with a soft brush, with reapplications recommended at 4- to 6-month intervals. A more intensive annual treatment regimen consisting of three applications within a 10-day period has been investigated, and this regimen was observed to be as effective as applications every 4 months.[104-106] Furthermore, single annual applications have been found to be without clinical benefit. The varnish has a brown color but is lost from the tooth surfaces within 24 to 48 hours. Because less than a milliliter of varnish is used for a professional treatment in preschool-aged children, the amount of fluoride that will ultimately be ingested when the varnish is lost from the tooth surfaces is less than 3 mg. Thus there are no practical concerns regarding safety, and this procedure is frequently recommended for use in young children in place of the traditional topical fluoride gel application.

Topical Fluorides for the General Anesthesia Patient. The application of fluoride to the teeth of children receiving dental care under a general anesthetic, after the placement of restorations, is certainly recommended. Thorough prophylaxis should precede the placement of the rubber dam for a quadrant of restorations. The fluoride should be applied after the restorative work has been completed for that quadrant but before removal of the rubber dam.

Home Fluoride Mouthrinses and Gels. The use of dilute oral fluoride rinses and/or gels as an additional dental caries control measure has become another helpful adjunct. Children under 4 years of age may not have full control over their swallowing reflexes; therefore, caution should be exercised in recommending these products for home use for this age group. However, some small children can expectorate rinses quite reliably under proper supervision, or the parent can brush on the gel and wipe away the excess. In non-fluoridated areas it may be appropriate to have the child swallow the rinse after "swishing" it to gain the systemic fluoride effect as well. Some rinses (acidulated or aqueous solutions that do not contain alcohol) are prepared to provide the necessary supplemental systemic dose of fluoride if the child does not drink fluoridated water. However, current Food and Drug Administration (FDA) regulations specify that fluoride rinses not be recommended for children under 6 years of age unless they are intended for use as a systemic fluoride supplement.

Radike et al observed schoolchildren who rinsed their mouths once each school day for 2 school years with a stannous fluoride mouthrinse containing 250 ppm fluoride (about 0.1% stannous fluoride).[107] There was a significant reduction in dental caries at the end of the first and second school years. Two independent examiners found caries reductions of 33% and 43% in DMFS scores. The anticaries benefit from the stannous fluoride mouthrinse was especially encouraging because the children already were receiving the optimum benefit of water fluoridation.

APF mouthwashes in concentrations of either 100 or 200 ppm fluoride ion used twice daily have been shown by Finn et al to be effective.[108] They reported that during a 26-month period the APF rinses containing relatively small amounts of fluoride were effective in reducing dental caries.

Miller made a preliminary report on results of the National Caries Program sponsored by the National Institute of Dental Research.[109] A nationwide school-based fluoride mouthrinse program that included 85,000 children in 17 states and Guam produced encouraging results. The schoolchildren rinsed their mouths for 60 seconds once weekly with 5 ml of a 0.2% neutral sodium fluoride solution. Children in the 7-, 11-, and 13-year-old groups experienced a reduction in dental decay. There was also evidence of caries decrease in the primary teeth.

Leske et al[110] and Leske, Ripa, and Green[111] have reported on results of a fluoride rinsing program that was begun in 1975 in the Three Village Central School District of Long Island, New York. The program was one of 17 demonstration projects sponsored by the National Institute of Dental Research, which initially enrolled approximately 4500 elementary schoolchildren (kindergarten through the sixth grade), who rinsed once a week with a 0.2% neutral sodium fluoride solution under the supervision of homeroom teachers. The prevalence of caries in the children who participated in the rinse program for 2 to 4 years was 20.4% DMFT and 24.4% DMFS lower than that of children who had never rinsed. The reduction in proximal caries was 49.6%. The reductions in occlusal and buccolingual caries were 21.0% and 18.8%, respectively. The examination of exfoliated teeth also indicated that fluoride rinsing may produce a residual benefit. The later report on children who had participated in the program for 7 years demonstrated caries prevalence reductions of 55.7% DMFT and 60.9% DMFS, with 85.4% reduction of proximal surface caries.

Extensive field research has been conducted on the use of fluoride mouthrinses. Most studies incorporate the use of a 0.2% sodium fluoride rinse once weekly or a 0.05% sodium fluoride rinse once daily. As does the work previously summarized, these other studies show unquestionable caries prevention benefits of the regular use of self-administered fluoride rinses when properly supervised. These benefits accrue to primary and permanent teeth, and seem to be helpful both in fluoridated areas and in areas with nonfluoridated water. The studies of Heifetz[112] and of Ripa and Leske[113] are cited in the references listed at the end of this chapter as good examples of clinical research with fluoride rinses. Based on numerous studies indicating the efficacy of fluoride rinses, some rinses were approved by the FDA in 1974 and by the ADA Council on Dental Therapeutics in 1975. Studies supporting the use of the dilute gels are not as numerous as those for the rinses, but some gels have also subsequently been approved.

Dietary Fluoride Supplements. A review of the literature on the value of fluorides administered during pregnancy fails to disclose any valid evidence to support such use even in nonfluoridated areas. In 1966 the FDA banned the manufacturers of fluoride supplements from marketing products bearing the claim that dental caries would be prevented in the offspring of women who used such products during pregnancy. The FDA took this action because of the insufficiency of clinical evidence to substantiate such a claim. There was no question of safety. Although some medical and dental practitioners have continued to prescribe dietary fluoride supplements for pregnant women since the FDA's advertising ban, generally there is unanimity among most research experts and public health officials that fluoride ingestion by gravid women does not benefit the teeth of their offspring, at least not the permanent teeth.

Participants in a symposium concerning the use of prenatal fluorides agreed that transfer of fluoride does occur from the mother to the fetus through the placenta.[114] Only in recent years has such a transfer been generally acknowledged. How much fluoride is transferred from the blood of the mother to the blood of the fetus, however, remains uncertain. Nevertheless, the members of the symposium generally agreed that some benefit of caries prevention accrues to the primary teeth when the fetus is subjected to fluoride. There was considerable doubt about the benefit to the permanent teeth. The symposium discussions seemed to lead to the conclusion that additional well-controlled research efforts are needed to define more clearly the possible benefits of prenatal fluoride administration. Some research into this issue continues, as does the controversy.

A study by Katz and Muhler suggested that the effect of fluoride on primary teeth is mainly postnatal.[115] In a study to determine the effect of waterborne fluoride on dental caries in primary teeth, 890 children from 4 to 7 years of age were examined in one Indiana city having a communal water supply with only 0.05 ppm fluoride and in three cities having a supply with a concentration of 1 ppm fluoride. Children living in the cities with fluoridated water had between 35% and 65% fewer dental caries in their primary teeth than those living in the fluoride-deficient city. Comparisons of dental caries incidence in the primary teeth of children living in the same city who were exposed either prenatally or postnatally or exclusively postnatally showed no difference between the groups.

Hennon, Stookey, and Muhler conducted a clinical study that included 815 children between 18 and 39 months of age residing in three fluoride-deficient Indiana communities.[116] The children received chewable tablets containing vitamins, vitamins plus fluoride, or fluoride alone (1 mg as sodium fluoride) and were examined for dental caries initially and at 6-month intervals. The findings during the first 2 years of the 5$^{1}/_{2}$-year study indicated a significant reduction of about 37% in the incidence of dental caries after 6 months in the children ingesting either the fluoride or vitamin-fluoride supplements.[117] This degree of protection increased to about 55% and 63%, respectively, after the children had used the supplement for 1 and 2 years. The important finding was the significant reduction in the incidence of dental caries after use of the tablets for only 6 months. This observation indicates a highly effective topical benefit of chewing the tablets, because most of the primary teeth had already erupted when the study began.

Many other studies have demonstrated the anticariogenic effectiveness of fluoride supplements. If children do not have the benefit of drinking water containing an optimum fluoride concentration, supplements should be prescribed in accordance with the dosages recommended in Table 10-3. The natural fluoride content of the water should first be determined. If the natural fluoride content is 0.6 ppm or higher, supplements should not be administered. If the fluoride content is below 0.6 ppm, the administration of fluoride

TABLE 10-3 Dietary Fluoride Supplementation Schedule			
AGE	LESS THAN 0.3 ppm F	0.3-0.6 ppm F	MORE THAN 0.6 ppm F
Birth-6 mos	0	0	0
6 mos-3 yrs	0.25 mg	0	0
3 yrs-6 yrs	0.50 mg	0.25 mg	0
6 yrs up to at least 16 yrs	1.00 mg	0.50	0

From American Academy of Pediatric Dentistry: Guideline on fluoride therapy, *Pediatr Dent* 24(7 suppl):66, 2002 (special issue: Reference manual 2002-2003).

supplements should commence as indicated in Table 10-3 and should continue through the time of the eruption of the second permanent molars.

A number of studies report the caries-preventive effects of adding fluoride to a variety of foods and beverages. Fluoride has been used as a caries-preventive additive in salt, milk, and even sugar. Some suppliers now offer controlled concentrations of fluoride in bottled water. Numerous reports show that these products can have measurable and favorable results when used as intended. Such products are designed for use by specific and targeted population groups. These products have not yet had widespread popularity, although there is growing interest in this concept and public acceptance seems to be growing for fluoridated bottled water for children who either do not have or do not use community fluoridated water.

Combinations of Fluoride Therapies. There is considerable evidence to suggest that using combinations of therapeutic fluoride agents often produces additive anticariogenic effects. The evidence also indicates that the earlier fluoride therapy is initiated in children the more effective the caries control will be. However, one must use caution in prescribing multiple therapies in very young children to avoid excessive fluoride ingestion.

Fluoride is the most effective caries-prevention agent commercially available today. Except in a patient who has a fluoride allergy (very rare), it is considered completely safe when properly used. The ingestion of high concentrations can lead to nausea, vomiting, dental fluorosis (mottling), or, in extreme cases, even death, especially in children. Extreme care must be used to safeguard the agents from inappropriate and/or inadvertent ingestion. It is imperative that the dental profession have full awareness of the hazards accompanying its use and yet be prepared to use it to the patient's maximum advantage through careful consideration of each patient's individual situation.

Chlorhexidine and Thymol. As an oral antimicrobial, chlorhexidine has been used in oral rinses, dentifrices, chewing gum, varnish, and gel. In the United States it is used most often in the form of a prescription oral rinse. Many children object to the taste of these products, but they have been shown to be effective against microorganisms causing both caries and periodontal disease. Thymol has also been included with chlorhexidine in some varnish preparations. To date, these products have not shown superior caries prevention results when compared to multiple fluoride therapies and they may require more frequent application to be effective. However, they should provide an additive effect and may be used in combination with fluoride, particularly in high-risk patients. In the rare situation in which a provider is trying to control or prevent caries in a patient with fluoride allergy, they could be very important therapies.

Povidone Iodine. Considerable data exist from laboratory and animal studies to confirm the dramatic suppression of mutans streptococci by iodine. Several studies reconfirm this observation in humans as well. Lopez et al published two human studies demonstrating that topical application of povidone iodine at 2-month intervals in dentate infants is effective in preventing S-ECC in children at high risk for the disease.[118,119] The authors called for more and larger in-depth clinical trials. If such trials prove as successful as these initial reports, they could hopefully lead to widespread implementation of an effective defense against this devastating disease for which minimal parental compliance is required.

Xylitol. Xylitol is a low-calorie sweetener that inhibits the growth of *S. mutans*. Numerous studies seem to confirm its anticariogenic capability. Xylitol has been tested as an additive to a variety of foods and to dentifrice. However, the vast majority of published data come from studies in which xylitol was incorporated into chewing gum. Makinen has reported numerous studies on the topic, most of them performed with many different coworkers in different parts of the world. In 2000, he published a concise summary titled "The Rocky Road of Xylitol to Its Clinical Application."[120] The available data not only show that xylitol chewing gum reduces caries activity but also provide evidence that it decreases the transmission of *S. mutans* from gum-chewing mothers to their children. The use of xylitol chewing gum seems to be gaining popularity as another caries prevention strategy. It should be readily accepted by many children.

RESTORATIVE DENTISTRY IN THE CONTROL PROGRAM

Excellent restorative dentistry is also valuable in the dental caries control program. For patients who do not comply with nonrestorative caries control recommendations (e.g., use of fluorides and/or antimicrobials, appropriate diet, and plaque control), the restorative

11

Mechanical and Chemotherapeutic Home Oral Hygiene

JEFFREY A. DEAN

CHRISTOPHER V. HUGHES

As the technological level of health care increases, it is important not to lose sight of the basics of patient care. In dentistry, this means establishing and maintaining effective preventive habits in our patients. No matter how sophisticated our dental techniques and procedures have become, preventive dentistry is the foundation on which all oral health care must be built.

In 1960 McDonald discussed how pediatric medicine had changed in the previous 30 years (1930 to 1960) from 90% treatment and 10% prevention to just the reverse.[1] He stated that preventive measures for dentistry were available and remained to be applied, as they had been in pediatrics. With this preventive philosophy, dentistry, particularly dentistry for children, has come a long way toward reaching this ratio of 90% prevention to 10% treatment.

At the core of this preventive foundation is home oral hygiene and plaque control. The area of oral hygiene has undergone recent developments that have turned a mundane subject into a field of surprising growth and research. Modern biology has made new inroads in the area of plaque control and will continue to exert a strong influence on how we look at oral hygiene and plaque in the future. The traditional focus of oral hygiene has been and will continue to be the control of the two most prevalent oral diseases, caries and periodontal disease. Although plaque control is essential to oral hygiene, it is important to realize that, unlike with periodontal disease, no clear relationship exists between plaque control and the prevention of caries. As discussed in Chapter 10, the complex etiology of decay centers on the following factors: tooth susceptibility, bacterial plaque, refined carbohydrates, and time. Many other variables, such as oral sugar clearance and salivary flow and pH, add to the complexity of this process. This complex etiology may help explain the difficulty in demonstrating a relationship between oral hygiene practices and caries prevention.

Despite this ambiguity, plaque control remains an essential element for oral health. Although Marsh has shown that the natural oral microflora confers several benefits on the host, in the absence of oral hygiene, dental plaque accumulates, which leads to shifts in bacterial populations away from those associated with health.[2] Treatment should therefore be designed to control rather than to eliminate dental plaque.

Not only have there been advances in biology, but the public's consciousness regarding home oral hygiene has been raised to new levels by the advertising of home health care products. The oral care market in the United States is expected to reach nearly $8 billion by 2007. Health and cosmetic awareness by patients is possibly at an all-time high; they are willing to pay for the best in health products.

This chapter addresses the broad area of home oral hygiene for the child and adolescent, from the biology of plaque development to plaque removal techniques and patient motivation. Dental health care professionals need to make home oral hygiene the core of their preventive foundation.

MICROBIAL ASPECTS OF ORAL HYGIENE AND PLAQUE FORMATION

Although Miller proposed in the late nineteenth century that microorganisms play a role in dental disease,[3] definitive evidence of the microbial etiology of dental caries and periodontal diseases did not appear until three quarters of a century later with the work of Keyes[4] and of Löe, Theilade, and Jensen.[5] Since these seminal studies were performed, the major focus of dental research has been to define the specific microorganisms in dental plaque that mediate these diseases. Although great progress has been made in identifying these pathogens, our primary tools in preventing dental diseases remain mechanical removal of plaque and promotion of the remineralization of the tooth surface. Therefore the following brief review of the timing, mechanisms, and biology of plaque formation provide a scientific rationale for any clinical program of oral hygiene and prevention.

Moore has demonstrated that the oral cavity naturally contains more than 300 bacterial species and numerous distinct bacterial habitats. Interestingly, only a limited number of species are found in high numbers in dental plaque.[6] These species are uniquely suited to this habitat. The formation of plaque on the tooth surface is characterized by progression from a limited number of pioneer species (mainly streptococci and other gram-positive organisms) to the complex flora of mature dental plaque. This maturation involves initial adherence of bacteria to the salivary pellicle and subsequent formation of a complex multispecies biofilm. Most oral bacteria have evolved specific adherence mechanisms that enable them to colonize the tooth surface. In addition, bacteria undergo a number of phenotypic changes as they initiate the formation of a biofilm. The molecular mechanisms that underlie these processes have been intensively studied. Kolenbrander has provided reviews of these areas.[7] Although their reports offer the possibility of new methods of plaque control, mechanical plaque removal with supplementation by chemotherapeutic agents currently offers the most practical method of controlling plaque.

Not only do microbial changes occur as plaque matures on the tooth surface, but mature dental plaques associated with oral diseases appear to differ from those associated with oral health. Many studies have demonstrated that, in dental caries, the pathogenicity of plaque is related to the numbers of *Streptococcus mutans* and related species present (see Balakrishnan et al[8]). In contrast, the plaques associated with gingival inflammation are characterized by a predominance of gram-negative bacteria rather than the predominantly gram-positive flora found in oral health. This transition seems to coincide with inflammatory changes that occur at the gingival margin. Plaque control efforts should be directed toward two goals: (1) limiting the numbers of mutans streptococci in dental plaques for prevention of caries by mechanical elimination of supragingival plaque and limitation of dietary sucrose, and (2) maintaining the predominantly gram-positive flora associated with gingival health by mechanical removal of plaque from the subgingival area on a regular basis. The use of chemotherapeutic agents, particularly chlorhexidine, can also play a role in maintenance of gingival health. The incorporation of these methods into the daily routines of patients and their parents is perhaps the greatest challenge facing the dentist.

MECHANICAL METHODS OF PLAQUE CONTROL

Mechanical methods of plaque control are the most widely accepted techniques for plaque removal. Toothbrushing and flossing are the essential elements of these mechanical methods; adjuncts include disclosing agents, oral irrigators, and tongue scrapers.

MANUAL TOOTHBRUSH

The toothbrush is the most common method for removing plaque from the oral cavity. A number of variables enter into the design and fabrication of toothbrushes. These include the bristle material; length, diameter, and total number of fibers; length of brush head; trim design of brush head; number and arrangement of bristle tufts; angulation of brush head to handle; and handle design. In addition, many features, such as the use of neon colors or familiar cartoon caricatures, are designed to attract the attention of potential purchasers (Fig. 11-1).

Today, most commercially available brushes are manufactured with synthetic (nylon) bristles. Park, Matis, and Christen identify the bristle and head of the toothbrush as the most important part of the brush, and note that the length of most bristles is 11 mm.[9] Brushes are classified as soft, medium, or hard based on the diameter of these bristles. The diameter ranges for these classifications are 0.16 to 0.22 mm for soft, 0.23 to 0.29 mm for medium, and 0.30 mm and higher for hard. In addition to the bristle diameter, the bristle end has been studied to determine the most beneficial

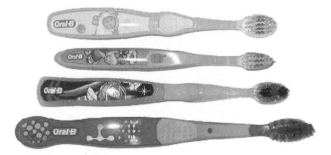

FIG. 11-1. Features such as neon colors or cartoon characters on toothbrushes are designed to attract the attention of purchasers.

type for plaque control. Of the three types of bristle ends (Fig. 11-2, *A* to *C*), coarse-cut, enlarged bulbous, and round, the round end is the bristle type of choice because it is associated with a lower incidence of gingival tissue irritation. However, even the coarse-cut bristles round off eventually with normal use (Fig. 11-2, *D*).

The soft brush is preferable for most uses in pediatric dentistry because of the decreased likelihood of gingival tissue trauma and increased interproximal cleaning ability. In evaluating the best toothbrush head and handle for children, Updyke concludes that it is best to use a brush with a smaller head and a thicker handle than on the adult-size brush to aid in access to the oral cavity and facilitate the child's grip of the handle.[10] However, no single brush design has been scientifically proved superior for removal of plaque. Multiple variables influence a brush's ability to remove plaque, and therefore the practitioner should make recommendations only after assessing a patient's individual needs.

Wear rates of toothbrush bristles and their subsequent ability to remove plaque raise another concern. Dean suggests that toothbrushes remain effective well after patients identify a brush as being worn out.[11] The cleansing effectiveness of toothbrushes is maintained until pronounced toothbrush wear has occurred. This implies that patients are much more likely to dispose of a brush well before its clinical usefulness actually ends than to continue to use a toothbrush that no longer cleans effectively. In this regard, one manufacturer claims that their commercial toothbrush* indicates when the brush should be replaced by means of centrally located tufts of bristles dyed with food colorant. When the blue band fades to halfway down the bristle, it is time to replace the brush (Fig. 11-3). The company states that on average this occurs after 3 months but that the time varies depending on the individual's brushing habits.

*Oral-B Indicator, Oral-B Laboratories, Inc., Belmont, Calif.

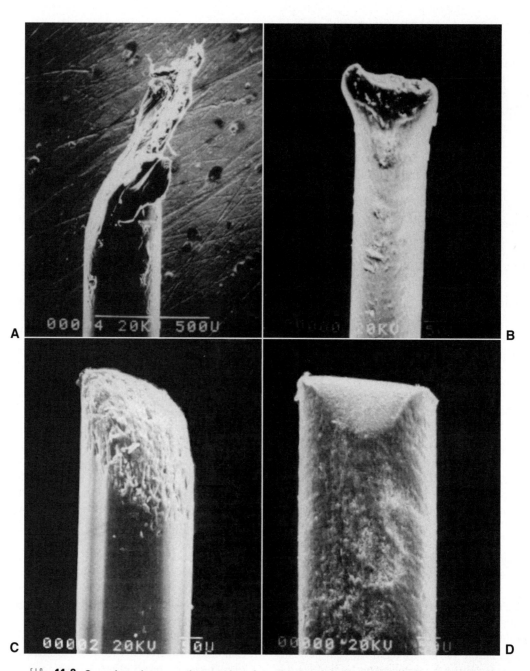

FIG. **11-2.** Scanning electron micrographs of toothbrush bristles manufactured by different processes. **A,** Coarse-cut bristle end, probably the result of an incomplete single-blade cut. **B,** Slightly enlarged, bulbous nylon bristle end, resulting from a double-blade or scissor cut. **C,** Tapered or round-end nylon toothbrush bristle produced by heat or a mechanical polishing process. **D,** Scrubbing, mechanical action of a toothbrush wear machine has nicely rounded off this bristle removed from a brush that was originally coarse-cut. *(From Park KK, Matis BA, Christen AG: Clin Prev Dent 7(4):5-10, 1985.)*

Parents frequently ask how often they should change a child's brush. Based on the studies just mentioned, the best advice is to replace the brush when it appears well worn. This can present some problems for parents, because some children, especially toddlers, chew their brushes when brushing, which rapidly gives the bristles a well-worn appearance.

FLOSS

Although toothbrushing is the most widely used method of mechanical plaque control, toothbrushing alone cannot adequately remove plaque from all tooth surfaces. In particular, it is not efficient in removing interproximal plaque, which means that interproximal cleaning beyond brushing is necessary. Many devices

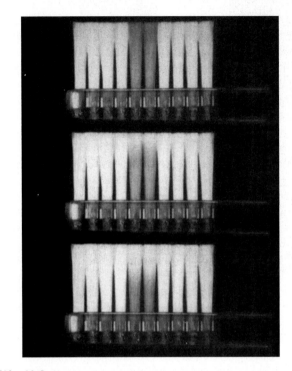

FIG. **11-3.** Blue dye in the center bristle tufts of this brush fades down from the end with use. When the dye reaches the half-way point *(bottom brush),* the manufacturer suggests replacing the brush.

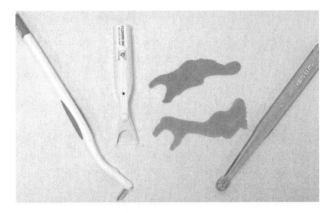

FIG. **11-4.** Several different methods for interproximal cleaning. *Left to right,* Interdental brush, Y-shaped floss holder, disposable floss holders, and end tuft brush.

have been suggested for interproximal removal of plaque, such as interdental brushes, floss holders and floss, and end tuft brush (Fig. 11-4). According to Mauriello et al, there appears to be no substantial difference between these devices in their ability to remove plaque and their tendency to produce gingival inflammation effects when they are used properly; however, floss is the standard device to which other devices are most often compared.[12] The other devices are more often recommended

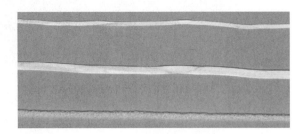

FIG. **11-5.** Several different types of dental floss are available: thin *(top),* tape *(middle),* and meshwork *(bottom).*

in certain unique circumstances, for example, the interdental brush may be recommended for orthodontic patients. Unfortunately, regular flossing does not occur daily in most households. Chen and Rubinson demonstrated that daily flossing was practiced by only 20% of mothers, 12% of fathers, and 6% of children within families.[13] In addition, 28% of mothers, 45% of fathers, and 48% of children never floss their teeth. This low compliance rate, particularly in children, is a problem requiring our attention as practitioners.

Several different types of floss are available: flavored and unflavored, waxed and unwaxed, and thin, tape, and meshwork* (Fig. 11-5). Almost all commercially available floss is made of nylon, although floss[†] made of Teflon material (polytetrafluoroethylene) is also available. The manufacturer claims that, because the material has a lower coefficient of friction than nylon, this floss does not shred, slides easily between tight contacts, and minimizes snapping of the floss.

Based on the work of Bass, unwaxed nylon-filament floss has generally been considered the floss of choice because of the ease of passing the floss between tight contacts, the lack of a wax residue, the squeaking sound effect produced by moving the floss over a clean tooth, and the fiber spread, which results in increased surface contact and greater plaque removal.[14] However, more recent work indicates clearly that individual patient needs and preferences should be taken into account before floss selection recommendations are made. Carr et al tested four different types of floss: waxed, unwaxed, woven, and shred resistant.[15] They studied the reductions in interproximal plaque scores for 24 dental hygiene students. Statistical analysis revealed no significant differences between floss types in cleaning efficacy, comfort of use, or the ease of use.

With these results kept in mind, it may prove beneficial in making floss recommendations to parents for their children to consider both the parent's and child's preferences and individual needs. From the perspective of patient acceptance, flavored waxed floss may be the

*Super Floss, Oral-B Laboratories, Inc., Belmont, Calif.
[†]Glide, W.L. Gore and Associates, Inc., Flagstaff, Ariz.

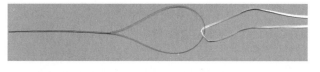

FIG. **11-6.** Floss-threading device with segment of thin floss attached.

most effective type. In addition, many parents complain that their fingers are too large for their child's mouth. Floss-holding devices (see Fig. 11-4) are an excellent alternative for parents when this complaint is voiced or when the dexterity of the parent or child prevents hand-holding of floss. For orthodontic patients, the use of Super Floss or a floss threader (Fig. 11-6) is helpful in negotiating the floss under the archwires to allow for interproximal cleaning. For orthodontic patients flossing is a tedious process but is nonetheless essential to maintenance of oral health.

POWERED MECHANICAL PLAQUE REMOVAL

The use of powered or electric toothbrushes has received considerable attention since the 1960s. The rationale for using powered brushes is that many patients remove plaque poorly because they lack adequate manual dexterity in manipulating the brush. The powered brushes should decrease the need for dexterity by automatically including some movement of the brush head. However, initial studies into the plaque removal effectiveness of powered toothbrushes failed to demonstrate greater efficacy for powered than for manual toothbrushes. Although improvement was seen initially, over time the level of cleaning achieved with power toothbrushes declined to the same level obtained using manual toothbrushes. Kerlinger refers to this as the Hawthorne effect: almost any change or experimental manipulation will induce an improvement in behavior, apparently because of a novelty effect.[16] The introduction of powered toothbrushes caused an initial increase in use, and therefore plaque and gingivitis were controlled. Over time, however, the results became comparable to those with manual brushes.

Despite these previous findings, use of the latest power brushes, such as the Sonicare* or the Braun Oral-B Kids' Power Toothbrush (D10),[†] may prove to be more beneficial than use of other brushes. The Sonicare uses sonic technology in the form of acoustic energy to improve the plaque removal ability of traditional toothbrush bristles. The brush has an electromagnetic device that drives the bristles' motions at 261 Hz, or 31,320 brush strokes per minute. Ho and Niederman found that the Sonicare brush was significantly more effective

than the manual brush in reducing the plaque index, gingival index, percentage of sites that bled on probing, pocket depth, and total gram-negative bacteria in a subgingival plaque sample.[17] Nowak et al have demonstrated a 40% improvement in the debris index component of the Simplified Oral Hygiene Index in children aged 4 to 9 years who were using the Braun Oral-B Kids' Power Toothbrush (D10).[18] Studies by Grossman and Proskin[19] and by Jongenelis and Wiedemann[20] also compared the effectiveness of electric versus manual toothbrushes when the toothbrushes were specifically designed for children. Both studies concluded that the powered toothbrushes removed significantly more plaque than the manual toothbrushes for children. Finally, Heanue et al performed a meta-analysis showing that power brushes with a rotation-oscillation action design removed more plaque and reduced gingivitis more effectively than manual brushes in both the short and the long term.[21] No other powered brush designs were consistently superior to manual toothbrushes.

The Toothbrush Acceptance Program Guidelines of the American Dental Association (ADA) Council on Scientific Affairs list several requirements for powered toothbrushes that are not imposed on manual toothbrushes.[22] Among these are evidence that the product can be employed under unsupervised conditions by the average layperson to provide a 15% statistically significant reduction over baseline in gingivitis and a statistically significant reduction in plaque.

Also noteworthy is the development of the Braun Oral-B Interclean.* This electrically powered cleaning device requires only single-handed usage while its filament rotates to undergo an elliptical movement, disrupting plaque attached to adjacent and proximate teeth. Gordon, Frascella, and Reardon compared the effect of Interclean use and manual flossing over a 4-week period on level of interproximal plaque, gingivitis, and papillary bleeding in 52 healthy volunteers.[23] The results demonstrated no statistically significant difference between manual flossing and use of the electric interdental cleaning device. Results from the personal preference phase of the study demonstrated that significantly more subjects preferred the interdental cleaning device (69.5%) to floss (24.5%). This new type of interdental cleaning device may be particularly helpful for adolescent orthodontic patients, and the promise for its future is bright.

DENTIFRICES

Dentifrices serve multiple functions in oral hygiene through the inclusion of a variety of agents. They act as plaque- and stain-removing agents through the use of abrasives and surfactants. Pleasant flavors and colors

*Philips Oral Healthcare, Inc., Snoqualmie, Wash.
†Oral-B Laboratories, Inc., Belmont, Calif.

*Braun GmbH, Kronberg, Germany.

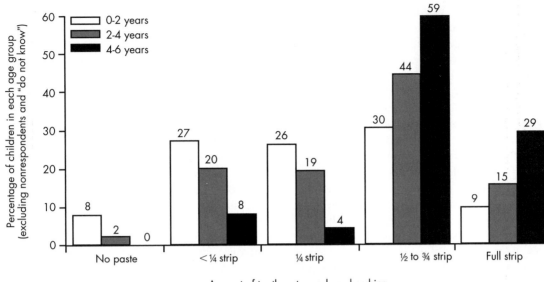

FIG. 11-7. Quantity of toothpaste used by children from birth to 6 years of age. *(From Levy SM, Zarei-M Z: J Dent Child 58(6):467-473, 1991.)*

encourage their use. They have tartar control properties because of the addition of pyrophosphates. Finally, dentifrices have anticaries and desensitization properties through the action of fluoride and other agents. A child's dentifrice should contain fluoride, rank low in abrasiveness, and carry the ADA seal of acceptance. In 2003, 36 different fluoride-containing dentifrices were listed as accepted dental therapeutic products by the Council on Scientific Affairs (http://ada.org/ada.seal.index.asp). Many of the 36 dentifrices are specifically designed and flavored to catch the attention of children.

These formulations are useful because a child is more likely to practice oral hygiene procedures if the tools to be used are pleasing to the child. Although the caries-preventive efficacy of fluoride toothpastes in children has been well documented, the impact of dentifrices on the total fluoride intake in children must be considered. Adair, Picitelli, and McKnight-Hanes confirmed that children tend to use larger amounts of dentifrice, brush for a longer period, and rinse and expectorate less when using a children's dentifrice than when using an adult dentifrice.[24] Levy and Zarei-M studied toothbrushing habits and quantities of toothpaste used on brushes in children from birth through 6 years. Fig. 11-7 shows their results.[25] This study did not quantify the amount of toothpaste, and therefore of fluoride, ingested from the use of this much paste on the brush. However, the investigators suggest that ingestion was likely a substantial source of systemic fluoride for these children during the years when a risk of dental fluorosis is present. It is interesting to note that many toothpaste advertisements show children with large amounts of toothpaste on their brushes. Clearly, this is not the perception dentists want the public to have when regarding the use of fluoridated toothpastes in young children.

Simard et al concluded from their study of 12- to 24-month-old children that 20% of the children ingested more than 0.25 mg of fluoride per day by toothbrushing alone.[26] They suggest the following to reduce the chance of dental fluorosis in children secondary to toothpaste ingestion. Manufacturers should market a low-fluoride dentifrice for infants or reduce the diameter of the tube orifice. Parents should be advised to delay the use of fluoride dentifrice until the child is older than 36 months and to use small, pea-sized quantities of toothpaste. Pediatricians should take into consideration all sources of fluoride before prescribing supplements. In the wake of these recommendations, one manufacturer has developed a dentifrice for children called Baby Orajel Tooth and Gum Cleanser.* The manufacturer states that it is nonabrasive, nonfoaming, without fluoride, safe for infants, and ideal for babies aged 4 months to 3 years. It contains a mild surfactant and simethicone, is sugar-free, and comes in vanilla and fruit flavors.

DISCLOSING AGENTS

In an effort to increase the patient's ability to remove plaque, several agents have been developed to allow for patient visualization of plaque. These include iodine, gentian violet, erythrosin, basic fuchsin, fast green, food

*Del Pharmaceuticals, Inc., Plainview, N.Y.

dyes, fluorescein, and a two-tone disclosing agent. Use of these agents is particularly helpful in teaching children toothbrushing techniques and educating them on the rationale for oral hygiene. FDC red No. 28 is a plaque-disclosing agent commonly used either as a liquid to be dabbed onto the teeth with a cotton swab or in the form of a chewable tablet (Fig. 11-8). Unfortunately, this dye stains the oral soft tissues and dental pellicle, as well as plaque, leaving an objectionable pink discoloration that lasts up to several hours after use. Most younger children do not appear to be bothered by the discoloration, but as children approach adolescence it can become a problem. Fluorescein disclosing agents were developed to address this problem because fluorescein is not visible under normal light. Their use does, however, require special equipment.

In a study by Lim et al, four different techniques were compared for clinically detecting plaque during different dietary regimes.[27] Subjects ranging in age from 18 to 27 years had their plaque levels assessed using a caries probe, a plaque-detection probe, erythrosin, and a two-tone disclosing agent at 3, 6, and 18 hours after thorough cleaning of their teeth. Thirty-eight patients

were assigned to a sucrose-restricted (SR) diet in the first part of the study, and 32 patients were assigned to a sucrose-supplemented (SS) diet in the second part of the study. At 3 hours, plaque was detectable on more than 12% of sites in those consuming the SR diet and up to 23% in those on the SS diet. After 18 hours, the proportion of plaque-covered surfaces had increased to between 52% (SR diet) and 73% (SS diet). For minimal amounts of plaque, the disclosing solutions were found to be the most sensitive assessment techniques. For moderate and abundant plaque deposits, however, the probe techniques were more sensitive.

The clinical significance of these data is that, in measuring a patient's oral hygiene abilities, one must assess plaque deposits immediately after the patient has cleaned his or her teeth. Otherwise, allowances must be made for factors such as the time elapsed since the teeth were cleaned and the patient's diet. If a patient is seen several hours after the teeth have been cleaned, the quality of plaque control may be deemed unsatisfactory regardless of the quality of the patient's performance. It is also interesting to note that disclosing

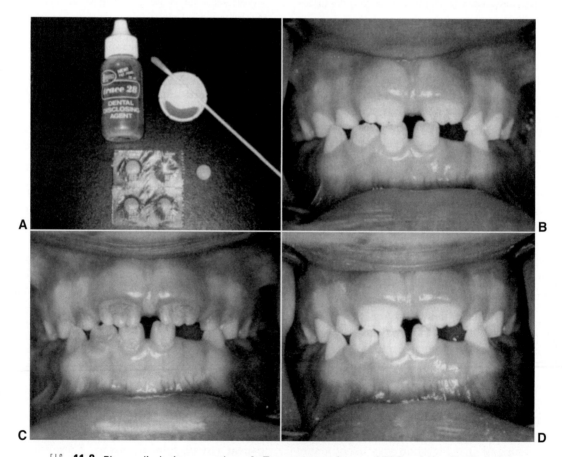

FIG. **11-8.** Plaque-disclosing procedure. **A,** Two common forms of FDC red No. 28 disclosing agent: a liquid that is dabbed on with a cotton swab and a chewable tablet. **B,** Mixed dentition in a patient before oral hygiene and disclosing. **C,** Patient before oral hygiene but after disclosing. **D,** Patient after oral hygiene and disclosing.

agents have some antimicrobial activity, according to Baab, Broadwell, and Williams.[28] Although short-term quantitative inhibition of plaque growth has not been observed clinically, long-term home use of disclosing agents may contribute to qualitative differences in plaque composition. Further studies are needed to measure the long-term in vivo effect of these agents.

OTHER ADJUNCTS FOR PLAQUE CONTROL

Several other devices, such as oral irrigators and tongue scrapers, have been suggested for routine oral hygiene. Oral irrigators use pulsed water or chemotherapeutic agents to dislodge plaque from the dentition. Tongue scrapers, which are flat, flexible plastic sticks, are used to remove bacterial and food deposits that accumulate within the rough dorsal surface of the tongue. In addition, gauze or special dental washcloths are useful in infants to massage the gums and to remove plaque on newly erupted teeth. Although these adjuncts add to our basic hygiene tools, toothbrushes and floss remain the most effective means of mechanical plaque removal. Professional recommendation of these adjuncts should be to suggest them as supplements to and not substitutes for the basic tools and should take into consideration the patient's and caregiver's individual needs, abilities, and preferences.

TECHNIQUES

As with toothbrush design, several different types of toothbrushing techniques for children have been advocated over the years. The more predominant techniques are the roll method, the Charters method, the horizontal scrubbing method, and the modified Stillman method. Anaise, in his study of the effectiveness of these four techniques in children 11 to 14 years of age, describes them as follows[29]:

Roll Method. The brush is placed in the vestibule, the bristle ends directed apically, with the sides of the bristles touching the gingival tissue. The patient exerts lateral pressure with the sides of the bristles, and the brush is moved occlusally. The brush is placed again high in the vestibule, and the rolling motion is repeated. The lingual surfaces are brushed in the same manner, with two teeth brushed simultaneously.

Charters Method. The ends of the bristles are placed in contact with the enamel of the teeth and the gingiva, with the bristles pointed at about a 45-degree angle toward the plane of occlusion. A lateral and downward pressure is then placed on the brush, and the brush is vibrated gently back and forth a millimeter or so.

Horizontal Scrubbing Method. The brush is placed horizontally on buccal and lingual surfaces and moved back and forth with a scrubbing motion.

Modified Stillman Method. The modified Stillman method combines a vibratory action of the bristles with a stroke movement of the brush in the long axis of the teeth. The brush is placed at the mucogingival line, with the bristles pointed away from the crown, and moved with a stroking motion along the gingiva and the tooth surface. The handle is rotated toward the crown and vibrated as the brush is moved.

Anaise concluded that the horizontal scrubbing method exhibited a more significant plaque-removing effect than the roll, Charters, and modified Stillman methods.[29] This finding supports the work done by McClure[30] and by Sangnes, Zachrisson, and Gjermo.[31]

In a study by Rugg-Gunn and Macgregor, uninstructed videotaped toothbrushing behavior in three age groups (5, 11, and 18 to 22 years) was analyzed.[32] The following conclusions were drawn:

- In the three age groups, the proportions of the areas that were brushed were 25%, 50%, and 67%, respectively.
- More time was spent brushing the lower than the upper teeth.
- The contralateral side (the left side in right-handed persons) was brushed more than the ipsilateral side in children, but equally in adults.
- Less than 10% of the time was spent brushing lingual areas.
- The most popular brushing strokes were the horizontal stroke in children and the vertical stroke in adults; the roll and circular strokes were seldom used.
- Eighty-four percent of subjects used more than one type of stroke.

The horizontal scrub technique removes as much or more plaque than the other techniques, regardless of how old the child is and whether the brushing is performed by the parent or the child. In addition, it is the technique most naturally adopted by children. Therefore, in most situations the horizontal scrubbing method can be recommended for brushing children's teeth. Regardless of the brushing method used, a systematic approach to brushing as advocated by Starkey should be employed.[33] By following a systematic approach, as shown in Fig. 11-9, the child or parent can help ensure that all areas of the mouth are cleaned. Notice also on this figure the positioning of the brush head on the lingual surfaces of the anterior teeth and on the distal aspect of the most posterior tooth in each quadrant.

For flossing, the following technique is recommended (Fig. 11-10):

1. A 46- to 61-cm (18- to 24-inch) length of floss is obtained, and the ends are wrapped around the

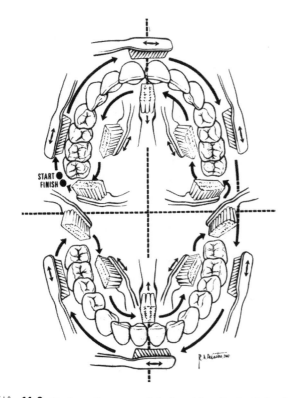

FIG. **11-9.** Systematic approach to brushing the teeth begins with the buccal aspects of the teeth in the maxillary right quadrant and follows the arrows. Bristles are held at a 45-degree angle to the long axis of the teeth and are directed to the gum line. Short back-and-forth strokes are used, allowing bristles to remain in the same place. The handle of the brush is placed parallel to the biting surfaces except when brushing the lingual aspects of the anterior teeth and the posterior aspects of the last tooth in each quadrant, when a heel-toe direction of brushing is used. *(Courtesy Dr. Paul Starkey.)*

patient's or parent's middle fingers. Floss should be long enough to allow the thumbs to touch each other when the hands are laid flat.

2. The thumbs and index fingers are used to guide the floss as it is gently sawed between the two teeth to be cleaned. Care must be taken not to snap the floss down through the interproximal contacts to avoid gingival trauma.

3. The floss is then manipulated into a C shape around each tooth individually and moved in a cervical-occlusal reciprocating motion until the plaque is removed. In between cleaning each pair of teeth the floss is repositioned on the fingers so that fresh, unsoiled floss is used at each new location.

Learning a flossing technique is difficult and takes some practice. Some children and their parents prefer to make a loop of floss. Tying the two ends of the floss together, instead of wrapping it around their fingers, assists them in holding and controlling the floss.

However, Rodrigues et al demonstrated that, even when the looped floss technique is used, a training program is required for children $6\frac{1}{2}$ to $7\frac{1}{2}$ years of age to accomplish significant reduction in proximal surface dental plaque indices.[34]

VISUAL-MOTOR SKILL MASTERY

Several attempts have been made to develop specific recommendations for when children can begin performing oral hygiene procedures themselves with adequate effectiveness. Terhune stated that the variables of age, gender, and eye-hand coordination could not precisely predict when particular children were ready to learn an effective dental flossing technique.[35] However, all 8- to 11-year-old children in his study learned how to use dental floss effectively within 10 days. Mescher, Brine, and Biller found that hand function was an age-related factor in children's ability to perform sulcular toothbrushing, but that hand function test scores were not accurate predictors of an individual's toothbrushing ability.[36]

Preisch, however, did find a significant relationship between developmental age and oral hygiene scores using a visual-motor integration developmental test.[37] With the use of this test, significant correlations have been shown between the ability of children to copy geometric forms and their academic achievement and motor skill level. Higher levels of thinking and behavior require integration among sensory inputs and motor action. A child can have well-developed visual and motor skills but may be unable to coordinate the two. Although both chronologic and developmental ages were found to be predictors of plaque removal ability, only developmental age demonstrated statistically significant predictive power. Unfortunately, because of the complexity of this test, we are left without a practical method for making recommendations to parents as to when their child can begin brushing on their own. As Preisch laments, many dentists use anecdotal accounts and tell parents to supervise their children's brushing until the children can color within the lines, tie their own shoelaces, or cut through a tough piece of meat.[37] However, this may still be our best practical recommendation.

TIME CONSIDERATIONS

Another of the important questions regarding home oral health care involves time considerations in oral hygiene practices. How often should patients brush and floss their teeth and for how long? In discussing frequency of oral hygiene procedures, Löe suggests that oral cleanliness should be regarded as a defined state in which all surfaces of all teeth are plaque free.[38] He states that it may not be surprising to find that complete removal of plaque once daily or every second day, or

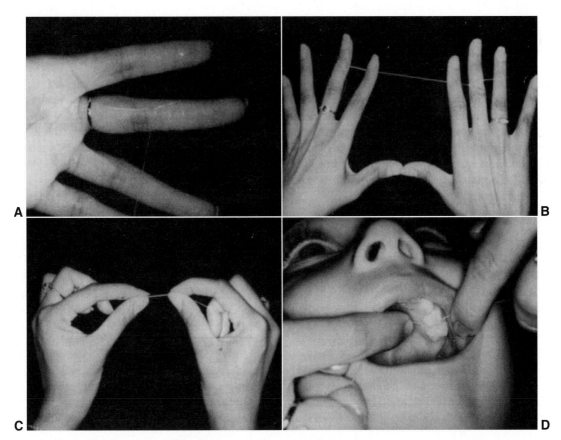

FIG. **11-10.** Flossing technique. **A,** The length of floss is wrapped around the middle fingers of each hand. **B,** Enough floss should be left between the middle fingers to allow the thumbs to touch when the hands are laid flat. **C,** The index fingers and thumbs are used to manipulate the floss. **D,** The floss is carefully placed in a C shape between the interproximal contacts and gently sawed up and down until each tooth surface is clean.

possibly even once every third day, is more valuable in preventing dental disease than performing two or three inadequate brushings per day. Indeed, Lang, Cumming, and Löe observed that completion of effective oral hygiene procedures at intervals of up to 48 hours is compatible with gingival health.[39] Studies addressing the relation between the frequency of hygiene procedures and caries experience in children have yielded inconclusive results.

In addition to optimal brushing frequency, the most efficacious length of brushing time has been investigated. In a study by Hodges, Bianco, and Cancro, 84 children aged 5 to 15 years brushed their teeth with a fluoridated dentifrice for 30, 60, 120, and 180 seconds.[40] The results of the study suggest that, statistically, a 1-minute brushing period provides the greatest plaque removal benefit of all time periods tested.

The following recommendations are made based on the preceding information. In children, thorough oral hygiene procedures should be performed at least once daily, preferably twice, with parental supervision. Teeth should be brushed for at least 1 minute with a fluoridated dentifrice; flossing and other plaque

removal activities are added to this time. If oral hygiene is accomplished only once per day, it should be the last thing the child does before bedtime at night. Because the flow of saliva and its buffering capacity are reduced during sleep, it is advantageous to remove plaque before bedtime. In addition, the development in children of a learned behavior performed at a specific time of day, each and every day, will prove beneficial throughout childhood and into adulthood.

CHEMOTHERAPEUTIC PLAQUE CONTROL

Although the use of mechanical therapy for plaque control can provide excellent results, it is clear that many patients are unable, unwilling, or untrained to practice routine effective mechanotherapy. In addition, certain patients with dental diseases (e.g., periodontitis) or medical diseases (e.g., immunocompromised conditions) require additional assistance beyond mechanotherapy to maintain a normal state of oral health. Because of this, chemotherapeutic agents have been developed as adjuncts in plaque control.

Van der Ouderaa has stated that the ideal chemotherapeutic plaque control agent should have the following characteristics[41]:

- Specificity only for the pathogenic bacteria
- Substantivity, the ability to attach to and be retained by oral surfaces and then be released over time without loss of potency
- Chemical stability during storage
- Absence of adverse reactions, such as staining or mucosal interactions
- Toxicologic safety
- Ecologic safety so as not to adversely alter the microbiotic flora
- Ease of use

No agent has yet been developed that has all of these characteristics.

There are several main routes of administration of antiplaque agents designed for home use. They are mouthwashes, dentifrices, gels, irrigators, floss, chewing gum, lozenges, and capsules. All of these are designed for local, supragingival administration, except the irrigator and capsule delivery methods. The irrigators can provide both supragingival and subgingival delivery. The capsules are designed for systemic distribution.

Both van der Ouderaa[41] and Mandel[42] have provided excellent reviews of the various chemotherapeutic agents and their uses. Box 11-1 is adapted from those reviews. Space does not allow a complete discussion of the agents listed in this box; however, a few pertinent subjects are addressed.

ANTISEPTIC AGENTS

The antiseptic agents used in chemotherapeutic plaque control have been shown to exhibit little or no oral or systemic toxicity in the concentrations used. Virtually no drug resistance is induced, and in most instances these agents have a broad antimicrobial spectrum. Chlorhexidine, a positively charged organic antiseptic agent, has received considerable attention and study because of its ability to reduce plaque and gingivitis scores. It has strong substantivity, binding well to many sites in the oral cavity and maintaining an ongoing antibacterial presence. Chlorhexidine binds with anionic glycoproteins and phosphoproteins on the buccal, palatal, and labial mucosa and the tooth-borne pellicle. Its antibacterial effects include binding well to bacterial cell membranes, increasing their permeability, initiating leakage, and precipitating intracellular components.

Grossman et al conducted a 6-month clinical trial in which 430 adults rinsed twice daily with either 0.12% chlorhexidine or a placebo.[43] Gingivitis and plaque scores were lower in the chlorhexidine group (34% to 41%) than in the placebo group (61%). Several

---

BOX 11-1   Chemotherapeutic Plaque Control Agents

ANTISEPTIC AGENTS
Positively Charged Organic Molecules:
Quaternary ammonium compounds—cetylpyridinium chloride
Pyrimidines—hexedine
Bis-biguanides—chlorhexidine, alexidine
Noncharged Phenolic Agents: Listerine (thymol, eucalyptol, menthol, and methylsalicylate), triclosan, phenol, and thymol
Oxygenating Agents: Peroxides and perborate
Bis-Pyridines: Octenidine
Halogens: Iodine, iodophors, and fluorides
Heavy Metal Salts: Silver, mercury, zinc, copper, and tin

ANTIBIOTICS
Niddamycin, kanamycin sulfate, tetracycline hydrochloride, and vancomycin hydrochloride

ENZYMES
Mucinases, pancreatin, fungal enzymes, and protease

PLAQUE-MODIFYING AGENTS
Urea peroxide

SUGAR SUBSTITUTES
Xylitol, mannitol

PLAQUE ATTACHMENT INTERFERENCE AGENTS
Sodium polyvinylphosphonic acid, perfluoroalkyl

---

studies have demonstrated the use and efficacy of chlorhexidine therapy in children as young as 8 years of age. Studies have examined its use in the form of a rinse, a spray, a varnish, and a chlorhexidine gel used in flossing.

Lang et al investigated the effects of supervised rinsing with chlorhexidine in 158 schoolchildren, aged 10 to 12 years.[44] The children were divided into four groups. Group A rinsed with a 0.2% solution of chlorhexidine digluconate (CHX) six times weekly. Group B rinsed with 0.2% CHX two times weekly. Group C rinsed with a 0.1% CHX solution six times weekly. Group D rinsed six times weekly with a placebo solution. All rinsing was performed under supervision, and no effort was made to change the children's oral hygiene habits. Fig. 11-11 shows the results of the study. All three experimental groups, A, B, and C, exhibited statistically significant reductions in the gingival index compared with the control group, Group D. The investigators concluded that gingivitis can be controlled successfully in children by regular rinsing with a chlorhexidine solution over an extended period.

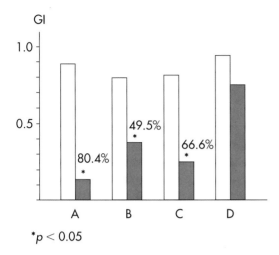

FIG. 11-11. Mean gingival index (GI) in four groups of school-children rinsing with chlorhexidine digluconate (CHX) or placebo solution for 6 months under supervision. *Clear bars,* Before treatment; *screened bars,* after treatment. Group A: 0.2% CHX 6 times weekly; Group B: 0.2% CHX 2 times weekly; Group C: 0.1% CHX 6 times weekly; Group D: Placebo 6 times weekly. *(From Lang NP et al: J Periodontal Res 17:101–111, 1982.)*

Chlorhexidine spray has stimulated interest regarding its use in disabled populations because of its effectiveness and ease of administration. Burtner et al demonstrated a 35% reduction in plaque levels with use of the spray compared with placebo use in a study of 16 institutionalized adult males with severe and profound mental retardation.[45] Chikte et al conducted a 9-week, double-blind, randomized crossover clinical trial involving 52 institutionalized mentally disabled individuals 10 to 26 years of age. By the end of the trial, plaque and gingival indices had been reduced by 48% and 52%, respectively, in the group treated with a stannous fluoride spray.[46] In the group treated with chlorhexidine spray, reductions in plaque and gingival indices were 75% and 78%, respectively.

In addition to its use in institutionalized patients with mental retardation, chlorhexidine has been studied for its use in immunocompromised patients. Ferretti et al found that the prophylactic use of chlorhexidine mouthrinse produced reductions in gingivitis and mucositis and oral microbial burden in patients undergoing bone marrow transplantation.[47] Raether et al, however, studying a similar patient population, found no significant difference between the group receiving chlorhexidine and that given a placebo in terms of number of oral ulcerations, development of bacteremia, and length of hospital stay.[48] Despite these findings, they suggested the use of a chlorhexidine mouthrinse as an antiplaque and antigingivitis agent in bone marrow transplant patients to augment their oral hygiene. Finally, chlorhexidine varnish has been shown by Fennis-le et al[49] and by Petersson et al[50] to suppress the level of mutans streptococci. However, recent clinical studies have failed to demonstrate a transfer of this effect into a decrease in caries on either smooth enamel surfaces or occlusal pits and fissures. Additional work is needed to conclusively demonstrate the value of chlorhexidine varnishes in reducing dental caries.

The use of positively charged antiplaque agents has been hampered by adverse reactions such as staining of teeth, impaired taste sensation, and increased supragingival calculus formation. Different attempts have been made to decrease these side effects, such as alteration of dietary habits, increase in mechanical plaque removal efforts, and use of hydrogen peroxide solutions in conjunction with the antiseptic agent. Continued research is needed to find methods to limit these adverse reactions.

The most widely known noncharged phenolic antiseptic agent is Listerine.* It has demonstrated a long history of efficacy and was among the original antiseptic agents studied by W.D. Miller in 1890.[3] In addition, it was the first over-the-counter mouthrinse to be accepted by the Council of Dental Therapeutics for its help in controlling plaque and gingivitis.[22] Despite its long history of use, studies by Clark et al[51] and by Brownstone et al[52] have shown chlorhexidine to be significantly more effective than Listerine in reducing plaque and gingivitis indices. Listerine tends to give patients a burning sensation, and it has a bitter taste. Lang and Brecx have summarized the changes in plaque index, gingival index, and discoloration index scores resulting from the use of four well-known chemotherapeutic plaque control agents (Fig. 11-12).[53] The effects of two daily 10-mL rinses with either 0.12% chlorhexidine digluconate, the quaternary ammonium compound cetylpyridinium chloride, the phenolic compound Listerine, or the plant alkaloid sanguinarine were compared with those of rinses with a placebo. All rinses were supervised by registered dental hygienists during these 21-day studies. The subjects were divided into five groups of eight individuals each and were instructed to refrain from oral hygiene during the 21 days. Although the sanguinarine, Listerine, and cetylpyridinium chloride inhibited plaque formation to some extent, they did not prevent gingivitis significantly more than the placebo. The chlorhexidine, however, maintained the preexperimental gingival index scores throughout the 21 days. Unfortunately, all of the antiseptics demonstrated higher discoloration index scores than the placebo. As can be seen in Fig. 11-12, *C,* chlorhexidine had the second highest discoloration score of the four agents.

*Pfizer Warner Lambert Division, Morris Plains, N.J.

couple, particularly if the child is their first, this is a time in their lives when they are most receptive to preventive health recommendations. These parents-to-be become acutely aware of their child's dependence on them for all of the child's nurturing and health care needs. Parents have a strong instinct to provide the best that they can for the child. Counseling them on their own hygiene habits and the effect they can have on their children as role models will aid in improving both the parents' and child's oral health. Discussing pregnancy gingivitis with the mother-to-be and dispelling some of the myths about childbirth and dental health can prove beneficial. In addition, a review of infant dental care (see next section) is useful for the expectant parents.

INFANTS (0 TO 1 YEAR OLD)

It is important that a few basic home oral hygiene procedures for the child begin during the first year of life. There is general agreement that plaque removal activities should begin on eruption of the first primary teeth. Some practitioners recommend cleaning and massaging of the gums before this to help in establishing a healthy oral flora and to aid in teething. This early cleaning must be done totally by the parent. It can be accomplished by wrapping a moistened gauze square or washcloth around the finger and gently massaging the teeth and gingival tissues. The child can be positioned in numerous ways during this procedure, but cradling the child with one arm while massaging the teeth with the hand of the other may be the simplest and provides the infant with a strong sense of security (Fig. 11-13). This procedure should be performed once daily. Generally, other plaque removal techniques are not necessary. The introduction of a moistened, soft-bristled, child- or infant-sized toothbrush during this age is advisable only if the parent feels comfortable using the brush. The use of a dentifrice is neither necessary nor advised as the foaming action of the paste tends to be objectionable

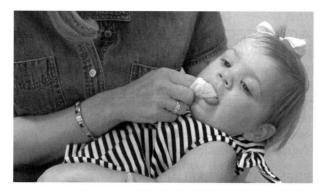

FIG. **11-13.** Arm-cradled position of child for effective cleansing of the oral cavity. This figure shows the use of a gauze square for wiping the child's dentition and gingival tissues.

to the infant. Because fluoride ingestion is possible, however, as mentioned earlier, use of a nonfluoridated tooth and gum cleanser may prove beneficial.

The child's first visit to the dentist should take place during this period. The American Academy of Pediatric Dentistry recommends that children have their first dental visit at approximately the time of eruption of the first tooth or, at the latest, by the age of 12 months.[61] When the child has special dental needs, such as medical problems or trauma, this visit can be sooner. Several objectives are accomplished at this visit. Certainly, instruction of the parents in the use of the oral hygiene practices just mentioned is necessary. In addition, an infant dental examination and fluoride status review should be accomplished, and dietary issues related to nursing and bottle caries as well as other health concerns are addressed. These subjects are discussed in more detail in other sections of this text. These first dental visits are also a time for the child to become familiar with the dental environment and the dental staff and the dentist, which makes any future dental treatment less anxiety provoking.

TODDLERS (1 TO 3 YEARS OLD)

During toddlerhood, the toothbrush should be introduced into the plaque removal procedure if this was not accomplished previously. Because of the inability of children in this age group to expectorate and the potential for fluoride ingestion, only a nonfluoridated dentifrice should be used. Most children enjoy imitating their parents and will readily practice toothbrushing. Unfortunately, adequate plaque removal is not usually accomplished by the child alone. Although the child should be encouraged to begin rudimentary brushing, the parent remains the primary caregiver in these hygiene procedures. The use of additional instruments for plaque control is generally unnecessary; however, flossing may be needed if any interproximal contacts are closed. The use of a flossing aid may also be indicated.

Positioning of the child and parent is again important. Although most children enjoy brushing their own teeth, many are resistant to allowing anyone else to do the brushing. Several positions can be used by the parent, but the lap-to-lap position, as shown in Fig. 11-14, allows one adult to control the child's body movements while the other adult brushes the teeth. Notice how the child's arms and legs are controlled with the hands and elbows of the adult responsible for body movements. The parents should be encouraged to make this a special time for the child and to praise the child as much as possible. For single-parent households, a one-adult position often becomes necessary. In this situation the parent sits on the floor with his or her legs stretched out in front and the child is positioned between the legs. The child's head is placed between the thighs of the parent, with the

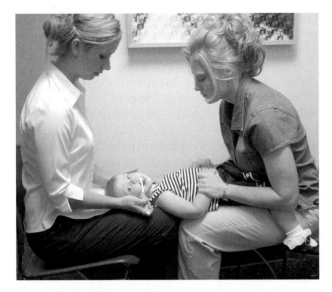

FIG. **11-14.** Lap-to-lap position of child. Two adults sit with knees touching, using their laps as a table on which to rest the child. The adult on the right holds the child's legs and arms while the adult on the left performs the oral hygiene procedures.

child's arms and legs carefully controlled by the legs of the parent. This position is a little awkward, but for a young child resistant to oral hygiene, it does allow these procedures to be accomplished.

PRESCHOOLERS (3 TO 6 YEARS OLD)

Although children in the preschool age range begin to demonstrate significant improvements in their ability to manipulate the toothbrush, it is still the responsibility of the parent to be the primary provider of oral hygiene procedures. All too often, parents of these children feel that the child has adequately achieved the skills necessary to clean the teeth. It is important to stress to the parents that they must continue to brush their child's teeth. A fluoride dentifrice can be introduced at 3 years of age. Although fluoride ingestion remains a concern for this age group, during this time, most children develop the skills to expectorate toothpaste adequately. Until this occurs, it is important for parents to continue to use only a pea-sized amount of toothpaste on the child's brush. In addition, it is during this age that flossing is most likely to begin. As mentioned previously, if the interproximal contacts are closed, the parent must begin flossing procedures. In the primary dentition, the posterior contacts may be the only areas where flossing is needed. The closure of the spaces between the primary molars tends to occur somewhere near the start of this age range. If any interproximal area has tooth-to-tooth contact, however, daily flossing of that area becomes necessary.

Proper positioning of the child continues to be useful for this age group in performing oral hygiene. One method advocated is that in which the parent stands behind the child and both face the same direction. The child rests his or her head back into the parent's nondominant arm. With the hand of this arm the cheeks can be retracted, and the other hand is used to brush. This position is also appropriate for flossing. To brush their child's teeth many parents use a frontal approach, which is awkward and provides little head support. This positioning technique should be discouraged.

It is also during this stage that fluoride gels and rinses for home use may be introduced. Because of the risk of ingestion, however, these agents should be employed in small quantities and their use should be limited to those patients demonstrating a moderate to high risk of caries. The use of other chemotherapeutic plaque control agents is generally not recommended.

SCHOOL-AGED CHILDREN (6 TO 12 YEARS OLD)

The 6- to 12-year stage is marked by acceptance of increasing responsibilities by the children. The need to assume responsibility for homework and household chores tends to occur during this time. In addition, the child can begin to assume more responsibility for oral hygiene. Parental involvement is still needed. However, instead of performing the oral hygiene, parents can switch to active supervision. By the second half of this stage, most children can provide their basic oral hygiene (brushing and flossing). Parents may find they only need to brush or floss their child's teeth in certain difficult-to-reach areas of the mouth or if there is a compliance problem. Parents do need to actively inspect their child's teeth for cleanliness on a regular basis. One helpful adjunct is the use of a disclosing agent. After the child has brushed, flossed, and used the disclosing agent on his or her teeth, the parent can easily visualize any remaining plaque and assist the child in removing it.

By this age, ingestion of fluoridated materials, such as dentifrices, gels, or rinses, is not as pronounced a concern because the children can now expectorate well. Certainly the use of fluoridated dentifrices is essential; however, fluoridated gels and rinses can be reserved for those children at risk for caries. In addition, the use of chlorhexidine or Listerine can be introduced to those at risk for periodontal disease and caries. Unfortunately, some children who might benefit from these chemotherapeutic agents will find their use objectionable.

Because early treatment of malocclusions has increased, this age group has undergone more of this treatment and experienced its accompanying increased risk for caries and periodontal disease. Special attention to oral hygiene is necessary for these patients. Increased frequency and adequacy of brushing and flossing becomes necessary. Although fluoridated dentifrices provide cost-efficient fluoride exposure, the use of fluoridated gels or rinses is strongly encouraged. In addition, as with other patients at risk for caries and periodontal disease, the use of chemotherapeutic agents and adjuncts such as oral irrigators is recommended. Feil et al published an interesting study on the intentional use if the Hawthorne effect to improve oral hygiene compliance in orthodontic patients.[62] Forty orthodontic adolescent patients with histories of poor oral hygiene were assigned to one of two groups. The experimental subjects were presented with a situation that stimulated participation in an experiment, whereas the control subjects had no knowledge of study participation. Although there were no statistically significant differences between the control and the experimental group at baseline, the experimental group showed significantly lower plaque scores at 3 months and again at 6 months. The experimental subjects had significantly improved oral hygiene, which suggests that the Hawthorne effect (participating in an "experimental study") caused the adolescent patients to pay more attention to oral hygiene and therefore to do a better job.

ADOLESCENTS (12 TO 19 YEARS OLD)

Although the adolescent patient usually has developed the skills for adequate oral hygiene procedures, compliance is a major problem during this age period. Griffin and Goepferd point out that motivating an adolescent to assume responsibility for personal oral hygiene may be complicated by reactions of rebellion against external authority and some incapacity to appreciate long-term consequences.[63] Macgregor and Balding's survey of 4075 children 14 years old suggests a positive relationship between self-esteem and toothbrushing behavior and motivation for mouth care in adolescents.[64] Because self-esteem declines between the ages of 11 and 14 and then shows a gradual improvement into adulthood, it is not hard to understand why plaque control in these patients declines. In addition, poor dietary habits and pubertal hormonal changes increase adolescents' risk for caries and gingival inflammation.

Therefore, it is important for practitioners and parents to continually help and guide adolescents as they progress through this difficult stage. Stressing their increased responsibility as young adults without appearing authoritarian can aid them in accepting their new role. The parents must be ready to adapt to their child's changing personality and to continue to reinforce the need for oral health care and hygiene. Increasing adolescents' knowledge regarding plaque control and oral diseases, as well as appealing to their appearance, may also help in motivating these patients.

IN-OFFICE ORAL HYGIENE PROGRAMS

As mentioned at the beginning of this chapter, preventive dentistry is the foundation on which all oral health care must be built. In establishing this foundation for their patients, practitioners must first look at themselves and their office environment. Each practice must establish a preventive philosophy that is evident throughout the patient's encounter with the dental office. This means that the dentist, the staff, and the practice systems and design must reflect this concept. All staff members must have a personal understanding and appreciation of the importance of this basic concept. This must be evident from their own personal hygiene and in their routine interactions with patients.

After this introspective look and adjustment, the practitioner can now turn to the patient directly. Ong discusses several basic concepts for developing a plaque control program in the dental office.[65] Gathering information from the child and parent is necessary for the practitioner to understand what their concerns are and to let them know that he or she understands these concerns. By discussing the patient's and parents' needs, and listening to and observing their reactions, the practitioner can gauge their readiness to begin the plaque control program. Dental education of the parent and child should be accomplished next with tailoring to the patient's individual problem. Describing exactly why oral hygiene is important in the patient's particular case can help with motivation. The information should be delivered in simple terms and with enthusiasm and conviction. It also needs to be conveyed to the child in age-appropriate language.

When specific age-appropriate oral hygiene instructions are given, it is important to be positive and reassuring, not critical. Use phrases like "Let me show you how to improve," rather than saying, "You're doing it all wrong." Be gentle but firm, and enlist the parent and patient's help in the treatment plan and therapy. Setting goals and complimenting achievements will assist in keeping the parent and patient's attitudes positive. It is very useful to be open to parental and patient feedback regarding their priorities and progress. As with many long-term commitments, cyclic participation can be expected and accepted to a certain extent. However, the parents and patient must know the consequences of neglect. Finally, establishment of a regular maintenance schedule is imperative. Along with prophylaxis, reinstruction and remotivation in the plaque control program is a necessary element for success. Recare intervals should be personalized to the individual patient's needs, with consideration of factors such as caries and periodontal disease risk; restorative, orthodontic, and prosthetic concerns; and individual patient and parental dental education and skill levels. It is the responsibility of every dental practitioner to make oral hygiene and prevention the core of his or her practice. By listening to, educating, adapting to, and motivating our patients and their parents, we can make our preventive practices successful and enjoyable.

REFERENCES

1. McDonald RE: Pediatrics allied with pedodontics, *Pediatr Herald* 1(5):1, 1960.
2. Marsh PD: The significance of maintaining the stability of the natural microflora of the mouth, *Br Dent J* 171(6):174-177, 1991.
3. Miller WD: *Microorganisms of the human mouth,* Philadelphia, 1890, SS White Dental Manufacturing.
4. Keyes PH: The infectious and transmissible nature of experimental dental caries, *Arch Oral Biol* 1:304-320, 1960.
5. Löe H, Theilade E, Jensen SB: Experimental gingivitis in man, *J Periodontol* 35:177-187, 1965.
6. Moore WE: Microbiology of periodontal disease, *J Periodontal Res* 22:335-341, 1987.
7. Kolenbrander PE: Oral microbial communities: biofilms, interactions, and genetic systems, *Annu Rev Microbiol* 54:413-437, 2000.
8. Balakrishnan M, Simmonds RS, Tagg JR: Dental caries is a preventable infectious disease, *Aust Dent J* 45(4):235-245, 2000.
9. Park KK, Matis BA, Christen AG: Choosing an effective toothbrush, *Clin Prev Dent* 7(4):5-10, 1985.
10. Updyke JR: A new handle for a child's toothbrush, *J Dent Child* 46:123-125, 1979.
11. Dean DH: Toothbrushes with graduated wear: correlation with in vitro cleansing performance, *Clin Prev Dent* 213(4):25-30, 1991.
12. Mauriello AM et al: Effectiveness of three interproximal cleaning devices, *Clin Prev Dent* 9(3):18-22, 1987.
13. Chen MS, Rubinson L: Preventive dental behavior in families: a national survey, *J Am Dent Assoc* 105:43-46, 1982.
14. Bass CC: An effective method of personal oral hygiene. Part II, *J La State Med Soc* 106:100, 1954.
15. Carr MP et al: Education of floss types for interproximal plaque removal, *Am J Dent* 13(4):212-214, 2000.
16. Kerlinger FN: *Foundations of behavioral research, educational and psychological injury,* New York, 1965, Holt, Rinehart and Winston.
17. Ho HP, Niederman R: Effectiveness of the Sonicare toothbrush on reduction of plaque, gingivitis, probing pocket depth and subgingival bacteria in adolescent orthodontic patients, *J Clin Dent* 8:15-19, 1997.
18. Nowak AJ et al: A practice based study of a children's power toothbrush: efficiency and acceptance, *Compendium* 23 (suppl 2):25-32, 2002.
19. Grossman E, Proskin H: A comparison of the efficacy and safety of an electric and a manual children's toothbrush, *J Am Dent Assoc* 128:469-474, 1997.
20. Jongenelis AP, Wiedemann W: A comparison of plaque removal effectiveness of an electric versus a manual toothbrush in children, *J Dent Child* 64:176-182, 1997.
21. Heanue M et al: Manual versus powered toothbrushing for oral health (Cochrane Review). *The Cochrane Library,* Issue 1, 2003.
22. American Dental Association, Council on Scientific Affairs: *Toothbrushes Acceptance Program Guidelines,* Chicago, 1998, The Association.
23. Gordon JM, Frascella JA, Reardon RC: A clinical study of the safety and efficacy of a novel electric interdental cleaning device, *J Clin Dent* 7:70-73, 1996.
24. Adair SM, Picitelli WP, McKnight-Hanes C: Comparison of the use of a child and an adult dentifrice by a sample of preschool children, *Pediatr Dent* 19:99-103, 1997.
25. Levy SM, Zarei-M Z: Evaluation of fluoride exposures in children, *J Dent Child* 58:467-473, 1991.
26. Simard PL et al: Ingestion of fluoride from dentifrices by children aged 12 to 24 months, *Clin Pediatr* 30:614-617, 1991.
27. Lim LP et al: A comparison of four techniques for clinical detection of early plaque formed during different dietary regimes, *J Clin Periodontol* 13:658-665, 1986.
28. Baab DA, Broadwell AH, Williams BL: A comparison of antimicrobial activity of four disclosant dyes, *J Dent Res* 62:837-841, 1983.
29. Anaise JZ: The toothbrush in plaque removal, *J Dent Child* 42:186-189, 1975.
30. McClure DB: A comparison of toothbrushing technics for the preschool child, *J Dent Child* 33:205-210, 1966.
31. Sangnes G, Zachrisson B, Gjermo P: Effectiveness of vertical and horizontal brushing techniques in plaque removal, *J Dent Child* 39:94-97, 1972.
32. Rugg-Gunn AJ, Macgregor ID: A survey of toothbrushing behavior in children and young adults, *J Periodontal Res* 13:382-389, 1978.
33. Starkey P: Instructions to parents for brushing the child's teeth, *J Dent Child* 28:42-47, 1961.
34. Rodrigues CR et al: The effect of training on the ability of children to use dental floss, *J Dent Child* 63:39-41, 1996.
35. Terhune JA: Predicting the readiness of elementary school children to learn an effective dental flossing technique, *J Am Dent Assoc* 86:1332-1336, 1973.
36. Mescher KD, Brine P, Biller I: Ability of elementary school children to perform sulcular toothbrushing as related to their hand function ability, *Pediatr Dent* 2:31-36, 1980.
37. Preisch JW: The relationship between visual motor integration and oral hygiene in children, master's thesis, Bloomington, 1984, Indiana University.
38. Löe H: How frequently must patients carry out effective oral hygiene procedures in order to maintain gingival health? *J Periodontol* 42:312-313, 1971.
39. Lang NP, Cumming BR, Löe H: Toothbrushing frequency as it relates to plaque development and gingival health, *J Periodontol* 44:396-405, 1973.
40. Hodges CA, Bianco JG, Cancro LP: The removal of dental plaque under timed intervals of toothbrushing, *J Dent Res* 60:425, 1981 (abstract 460).
41. van der Ouderaa FJ: Anti-plaque agents: rationale and prospects for prevention of gingivitis and periodontal disease, *J Clin Periodontol* 18:447-454, 1991.
42. Mandel ID: Chemotherapeutic agents for controlling plaque and gingivitis, *J Clin Periodontol* 15:488-498, 1988.
43. Grossman E et al: Six-month study of the effects of a chlorhexidine mouthrinse on gingivitis in adults, *J Periodontal Res* 16(21 suppl):33-43, 1986.
44. Lang NP et al: Effects of supervised chlorhexidine mouthrinses in children, *J Periodontal Res* 17:101-111, 1982.
45. Burtner AP et al: Effects of chlorhexidine spray on plaque and gingival health in institutionalized persons with mental retardation, *Spec Care Dentist* 11(3):97-100, 1991.
46. Chikte UM et al: Evaluation of stannous fluoride and chlorhexidine sprays on plaque and gingivitis in handicapped children, *J Clin Periodontol* 18:281-286, 1991.
47. Ferretti GA et al: Control of oral mucositis and candidiasis in marrow transplantation: a prospective, double-blind trial of chlorhexidine gluconate oral rinse, *Bone Marrow Transplant* 3:483-493, 1988.

48. Raether D et al: Effectiveness of oral chlorhexidine for reducing stomatitis in a pediatric bone marrow transplant population, *Pediatr Dent* 11:37-42, 1989.

49. Fennis-le YL et al: Effect of 6-month application of chlorhexidine varnish on evidence of occlusal caries in permanent molars: a three-year study, *J Dent* 26:233-238, 1998.

50. Petersson LG et al: Effect of semi-annual applications of a chlorhexidine/fluoride varnish mixture on approximal caries incidence in schoolchildren: a three-year radiographic study, *Eur J Oral Sci* 106:623-627, 1998.

51. Clark MJ et al: The effect of 3 mouthrinses on plaque and gingivitis development, *J Clin Periodontol* 19:19-23, 1992.

52. Brownstone BM et al: Efficacy of Listerine, Meridol, and chlorhexidine mouthrinses as supplements to regular tooth-cleaning measures, *J Clin Periodontol* 19:202-207, 1992.

53. Lang NP, Brecx MC: Chlorhexidine digluconate: an agent for chemical plaque control and prevention of gingival inflammation, *J Periodontal Res* 16(21 suppl):74-89, 1986.

54. Selbst AM, DeMaio JG, Boenning D: Mouthwash poisoning, *Clin Pediatr* 24:162-163, 1985.

55. Park K et al: Comparison of plaque pH response from a variety of sweeteners, *J Dent Res* 71(AADR Abs):269, 1992.

56. Hoerman KC et al: Effect of gum chewing on plaque accumulation, *J Clin Dent* 2(1):17-21, 1990.

57. Isokangas P et al: Xylitol chewing gum in caries prevention: a field study in children, *J Am Dent Assoc* 117:315-320, 1988.

58. O'Mullane D: New agents in the chemical control of plaque and gingivitis: reaction paper, *J Dent Res* 71:1455-1456, 1992.

59. Jakober RL, Perritt AM: Comparative evaluation of test parameters in plaque removal: a preliminary report, *Clin Prev Dent* 13(2):29-31, 1991.

60. Ciancio SG: Agents for the management of plaque and gingivitis, *J Dent Res* 71:1450-1454, 1992.

61. American Academy of Pediatric Dentistry: Guidelines on Infant Oral Health Care, *Pediatr Dent* (supplemental issue: reference manual 2002-2003) 24:47, 2002.

62. Feil PH et al: Intentional use of the Hawthorne effect to improve oral hygiene compliance in orthodontic patients, *J Dent Educ* 66(10):1129-1135, 2002.

63. Griffen AL, Goepferd SJ: Preventive oral health care for the infant, child, and adolescent, *Pediatr Clin North Am* 38(5):1209-1226, 1991.

64. Macgregor ID, Balding JW: Self-esteem as a predictor of toothbrushing behavior in young adolescents, *J Clin Periodontol* 18:312-316, 1991.

65. Ong G: Practical strategies for a plaque-control program, *Clin Prev Dent* 13(3):8-11, 1991.

SUGGESTED READINGS

Brightman LJ et al: The effects of a 0.12% chlorhexidine gluconate mouthrinse on orthodontic patients aged 11 through 17 with established gingivitis, *Am J Orthod Dentofacial Orthop* 100:324-329, 1991.

Coontz EJ: The effectiveness of a new oral hygiene device on plaque removal, *Quintessence Int* 7:739-742, 1983.

de la Rosa M, Sturzenberger OP, Moore DJ: The use of chlorhexidine in the management of gingivitis in children, *J Periodontol* 59:387-389, 1988.

Glass RT: The infected toothbrush, the infected denture, and transmission of disease: a review, *Compendium* 8:592-598, 1992.

Hancock E, Nowell D: Preventive strategies and supportive treatment, *Periodontology* 2000 25:59-76, 2001.

Kallio, PJ: Health promotion and behavioral approaches in the prevention of periodontal disease in children and adolescents, *Periodontology* 2000 26:135-145, 2001.

Kimmelman BB, Tassman GC: Research in designs of children's toothbrushes, *J Dent Child* 27:60-64, 1960.

Loesche WJ: Role of Streptococcus mutans in human dental decay, *Microbiol Rev* 50:353-380, 1986.

Pinkham JR: Oral hygiene in children: relationship to age and brushing time, *J Prev Dent* 2(2):28-31, 1975.

Sandham HJ, Nadeau L, Phillips, HI: The effect of chlorhexidine varnish treatment on salivary mutans streptococcal levels in child orthodontic patients, *J Dent Res* 71:32-35, 1992.

Whittaker CJ, Klier CM, Kolenbrander PE: Mechanisms of adhesion by oral bacteria, *Annu Rev Microbiol* 50:513-552, 1996.

12

Nutritional Considerations for the Pediatric Dental Patient

JAMES L. McDONALD, JR.

CHAPTER OUTLINE

When the leading causes of death in the United States are tabulated (Table 12-1), the list is headed by heart disease and cancer, with stroke a distant third. When the focus is instead on the root causes of death, three major underlying factors related to lifestyle choices can be identified: cigarette smoking, a sedentary lifestyle, and inappropriate dietary choices. It has become increasingly clear that what we eat (and don't eat) is a major factor in determining both the quantity and quality of our lives. The basis of our dietary choices, and thus our nutritional status, is established early in life. It follows that food choices and patterns of eating initiated in childhood affect our health and well-being at every stage of life. There are many ways in which health professionals can promote the health of their patients. A major one is to educate them regarding the importance of following good nutritional principles. This chapter focuses on those nutritional factors that have the greatest potential influence on the health of the pediatric dental patient.

Several decades ago it was recognized that our health is profoundly affected by our dietary choices; since then, an evolution has occurred in efforts to promote healthy food choices in the United States. In 1977, the Senate Select Committee on Nutrition and Human Needs first published the *Dietary Goals for the United States*. This was followed in 1979 by *Healthy People: The Surgeon General's Report on Health Promotion and Disease Prevention* and again in 1988 by *The Surgeon General's Report on Nutrition and Health*. This latter document concluded that 5 of the 10 leading causes of death in the United States were related to poor dietary choices. In 1990, the U.S. Department of Health and Human Services released *Healthy People 2000*, a report that described the general goals for increasing life span, reducing health disparities, and achieving better access to preventive services for all Americans over the following decade. Numerous nutritional goals were outlined in this report. The latest report, *Healthy People 2010*, was released in January 2000. Its overall nutritional focus is to promote health and to reduce chronic disease associated with diet and weight. Chapter 19 of the report discusses a number of these objectives, many of which are related to pediatric nutrition; the latter are summarized in Table 12-2, which shows both the current status and target level for each.

Other nutrition-related objectives for children include reducing sodium consumption, increasing calcium intake, and reducing iron-deficiency anemia. As can be noted from Table 12-2, some of the nutrition objectives (19-5, 19-6, 19-7) are particularly ambitious and require major changes in eating behavior. Whether these objectives realistically can be met is another issue.

The *Dietary Guidelines for Americans* (the ABCs) promulgated by the U.S. Department of Agriculture (USDA) include the following recommendations and support the objectives in *Healthy People 2010*:

*A*im for fitness.

- Aim for a healthy weight.
- Be physically active each day.

*B*uild a healthy base.

- Let the Food Guide Pyramid guide your food choices.
- Choose a variety of grains daily, especially whole grains.
- Choose a variety of fruits and vegetables daily.
- Keep food safe to eat.

*C*hoose sensibly.

- Choose a diet low in saturated fat and cholesterol and moderate in fat.
- Choose beverages and foods so as to moderate your intake of sugars.
- Choose and prepare foods with less salt.
- If you drink alcoholic beverages, do so in moderation.

FOOD GUIDE PYRAMID

The Food Guide Pyramid (see Fig. 10-6 on p. 221) was introduced by the USDA in 1992 as a pictorial representation for the USDA's Daily Food Guide. It is a tool commonly used to help plan a healthful diet. It organizes the foods we eat into five major food groups and one miscellaneous category. The latter category includes

TABLE 12-1	Leading Causes of Death in the United States (Final 2000 Data)
CAUSE	**NUMBER OF DEATHS**
Heart disease	710,760
Cancer	553,091
Stroke	167,661
Chronic lower respiratory disease	122,009
Accidents	97,900
Diabetes	69,301
Pneumonia/influenza	65,313
Alzheimer disease	49,558
Nephritis, nephritic syndrome, and nephrosis	37,251
Septicemia	31,224

From US Department of Health and Human Services, Centers for Disease Control and Prevention: *Natl Vital Stat Rep* 50(16), 2002.

TABLE **12-2** *Healthy People 2010 Selected Nutritional Goals*

NUMBER	OBJECTIVE	CURRENT	TARGET
19-3	Reduce the proportion of children and adolescents who are overweight or obese	11%	5%
19-4	Reduce growth retardation among low-income children under 5 years of age	8%	5%
19-5	Increase the proportion of persons aged 2 and older who consume at least two daily servings of fruit	28%	75%
19-6	Increase the proportion of persons aged 2 and older who consume at least three daily servings of vegetables, with at least one third being dark green or deep yellow vegetables	3%	50%
19-7	Increase the proportion of persons aged 2 and older who consume at least six daily servings of grain products, with at least three being whole grains	7%	50%
19-8	Increase the proportion of persons aged 2 and older who consume less than 10% of calories from saturated fat	36%	75%
19-9	Increase the proportion of persons aged 2 and older who consume no more than 30% of calories from fat	33%	75%
19-15	Increase the proportion of children and adolescents age 6 to 19 whose intake of meals and snacks at schools contributes proportionally to good overall dietary quality	*	*

*No target established.

TABLE **12-3** Number of Servings of Major Food Groups Needed Each Day

	CHILDREN (2-6 YEARS)	OLDER CHILDREN OR TEENAGED GIRLS	TEENAGED BOYS
1. Milk and milk products	2	3	3
2. Meat and meat alternatives	2	2	3
3. Vegetables	3	4	5
4. Fruits	2	3	4
5. Bread and cereals	6	9	11

fats, oils, and sweets, all of which are to be used sparingly. The major food groups and recommended daily servings for children and adolescents are presented in Table 12-3.

Two cautions should be kept in mind in using the Food Guide Pyramid. One caution is that teens, young adults, pregnant and nursing women, and women concerned about osteoporosis prevention need at least four daily servings from the milk products group or additional calcium from alternative sources. The second caution is that "one serving" does not equal the exaggerated serving sizes often presented at commercial eating establishments, but rather represents a smaller, more conservative food serving size. If one were to use as the standard the large serving sizes typical of today's American culture, then it would be impossible to meet these recommendations without consuming a large excess of calories.

MALNUTRITION AMONG U.S. CHILDREN

Malnutrition may take the form of either undernutrition (inadequate intake of nutrients that potentially leads to

deficiency diseases) or overnutrition (excessive dietary intake of energy, fat, or cholesterol that predisposes individuals to chronic diseases later in life). The latter excessive consumption pattern is probably quantitatively more relevant to overall mortality and morbidity rates in contemporary U.S. society than are nutrient deficiencies.

In March 2002, the U.S. Department of Health and Human Services released the infant mortality data as of 2000. These data showed some positive gains compared to the past. The rate at which infants die before their first birthday reached a historic low of 6.9 deaths per 1000 live births. Moreover, the proportion of mothers receiving early prenatal care is at a record high. Malnutrition as measured by low weight for age and low growth rates has also declined. Some of this decline has been attributed to better nutrition. By the same token, the U.S. infant mortality rate continues to rank among the highest of the industrialized nations. The infant mortality rate among black children is more than double that among white children. Also, more than 13 million children in the United States are estimated to be living below the poverty level, and some estimates indicate that approximately 10% suffer to some degree from clinical malnutrition. Certainly, all poor children are at risk for the long-term consequences of malnutrition.[1]

DIETARY PATTERNS

Numerous national surveys measuring nutritional status and dietary patterns of children and adolescents were conducted in the 1970s and 1980s. More recent information shows some intriguing trends. In comparing food intake trends among children aged 6 to 11 over approximately a 20-year period from 1977 through 1998, Enns, Mickle, and Goldman reported increases in consumption of soft drinks, grain products as a whole, grain mixtures (crackers, popcorn, pretzels, corn chips), fried potatoes, noncitrus juices and nectars, cheese, candy, and fruit drinks and ades.[2] Decreases were noted in intake of milk in general and whole milk, various vegetables and legumes, beef, pork, and eggs. For any given pyramid group, less than one half of the children consumed the recommended number of servings, and their intakes of discretionary fat and added sugars were much higher than recommended.

Similar findings were reported by Cullen et al, who evaluated the intake of soft drinks, fruit-flavored beverages, and fruits and vegetables by children in grades 4 through 6.[3] Lower parental education level was associated with higher consumption of soft drinks and sweetened beverages, and students who had a high consumption of sweetened beverages reported low fruit and high calorie intakes. Troiano et al have also reported that beverages contribute 20% to 24% of energy intake among youth aged 2 to 19 years and that soft drinks provide 8% of energy intake among adolescents.[4]

An additional disturbing trend is an increase in away-from-home eating as well as expanding portion sizes in the U.S. marketplace. Again, in examining the changes in dietary intake patterns between 1977 and 1996, Guthrie, Lin, and Frazao reported that food prepared away from home increased from 18% to 32% of total calories consumed.[5] Both meals and snacks prepared away from home contained more calories per eating occasion. Food eaten outside the home was also higher in both total and saturated fat on a percentage basis, and contained less dietary fiber, calcium, and iron per calorie. Based on this information, eating away from home is associated with a compromised quality of nutritional intake.

As touched upon earlier, another major trend being reported is that most marketplace portions of foods exceed standard serving sizes by at least a factor of 2 (bagels and sodas) and sometimes by a factor of 8 (cookies).[6] Fast-food chains offer larger sizes of hamburgers, sodas, and french fries. The current sizes are often two to five times larger than the original size marketed. These changes in dietary patterns parallel the progressive increase in obesity seen in the United States.

PROBLEMS OF UNDERCONSUMPTION

IRON DEFICIENCY

Although the prevalence of iron deficiency has declined in recent years, it remains an important pediatric public health problem in the United States. Many of the adverse consequences of iron deficiency are associated with its most severe form, iron-deficiency anemia.[7-9] However, iron deficiency without anemia has been linked to negative impacts on cognitive development in children and adolescents.[10] Typically, the high iron needs for growth, when combined with a low dietary intake, produce a low iron status in children. Iron deficiency early in life appears related to behavioral problems in infants who score significantly lower on various tests measuring intellectual and motor functioning. It has long been recognized that toddlers and adolescent females are among the most susceptible groups. The prevalence of iron deficiency has been estimated to be higher among non-Hispanic black and Mexican-American females than among non-Hispanic white females. To prevent iron deficiency, vulnerable populations should be encouraged to eat iron-rich foods and breast-feed or use iron-fortified formula for infants. Iron is found primarily in meat, poultry, and fish. However, other foods such as beans, lentils, fortified cereal grain products, and certain vegetables can make a significant contribution to dietary intake of iron.

Clinical signs of iron-deficiency anemia may include weakness, fatigue, pallor, and numbness and tingling of the extremities. Common oral manifestations are glossitis and fissures at the corners of the mouth (*angular cheilitis*). The papillae of the tongue may be atrophied, which gives the tongue a smooth, shiny, red appearance.

CALCIUM INADEQUACY

Osteoporosis is a bone disease of older individuals and is primarily seen in postmenopausal women. It is characterized by a reduction in the quantity of skeletal tissue, and thus is often considered to be a geriatric disorder. Education for its prevention, however, is legitimately within the domain of pediatricians and pediatric dentists. Childhood and adolescence are crucial times for development of the skeletal system, and the dietary requirement for calcium peaks during the teenage years. The Food and Nutrition Board of the Institute of Medicine recommends an intake of 1300 mg per day of calcium during adolescence. This equals roughly the amount of calcium present in $4^{1}/_{3}$ cups of milk, so this is not a particularly easy recommendation to meet.

Achieving a high peak bone mass is the first line of defense against osteoporosis. Low calcium intake, particularly in combination with low levels of physical activity, may compromise the attainment of optimal peak bone mass. This is a particularly important consideration for adolescent girls, because almost half of the adult skeletal mass is formed during the second decade of life and calcium accumulation normally triples during the pubertal growth spurt.[11] Unfortunately, this is the very age group that is at highest risk for low calcium intakes. Only 30% of adolescent girls reach 75% of the recommended daily allowance for calcium, and calcium intake appears to be declining among 6- to 11-year-olds.[12] This problem may be alleviated by educating youth to select more calcium-rich foods (dairy products, fortified breakfast cereals, fortified orange juice concentrates) or to consider using calcium supplements. Calcium carbonate has a good absorption rate and has been characterized as a relatively inexpensive supplement containing a high percentage level of calcium.[13]

VITAMIN D DEFICIENCY

Fortified milk serves as the primary dietary source of vitamin D in the United States. Few other commonly consumed foods contain appreciable quantities of this vitamin. Exposure to sunlight is another important source of vitamin D, because ultraviolet rays from the sun trigger vitamin D synthesis in the skin. Vitamin D is an essential nutrient for proper bone growth, and children who receive too little can develop the bone disease rickets. During the first half of the twentieth century, thousands of cases of vitamin D–deficiency rickets were reported in the United States, particularly in the northern climates during the winter months when exposure to sunlight was minimal. This disease was virtually eradicated once vitamin D began to be added to milk. In recent years, however, somewhat of a resurgence of rickets has been seen, particularly in dark-skinned, breast-fed babies. There appear to be two major reasons for this resurgence. First, heavily pigmented skin is less efficient than is light skin in synthesizing vitamin D from sunlight. Second, many nonwhite people are unable to efficiently digest the lactose in milk, which leads to a significant reduction in milk intake and consequently in vitamin D levels. O'Dell et al reported that, of 1546 black women studied, 42% had blood vitamin D levels below the value considered to reflect a vitamin D deficiency.[14] In contrast, only 4% of white women demonstrated blood concentrations below that threshold. Thus, vitamin D deficiency appears to be a major unrecognized disease in certain populations of adult women of childbearing age. The recommended intake of vitamin D for adults who do not receive sufficient exposure to sunlight should be reevaluated in light of these findings.

VITAMIN B$_{12}$ DEFICIENCY

Vitamin B$_{12}$ is one of the B-complex vitamins, and it contains cobalt in the molecule; thus it is the only vitamin that contains a mineral. Vitamin B$_{12}$ is essential for the synthesis of red blood cells and for myelin synthesis in the nervous system. This vitamin is not thought to be present in plant foods, and as a result strict vegetarians are considered to be at risk for a dietary deficiency of this vitamin. During 2001, neurologic impairment resulting from a vitamin B$_{12}$ deficiency was reported in two children breast-fed by mothers who followed vegetarian diets (consumption of limited food of animal origin).[15] In one of these cases, the diagnosis was made at 15 months, and vitamin B$_{12}$ therapy was initiated. At age 28 months, the child's developmental skill levels ranged from 9 months for fine motor skills to 18 months for gross motor skills. Her expressive language was at a 10-month level. Health care providers should be alert to the possibility of B$_{12}$ deficiency under these circumstances. Patients following vegetarian diets should ensure an adequate intake of vitamin B$_{12}$. The only reliable unfortified sources of this vitamin are animal products, including meat, dairy products, and eggs. Plant foods fortified with this vitamin, such as some cereals, meat analogues, soy or rice beverages, and nutritional yeast, can be reliable and regular sources.

PROBLEMS OF OVERCONSUMPTION

For most children and adolescents in the United States, compromised health brought on by malnutrition is much more likely to be related to overconsumption than to underconsumption. The eating environment in contemporary America has been characterized as consisting of convenient, relatively inexpensive, highly palatable foods served in large portions.[16] The chronic adherence to this type of eating pattern from childhood through adult life contributes to obesity and to numerous diseases, including diabetes, hypertension, coronary heart disease, and certain types of cancer. Those diseases that become evident during adulthood but have their origins in childhood and adolescence provide the health care professional with a potential avenue for preventive medicine. Atherosclerotic heart disease is such a case. Modifiable risk factors can be identified and addressed in the pediatric population, with the goal of preventing or ameliorating heart disease in later life. Thus, prevention of coronary heart disease is a pediatric health issue, as is prevention of the other diseases mentioned earlier.

OBESITY AND PHYSICAL ACTIVITY LEVELS

Data from a variety of sources strongly indicate that we are in the midst of an obesity epidemic among children, adolescents, and adults in the United States. Obesity results from a chronic imbalance between energy intake and energy expenditure. Although obesity is defined as the excessive accumulation of fat in the body, it is typically diagnosed based on weight and weight-for-height measures. As mentioned previously, a major focus of the nationwide health promotion and disease prevention agenda in *Healthy People 2010* is to reduce the proportion of children and adolescents who are overweight or obese. Unfortunately, a large disparity is found between the existing prevalence rates of obesity and the prevalence rate goals targeted in *Healthy People 2010*.[17] The percentage of overweight young people in the United States has doubled since 1980, and currently one in seven children and adolescents is affected.[18]

The consequences of obesity are many and are both immediate and long-term. The current epidemic of type 2 diabetes in children and adolescents is associated with obesity and a persistently elevated body mass index (BMI). The BMI is calculated by dividing the individual's weight in kilograms by the square of height in meters. A BMI of 30 or higher generally is considered to indicate obesity and may be a critical etiologic factor in the high prevalence of type 2 diabetes among an increasingly younger population. A recent study found that 25% of obese children (aged 4 to 10 years) were glucose intolerant.[19] This figure is noteworthy because glucose intolerance is a precursor to diabetes. Other obesity-related disorders, such as obstructive sleep apnea, have been observed in as many as one in six obese children. This condition can lead to daytime somnolence, neuro-cognitive abnormalities, and impaired learning.

Aside from the obvious health risks associated with obesity in childhood and adolescence, there are also significant psychologic and quality-of-life issues to be considered. Ackard et al reported that objective overeating with loss of control in adolescents was associated with lower scores on measures of body satisfaction and self-esteem and higher scores on a measure of depressive mood.[20] Overeating was also associated with suicide risk. Thus, objective overeating among adolescents is linked to a number of adverse behaviors and negative psychologic experiences. It remains to be determined whether objective overeating is an early warning sign of psychologic distress or rather a potential consequence of compromised psychologic health.

Schwimmer, Burwinkle, and Varni compared the health-related quality of life of obese children and adolescents with that of both their healthy, nonobese counterparts and a cohort of children and adolescents diagnosed as having cancer.[18] They found that quality-of-life ratings of severely obese children and adolescents were lower than those of children and adolescents who are healthy and similar to those of children and adolescents diagnosed with cancer. An impaired self-image and perception of low quality of life in this population

group is not terribly surprising, because obesity is one of the most stigmatizing and least socially acceptable conditions in childhood. These and similar findings emphasize how critical it is for health professionals, teachers, and parents to be aware not only of the medical risks of obesity in children but also of the potential psychologic significance of this condition.

Because obese children tend to become obese adults, the potential impact of childhood obesity on the health care system is enormous. It has been suggested that the increased medical care costs associated with obesity may be greater than those associated with smoking and drinking.[21] Severe obesity has long been thought to reduce life expectancy. A recent report states that white men aged 20 years with BMI greater than 45 (extreme obesity) are estimated to lose 13 years of life because of their obesity.[22] If one assumes a life expectancy of 78 years, this translates into a 22% reduction in remaining years of life for these individuals. Despite several decades of various public health efforts to educate the population regarding the dangers of obesity, the trend toward progressively increasing body weight has not been reversed or even slowed. The time has clearly come for identifying new strategies to deal with this issue. To focus on reversing this alarming obesity trend in children and adolescents and devising more effective strategies for dealing with it, all the major etiologic factors must be identified.

One such factor is the possible influence of the mass media on childhood health behaviors. Sometimes the media appear to receive the blame for almost every ill present in contemporary society. Nevertheless, the fact remains that a typical teenager's life today is increasingly saturated with the mass media, which often depict an array of unhealthy behaviors, including physical aggression, unprotected sex, smoking, drinking, and poor nutritional choices.[23] Chronic behaviors involving poor nutritional choices inevitably will lead to obesity, high disease risks, or eating disorders such as anorexia nervosa and bulimia.

Clearly more teens than ever are obese, primarily because they eat food of low nutritional density at the expense of fruits and vegetables, and they do not get enough exercise. A 2000 report to the President from the Secretary of Health and Human Services and the Secretary of Education describes our nation's youth as "in large measure, inactive, unfit, and increasingly overweight. This increasingly sedentary lifestyle threatens to reverse the decades of progress achieved in reducing deaths from cardiovascular diseases." Physical activity is a major determinant of both morbidity and mortality. It has been identified as a national priority area for promoting the health of the U.S. population. In spite of the documented benefits of an active lifestyle, however, many Americans, including children and adolescents, do not meet the recommendations for physical activity. This fact is particularly sobering because the adolescent years are thought to be the period during which adult health-related behaviors such as dietary and physical activity patterns begin to develop. Thus, childhood may be a critical time for promoting physical activity. Studies indicate that the current levels of physical activity in children and adolescents have declined in recent years. For example, walking and bicycling among 5- to 15-year-olds decreased by 40% between 1977 and 1995. The reduction in total physical activity that occurs from mid to late adolescence appears to be related more to a reduction in the number of activities in which adolescents choose to participate than in a decline in the time spent on each activity.[24] This finding supports other evidence that physical activity declines during adolescence.

The following are some general findings concerning physical activity and health that have emerged over the past decade or two:

1. People who tend to be inactive can improve their health and well-being by becoming even moderately active on a regular basis.
2. Physical activity need not be strenuous to provide some health benefits.
3. Greater health benefits can be achieved by increasing the intensity, frequency, or duration of the physical activity.

Current physical activity recommendations generally state that children and adults should strive for at least 30 minutes daily of physical activity of moderate intensity. The approximate energy expenditure of various physical activities is shown in Table 12-4. An alternate approach might be to engage in separate 5- to 10-minute periods of moderately intense activity throughout the day for a total of at least 30 minutes for adolescents and 60 minutes for children. Walking briskly, biking, swimming, engaging in games and sports, participating in physical education classes, and doing tasks at home or in the garden may all contribute to accumulated physical activity. Walking programs are increasingly being promoted for our youth in selected school systems. Many of these programs are using pedometers to register the number of steps being taken. These small units, which clip onto waistbands, resemble tiny pagers and are reasonably accurate in counting all the steps taken over a given period of time. For some programs, the goal is to reach 12,000 steps per day, but for all the programs, a general objective is to motivate the person wearing the pedometer to progressively increase the step count over time and perhaps to maintain a minimally acceptable level of steps per day.

It seems intuitive that the more time children (and adults for that matter) spend watching television and playing video games, the more likely they are to be obese. Research shows that the prevalence of obesity is lowest among children watching 1 or fewer hours of television a day and highest among those watching 4 or more hours of television a day.[25] Not only will sedentary children expend less energy, but they will invariably be increasing their consumption of high-fat, high-sugar, high-caloric snack foods during these sedentary periods. Research from more than a decade ago indicates that food (typically sweet snacks) is consumed or referred to three to five times per half-hour on prime-time programming.[26] Also, the majority of commercials shown during children's programming promote foods with low nutritional value, including candy, soft drinks, sugared cereals, and potato chips, as well as other high-salt, high-fat snacks.[27]

EATING DISORDERS

Looking good is certainly a high priority for most teenagers, and for some adolescent girls in particular, getting "thin enough" can become an obsession. Estimates are that 5 million Americans suffer from eating disorders and that 5% of female and 1% of male Americans have anorexia nervosa, bulimia nervosa, or binge-eating disorder. Because women and men are often secretive about their eating disorders, existing epidemiologic studies may underestimate the true prevalence of these conditions.[28] Some personality traits, such as perfectionism and concern with weight and shape, may cluster in families of women with eating disorders. Perfectionism may be an environmentally transmitted or genetically mediated trait that flows down to offspring.[29]

Again, the mass media are viewed by many as a major contributor to the mixed messages regarding desirable eating behaviors and desirable looks. Given

TABLE 12-4	Approximate Energy Expenditure of Various Types of Exercise
TYPE OF EXERCISE	**CALORIES USED PER 30 MINUTES***
Raking leaves	100
Walking (15-minute miles)	200
Playing singles tennis	210
Stationary cycling	300
Stair climbing	300
Jogging (10-minute miles)	330
Shoveling snow	350
Rowing	350

Data from National Institute of Sports Medicine.
*These values will be higher for larger individuals, lower for smaller individuals.

all the unhealthy food consumption depicted in the media, how is it that most of the people in the media, especially white women, are so thin and apparently healthy? Content analyses show that more than two thirds of the women characters on television, but only 18% of the men, are thin. Analyses of body measurements of 500 models listed on modeling agency web sites and of *Playboy* centerfolds from 1985 to 1997 showed that nearly all the centerfolds and three quarters of the models had BMIs of 17.5 or below, a figure that meets the American Psychological Association's criterion for anorexia nervosa.[23] Although boys may be increasingly influenced by the portrayals of muscular men in the media, most research has focused on the effects of media portrayals on girls' eating and dietary habits. Teenaged girls are most at risk for developing eating disorders as they struggle with bodies that are getting larger in a culture that simultaneously attempts to sell them junk food and tells them that they should be thin. For some girls, bulimia must appear as a rational response to these contradictory messages: splurge and then purge.[23]

ANOREXIA NERVOSA

Preoccupation with appearance and body weight during adolescence often leads to restriction in food intake. Anorexia nervosa results when this behavior is carried to the point of starvation. This illness, which is much less common in males and is also less common than bulimia nervosa, is characterized by self-imposed weight loss, amenorrhea, and a distorted attitude toward eating and body weight. In some instances this behavior is used as a means of establishing a sense of identity and control. Anorexia nervosa has captured the interest of psychoanalysts, behavior therapists, family therapists, nutritionists, and endocrinologists alike because of the interplay between the powerful psychologic and physiologic components of the disease. Anorexia nervosa rarely begins before puberty and probably is manifest across a wide range of severity levels. Affected individuals often lack the ability to recognize that their emaciated bodies are too thin. Despite their advanced state of wasting, they may continue to believe that they are overweight. The four diagnostic criteria for anorexia nervosa are the following[30]:

- Refusal to maintain a body weight equal to or greater than 85% of that expected for the patient's age and height.
- An intense fear of gaining weight or becoming fat, even though the individual is underweight.
- A distorted view of one's body weight, size, or shape; the emaciated anorexic individual actually feels fat.
- In postmenarcheal women and girls, the absence of at least three consecutive menstrual cycles.

A wide range of complications, including many of the consequences of starvation, is possible in anorexia nervosa. Fat depletion is the most obvious physical consequence. Qualitative deficiencies in the diet may lead to anemia, to hypoproteinemia, and sometimes to vitamin deficiencies. Serious electrolyte imbalances, notably hypokalemia, can occur when vomiting or laxative or diuretic abuse are practiced. Anorexia may be accompanied by enlargement of the parotid glands, edema of the legs, increased facial hair, and reductions in blood pressure and pulse rate. Nutritional deficiencies may lead to a reduction in the amount and pH of the saliva and an increase in dental caries susceptibility. Gingivitis may also be noted. Long-term studies have demonstrated diverse outcomes ranging from full recovery to chronicity and death. Outpatient treatment is preferred for most individuals. If the illness is severe and family and environmental circumstances are too damaging or if there is little response to outpatient treatment, then hospitalization is indicated. Fluoxetine hydrochloride appears to help control the obsessive-compulsive behavior involved in both anorexia nervosa and bulimia. This drug raises the brain levels of serotonin, and as a consequence the urge to binge and the preoccupation with food appears to lessen.

BULIMIA

Another eating disorder, bulimia nervosa, is characterized by binge eating and invariably by self-induced vomiting. It also is more prevalent in young women and is more common than is anorexia nervosa. It usually begins during late adolescence or early adult life. Its prevalence among males is probably vastly underestimated because of underreporting. The American Psychiatric Association diagnostic criteria for bulimia nervosa are the following[30]:

- Consumption of an unusually large amount of food in a discrete time period (within 2 hours)
- A perceived lack of control over eating during an episode
- Compensatory behavior to rid the body of excess calories and prevent weight gain
- The occurrence of binge eating and compensatory behaviors at least twice a week for 3 months
- A persistent concern with body shape and size

Bulimia nervosa is associated with significant health consequences, although it is more medically benign than is anorexia nervosa. Approximately half of patients with this disorder have fluid and electrolyte abnormalities. A small percentage develop hypokalemia. Enlargement of the parotid glands, esophagitis, and gastric necrosis may also occur. Enamel erosion is common among bulimia nervosa patients because of the exposure of the tooth surfaces to the highly acidic regurgitated gastric contents. The degree of enamel damage can be extensive. Although unanimity of opinion does not exist, the suggestion has been made that toothbrushing after vomiting actually promotes enamel loss and that, instead, patients should be instructed to rinse with an alkaline solution such as sodium bicarbonate dissolved in water. Other suggestions include use of liquid sugar-free antacids, water, or milk. Fluoride treatment should be considered because of its potential for remineralizing previously demineralized areas of the dentition. Daily rinses with 0.5% sodium fluoride and administration of a 1.1% neutral fluoride gel in custom trays can be recommended.

Most bulimic patients can be treated effectively as outpatients. Multidisciplinary treatment approaches seem indicated, although indications exist that antidepression medications may be helpful in some cases. There is some evidence that individuals who eat dinner with their families regularly score significantly lower on the bulimia-risk scale.[31] Family meals may serve a protective function against disordered eating as well as other problems by acting as a forum for working through various issues.

As health care professionals deal with eating disorders in their patients, they recognize that primary prevention combined with early detection and treatment clearly helps reduce morbidity and mortality in affected adolescents.[32]

NUTRITIONAL CONSIDERATIONS FROM INFANCY THROUGH ADOLESCENCE

During postnatal life, childhood exposure to environmental factors, primarily via dietary intake, will slowly begin to condition adult susceptibility to diseases both positively and negatively.[33] Some examples of dietary factors include calories, saturated fat, sodium, calcium, and antioxidants. Although dietary intervention for disease prevention is possible in adult life, it is difficult and the beneficial results are sometimes limited. A better option is to promote intake of a diet with high nutritional quality early in life; this can reduce risk factors and potentially accomplish major reductions in the incidence of several diseases of adults.

INFANT AND TODDLER (0 TO 3 YEARS OLD)

Except for prenatal existence, the period of most rapid growth in humans occurs during the first 6 months of life. Thus, energy and nutrient requirements are high during this time. A full-term infant is capable of digesting and absorbing protein, a moderate amount of fat, and simple carbohydrates. Starch presents some digestive challenges, however, because amylase, the starch-splitting enzyme, is not produced in significant quantities

until approximately the age of 3 months. Moreover, the immature kidneys of an infant cannot concentrate waste efficiently. As a result, the infant must excrete relatively more water than does an adult to eliminate a comparable amount of waste. When dealing with infants, one must always be on guard against dehydration, which has potentially very serious consequences.

Liquid or semiliquid foods are the choice until the teeth begin to erupt. Breast-feeding continues to be the best overall method of infant feeding, and breast milk could well be the infant's only food source for the first 4 to 6 months. Observational studies in affluent populations generally show no difference in weight or length gain between exclusively breast-fed and partially breast-fed infants during the first 4 to 6 months of life. Thereafter, milk can be supplemented with various pureed foods, either homemade or commercially prepared. Breast milk complemented by the infant's own internal stores will meet most of the nutrient needs until the first 6 months have elapsed. Supplements of substances such as vitamin D, iron, and fluoride should be considered after consulting with the child's pediatrician and pediatric dentist. Evidence suggests that low tissue levels of iron adversely affect brain and intellectual development and performance. Whether breast-fed infants should receive iron supplements is still the subject of debate. Although infants who are exclusively breast-fed appear to be iron sufficient at 6 months of age, some breast-fed infants who do not receive iron supplements are in negative iron balance between the ages of 3 and 6 months. Therefore, it may be desirable to begin iron supplementation (often with ferrous sulfate) for the breast-fed infant at about 4 months of age. If the baby is formula-fed, the makeup of the formula determines what additional supplementation is indicated. If an iron-fortified formula is not used, iron supplements again may be recommended after 4 months of age. The use of infant fluoride supplements to maximize caries resistance is discussed elsewhere in this text. The pediatrician and pediatric dentist may be consulted regarding specific situations and local circumstances.

There is no nutritional need for introducing solid foods to infants prior to 6 months of age.[34] Earlier use may contribute to the development of allergies or increased risk of obesity. New foods should be introduced singly to permit detection of allergies. For the first 6 months of life, the optimal single food for the infant is human milk, or alternative formula when indicated. Some concerns have been expressed over inclusion of egg yolk when solid foods begin to be added to the weanling diet because of the potential for elevation of blood cholesterol levels. However, a recent study indicates that egg yolk may be safely introduced into the weanling diet with no elevation in plasma cholesterol level nor increase in the prevalence of egg allergies.[35]

Regular unmodified cow's milk is not considered suitable for infants. It is an insufficient source of vitamin C and iron. Moreover, it may cause gastrointestinal bleeding, and its solute load is too heavy for the infant's renal system to handle. In addition, low-fat milks should not be used by infants because of their insufficient energy provision and their lack of essential fatty acids.

When the infant becomes a toddler and the rapid growth rate of the first year declines, parents are frequently concerned about a very noticeable reduction in appetite. This is a normal occurrence. Although fewer calories may be needed for growth at this stage, the dietary needs for protein and minerals to promote muscle and skeletal development remain high. Thus, a variety of foods should be offered in smaller amounts several times a day to provide these key nutrients. Attractive, brightly colored foods seem to be particularly appealing to children.

PRESCHOOLER (3 TO 6 YEARS OLD)

Physical growth occurs in spurts between 3 and 6 years of age. The child is not growing as rapidly as in the first years of life. Thus, fewer calories are required but relatively high protein and mineral needs remain. A variety of foods should be offered but in lesser amounts. Parents sometimes provide adult-sized food servings to a child who may be only one fifth the size of an adult. Care must be taken not to turn mealtimes into major struggles for control over what to eat, how much to eat, and when to eat.

Although it is important to keep the total fat, saturated fat, and cholesterol at recommended levels in the diet, care must be taken not to overdo this approach. With insufficient intake of calories and nutrients, the child cannot grow and develop to full potential. The child of this age should be helped to grow out of fatness by increasing physical activity rather than by severely restricting calories. Providing wholesome, nutritious snacks can promote adequate intake of essential nutrients without adding excessive calories.

SCHOOL-AGED CHILD (6 TO 12 YEARS OLD)

The 6- to 12-year stage is generally accompanied by a reduced rate of growth, which results in a decline in food requirements per unit of body weight. As a result, there is some need to be more discriminatory in food selection, with emphasis on high nutrient density (foods having a high ratio of nutrients to calories). Vegetables are generally among the least-favored foods in this age group, but fruits are usually liked and provide many of the same nutrients. In this age group, regular eating patterns should be established; at the same time, consumption of nutritious snacks should be stressed and the use of foods, particularly sweets, as rewards should be minimized. Children should be encouraged to eat breakfast.

This long-standing advice delivered by mothers from time immemorial seems consistent with the research literature. Reddan, Wahlstrom, and Reicks found in a study of fourth- through sixth-graders in a school with a universal school breakfast program that the majority of students felt that eating breakfast provides benefits of increased energy and ability to pay attention in school.[36] Barriers to eating breakfast cited by students were not having time and not being hungry in the morning. A focus on eating foods with high nutrient value and maintaining sufficient physical activity levels is important throughout this age range, because obesity problems often begin in this period.

ADOLESCENT (12 TO 18 YEARS OLD)

The nutritional requirements of adolescents are influenced primarily by the onset of puberty and the final growth spurt of childhood. This profound increase in growth rate is accompanied by increased needs for energy, protein, vitamins, and minerals. In general, girls consume far less food than do boys and must meet their needs for individual nutrients within a smaller range of caloric intakes. As a result, adolescent females are at high risk for nutritional inadequacies. In addition, girls often encounter significant social and peer pressure to restrict food intake for weight-control purposes. A multitude of fad weight-loss diets may be tried at this time. Some adolescent girls also turn to cigarette smoking to help control their body weight. The nutritional status of adolescent girls remains of concern because of low dietary intakes and attendant marginal iron, calcium, and folic acid status. Generally, as girls progress through adolescence, their average intake of vitamins and minerals and calories declines, while their nutritional requirements actually increase. Particularly among adolescent female athletes in sports that emphasize leanness, research indicates that reported energy and nutrient intakes are generally well below recommended levels and lower than those of typical teenage girls.[37]

Teenagers, particularly boys, receive a greater proportion of their total energy intake from snacks than do other population groups. Although these snack items may have significant nutritional value, more often than not they are high in fat and sugar and thus contribute relatively low quantities of essential nutrients compared with their caloric content. The result may be the establishment of lifetime eating patterns that promote future risk of heart disease, obesity, hypertension, and cancer.

Table 12-5 summarizes some major gender differences in adolescent nutrition issues.

DRUG AND ALCOHOL USE IN ADOLESCENCE

The teenage years are typically a period of search for identity, independence, and peer acceptance. Enmeshed

TABLE 12-5 Gender Differences in Adolescent Nutritional Issues	
FEMALES	**MALES**
Lower energy needs	Higher energy needs
Thinness considered important	Strength considered important
Concern about peak bone mass	Less concern about peak bone mass
Higher risk for eating disorders	Lower risk for eating disorders
Higher risk for nutritional deficiencies	Lower risk for nutritional deficiencies

within this search are a myriad of personal choices to be made, including decisions concerning the use of drugs, alcohol, and tobacco. If the choice is made to use these types of substances, the individual should recognize that all have significant negative impacts on fitness and health. Aside from the dangers of establishing a lifetime addiction and increasing the risk of numerous diseases, the use of alcohol, nicotine, and other drugs has a significant negative impact on the nutrient status of the affected individual.

Nicotine is the psychoactive substance in tobacco products. Based on the fact that 90% of tobacco users become addicted to the use of tobacco, nicotine may be considered one of the most addictive substances known. Cigarette smoking affects nutrition in numerous ways. Studies have shown that smokers have a lower intake than nonsmokers of numerous essential nutrients, including vitamins C and A, β-carotene, folic acid, and dietary fiber. Moreover, several of these nutrients have been associated with a reduced risk of lung cancer, a disease for which cigarette smokers are at high risk. Therefore, the typical smoker is receiving less of the very nutrients most needed. Evidence also exists that smokers metabolize vitamin C more rapidly than do nonsmokers. The result is that smokers require approximately twice as much vitamin C as do nonsmokers to maintain similar blood levels. Smoking also influences both hunger and body weight, tending to postpone feelings of hunger and to reduce weight. In spite of the fact that smokers as a group weigh less than nonsmokers, there are strong indications that smoking is associated with greater fat accumulations in the central portion of the body (a higher waist-to-hip ratio).

Tobacco use in youth has long been considered to be a gateway to the subsequent introduction and use of other drugs. For example, in a study of 20,000 children and adolescents, those who were pack-a-day smokers were more likely to drink alcohol, were 7 times more likely to use smokeless tobacco, and were 10 to 30 times

more likely to use illicit drugs than were nonsmokers.[38] Moreover, there was a strong dose-dependent relationship between smoking behavior and binge drinking, as well as between smoking and the use of alcohol and illicit drugs.

Alcohol is a very popular substance among many of the nation's youth and is not difficult to obtain for the vast majority of them. Some adolescents, as well as adults, use alcohol as an inappropriate way to cope with problems and stress. Nutritionally speaking, alcohol is a relatively high energy substance (7 kcal/g versus 4 kcal/g for carbohydrates) that is devoid of any nutritional value. Alcohol use displaces the intake of essential nutrients. With chronic, excessive use it adversely affects the absorption, transport, and metabolism of nutrients, which sometimes leads to serious nutritional inadequacies.

The long-term use of other drugs, such as cocaine and heroin, often produces numerous adverse physiologic effects, many of which compromise the nutritional state of the user and may result in multiple nutritional problems. Chronic abuse of these drugs may lead to eating disorders, in part because of chronic loss of appetite produced by the drugs. Often, during the "highs" produced by drugs, the individual loses interest in food, eating, and nutrient intake. The nutritional quality of the diet suffers under these circumstances.

REFERENCES

1. Karp R: Malnutrition among children in the United States: the impact of poverty. In Shils M et al, editors: *Modern nutrition in health and disease.* Philadelphia, 1999, Lippincott Williams & Wilkins, chap 60.
2. Enns CW, Mickle SJ, Goldman JD: Trends in food and nutrient intakes by children in the United States, *Fam Econ Nutr Rev* 14(2):56-68, 2002.
3. Cullen KW et al: Intake of soft drinks, fruit-flavored beverages, and fruits and vegetables by children in grades 4 through 6, *Am J Public Health* 92(9):1475-1478, 2002.
4. Troiano RP et al: Energy and fat intakes of children and adolescents in the United States: data from the National Health and Nutrition Examination Surveys, *Am J Clin Nutr* 72(5 suppl):1343S-1353S, 2000.
5. Guthrie J, Lin B, Frazao E: Role of food prepared away from home in the American diet, 1977-78 versus 1994-96: changes and consequences, *J Nutr Educ Behav* 34:140-150, May-June 2002.
6. Young L, Nestle M: Expanding portion sizes in the U.S. marketplace: implications for nutrition counseling, *J Am Diet Assoc* 103(2):231-234, Feb 2003.
7. Haas JD, Brownlie T: Iron deficiency and reduced work capacity: a critical review of the research to determine a causal relationship, *J Nutr* 131:676S-688S, 2001.
8. Rasmussen KM: Is there a causal relationship between iron deficiency or iron-deficiency anemia and weight at birth, length of gestation and perinatal mortality? *J Nutr* 131: 590S-601S, 2001.
9. Iron deficiency—United States, 1999-2000, *MMWR Morb Mortal Wkly Rep* 51(40):897-899, Oct 11, 2002.

10. Grantham-McGregor S, Ani C: A review of studies on the effect of iron deficiency on cognitive development in children, *J Nutr* 131:649S-666S, 2001.

11. Kreipe RE: Bones of today, bones of tomorrow, *Am J Dis Child* 146:22-25, 1992 (editorial).

12. Committee on Nutrition, American Academy of Pediatrics: Policy statement on calcium requirements of infants, children, and adolescents (RE9904*), Pediatrics* 104(5):1152-1157, 1999.

13. Keller J, Lanou A, Barnard N: The consumer cost of calcium from food and supplements, *J Am Diet Assoc* 102:1669-1671, Nov 2002.

14. O'Dell SN et al: Hypovitaminosis D prevalence and determinants among African American and white women of reproductive age: third National Health and Nutrition Examination Survey, 1988-1994, *Am J Clin Nutr* 76:187-192, July 2002.

15. Neurologic impairment in children associated with maternal dietary deficiency of cobalamin—Georgia, 2001, *MMWR Morb Mortal Wkly Rep* 52(4):61-64, Jan 31, 2003.

16. Rolls B, Morris E, Roe L: Portion size of food affects energy intake in normal-weight and overweight men and women, *Am J Clin Nutr* 76:1207-1213, 2002.

17. Neumark-Sztainer D et al: Overweight status and eating patterns among adolescents: where do youths stand in comparison with the *Healthy People 2010* objectives? *Am J Public Health* 92(5):844-851, 2002.

18. Schwimmer JB, Burwinkle TM, Varni JW: Health-related quality of life of severely obese children and adolescents, *JAMA* 289(14):1813-1819, 2003.

19. Sinha R et al: Prevalence of impaired glucose tolerance among children and adolescents with marked obesity [erratum in *N Engl J Med* 346(22):1756, 2002], *N Engl J Med* 346(11):802-810, 2002.

20. Ackard DM et al: Overeating among adolescents: prevalence and associations with weight-related characteristics and psychological health, *Pediatrics* 111(1):67-74, 2003.

21. Sturm R: The effects of obesity, smoking, and drinking on medical problems and costs: obesity outranks both smoking and drinking in its deleterious effects on health and health costs, *Health Aff (Millwood)* 21:245-253, 2002.

22. Fontaine K et al: Years of life lost due to obesity, *JAMA* 289:187-193, 2003.

23. Brown JK, Witherspoon EM: The mass media and American adolescents' health, *J Adolesc Health* 31(6 suppl):153-170, 2002.

24. Aaron DJ et al: Longitudinal study of the number and choice of leisure time physical activities from mid to late adolescence: implications for school curricula and community recreation programs, *Arch Pediatr Adolesc Med* 156(11):1075-1080, 2002.

25. Crespo CJ et al: Television watching, energy intake, and obesity in U.S. children: results from the third National Health and Nutrition Examination Survey, 1988-1994, *Arch Pediatr Adolesc Med* 155(3):360-365, 2001.

26. Story M, Faulkner P: The prime time diet: a content analysis of eating and food messages in television content and commercials, *Am J Public Health* 80:738-740, 1990.

27. Taras HL, Gage M: Advertised foods on children's television, *Arch Pediatr Adolesc Med* 149:649-652, 1995.

28. Faine MP: Recognition and management of eating disorders in the dental office, *Dent Clin North Am* 47(2):395-410, 2003.

29. Woodside D et al: Personality, perfectionism, and attitudes toward eating in parents of individuals with eating disorders, *Int J Eat Disord* 31:290-299, 2002.

30. American Psychiatric Association: *Diagnostic and statistical manual for mental disorders,* 4th ed, Washington, DC, 2000, The Association.

31. Ackard D, Neumark-Sztainer D: Family mealtime while growing up: associations with symptoms of bulimia nervosa, *Eat Disord* 9:239, 2001.

32. Rome ES et al: Children and adolescents with eating disorders: the state of the art, *Pediatrics* 111(1):e98-e108, 2003.

33. Caballero B: Early nutrition and risk of disease in the adult, *Public Health Nutr* 4(6a):1335-1336, 2001.

34. WHO Working Group on the Growth Reference Protocol and WHO Task Force on Methods for the Natural Regulation of Fertility: Growth of healthy infants and the timing, type and frequency of complementary foods, *Am J Clin Nutr* 76:620-627, 2002.

35. Makrides M et al: Nutritional effect of including egg yolk in the weaning diet of breast-fed and formula-fed infants: a randomized controlled trial, *Am J Clin Nutr* 75:1084-1092, 2002.

36. Reddan J, Wahlstrom K, Reicks M: Children's perceived benefits and barriers in relation to eating breakfast in schools with or without Universal School Breakfast, *J Nutr Educ Behav* 34(1):47-52, 2002.

37. Beals K: Eating behaviors, nutritional status, and menstrual function in elite female adolescent volleyball players, *J Am Diet Assoc* 102(9):1293-1296, Sep 2002.

38. Waldman HB: Do your pediatric patients drink alcohol? Are they heavy or binge drinkers? *J Dent Child* 65:194-197, 1998.

SUGGESTED READING

US Department of Health and Human Services, Centers for Disease Control and Prevention, *Natl Vital Stat Rep* 50(16), 2002.

13

Local Anesthesia and Pain Control for the Child and Adolescent

RALPH E. McDONALD

DAVID R. AVERY

JEFFREY A. DEAN

It is generally agreed that one of the most important aspects of child behavior guidance is the control of pain. If children experience pain during restorative or surgical procedures, their future as dental patients may be damaged. Therefore it is important at each visit to reduce discomfort to a minimum and to control painful situations. There are many pharmacologic pain control strategies to help children cope with these situations, both preoperatively and postoperatively. Most of these strategies involve the use of local anesthetics and/or analgesics.

Because there is usually some discomfort associated with the procedure, use of a local anesthetic is generally indicated when operative work is to be performed on the permanent teeth, and the same is true of cavity preparations in primary teeth. Dental procedures can be carried out more effectively if the child is comfortable and free of pain. The local anesthetic can prevent discomfort that may be associated with placing a rubber dam clamp, ligating teeth, and cutting tooth structure. Even the youngest child treated in the dental office normally presents no contraindications for the use of a local anesthetic.

Investigators have found that injection is the dental procedure that produces the greatest negative response in children. Responses become increasingly negative over a series of four or five injections. Venham and Quatrocelli[1] have reported that a series of dental visits sensitized children to the stressful injection procedure while reducing their apprehension toward relatively nonstressful procedures. Thus dentists should anticipate the need for continued efforts to help the child cope with dental injections.

TOPICAL ANESTHETICS

Topical anesthetics reduce the slight discomfort that may be associated with the insertion of the needle before the injection of the local anesthetic. Some topical anesthetics, however, present a disadvantage if they have a disagreeable taste to the child. Also, the additional time required to apply them may allow the child to become apprehensive concerning the approaching procedure.

Topical anesthetics are available in gel, liquid, ointment, and pressurized spray forms. However, the pleasant-tasting and quick-acting liquid, gel, or ointment preparations seem to be preferred by most dentists. These agents are applied to the oral mucous membranes with a cotton-tipped applicator. A variety of anesthetic agents have been used in topical anesthetic preparations, including ethyl aminobenzoate, butacaine sulfate, cocaine, dyclonine, lidocaine, and tetracaine.

Ethyl aminobenzoate (benzocaine) liquid, ointment, or gel preparations are probably best suited for topical

anesthesia in dentistry. They offer a more rapid onset and longer duration of anesthesia than other topical agents. They are not known to produce systemic toxicity as oral topical anesthetics, but a few localized allergic reactions have been reported from prolonged or repeated use. Examples of commercially available products are Hurricaine,[*] Topicale,[†] and Gingicaine.[‡] All three products are available in gel form. Gingicaine is also available in liquid and spray forms, and Hurricaine is available as a liquid. Topicale is available in ointment form.

The mucosa at the site of the intended needle insertion is dried with gauze, and a small amount of the topical anesthetic agent is applied to the tissue with a cotton swab. Topical anesthesia should be produced in approximately 30 seconds.

During the application of the topical anesthetic, the dentist should prepare the child for the injection. The explanation should not necessarily be a detailed description but simply an indication that the tooth is going to be put to sleep so that the treatment can proceed without discomfort.

A more recently developed product for achieving topical anesthesia is known as DentiPatch[§] (lidocaine transoral delivery system). This system seems to be designed primarily for situations in which superficial oral tissue anesthesia is desired for several minutes rather than the shorter time required for local anesthetic injections. The use of this product has not yet been shown to be convenient or efficacious in young children.

JET INJECTION

The jet injection instrument is based on the principle that small quantities of liquids forced through very small openings under high pressure can penetrate mucous membrane or skin without causing excessive tissue trauma. One jet injection device, the Syrijet Mark II,[‖] holds a standard 1.8-ml cartridge of local anesthetic solution. It can be adjusted to expel 0.05 to 0.2 ml of solution under 2000 psi pressure.

Jet injection produces surface anesthesia instantly and is used by some dentists instead of topical anesthetics. The method is quick and essentially painless, though the abruptness of the injection may produce momentary anxiety. This technique is also useful for obtaining gingival anesthesia before a rubber dam clamp is placed for isolation procedures that otherwise do not require local anesthetic. Similarly, soft tissue anesthesia may be obtained before band adaptation of

*Beutlich L.P. Pharmaceuticals, Inc., Chicago, Ill.
†Premier Dental Products, Inc., Plymouth Meeting, Penn.
‡Gingi-Pak, Inc., Camarillo, Calif.
§Noven Pharmaceuticals, Inc., Miami, Fla.
‖Mizzy, Inc., Cherry Hill, N.J.

partially erupted molars or for the removal of a very loose (soft tissue–retained) primary tooth. O'Toole has reported that the Syrijet may be employed in place of needle injections for nasopalatine, anterior palatine, and long buccal nerve blocks.[2]

A more recently developed jet injection device reported by Duckworth et al delivers a dose of dry powdered anesthetic to the oral mucosa.[3] In this study, an initial trial with 14 adult subjects, successful topical analgesia without tissue damage was reported. Of course, more clinical trials are required before substantial claims can be made regarding how efficacious the technique is and whether its routine use for topical anesthesia is warranted.

LOCAL ANESTHESIA BY CONVENTIONAL INJECTION

Wittrock and Fischer[4] and later Trapp and Davies[5] demonstrated that human blood can be readily aspirated with the smaller-gauge needles. Trapp and Davies reported positive aspiration through 23-, 25-, 27-, and 30-gauge needles without a clinically significant difference in resistance to flow. Malamed recommends the use of larger-gauge needles (i.e., 25 gauge) for injection into highly vascular areas or areas where needle deflection through soft tissue may be a factor.[6] Regardless of the size of the needle used, it is generally agreed that the anesthetic solution should be injected slowly and that the dentist should watch the patient closely for any evidence of an unexpected reaction.

The injections that are most commonly used in the treatment of children are described in the following sections.

ANESTHETIZATION OF MANDIBULAR TEETH AND SOFT TISSUE

INFERIOR ALVEOLAR NERVE BLOCK (CONVENTIONAL MANDIBULAR BLOCK)

When deep operative or surgical procedures are undertaken for the mandibular primary or permanent teeth, the inferior alveolar nerve must be blocked. The supraperiosteal injection technique may sometimes be useful in anesthetizing primary incisors, but it is not as reliable for complete anesthesia of the mandibular primary or permanent molars.

Olsen reported that the mandibular foramen is situated at a level lower than the occlusal plane of the primary teeth of the pediatric patient.[7] Therefore the injection must be made slightly lower and more posteriorly than for an adult patient. An accepted technique is one in which the thumb is laid on the occlusal surface of the molars, with the tip of the thumb resting on the internal oblique ridge and the ball of the thumb resting

in the retromolar fossa. Firm support during the injection procedure can be given when the ball of the middle finger is resting on the posterior border of the mandible. The barrel of the syringe should be directed on a plane between the two primary molars on the opposite side of the arch. It is advisable to inject a small amount of the solution as soon as the tissue is penetrated and to continue to inject minute quantities as the needle is directed toward the mandibular foramen.

The depth of insertion averages about 15 mm but varies with the size of the mandible and its changing proportions depending on the age of the patient. Approximately 1 ml of the solution should be deposited around the inferior alveolar nerve (Figs. 13-1 and 13-2).

LINGUAL NERVE BLOCK

One can block the lingual nerve by bringing the syringe to the opposite side with the injection of a small quantity of the solution as the needle is withdrawn. If small amounts of anesthetic are injected during insertion and withdrawal of the needle for the inferior alveolar nerve block, the lingual nerve will invariably be anesthetized as well.

LONG BUCCAL NERVE BLOCK

For the removal of mandibular permanent molars or sometimes for the placement of a rubber dam clamp on these teeth, it is necessary to anesthetize the long buccal nerve. A small quantity of the solution may be deposited in the mucobuccal fold at a point distal and buccal to the indicated tooth (Fig. 13-3).

All facial mandibular gingival tissue on the side that has been injected will be anesthetized for operative procedures, with the possible exception of the tissue facial to the central and lateral incisors, which may receive

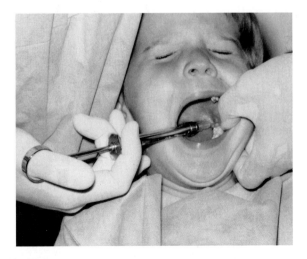

FIG. **13-1.** The mandible is supported by the thumb and middle finger, while the needle is directed toward the inferior alveolar nerve.

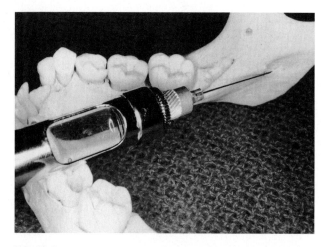

FIG. **13-2.** Anesthetic solution is deposited around the inferior alveolar nerve.

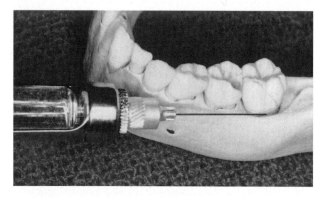

FIG. **13-3.** In anesthetizing the long buccal nerve, a small quantity of the solution may be deposited in the mucobuccal fold adjacent to the first permanent molar.

innervation from overlapping nerve fibers from the opposite side.

INFILTRATION ANESTHESIA FOR MANDIBULAR PRIMARY MOLARS

Wright et al have studied the effectiveness of injecting local anesthetic solution in the mucobuccal fold between the roots of primary mandibular molars.[8] Based on observational data, little or no pain was experienced by 65% of the children during cavity preparation. It was also noted that children who demonstrate comfort at the time of injection are likely to exhibit no pain during successive procedures.

Oulis, Vadiakas, and Vasilopoulou,[9] as well as Sharaf,[10] reported very similar studies comparing the effectiveness of mandibular infiltration anesthesia to mandibular block anesthesia in children 3 to 9 years of age for restorative pulpotomy and extraction therapies in primary mandibular molars. Eighty-nine and 80 children, respectively, were included in their studies. Oulis, Vadiakas, and Vasilopoulou found that

the two anesthesia techniques were equally effective for restorative procedures, but the mandibular infiltration technique was less effective than mandibular block for extraction and pulpotomy.[9] Sharaf reported that the infiltration anesthesia was as effective as block anesthesia for all the performed therapies except for pulpotomy in mandibular second primary molars.[10] From these reports, one may infer that mandibular block anesthesia produces more profound anesthesia of mandibular primary molars, but infiltration may produce adequate anesthesia in mandibular primary molars for most restorative procedures.

INFILTRATION FOR MANDIBULAR INCISORS

The terminal ends of the inferior alveolar nerves cross over the mandibular midline slightly and provide conjoined innervation of the mandibular incisors. Therefore a single inferior alveolar nerve block may not be adequate for operative or surgical procedures on the incisors, even on the side of the block anesthesia. The labial cortical bone overlying the mandibular incisors is usually thin enough for supraperiosteal anesthesia techniques to be effective.

If only superficial caries excavation of mandibular incisors is needed or if the removal of a partially exfoliated primary incisor is planned, infiltration anesthesia alone may be adequate. Incisor infiltration is most useful as an adjunct to an inferior alveolar nerve block when total anesthesia of the quadrant is desired. In this case the infiltration injection is made close to the midline on the side of the block anesthesia, but the solution is deposited labial to the incisors on the opposite side of the midline. For example, if block anesthesia is used for the mandibular right quadrant, anesthetic solution is infiltrated over the left mandibular incisors by insertion of the needle just to the right of the midline diagonally toward the left incisors.

MANDIBULAR CONDUCTION ANESTHESIA (GOW-GATES MANDIBULAR BLOCK TECHNIQUE)

In 1973 Gow-Gates introduced a new method of obtaining mandibular anesthesia, which he referred to as *mandibular conduction anesthesia*.[11] This approach uses external anatomic landmarks to align the needle so that anesthetic solution is deposited at the base of the neck of the mandibular condyle. This technique is a nerve block procedure that anesthetizes virtually the entire distribution of the fifth cranial nerve in the mandibular area, including the inferior alveolar, lingual, buccal, mental, incisive, auriculotemporal, and mylohyoid nerves. Thus with a single injection the entire right or left half of the mandibular teeth and soft tissues can be anesthetized, except possibly the mandibular incisors, which may receive partial innervation from the incisive nerves of the opposite side. Gow-Gates suggested that, once the

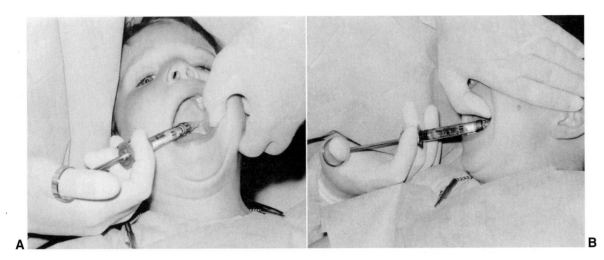

FIG. **13-4. A,** Injection site for the Gow-Gates mandibular block technique. **B,** Barrel of the syringe is aligned with a line from the corner of the mouth to the intertragic notch.

technique is learned properly, it rarely fails to produce good mandibular anesthesia.[11] He had used the technique in practice more than 50,000 times. The technique has become increasingly popular and is often referred to as the *Gow-Gates technique.*

The external landmarks to help align the needle for this injection are the tragus of the ear and the corner of the mouth. The needle is inserted just medial to the tendon of the temporal muscle and considerably superior to the insertion point for conventional mandibular block anesthesia. The needle is also inclined upward and parallel to a line from the corner of the patient's mouth to the lower border of the tragus (intertragic notch). The needle and the barrel of the syringe should be directed toward the injection site from the corner of the mouth on the opposite side (Fig. 13-4).

ANESTHETIZATION OF MAXILLARY PRIMARY AND PERMANENT INCISORS AND CANINES

SUPRAPERIOSTEAL TECHNIQUE (LOCAL INFILTRATION)

Local infiltration (supraperiosteal technique) is used to anesthetize the primary anterior teeth. The injection should be made closer to the gingival margin than in the patient with permanent teeth, and the solution should be deposited close to the bone. After the needle tip has penetrated the soft tissue at the mucobuccal fold, it needs little advancement before the solution is deposited (2 mm at most) because the apices of the maxillary primary anterior teeth are essentially at the level of the mucobuccal fold. Some dentists prefer to pull the upper lip down over the needle tip to penetrate the tissue rather than advancing the needle upward. This approach works quite well for the maxillary anterior region (Figs. 13-5 to 13-7).

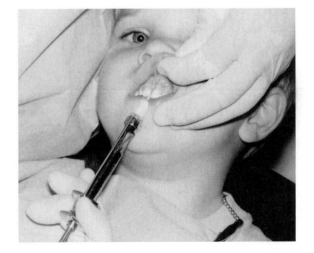

FIG. **13-5.** Anesthetizing a primary central incisor. The supraperiosteal injection should be close to the bone and adjacent to the apex of the tooth.

In anesthetizing of the permanent central incisor teeth the puncture site is at the mucobuccal fold, so that the solution may be deposited slowly and slightly above and close to the apex of the tooth. Because nerve fibers may be extending from the opposite side, it may be necessary to deposit a small amount of the anesthetic solution adjacent to the apex of the other central incisor to obtain adequate anesthesia in either primary or permanent teeth. If a rubber dam is to be applied, it is advisable to inject a drop or two of anesthetic solution into the lingual free marginal tissue to prevent the discomfort associated with the placement of the rubber dam clamp and ligatures.

Before extraction of the incisors or canines in either the primary or permanent dentition, it will be necessary to anesthetize the palatal soft tissues. The nasopalatine injection provides adequate anesthesia for the palatal

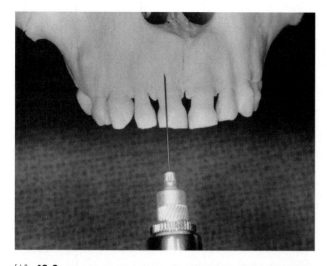

FIG. **13-6.** Needle point is opposite the apex of the maxillary primary incisor.

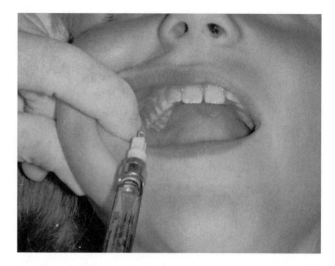

FIG. **13-8.** Injection of the anesthetic solution to anesthetize the maxillary first primary molar for operative procedures.

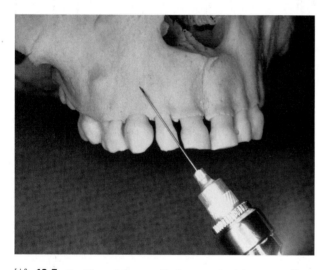

FIG. **13-7.** Position of the needle for anesthetizing a maxillary primary canine.

tissues of all four incisors and at least partial anesthesia of the canine areas. Nerve fibers from the greater (anterior) palatine nerve usually extend to the canine area as well. If only a single anterior tooth is to be removed, adequate palatal anesthesia may also be obtained when anesthetic solution is deposited in the attached palatal gingiva adjacent to the tooth to be removed. If it is observed that the patient does not have profound anesthesia of anterior teeth during the operative procedures with the supraperiosteal technique, a nasopalatine injection is advisable.

ANESTHETIZATION OF MAXILLARY PRIMARY MOLARS AND PREMOLARS

Traditionally, dentists have been taught that the middle superior alveolar nerve supplies the maxillary primary molars, the premolars, and the mesiobuccal root of the first permanent molar. There is no doubt that the middle superior alveolar nerve is at least partially responsible for the innervation of these teeth. However, Jorgensen and Hayden have demonstrated plexus formation of the middle and posterior superior alveolar nerves in the primary molar area on child cadaver dissections.[12] The role of the posterior superior alveolar nerve in innervating the primary molar area has not previously received adequate attention. In addition, Jorgensen and Hayden have demonstrated maxillary bone thickness approaching 1 cm overlying the buccal roots of the first permanent and second primary molars in the skulls of children.[12]

The bone overlying the first primary molar is thin, and this tooth can be adequately anesthetized by injection of anesthetic solution opposite the apices of the roots (Figs. 13-8 and 13-9). However, the thick zygomatic process overlies the buccal roots of the second primary and first permanent molars in the primary and early mixed dentition. This thickness of bone renders the supraperiosteal injection at the apices of the roots of the second primary molar much less effective; the injection should be supplemented with a second injection superior to the maxillary tuberosity area to block the posterior superior alveolar nerve as has been traditionally taught for permanent molars (Figs. 13-10 and 13-11). This supplemental injection helps compensate for the additional bone thickness and the posterior middle superior alveolar nerve plexus in the area of the second primary molar, which compromise the anesthesia obtained by injection at the apices only.

To anesthetize the maxillary first or second premolar, a single injection is made at the mucobuccal fold to allow the solution to be deposited slightly above the apex of the tooth. Because of the horizontal and vertical

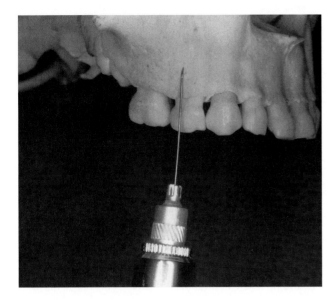

FIG. **13-9.** Anesthetic solution is injected opposite the apices of the buccal roots of the first primary molar.

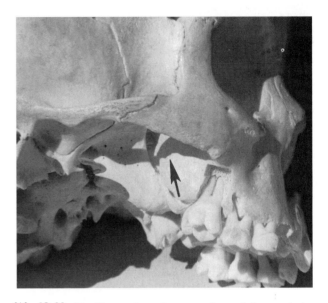

FIG. **13-11.** Maxillary tuberosity area *(arrow)* for posterior superior alveolar injection. *(Courtesy Dr. Paul E. Starkey.)*

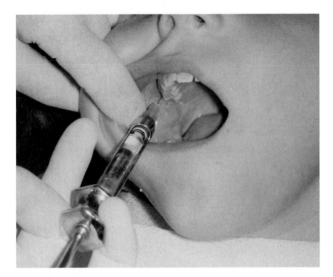

FIG. **13-10.** Posterior superior alveolar injection for maxillary permanent molars and second primary molar.

growth of the maxilla that has occurred by the time the premolars erupt, the buccal cortical bone overlying their roots is thin enough to permit good anesthesia with this method. The injection should be made slowly, and the solution should be deposited close to the bone; these recommendations hold true for all supraperiosteal and block anesthesia techniques in dentistry.

Before operative procedures for maxillary primary molars and maxillary premolars, the appropriate injection technique(s) for the buccal tissues, as just described, should be performed. If the rubber dam clamp impinges on the palatal tissue, injection of a drop or two of the anesthetic solution into the free marginal tissue lingual to the clamped tooth will alleviate the discomfort and

will be less painful than the true greater (anterior) palatine injection. The greater palatine injection is indicated if maxillary primary molars or premolars are to be extracted or if palatal tissue surgery is planned.

ANESTHETIZATION OF MAXILLARY PERMANENT MOLARS

To anesthetize the maxillary first or second permanent molars, the dentist instructs the child to partially close the mouth to allow the cheek and lips to be stretched laterally. The tip of the dentist's left forefinger (for a right-handed dentist) will rest in a concavity in the mucobuccal fold and is rotated to allow the fingernail to be adjacent to the mucosa. The ball of the finger is in contact with the posterior surface of the zygomatic process. Bennett suggests that the finger be on a plane at right angles to the occlusal surfaces of the maxillary teeth and at a 45-degree angle to the patient's sagittal plane.[13] The index finger should point in the direction of the needle during the injection. The puncture point is in the mucobuccal fold above and distal to the distobuccal root of the first permanent molar. If the second molar has erupted, the injection should be made above the second molar. The needle is advanced upward and distally, depositing the solution over the apices of the teeth. The needle is inserted for a distance of approximately ³/₄ inch (2 cm) in a posterior and upward direction; it should be positioned close to the bone, with the bevel toward the bone (see Figs. 13-10 and 13-11).

To complete the anesthesia of the first permanent molar for operative procedures, the supraperiosteal injection is made by insertion of the needle in the mucobuccal fold and deposition of the solution at the apex of the mesiobuccal root of the molar.

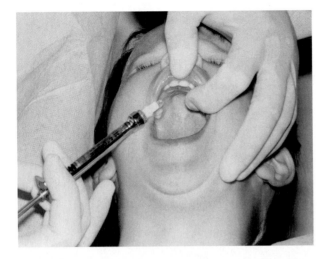

FIG. **13-12.** Blocking of the nasopalatine nerve may be accomplished by injecting alongside the incisive papilla.

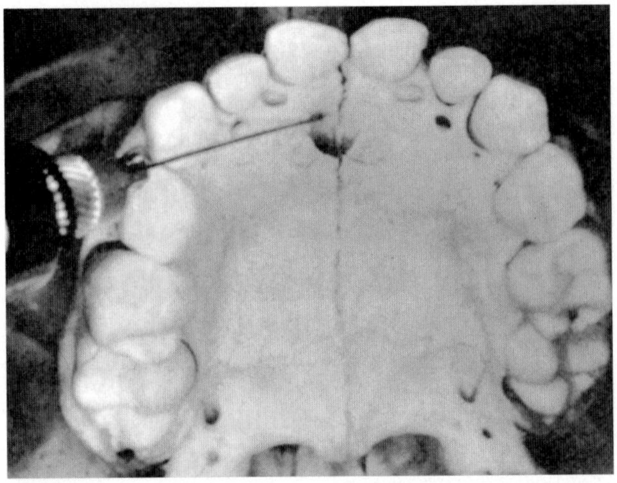

FIG. **13-13.** The needle is directed upward into the incisive canal when anesthetizing the nasopalatine nerve.

ANESTHETIZATION OF THE PALATAL TISSUES

Anesthesia of the palatal tissues can be one of the more exquisitely painful procedures performed in dentistry. Ramirez, Lee, and Takara discuss methods for achieving profound anesthesia with minimal pain in the palatal and lingual aspects.[14] After buccal infiltration, they suggest interdental (interpapillary) infiltration, with slow injection of the anesthetic solution as the needle is penetrating the papilla. The interdental infiltration allows diffusion of the anesthetic to the palatal aspect via the craterlike area of the interproximal oral mucosa joining the lingual and buccal interdental papillae, known as the col. Blanching of the area is indicative of sufficient anesthesia of the superficial soft tissues; however, additional palatal infiltration may be given as needed.

NASOPALATINE NERVE BLOCK

Blocking the nasopalatine nerve will anesthetize the palatal tissues of the six anterior teeth. If the needle is carried into the canal, it is possible to anesthetize the six anterior teeth completely. However, this technique is painful and is not routinely used before operative procedures. If the patient experiences incomplete anesthesia after supraperiosteal injection above the apices of the anterior teeth on the labial side, it may be necessary to resort to the nasopalatine injection. The path of insertion of the needle is alongside the incisive papilla, just posterior to the central incisors. The needle is directed upward into the incisive canal (Figs. 13-12 and 13-13). The discomfort associated with the injection can be reduced by deposition of the anesthetic solution in advance of the needle. When anesthesia of the canine

area is required, it may be necessary to inject a small amount of anesthetic solution into the gingival tissue adjacent to the lingual aspect of the canine to anesthetize overlapping branches of the greater palatine nerve.

GREATER (ANTERIOR) PALATINE INJECTION

The greater palatine injection will anesthetize the mucoperiosteum of the palate from the tuberosity to the canine region and from the median line to the gingival crest on the injected side. This injection is used with the middle or posterior alveolar nerve block before surgical procedures. The innervation of the soft tissues of the posterior two thirds of the palate is derived from the greater and lesser palatine nerves.

Before the injection is made, it is helpful to bisect an imaginary line drawn from the gingival border of the most posterior molar that has erupted to the midline. Approaching from the opposite side of the mouth, the dentist makes the injection along this imaginary line and distal to the last tooth (Figs. 13-14 and 13-15). In the child in whom only the primary dentition has erupted, the injection should be made approximately 10 mm posterior to the distal surface of the second primary molar. It is not necessary to enter the greater palatine foramen. A few drops of the solution should be injected slowly at the point where the nerve emerges from the foramen.

SUPPLEMENTAL INJECTION TECHNIQUES

INFRAORBITAL NERVE BLOCK AND MENTAL NERVE BLOCK

The infraorbital nerve block and the mental nerve block are two additional local anesthetic techniques used by many dentists. The infraorbital nerve block anesthetizes

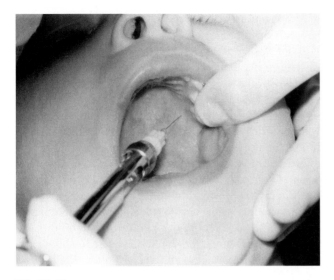

FIG. **13-14.** Greater palatine injection is used in conjunction with the middle or posterior alveolar nerve block before removal of a maxillary primary molar.

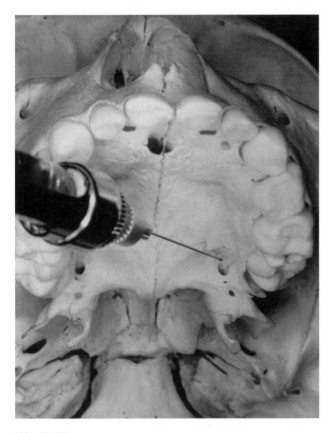

FIG. **13-15.** The needle is inserted approximately 10 mm posterior to the distal surface of the second primary molar.

the branches of the anterior and middle superior alveolar nerves. It also affects innervation of the soft tissues below the eye, half of the nose, and the oral musculature of the upper lip on the injected side of the face. This leaves the child with a feeling of numbness above the

mouth similar to that below the mouth when an inferior alveolar nerve is blocked. In addition, there is temporary partial oral paralysis. These effects do not contraindicate use of the technique when it is truly needed. However, we find its use difficult to justify in routine operative and extraction procedures for teeth innervated by the anterior and middle superior alveolar nerves, since the supraperiosteal techniques are more localized and just as effective. The infraorbital block technique is preferred when impacted teeth (especially canines or first premolars) or large cysts are to be removed, when moderate inflammation or infection contraindicates use of the supraperiosteal injection site, or when longer duration or a greater area of anesthesia is needed.

The mental nerve block leaves the patient with essentially the same feelings of numbness as the inferior alveolar nerve block. Blocking the mental nerve anesthetizes all mandibular teeth in the quadrant except the permanent molars. Thus the mental nerve block makes it possible to perform routine operative procedures on all primary teeth without discomfort to the patient. However, we believe that the inferior alveolar nerve block should be favored unless there is a specific contraindication to its use at the inferior alveolar nerve injection site. The mental nerve block is no more comfortable for the patient, and the technique puts the syringe in clear view of the patient, whereas the inferior alveolar nerve block may be performed with the syringe out of the child's direct vision.

The reader is referred to the textbooks by Jorgensen and Hayden[12] and by Malamed[6] listed at the end of this chapter for more detailed information concerning the infraorbital block, the mental block, and other local anesthetic techniques.

PERIODONTAL LIGAMENT INJECTION (INTRALIGAMENTARY INJECTION)

The periodontal ligament injection has been used for many years as an adjunctive method of obtaining more complete anesthesia when supraperiosteal or block techniques failed to provide adequate anesthesia. This technique has also gained credibility as a good method of obtaining primary anesthesia for one or two teeth.

The technique is simple, requires only small quantities of anesthetic solution, and produces anesthesia almost instantly. The needle is placed in the gingival sulcus, usually on the mesial surface, and advanced along the root surface until resistance is met. Then approximately 0.2 ml of anesthetic is deposited into the periodontal ligament. For multirooted teeth, injections are made both mesially and distally. Considerable pressure is necessary to express the anesthetic solution.

A conventional dental syringe may be used for this technique. However, the great pressure required to express the anesthetic makes it desirable to use a syringe with a closed barrel to offer protection in the unlikely event that the anesthetic cartridge should break. Some syringes are equipped with a metal or Teflon sleeve that encloses the cartridge and provides the necessary protection should breakage occur.

Syringes designed specifically for the periodontal ligament injection technique have been developed. One syringe, the Peri-Press,* is designed with a lever-action "trigger" that enables the dentist to deliver the necessary injection pressure conveniently. The Peri-Press syringe has a solid metal barrel and is calibrated to deliver 0.14 ml of anesthetic solution each time the trigger is completely activated.

There are some possible psychologic disadvantages to use of the periodontal ligament injection technique, especially for the inexperienced pediatric patient. The technique provides the patient with an opportunity to see the syringe and to watch the administration of the anesthetic. This may not be a significant problem for the experienced, well-adjusted dental patient, but it may contribute to the anxiety reaction of the new or anxiety-prone patient. In addition, the very design of the Peri-Press (which resembles a handgun) probably has some adverse psychologic effects.

There are two types of syringes designed specifically for intraligamentary injections. One is gunlike and the other is penlike. They both have the additional disadvantage of being quite expensive compared to a good, conventional aspirating syringes. The penlike syringe would be preferred in pediatric dentistry, but unfortunately it is even more expensive than the gunlike instrument.

Nevertheless, the periodontal ligament injection technique seems to offer a valuable adjunctive method of achieving dental anesthesia.

Malamed has reported a clinical study in which impressive results were obtained for certain procedures when the periodontal ligament injection technique was used.[15] The sample size was small for some procedures, and he pointed out that additional research was warranted. However, seven periodontal procedures (curettage and root planing) were performed with 100% effective anesthesia, and two teeth were extracted with 100% effective anesthesia (injections were administered to the mesial, distal, buccal, and lingual areas for these procedures). Seventy-one routine restorative procedures were performed under periodontal ligament anesthesia, with 91.5% effectiveness. The technique proved 66.6% effective for crown preparation procedures on 12 teeth, and for eight endodontic procedures adequate

*University Dental Implements, Fanwood, N.J.

anesthetization was achieved only 50% of the time. Several different anesthetics were used, with and without vasoconstrictors, yet there seemed to be little difference in success rates or duration of pulpal anesthesia with the various agents. Because of the confined space and the limited blood circulation at the injection site for the periodontal ligament technique, the use of vasoconstrictors as an additive to the anesthetic solution may not be warranted. In fact, vasoconstrictors might conceivably contribute to ischemia of the periodontal ligament, which could at least add to localized postoperative discomfort or possibly cause more serious damage to the periodontal ligament. Walton and Abbott have also reported a clinical evaluation of the technique that showed a 92% success rate.[16]

The periodontal ligament injection offers the following advantages for either primary or adjunctive anesthesia:

1. It provides reliable pain control rapidly and easily.
2. It provides pulpal anesthesia for 30 to 45 minutes, long enough for many single-tooth procedures without an extended period of postoperative anesthesia.
3. It is no more uncomfortable than other local anesthesia techniques.
4. It is completely painless if used adjunctively.
5. It requires very small quantities of anesthetic solution.
6. It does not require aspiration before injection.
7. It may be performed without removal of the rubber dam.
8. It may be useful in patients with bleeding disorders that contraindicate use of other injections.
9. It may be useful in young or disabled patients in whom the possibility of postoperative trauma to the lips or tongue is a concern.

INTRAOSSEOUS INJECTION, INTERSEPTAL INJECTION, AND INTRAPULPAL INJECTION

Intraosseous, interseptal, and intrapulpal injection techniques have been known for many years, but they have recently received renewed attention. The intrapulpal injection is an adjunctive anesthesia technique designed to obtain profound pulpal anesthesia during direct pulp therapy when other local anesthesia attempts have failed. The intrapulpal injection often provides the desired anesthesia, but the technique has the disadvantage of being painful initially, although the onset of anesthesia is usually rapid.

Intraosseous injection techniques (of which the interseptal injection is one type) require the deposition of local anesthetic solution in the porous alveolar bone. One may do this by forcing a needle through the cortical plate and into the cancellous alveolar bone, or a small,

TABLE 13-1 Maximum Recommended Doses of Local Anesthetics

DRUG	PROPRIETARY NAME	PERCENT OF LOCAL ANESTHETIC	VASOCONSTRICTOR	DURATION OF ANESTHETIC	MAXIMUM RECOMMENDED DOSE (MALAMED)
Lidocaine	Xylocaine	2	Epinephrine 1:100,000	Pulpal: 60 min Soft tissue: 3-5 hr	4.4 mg/kg
Mepivacaine	Carbocaine	3	—	Pulpal: 20-40 min Soft tissue: 2-3 hr	4.4 mg/kg
Prilocaine	Citanest Forte	4	Epinephrine 1:200,000	Pulpal: 60-90 min Soft tissue: 3-8 hr	6.0 mg/kg
Bupivacaine	Marcaine HCl	0.5	Epinephrine 1:200,000	Pulpal: 90-180 min Soft tissue: 4-9 hr	1.3 mg/kg

Adapted from Malamed SF: *Handbook of local anesthesia*, ed 4, St Louis, 1997, Mosby.

round bur may be used to make an access in the bone for the needle. A small, reinforced intraosseous needle may be used to penetrate the cortical plate more easily. This procedure is not particularly difficult in children because they have less dense cortical bone than adults. The intraosseous techniques have been advocated for both primary anesthesia and adjunctive anesthesia when other local injections have failed to produce adequate anesthesia. These techniques have been reported by Lilienthal to produce profound anesthesia.[17] They do not seem to offer any advantages over the periodontal ligament injection except when use of the latter is contraindicated by infection in the periodontal ligament space.

COMPUTER-CONTROLLED LOCAL ANESTHETIC DELIVERY SYSTEM (WAND)

Reports by Friedman and Hochman[18] and by Krochak and Friedman[19] emphasize the advantages of a computer-controlled local anesthetic delivery system known as the Wand.* The system includes a conventional local anesthetic needle and a disposable, wandlike syringe held by a pen grasp when used for oral local anesthetic injections. A microprocessor with a foot control regulates the delivery of anesthetic solution through the syringe at a precision-metered flow rate, constant pressure, and controlled volume. The system includes an aspiration cycle for use when necessary. Block, infiltration, palatal, and periodontal ligament injections are all reported to be more comfortable for the patient with the Wand than with conventional injection techniques. In a randomized clinical trial comparing the Wand with the traditional anesthetic delivery system, Allen et al demonstrated that use of the Wand led to significantly fewer disruptive behaviors ($p < 0.1$) in preschool-aged children.[20] None of the preschool-aged children exposed to the Wand required restraint during the initial interval while nearly half of the children

receiving a traditional injection required some type of immediate restraint.

COMPLICATIONS AFTER A LOCAL ANESTHETIC

ANESTHETIC TOXICITY

Systemic toxic reactions from the anesthetics are rarely observed in adults. However, young children are more likely to experience toxic reactions because of their lower body weight. Young children are also often sedated with pharmacologic agents before the treatment. The potential for toxic reactions increases when local anesthetics are used in conjunction with sedation medications. Aubuchon found a direct lineal relationship between the number of cartridges of local anesthetic administered and the frequency of severe reactions.[21] It is most important for dentists who treat children to be acutely aware of the maximum recommended dosages of the anesthetic agents they use, because allowable dosages are based on the patient's weight (Table 13-1). For example, the toxic dose of lidocaine would be attained if hardly more than 1½ cartridges (3 ml) of 2% lidocaine with 1:100,000 epinephrine were injected at one time in a patient weighing 14 kg (30 lb). Yet 5½ cartridges of the same anesthetic agent would be required to reach the toxic level in an adolescent patient weighing 46 kg (100 lb).

Because there is the possibility of toxic reaction to local anesthetic in some children, Wilson et al have studied and reported on the clinical effectiveness of 1% and 2% lidocaine.[22] They found that 1% and 2% lidocaine were equally effective when performing minor procedures on primary molars.[22] The 1% lidocaine had a slightly lower effectiveness for major procedures, including pulpotomies and extractions.

TRAUMA TO SOFT TISSUE

Parents of children who receive regional local anesthesia in the dental office should be warned that the soft tissue in the area will be without sensation for a period

*Milestone Scientific, Livingston, N.J.

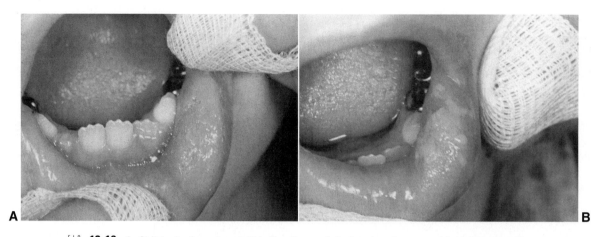

FIG. **13-16. A,** Child who has chewed his lip after an inferior alveolar nerve block for operative procedures. **B,** Twenty-four hours after the initial trauma, a large ulcerated area is evident.

of 1 hour or more. These children should be observed carefully so that they will not purposely or inadvertently bite the tissue. Children who receive an inferior alveolar injection for routine operative procedures may bite the lip, tongue, or inner surface of the cheek. Sometimes a parent calls the dentist's office an hour or two after a dental appointment to report an injury to the child's oral mucous membrane. The parent may wonder if the accident occurred during the dental appointment; in all probability the child has chewed the area, and the result 24 hours later is an ulceration, often termed a *traumatic ulcer* (Fig. 13-16). Complications after a self-inflicted injury of this type are rare. However, the child should be seen in 24 hours, and a warm saline mouth rinse is helpful in keeping the area clean.

In a prospective study, College et al evaluated unilateral versus bilateral mandibular nerve block anesthesia with regard to postoperative soft tissue trauma and other complications in a pediatric population.[23] Their results showed that after unilateral and bilateral blocks, 13% of patients experienced postoperative soft tissue trauma, with the younger patients (less than 4 years of age) experiencing over twice as many problems as the older patients (over 12 years of age). Interestingly, the study showed that, in the group younger than age 4, patients receiving the unilateral nerve blocks had a statistically significantly higher incidence of trauma than the patients receiving the bilateral nerve blocks (35% versus 5%). Although the use of bilateral mandibular nerve blocks has been discouraged in the past, College et al concluded that there is no contraindication to the use of bilateral mandibular block anesthesia in pediatric patients.

ELECTRONIC DENTAL ANESTHESIA

Although an excellent record of effective and safe local anesthesia has been achieved in dentistry and medicine

by injection, it is common knowledge that many children and adults have acquired a significant aversion to any form of therapy requiring injection with a needle. This aversion has prompted the investment of much time, energy, and resources in the search for effective and practical local anesthesia techniques that do not require the use of needles. During the late twentieth century, renewed interest in electronic dental anesthesia (EDA) as a viable alternative to conventional local injections occurred. At least six clinical studies have been completed to evaluate the efficacy of EDA in children.[24-29] In general, these studies show that EDA can produce sufficient oral local anesthesia and analgesia to comfortably allow many invasive dental procedures in children. However, the procedures cannot be performed as efficiently, and the effectiveness of anesthesia is not consistently as reliable as with conventional techniques. Further research on EDA and the refinement of EDA delivery systems are required before EDA can be recommended as a superior substitute for conventional procedures.

ANALGESICS

In addition to local administration of anesthetics to aid in pain control, occasionally systemic administration of analgesics is necessary to help control pain. These analgesics may be needed in instances of moderate to severe pain associated with trauma or infectious processes such as abscessed teeth, or they may be administered preoperatively or postoperatively in association with a dental procedure that may cause pain for the child. The rationale for preoperative administration of analgesics draws on the theory that giving the drug before the procedure provides effective analgesia because it precedes the inflammatory response and subsequent pain incurred during the operative procedure. This theory is not without controversy, however, and there are conflicting reports within the literature as to the efficacy of this technique.

TABLE **13-2** Medications and Dosages for Oral Pediatric Postoperative Pain Management				
MEDICATION	AVAILABILITY	DOSAGE	40-LB CHILD	80-LB CHILD
Acetaminophen	Elixir: 160 mg/5 ml Tablets: 325 mg tab Chewable: 160 mg	10-15 mg/kg/dose given at 4-6 hr intervals	160 mg = 1 tsp 160 mg = 1 chewable	325 mg = 1 tablet 320 mg = 2 chewables
Ibuprofen	Suspension: 100 mg/5 ml Tablets: 200, 300, 400, 600, 800 mg	4-10 mg/kg/dose given at 6-8 hr intervals	100 mg = 1 tsp	200 mg = 2 tsp 200 mg = 1 tablet
Tramadol	Tablets: 50, 100 mg	1-2 mg/kg/dose given at 4-6 hr intervals— maximum 100 mg	25 mg = 1/2 tablet	50 mg = 1 tablet
Codeine and acetaminophen	Suspension: 12 mg/5 ml	0.5-1.0 mg codeine/ kg/dose given at 4-6 hr intervals	12 mg = 1 tsp	24 mg = 2 tsp
Meperidine	Syrup: 50 mg/5 ml Tablets: 50 mg, 100 mg	1-2 mg/kg/dose given at 4-6 hr intervals	25 mg = 1/2 tsp	50 mg = 1 tsp

Adapted from Tate AR, Acs G: *Dent Clin North Am* 46:707-717, 2002.

Tate and Acs suggest that the selection and dosages of analgesics vary because of the change in body weight and composition that occur throughout childhood.[30] Of course, the first choice in most cases is the least potent analgesic with the fewest side effects. Table 13-2, adapted from Tate and Acs, shows common pediatric pain management agents and their appropriate dosage schedules.[30] Tate and Acs suggest that only rarely does the recommended dosage of acetaminophen or nonsteroidal antiinflammatory drugs fail to control the dental pain. In the rare cases in which acetaminophen or nonsteroidal antiinflammatory drugs are not sufficient to manage the pain, the combination of codeine and acetaminophen provides the needed pain relief. Finally, in cases of severe pain in which codeine and acetaminophen are not effective, meperidine may be indicated.

REFERENCES

1. Venham L, Quatrocelli S: The young child's response to repeated dental procedures, *J Dent Res* 56:734-738, 1977.
2. O'Toole TJ: Administration of local anesthesia. In Snawder KD: *Handbook of clinical pedodontics*, St Louis, 1980, Mosby.
3. Duckworth GM et al: Oral PowderJect: a novel system for administering local anaesthesia to the oral mucosa, *Br Dent J* 185:536-539, 1998.
4. Wittrock JW, Fischer WE: The aspiration of blood through small-gauge needles, *J Am Dent Assoc* 76:79-81, 1968.
5. Trapp LD, Davies RO: Aspiration as a function of hypodermic needle internal diameter in the in vivo human upper limb, *Anesth Prog* 27:49-51, 1980.
6. Malamed SF: *Handbook of local anesthesia*, ed 4, St Louis, 1997, Mosby.
7. Olsen NH: Anesthesia for the child patient, *J Am Dent Assoc* 53:548-555, 1956.
8. Wright GZ et al: The effectiveness of infiltration anesthesia in the mandibular molar region, *Pediatr Dent* 13:278-283, 1991.
9. Oulis CJ, Vadiakas GP, Vasilopoulou A: The effectiveness of mandibular infiltration compared to mandibular block anesthesia in treating primary molars in children, *Pediatr Dent* 18:301-305, 1996.
10. Sharaf AA: Evaluation of mandibular infiltration versus block anesthesia in pediatric dentistry, *J Dent Child* 64:276-281, 1997.
11. Gow-Gates GAE: Mandibular conduction anesthesia: a new technique using extraoral landmarks, *Oral Surg* 36:321-328, 1973.
12. Jorgensen NB, Hayden J Jr: *Sedation, local and general anesthesia in dentistry*, ed 3, Philadelphia, 1980, Lea & Febiger.
13. Bennett CR: *Monheim's local anesthesia and pain control in dental practice*, ed 7, St Louis, 1984, Mosby.
14. Ramirez K, Lee JK, Takara JT: Painless pediatric local anesthesia, *Gen Dent* 49(2):174-176, 2001.
15. Malamed SF: The periodontal ligament (PDL) injection: an alternative to inferior alveolar nerve block, *Oral Surg* 53:117-121, 1982.
16. Walton RE, Abbott BJ: Periodontal ligament injection: a clinical evaluation, *J Am Dent Assoc* 103:571-575, 1981.
17. Lilienthal B: A clinical appraisal of intraosseous dental anesthesia, *Oral Surg* 39:692-697, 1975.
18. Friedman MJ, Hochman MN: A 21st century computerized injection system for local pain control, *Compend Contin Educ Dent* 18:995-1000, 1002-1004, 1997.
19. Krochak M, Friedman N: Using a precision-metered injection system to minimize dental injection anxiety, *Compend Contin Educ Dent* 19:137-143, 146-150, 1998.
20. Allen KD et al: Comparison of a computerized anesthesia device with a traditional syringe in preschool children, *Pediatr Dent* 24(4):315-320, 2002.
21. Aubuchon RW: Sedation liabilities in pedodontics, *Pediatr Dent* 4:171-180, 1982.

BOX 14-1   American Society of Anesthesiologists' Physical Status Classification System

P1 A normal healthy patient
P2 A patient with mild systemic disease
P3 A patient with severe systemic disease
P4 A patient with severe systemic disease
P5 A moribund patient who is not expected to survive without the operation
P6 A declared brain-dead patient whose organs are being removed for donor purposes

may actually benefit from this approach, but this must be determined in consultation with the child's physician. Generally, patients categorized into classes III and IV are better managed in a hospital setting.

The medical history should include information regarding the following:

1. Allergies and previous allergic or adverse drug reactions
2. Current medications, including dosage, time, route, and site of administration
3. Diseases or abnormalities in the patient, including pregnancy status of adolescents
4. Previous hospitalizations, including the date, purpose, and hospital course
5. History of general anesthesia or sedation and any associated complication
6. Family history of diseases and anesthetic complications
7. Review of body systems
8. Age in years and months and weight in kilograms

The physical evaluation should include the following:

1. Vital signs, including heart and respiratory rates and blood pressure. If determination of baseline vital signs is prevented by the patient's physical resistance or emotional condition, the reason(s) should be documented.
2. Evaluation of airway patency.
3. ASA classification (see Box 14-1).

INFORMED CONSENT

The parent or legal guardian must be agreeable to the use of conscious sedation for the child. These individuals are entitled to receive complete information regarding the reasonably foreseeable risks and the benefits associated with the particular technique and agents being used, as well as any alternative methods available. Therefore the explanation should be in clear, concise terms that are familiar to them (Fig. 14-2). The consent form can be on or part of a sedation record with space provided for the signatures of all parties.

Because conscious sedation is not considered a routine part of every dental visit, this consent should be separate and distinct from permission to treat the patient.

INSTRUCTIONS TO PARENTS

Information in written form should be reviewed with the person caring for the child and given to this person along with the notice of the scheduled appointment (Fig. 14-3). This information should include a 24-hour contact number for the practitioner.

Dietary instructions should be as follows:

1. No milk or solids for 6 hours for children 6 to 36 months old and for 6 to 8 hours for children 36 months and older
2. Clear liquids up to 3 hours before the procedure for children aged 6 months and older.

The reasons for these recommendations are twofold. First, emesis during or immediately after a sedative procedure is a potential complication that can result in aspiration of stomach contents leading to laryngospasm or severe airway obstruction. Aspiration may even present difficulties later in the form of aspiration pneumonia. At the very least, it creates an unfavorable disruption of the office routine. Second, because most conscious sedation agents are administered by the oral route, drug uptake is maximized when the stomach is empty.

The parent or guardian should also be advised that he or she will be expected to remain in the area of the office during the sedation appointment. With regard to transportation, the instructions should request that a second person accompany the parent so that the person caring for the child may be free to attend to the child's needs during the trip home.

The caregiver should be advised that, on arriving home, the child may sleep for several hours and may be drowsy and irritable for up to 24 hours after the sedation. It is important to stress the need for frequent observation if the child is sleeping, to ensure an open airway. Activity should be restricted to quieter pursuits and closely supervised for the remainder of the day.

Following treatment the child should first be offered clear liquids and may advance to solid foods as tolerated. Once solids are tolerated, there are no dietary restrictions other than those imposed as a result of the dental procedure performed. Nausea and vomiting may occur, especially when narcotics have been used, which may thus prolong the delay before beginning solid food intake. In this event, special attention should be paid to the fluid intake to ensure adequate hydration.

Knowledge on the part of the parent of what to expect is the most reliable way to ensure a calm, comfortable,

**CONSENT FOR THE USE OF SEDATION OR GENERAL ANESTHESIA
FOR
PEDIATRIC DENTAL TREATMENT**

I _____, as the legally responsible parent or guardian of _____, give my consent to the use of local anesthetics, sedative drugs, or general anesthetic agents that Dr(s). _____ may deem necessary on the child's examination chart, as previously explained to me, and any other procedure deemed necessary or advisable as a corollary to the planned treatment for _____, except for: (if none, so state) _____.

I have been informed and understand that occasionally there are complications of the treatment, drugs, or anesthetic agents, including but not limited to: numbness, infection, swelling, bleeding, discoloration, nausea, vomiting, allergic reactions, brain damage, stroke, or heart attack. I further understand and accept that complications may require hospitalization and may even result in death.

Dr(s). _____ discussed with me, to my satisfaction, these complications. I acknowledge the receipt of and understand the preoperative and postoperative instructions. The treatment and sedation or anesthesia procedures have been explained to me, to my satisfaction, along with possible alternative methods and their advantages and disadvantages, risks, consequences, and probable effectiveness of each, as well as the prognosis if no treatment is provided.

I have read this consent and understand, to my satisfaction, the procedures to be performed and accept the possible risks.

Legally responsible parent or guardian: _____ Date: _____

Address: _____

Witness: _____
I certify that I explained the above procedures to the parent or guardian before requesting his or her signature.

_____ Date: _____
Signature of dentist

FIG. **14-2.** Example of form for informed consent. *(Courtesy Dr. Kenneth C. Troutman)*

and uncomplicated postsedation period. Therefore these instructions and recommendations should be in written form and should be reviewed again with the person responsible for the patient and given to this person at the time of discharge from the office (Fig. 14-4).

DOCUMENTATION

Meticulous and accurate documentation of the sedation experience is imperative. In the event of an adverse reaction, the best insurance is an accurate, clear, continuous, documented account of what occurred before, during, and after the encounter.

Preprocedural records should document (1) proper adherence to food and liquid intake restrictions; (2) the preoperative health evaluation, including the patient's health history and a complete physical assessment along with the patient's current weight, age, and baseline vital signs; (3) name and address of the physician who usually cares for the child; (4) a note as to why the particular method of management was chosen; (5) the presence of informed consent; and (6) the delivery of instructions to the caregiver.

Intraoperatively the appropriate vital signs should be recorded as they are assessed (Table 14-2). Timed notations regarding the patient's appearance should be included. The type of drug, the dose given, and the route, site, and time of administration should be clearly indicated. If a prescription is used, either a copy of the prescription or a note as to what was prescribed should also be a part of the permanent record.

INSTRUCTIONS TO FOLLOW BEFORE YOUR CHILD'S SEDATION

EATING AND DRINKING
1. No milk or solid foods 6 hours before the sedation appointment.
2. Clear liquids such as water, clear juices, gelatin, Popsicles, or broth, may be given up to 3 hours before the appointment.
3. Let everyone in the home know the above information, because siblings or others living in the home often unknowingly feed the child.

ACTIVITY
1. Plan the child's sleep and awakening times to encourage the usual amount of sleep the day before the sedation appointment.
2. Please arrive on time for your scheduled appointment. This is a long appointment, and you may be here for several hours.
3. The legal guardian must accompany the child to the sedation appointment.
4. A second responsible adult must join you and your child at the time of discharge. This enables one adult to drive the car while the second adult focuses attention on your child after the treatment is completed. The child should be carefully secured in a car seat belt during transportation.
5. Make sure your child uses the restroom before the sedation.

ACTIVITY AFTER THE SEDATION
1. Your child may take a long nap. He/she may sleep from 3 to 8 hours and may be drowsy and irritable for up to 24 hours after sedation. When your child is asleep, you should be able to awaken him/her easily.
2. Your child may be unsteady when walking or crawling and will need support to protect him/her from injury. An adult must be with the child at all times until the child has returned to his/her usual state of alertness and coordination.
3. Closely supervise any activity for the remainder of the day.

CHANGE IN HEALTH
It is important that you notify the office of the development of a cold, cough, fever, or any illness within 14 days before the sedation appointment. For your child's safety, the sedation may need to be rescheduled.

FIG. **14-3.** Example of presedation instructions to the parent or caregiver.

After completion of treatment, the patient should be continuously observed in an appropriately equipped recovery area. The patient should remain under direct observation until respiratory and cardiovascular stability have been ensured. The patient should not be discharged until the presedation level of consciousness or a level as close as possible for that child has been achieved (Box 14-2). At the time of discharge, the condition of the patient should be noted.

SEDATION TECHNIQUES

A variety of methods are available for producing sedation or alteration of mood in the pediatric patient. These systemic procedures are based on the thoughtful use of various drugs that produce sedation as one of their principal effects, as well as the use of differing routes of administration. Sedative drugs may be administered by inhalation or by oral, rectal, submucosal, intramuscular,

or intravenous routes. The use of combinations of drugs and specific selection of routes of administration to maximize effect and increase safety, as well as maximize patient acceptability, are common. Inhalation of a nitrous oxide–oxygen mixture is often coupled with administration of an agent by any of the other routes.

Another very practical and efficient technique is the timed sequencing of a combination of drugs. The only classification of sedative drugs acceptable for administration preprocedurally outside of the treatment facility is the minor tranquilizers (e.g., diazepam, hydroxyzine). Minor tranquilizers do not include chloral hydrate or narcotics.[2] These agents can be given well before the actual procedure by the parent at home, or on arrival at the office to calm the apprehensive patient. Doing so may aid in the administration of other agents as the procedure begins. This sequencing of drugs may in fact reduce the quantity of subsequently administered

CARE OF YOUR CHILD AFTER SEDATION

Today your child had dental treatment under conscious sedation.

He/she received the following medicine(s) for sedation:

☐ Chloral hydrate   ☐ Meperidine (Demerol)   ☐ Hydroxyzine (Vistaril)
☐ Diazepam (Valium)   ☐ Midazolam   ☐ Other_____

Children repond to sedation in their own way, but the following guidelines will help you know what to expect at home:

GOING HOME
1. Your child will not be able to walk well, so we suggest that you carry your child or use a wheelchair to transport your child to the car.
2. Young children must be restrained in a car safety seat and older children must be restrained with a seat belt during transportation.

ACTIVITY
1. Your child may take a long nap. He/she may sleep from 3 to 8 hours and may be drowsy and irritable for up to 24 hours after sedation. When your child is asleep, you should be able to awaken him/her easily.
2. Your child may be unsteady when walking or crawling and will need support to protect him/her from injury. An ADULT must be with the child at all times until the child has returned to his/her usual state of alertness and coordination.
3. Your child should not perform any potentially dangerous activities, such as riding a bike, playing outside, handling sharp objects, working with tools, or climbing stairs until he/she is back to his/her usual alertness and coordination for at least 1 hour.
4. We advise you to keep your child home from school or daycare after treatment and possibly the next day if your child is still drowsy or unable to walk well. Your child should return to his/her usual state of alertness and coordination within 24 hours.

EATING AND DRINKING INSTRUCTIONS
Begin by giving clear liquids such as clear juices, water, gelatin, Popsicles, or broth. If your child does not vomit after 30 minutes, you may continue with solid foods.

REASONS TO CALL THE DOCTOR
1. You are unable to arouse your child.
2. Your child is unable to eat or drink.
3. Your child experiences excessive vomiting or pain.
4. Your child develops a rash.

FOR THESE OR ANY OTHER CONCERNS about your child's sedation, please contact our office at_____.

FIG. **14-4.** Example of postsedation instructions to the parent or caregiver.

agents. In some instances, this preprocedural administration may be all that is required for a particular patient.

The selection of technique is often made as a matter of clinical judgment. It is a question of successfully matching a method to a specific objective.

The primary goal of these techniques is to produce a quiescent patient to ensure the best quality of care. Another goal might be to accomplish a more complex or lengthy treatment plan in a shorter period by lengthening appointment times and thereby reducing the number of repeat visits required. Children presenting with a dental injury or acute pain may require sedation for completion of treatment as well as postoperative analgesia. In fact, the reduction in anxiety may reduce the amount of analgesia required. Conscious sedation may also allow for more comfortable and acceptable treatment for physically impaired or cognitively disabled patients. Often these patients may benefit from parenteral sedation.

TABLE **14-2** Template of Definitions and Characteristics for Levels of Sedation and General Anesthesia

| | FUNCTIONAL LEVEL OF SEDATION | | | |
| | CONSCIOUS SEDATION | | | DEEP SEDATION |
	MILD SEDATION (ANXIOLYSIS)	INTERACTIVE	NONINTERACTIVE/AROUSABLE WITH MILD/MODERATE STIMULUS	NONINTERACTIVE/NON-AROUSABLE EXCEPT WITH INTENSE STIMULUS
	(Level 1)	**(Level 2)**	**(Level 3)**	**(Level 4)**
Goal	Decrease anxiety; facilitate coping skills	Decrease or eliminate anxiety; facilitate coping skills	Decrease or eliminate anxiety; facilitate coping skills; promote sleep	Eliminate anxiety; coping skills overridden
Responsive-ness	Uninterrupted interactive ability; totally awake	Minimally depressed level of consciousness; eyes open or temporarily closed; responds appropriately to verbal commands	Moderately depressed level of consciousness; state mimics physiologic sleep (vital signs not different from those during sleep); eyes closed most of time; may or may not respond to verbal prompts alone; responds to mild/moderate stimuli (e.g., repeated trapezius pinching or needle insertion in oral tissues elicits reflex withdrawal and appropriate verbalization [complaint, moan, crying]); airway only occasionally may require readjustment via chin thrust	Deeply depressed level of conscious-ness; sleeplike state, but vital signs may be slightly depressed compared with physiologic sleep; eyes closed; does not respond to verbal prompts alone; reflex withdrawal with no verbalization when intense stimulus occurs (e.g., repeated, prolonged, and intense pinching of the trapezius); airway expected to require constant monitoring and frequent management
Personnel required	2	2	2	3
Monitoring equipment	Clinical observation*	PO; precordial recommended†	PO, precordial, BP; capno desirable†	PO and capno, precordial, BP, ECG; defibrillator desirable
Monitoring informa-tion	None	HR, RR, O$_2$ before, during (q15min), after, as needed	HR, RR, O$_2$, BP; [CO$_2$] if available; before, during (q10min), after until stable/discharge criteria met	HR, RR, O$_2$, [CO$_2$], BP before, during (q5min), after until stable/discharge criteria met

American Academy of Pediatric Dentistry: Guidelines on the elective use of conscious sedation, deep sedation and general anesthesia in pediatric dental patients, *Pediatr Dent* 24(7):74-80, 2003.

BP, Blood pressure; *capno,* capnography; *ECG,* electrocardiography; *HR,* heart rate; *PO,* pulse oximetry; *precordial,* precordial (pretracheal) stethoscope; *RR,* respiratory rate.

*It should be noted that clinical observation should accompany any level of sedation and general anesthesia.

†"Recommended" and "desirable" should be interpreted as not a necessity but an adjunct in assessing patient status.

Although the presence of a compromising medical condition is generally a contraindication to sedation, some patients in this category may in fact benefit from its use.[6] This would, of course, include patients for whom stress reduction would reduce the likelihood of complication. These children should be managed in close cooperation with the physicians who regularly cares for them.

NITROUS OXIDE AND OXYGEN SEDATION

Eighty-five percent of pediatric dentists use nitrous oxide and oxygen for sedation of patients. This makes it the most frequently used sedative agent.

Nitrous oxide is a slightly sweet-smelling, colorless, inert gas. It is compressed in cylinders as a liquid that vaporizes on release. This is an endothermic reaction

BOX 14-2 Discharge Criteria

1. Cardiovascular function is satisfactory and stable.
2. Airway patency is uncompromised and satisfactory.
3. Patient is easily arousable and protective reflexes are intact.
4. State of hydration is adequate.
5. Patient can talk, if applicable.
6. Patient can sit unaided, if applicable.
7. Patient can ambulate, if applicable, with minimal assistance.
8. If the child is very young or disabled, incapable of the usually expected responses, the presedation level of responsiveness or the level as close as possible for that child has been achieved.
9. Responsible individual is available.

that pulls heat from the cylinder and environment; consequently the cylinder will become cool or even cold when in use. The gas is nonflammable but will support combustion.

Pharmacokinetics. Nitrous oxide is slightly heavier than air, with a specific gravity of 1.53, and has a blood to gas partition coefficient of 0.47. Because of its low solubility in blood, it has a very rapid onset and recovery time. Nitrous oxide will become saturated in blood within 3 to 5 minutes following administration and is physically dissolved in the serum fraction of the blood. There is no biotransformation, and the gas is rapidly excreted by the lungs when the concentration gradient is reversed. Very small amounts may be found in excreted body fluids and intestinal gas.

A phenomenon termed *diffusion hypoxia* may occur as the sedation is reversed at the termination of the procedure. The nitrous oxide escapes into the alveoli with such rapidity that the oxygen present becomes diluted; thus the oxygen–carbon dioxide exchange is disrupted and a period of hypoxia is created. However, this phenomenon is reported not to occur in healthy pediatric patients.[7] Nonetheless, to minimize this effect, the patient should be oxygenated for 3 to 5 minutes after a sedation procedure, if for no other reason than to allow for proper nasal hood evacuation of the exhaled gas.

Pharmacodynamics. Nitrous oxide produces nonspecific central nervous system (CNS) depression. Although it is classed with inhalational general anesthetics, it produces limited analgesia, and thus surgical anesthesia is unlikely unless concentrations producing anoxia are reached. Nitrous oxide is the weakest of all inhalation agents, with a minimum alveolar concentration of 105. The minimum alveolar concentration of an inhalation agent is a measure of its potency. It is the concentration required to produce immobility in 50% of patients. At concentrations between 30% and 50%, nitrous oxide will produce a relaxed, somnolent patient who may appear dissociated and easily susceptible to suggestion. Amnesia may occur in some patients, but there is little alteration of learning or memory. At concentrations greater than 60%, patients may experience discoordination, ataxia, giddiness, and increased sleepiness. It is not recommended that concentrations greater than 50% be used in dental practice.

Nitrous oxide reduces hypoxic-driven ventilation and has minimal effect on the hypercapnic respiratory drive. When used as a single agent, nitrous oxide will not cause hypoxemia. It should be avoided, however, in patients who rely significantly on hypoxia-driven ventilation, in whom exposure to high levels of oxygen can result in respiratory depression. When combined with other agents that depress respiration, nitrous oxide decreases the body's normal response to low oxygen tension. These effects are usually negligible, however, because of the high concentration of oxygen administered with the combination. Nitrous oxide slightly increases the respiratory minute volume. As the patient becomes more relaxed from the effects of nitrous oxide, the respiratory rate may decrease slightly. The gas is nonirritating to the respiratory tract and can be given to patients with asthma without fear of bronchospasm. Problems can arise, however, from the added respiratory effects when it is given in combination with narcotics or other CNS depressants.

Cardiac output is decreased and peripheral vascular resistance is increased when nitrous oxide is used. This is generally of insignificant degree and is a consideration only in patients with severe cardiac disease. The respiratory and cardiac effects may be secondary to the high concentration of oxygen administered in conjunction with nitrous oxide.

Adverse Effects and Toxicity. Nausea and/or vomiting is the most common adverse effect experienced with nitrous oxide sedation. The incidence increases significantly with concentrations in excess of 50%, with lengthy procedures, with rapid fluctuations in concentrations, and with rapid induction and reversal.

Nitrous oxide will become entrapped in gas-filled spaces such as the middle ear, sinuses, and the gastrointestinal tract. Middle ear pressure will increase significantly, and although it is of little significance in a patient with normal patency of eustachian tubes, it can induce pain in patients with acute otitis media. Because of this, use of nitrous oxide should be avoided in patients with acute otitis media.

Other contraindications include severe behavioral problems and emotional illness, uncooperativeness, fear of "gas," claustrophobia, maxillofacial deformities that prevent nasal hood placement, nasal obstruction (e.g., upper respiratory infection, nasal polyps, deviated septum), chronic obstructive pulmonary disease, pregnancy, and situations in which high oxygenation is inadvisable (e.g., bleomycin therapy).

In clinical use for sedation at proper concentrations of medical-quality nitrous oxide and oxygen, the gas has no toxic effects. The greatest concern regarding toxicity centers on exposure of dental personnel to high ambient air levels of the gas for periods of time during its use for patient sedation. Chronic exposure to nitrous oxide, including recreational abuse, can over time produce neurotoxicity, impotence, and renal and/or liver toxicity. The rate of spontaneous abortion is known to be higher in operating room personnel and in the spouses of operating room personnel.[8] In addition, chronically exposed individuals may experience a decrease in fertility.[9] An increase in hepatic disease was found in dentists and dental personnel exposed to high levels of nitrous oxide for periods longer than 3 hours per week. Because of these facts, leakage from open systems, such as those used in the dental office, should be reduced as much as possible. This can be accomplished by limiting the amount of mouth breathing by the patient and using an efficient scavenging system. The installation of laminar air-flow systems might also be considered in new office constructions when it is known that considerable amounts of nitrous oxide will be in use. In addition, the office as well as office personnel should be periodically monitored for exposure to unscavenged nitrous oxide. A variety of units are available that use infrared spectrophotometry to measure ambient levels. These machines can detect levels as low as 1 ppm and are particularly useful for uncovering leaks around tanks and flowmeters. A less costly and more practical approach is the use of dosimetry badges that are worn by office personnel when using nitrous oxide. These units are generally worn for an 8-hour period and report exposure as time-weighted averages. Exposure-limiting methods are listed in Box 14-3.

Equipment. Several manufacturers produce machines for the safe delivery of nitrous oxide–oxygen mixtures for use in conscious sedation in the dental office. The machine should be of the continuous-flow design, with flowmeters capable of accurate regulation. A fail-safe mechanism that provides automatic shutdown if oxygen falls below 25% and audible and visual alarms that are activated by oxygen failure are important design features. There should be a flush lever for easy and immediate flushing of the system with 100% oxygen.

Mobile, self-contained units are available, as well as those operating from a central supply. A major safety consideration with either type is the presence of a good pin-indexed yoke system to absolutely prevent crossover of the cylinder hookup. One should be continuously

---

BOX 14-3   Controlling Ambient Nitrous Oxide Levels

VENTILATION
- Operatories must have good cross ventilation. Exhaust vents should preferably be located in the ceiling as close to the head of the chair as possible.
- Nitrous oxide exhaust must be vented to the outside.
- Room air exchanges of 10 or more per hour are recommended.

WORK PRACTICES
- Inspect equipment each day to ensure that all connectors are tight and that tubing and bags are free of holes and cracks.
- Always use a scavenger system when administering nitrous oxide and oxygen. Adjust the scavenger flow rate to 45 L/min.
- Select an appropriately sized mask to ensure a sealed but comfortable fit.
- Instruct patients to refrain from mouth breathing and talking during the procedure.
- Adjust the nitrous oxide and oxygen flow rate to keep the bag from overfilling. The bag should collapse and expand as the patient breathes.
- After administration, flush the patient and system by administering 100% oxygen to the patient for at least 5 minutes.

MAINTENANCE
- Schedule periodic inspections every 3 months of all aspects of the system, with particular attention to areas of potential leaks.
- Document results of inspections as well as all corrective actions taken.
- Ensure that repairs and modifications are performed only by authorized dealers.
- Consider periodic personal sampling of dental personnel with a dosimeter.

Adapted from American Dental Association Council on Scientific Affairs, Council on Dental Practice: *J Am Dent Assoc* 128:364-365, 1997; and Howard WR: *J Am Dent Assoc* 128:356-360, 1997.

---

aware of the danger of crossed lines or cylinders. Such crossover becomes possible when office renovations are done and when fittings wear with age and use.

An efficient scavenger system is an important component of any hose-mask system. The double-mask type is the most efficient type of scavenger (Fig. 14-5). These systems exhaust into the vacuum waste system, which should be vented to the outside to prevent dispersal of gases to other areas of the office or building. Nasal hoods should be of good design and should be available in pediatric and adult sizes to ensure adequate fit, which further reduces leakage (Fig. 14-6).

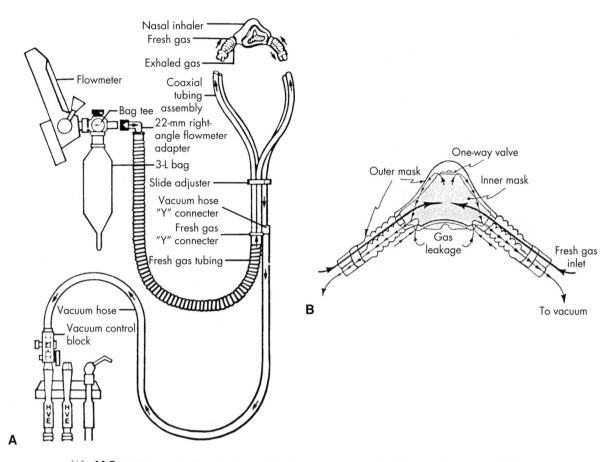

FIG. **14-5. A,** Schematic drawing illustrating the components of a nitrous oxide–oxygen delivery and scavenging system. **B,** Components of the system's nasal hood. *(Courtesy Porter Instrument Co., Hatfield, Pa.)*

Technique. After a thorough inspection of the equipment, the mask should be introduced to the patient with an explanation delivered at the appropriate level of understanding, and then the mask should be carefully placed over the nose. The delivery tubes are tightened behind the chair back in a comfortable position. The bag is filled with 100% oxygen and delivered to the patient for 2 or 3 minutes at an appropriate flow rate, typically between 4 and 6 L per minute. With an appropriate flow rate, slight movement of the mixing bag should be apparent with each inhalation and exhalation. With too high a flow rate, the bag will be overinflated, movement will not be seen with each breath, and leakage will occur from around the mask. In this instance, the flow rate should be adjusted downward. Too low a flow rate will deplete the bag of mixed gases. Once the proper flow rate is achieved, the nitrous oxide can be introduced by slowly increasing the concentration at increments of 10% to 20% to achieve the desired level. The operator should encourage the patient to breathe through the nose with the mouth closed. The sensations should be explained as they begin to be felt.

They are best described as a floating, giddy feeling with tingling of the digits. The eyes will take on a distant gaze with sagging eyelids. When this state is reached, the local anesthetic may be given. Once this is completed, the concentration can be reduced to 30% nitrous oxide and 70% oxygen or lower. The patient can now be maintained and monitored, and the contemplated procedure carried out. The dentist should communicate with the patient throughout the procedure, paying particular attention to the maintenance of an open, relaxed airway. The level of nitrous oxide may be periodically reduced to determine the minimum level required for that patient. This should be recorded for future reference. An emesis basin should be readily available, and in the event that vomiting does occur, the head should be rotated to the side. However, the laryngeal reflex is not obtunded with nitrous oxide, and so aspiration of vomitus is unlikely.[10]

Recovery can be achieved quickly by reverse titration. Once the sedation is reversed, the patient should be allowed to breathe 100% oxygen for 3 to 5 minutes. Oxygenation will purge the patient and the nitrous

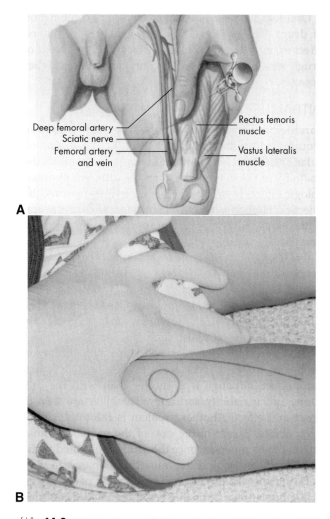

Deep femoral artery
Sciatic nerve
Femoral artery
and vein

Rectus femoris
muscle

Vastus lateralis
muscle

A

B

FIG. **14-8. A,** Anatomy of the anterior thigh of a child. **B,** Demonstration of patient injection site. (**A** *courtesy Wyeth Laboratories, Philadelphia;* **B** *courtesy Dr. David R. Avery.*)

SUBMUCOSAL SEDATION

Submucosal sedation involves the deposition of the drug beneath the mucosa. Its use is almost exclusively the province of dentistry. Although the effectiveness of oral local anesthetics is best if they are placed subperiosteally, most infiltrations are in fact submucosal injections. As is the case with local anesthetics, care must be taken that sedatives are not injected into any of the muscles of the face and jaw lest the absorption and effect of the drug be unduly and unexpectedly prolonged. The site usually chosen for injection is the buccal vestibule, particularly in the area of the maxillary primary molar or canine teeth.

The term *submucosal* is often used interchangeably with *subcutaneous*. This usage may be erroneous, because research has shown the serum level of a drug to rise very quickly after injection into the vessel-rich areas just described. The response time probably should be

considered to be somewhere between those of the intramuscular and the intravenous administration of a drug. This fact makes the method suitable for the pediatric patient for whom quick administration and onset is desirable. Caution should be exercised, however, to select a drug that is not irritating to tissue. The information provided with the drug will indicate its suitability for tissue injection. It is important to remember that this is a parenteral route of administration, and adherence to all of the necessary precautions and requirements must be ensured.

Technique. The technique requires only a syringe suitably sized for the volume of drug affixed with a 27- or 30-gauge, ½-inch needle. A tuberculin syringe is recommended for volumes less than 1 ml. Some patient restraint is usually required. Placement of a small quantity of local anesthesia without vasoconstrictor in the area of injection is preferred if the drug being used is known to be painful on injection. The local anesthetic required for pain control of the procedure should not be given in the same area after the injection of the sedative drug, because the action of the vasoconstrictor will slow the uptake of the sedative drug. Also, the physiochemical properties of the sedative agent may interfere with the effectiveness of the local anesthetic agent.

The drugs most commonly administered by the submucosal technique are the narcotics meperidine and fentanyl.

INTRAVENOUS SEDATION

Sedation levels in which the patient remains conscious are readily achievable through the use of intravenous techniques. In the hands of properly trained professionals this method can be the easiest, most efficient, and safest next to sedation by inhalation. Controversy has existed for several years over what constitutes adequate training in the use of this modality. The individual state boards are resolving this controversy by writing requirements in terms of didactic and clinical hours required to be certified by the board to use intravenous sedation. Generally, these requirements are following those set forth by the American Dental Association's Guidelines for the Use of Conscious Sedation, Deep Sedation, and General Anesthesia for Dentists.[1]

The use of intravenous conscious sedation in pediatric dentistry is somewhat restricted to certain types and ages of patients. Venipuncture is difficult to accomplish in the very young or the combatant child. Such difficulty is attributable to smaller vein size and availability together with the need to restrain the patient. Because of this, the technique is often more suitable for the apprehensive preteen and adolescent patient.

The attribute that makes intravenous sedation desirable for some patients also makes it undesirable for others in the hands of the untrained practitioner. In very young children, the incidence of untoward effects is increased. The onset of action of the drug or drugs used is approximately 20 to 25 seconds, which is the most rapid among all techniques. Thus the opportunity to render the patient unconscious unintentionally is much greater. A practitioner with limited training in management of the airway or of the unconscious patient should never consistently crowd this line between consciousness and unconsciousness.

The possibility of phlebitis is also a disadvantage, particularly with drugs insoluble in water. Hematoma at the site of venipuncture is a complication. There is also an increased need to monitor the patient more closely on a continuous basis, and this usually means the use of an assistant who has had extensive training in the monitoring of sedated patients. In fact, current sedation guidelines require the presence of a third person for the sole purpose of monitoring.

With the intravenous method of sedation one must also consider that, although the onset of effect is very rapid, the reversal of effect is not.

Techniques. There are basically two techniques for using intravenous sedation. The first employs a single drug, usually a benzodiazepine, whereas the second requires a sophisticated combination of several drugs, usually including a narcotic. The single-drug technique is probably the most adaptable to pediatric practice. Unless extensive training opportunities exist, the multiple-drug method should not be considered.

COMBINATIONS OF METHODS AND AGENTS

It is often advantageous to consider combining methods and agents to produce a state of balanced conscious sedation. A goal of combining agents should be to establish a balance between sedation, analgesia, and amnesia, all while minimizing adverse effects and maintaining physiologic homeostasis. When agents are combined, often one drug will be potentiated by another. Their combination thus enables the operator to reduce the dosage of a stronger drug, such as a narcotic, and thus reduce the possibility or degree of an adverse effect, such as severe respiratory depression. Another goal in combining agents might be to quiet the behavior of the patient for the introduction of a method requiring more patient cooperation, such as placement of an intravenous line.

Conscious sedation is usually most effective when combined with the use of local anesthesia. Sedation techniques are not pain-control techniques, and the sedative effects are often overridden when intraoperative pain is experienced by the patient. To overcome this circumstance with the use of sedative agents alone requires the use of very high doses or the addition of a narcotic to the regimen; this produces a deeper level of sedation than might be required and increases the possibility of adverse effects. Sedation techniques should not be used simply to escape the need to inject a local anesthetic. One should also remember that local anesthetic agents are CNS depressants, and effects will be additive. Occasionally a drug with a known capacity to improve postoperative comfort also may be used, particularly if surgical procedures are required.

Inhalation sedation is the next most frequently combined technique. Nitrous oxide and oxygen can be combined with all other methods of conscious sedation. Not only does this combination provide increased sedation, but it also increases the availability of oxygen for the patient. In fact, inhalation sedation is so often used in combination that one should be reminded that nitrous oxide is also a CNS depressant and should be the first agent to be reduced or reversed when the sedation level becomes deeper than desired.

The orally administered sedatives are the next most commonly employed in combination. Most frequently combined include sedative hypnotics, narcotics, and/or antihistamines. A great deal of care must be taken when combining oral agents to avoid deepening the patient's state from conscious sedation to unconscious sedation or general anesthesia. It is important to appreciate that oral agents are potent and that combinations are capable of deepening the patient's sedation to the point that protective reflexes may be lost.

The oral premedication of the patient with minor tranquilizers in advance of the use of inhalation or parenteral sedation methods is a common practice. This technique works especially well to calm the patient for a smoother beginning of a sedative appointment. When parenteral agents are used, unless the result of admixture is definitely known, it is not good practice to mix the agents before administration to the patient, because they may be incompatible in mixed solution. Combining drugs complicates their use because of their additive, synergistic, or potentiating effects. This makes recognition of the causative agent of the untoward effect and subsequent efficient management very difficult. The combination of methods or agents should be viewed as a balancing technique and should always be manipulated so as to produce a maximum result with minimum risk of complication.

Multiple-drug use is also common with intravenous methods of conscious sedation. All the previous cautions pertain in these situations as well. Because of the great potential for swiftly occurring, serious adverse reactions, these multiple-drug intravenous techniques should *never* be used by anyone who is *not* specifically trained in their use.

Regardless of the method of administration, the combining of agents should be approached with great caution because of the possibility of additive effects. Individual drug doses should be reduced by 20% to 50% when the drugs are given in combination.

which is believed to be influenced by the rapidity with which the drug is administered.[12] Apnea is more likely to occur when midazolam is used with narcotics.[13] Hypotension also occurs more frequently with this combination. Doses should be adjusted downward when midazolam is used with any other CNS depressant, especially the narcotics. These effects are not usually seen if the drug is appropriately titrated.

Compared with diazepam, midazolam produces better anxyolysis and amnesia. In fact, between 75% and 90% of patients will experience retrograde amnesia for up to 4 hours when given midazolam. Midazolam is three to four times more potent than diazepam and has twice the affinity for the benzodiazepam receptor.

DOSAGE: Oral—0.25 to 1.0 mg/kg to a maximum single dose of 20 mg
IM—0.1 to 0.15 mg/kg to a maximum dose of 10 mg
IV—slow IV titration; see manufacturer's recommended dosage guidelines
SUPPLIED: Syrup—2 mg/ml
Injectable—1 mg/ml and 5 mg/ml vials

BENZODIAZEPINE ANTAGONIST
■ *Flumazenil* (Romazicon)

Flumazenil is a benzodiazepine receptor antagonist. The drug selectively inhibits the CNS effects of the benzodiazepines by a competitive, high-affinity interaction with benzodiazepine receptors. It has no antagonistic properties against the opioids. When carefully titrated, flumazenil has been shown to be effective in reversing the sedative effects but not necessarily the amnesic or anxiolytic qualities of benzodiazepines.

Flumazenil is well tolerated in patients having no dependence on or increased tolerance to benzodiazepines. In patients with benzodiazepine dependency, withdrawal symptoms will occur when flumazenil is given. Induced seizure activity will occur in patients receiving benzodiazepines for control of convulsive disorders when flumazenil is used. The drug is recommended for intravenous use only and is not recommended for use in children younger than 18 years of age.

For reversal of conscious sedation, the initial dose should be 0.2 mg given over 15 seconds. Should the desired level of consciousness not occur after waiting an additional 45 seconds, another dose of 0.2 mg should be administered and dosing repeated at 60-second intervals to a maximum total dose of 1 mg. Most patients will respond to doses in the range of 0.6 to 1.0 mg. A series of injections is preferable to a single bolus to titrate to a desired end point and thus manage the problem with the minimally effective amount of drug. Onset of reversal is usually seen within 1 to 2 minutes. The duration and degree of reversal are related to dose and plasma concentration of the sedating benzodiazepine, as well as that of the antagonist given. This, coupled with the fact that the duration of effect is shorter for flumazenil than for most benzodiazepines, means that resedation can occur. Patients should be carefully monitored for resedation and respiratory depression throughout the period of reversal. The longer the period of sedation, the longer the period required for monitoring and surveillance for resedation. If resedation should occur, repeated doses of flumazenil at no less than 20-minute intervals may be used.

DOSAGE: IV—as just described
SUPPLIED: 5- and 10-ml multiple-use vials containing 0.1 mg/ml in boxes of 10

SEDATIVE HYPNOTICS
■ Barbiturates

Barbiturates can produce all levels of CNS depression, ranging from mild sedation to general anesthesia and deep coma. Their use has fallen out of favor, however, with the availability of sedatives and hypnotics with fewer adverse effects. Consequently, barbiturates are of very limited value for pediatric patients.

■ *Chloral Hydrate* (Noctec, Aquachloral Supprettes)

Chloral hydrate is an extremely well known and widely used drug for pediatric sedation. It has an onset of action of 30 to 60 minutes when given orally. It has a duration of action between 4 and 8 hours and a half-life of 8 to 11 hours as a result of the formation of active metabolites. The primary metabolite of choral hydrate is trichloroethanol, which is responsible for most of the CNS effects that occur.

Chloral hydrate is irritating to gastric mucosa and unless diluted in a flavored vehicle will frequently cause nausea and vomiting. Children given chloral hydrate often enter a period of excitement and irritability before becoming sedated. The drug causes prolonged drowsiness or sleep and respiratory depression. In large doses it produces general anesthesia. Large doses also depress the myocardium and can produce arrhythmias, and thus should be avoided in patients with cardiac disease.[14,15] The lethal dose of chloral hydrate is stated to be 10 g in adults, yet ingestion of 4 g has caused death.

Because the drug does not reliably produce sedation of a degree to permit operative procedures at lower doses, the tendency is to push the dosage higher to achieve the necessary sedation. With such a wide range of reported toxicity, this drug may be an unwise choice for many pediatric patients. It is recommended that young children receive not more than 1 g as a total dose. Risks are increased when chloral hydrate is combined with nitrous oxide, narcotics, or local anesthetic agents.

At higher doses and in combination with other agents, loss of a patent airway is a common problem.[16]

DOSAGE: Must be individualized for each patient
RECOMMENDED: 25 to 50 mg/kg to a maximum of 1 g
SUPPLIED: Oral capsules—500 mg
        Oral solution—250 and 500 mg/5 ml
        Rectal suppositories—324 and 648 mg

NARCOTICS

Narcotics are the "heavy artillery" of pediatric conscious sedation. They are not employed with any great consideration for their analgesic properties. They do produce sedation and euphoria to a greater degree in children than in adults. Local anesthesia is still required for intraoperative pain control. One should remember that local anesthetics are also CNS depressants.

A significant drug-drug and drug-physiologic interaction can occur when narcotics or other drugs that depress respiration are combined with local anesthetics. In usual doses, local anesthetics are CNS depressants and will provide additive depression when combined with other CNS depressants. In addition, when drugs that depress respiration are used (particularly narcotics), varying degrees of hypercarbia can occur, with a resultant decrease in serum pH. As the respiratory depression continues to deepen, metabolic acidosis will result in an increase in the availability of lidocaine to the CNS. This occurs as a result of less serum protein binding of lidocaine along with central vasodilation and an increase in blood flow to the CNS in an acidotic state. Consequently the threshold for CNS lidocaine toxicity is lowered. Lidocaine toxicity will result in CNS excitation and seizures and ultimately coma and death. As a result, *the maximum dosage of local anesthetic must be reduced when used in combination with a CNS and/or respiratory depressant.* This very important and significant interaction is often overlooked and in fact is the cause of many of the adverse incidents reported in pediatric sedation. It is important to remember that the maximum local anesthetic dose in children may allow for the use of only one or two dental cartridges, which is quite different than for adult patients.

Combination with other sedative drugs, including nitrous oxide–oxygen, will reduce the need for larger doses of narcotics and thus reduce the potential for unwanted effects from these potent drugs. A practitioner employing the narcotics should be thoroughly familiar with their actions and interactions and should have had some supervised experience in their use as well as in management of the airway and patient resuscitation procedures.

■ *Meperidine* (Demerol)

A synthetic opiate agonist. It is very water soluble but is incompatible with many other drugs in solution. Meperidine may be administered orally or by subcutaneous, intramuscular, or intravenous injection. It is least effective by mouth. It is very bitter and requires masking by a flavoring agent. By the oral route, peak effect occurs in 1 hour and lasts about 4 hours. Parenteral administration shortens the time of onset and duration. High doses that lead to an accumulation of normeperidine, a primary metabolite of meperidine, have resulted in seizures. Meperidine should be used with extreme caution in patients likely to accumulate or be sensitive to this metabolite (e.g., patients with hepatic or renal disease, or history of seizures).

DOSAGE: Oral, SC, or IM—1.0 to 2.2 mg/kg, not to exceed 100 mg
SUPPLIED: Oral tablets—50 and 100 mg
        Oral syrup—50 mg/5 ml
        Parenteral solution—25, 50, 75, and 100 mg/ml

■ *Fentanyl* (Sublimaze)

A synthetic opiate agonist in the same chemical class as meperidine. It is a very potent narcotic analgesic. A dose of 0.1 mg is approximately equivalent to 10 mg of morphine or 75 mg of meperidine. Fentanyl has a rapid action, and after a submucosal or intramuscular injection the onset will occur in 7 to 15 minutes; duration of effects is 1 to 2 hours. The drug is metabolized by the liver and is excreted in the urine.

Respiratory depression is the same as with other narcotics. Respiratory rate decreases but returns to near normal quite rapidly. Tidal volume, however, remains depressed. The response to carbon dioxide can be depressed for extended periods, long after the analgesic effect has disappeared. It is believed that this characteristic is attributable to redistribution of the drug. When fentanyl is used, one should be attentive to and competent in airway management. With higher doses administered rapidly by vein, rigidity of skeletal muscle has been reported. Apnea has also occurred under these circumstances. This effect can be reversed by administration of naloxone along with a skeletal muscle relaxant and/or managed by assisted or controlled ventilation. Bradycardia has been reported. Atropine can be used to normalize heart rate.

Fentanyl produces little histamine release and has much less emetic effect than morphine or meperidine.

Fentanyl can be administered by the intramuscular, intravenous, or submucosal route. When it is used with other CNS depressants, the dose should be reduced. The drug works well with orally administered diazepam and nitrous oxide–oxygen. It is not recommended for use in children under 2 years of age.

DOSAGE: 0.002 to 0.004 mg/kg
SUPPLIED: 0.05 mg/ml in 2- and 5-ml ampules

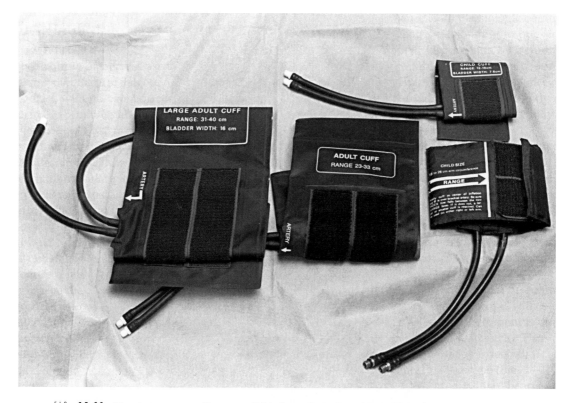

FIG. **14-11.** Blood pressure cuffs are available in various sizes. The width of the cuff should cover approximately two thirds of the upper arm.

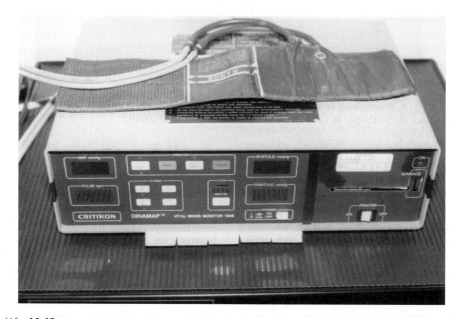

FIG. **14-12.** Automated vital signs monitor. *(Courtesy Dinamap by Critikon, Inc., Tampa, Fla.)*

of diodes on the same limb as a blood pressure cuff, (4) fingernail polish on the digit to which the sensor is attached, (5) cold limbs, (6) profound tissue pigmentation, (7) reuse of disposable oxisensors, and (8) motion artifact. Sensor displacement is the most common cause

for false readings in children and can be minimized by using a sensor with adhesive tabs rather than a clip-on sensor. Securing the sensor with additional tape and using a toe rather than a finger may also help minimize displacement.

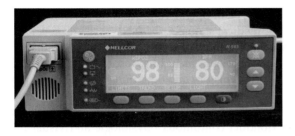

FIG. **14-13.** Pulse oximeter. *(Courtesy Nellcor, Pleasanton, Calif.)*

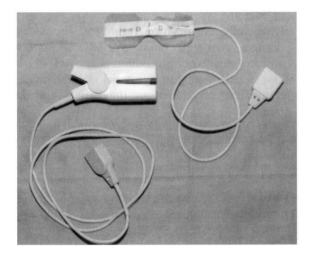

FIG. **14-14.** Two types of optical sensors. Sensors with adhesive tabs are less likely to dislodge in pediatric patients than are clip-on sensors.

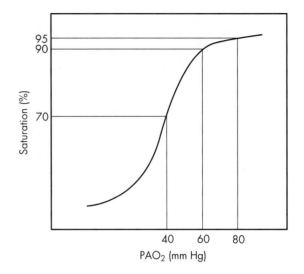

FIG. **14-15.** Oxyhemoglobin dissociation curve, which shows the saturation of hemoglobin with oxygen (SaO_2) relative to the oxygen tension (PaO_2). Hypoxemia is defined as PaO_2 below 80 mm Hg (95% SaO_2). *(From Dionne R, Phero, J, Becker D: Management of pain and anxiety in the dental office, Philadelphia, 2002, WB Saunders.)*

Knowing the peripheral oxygen saturation from moment to moment is important to detect sudden deterioration of the patient's physiologic status during conscious sedation. Hypoxia is almost always the primary complication with these techniques of patient management. Oxygen saturation measures oxygenation, the transport of oxygen to metabolically active tissues. It does not, however, reflect ventilation—the movement of gases from the atmosphere to alveoli. Thus, oxygenation represents only half of the results of ventilation. Ventilation must be evaluated independently from oxygenation.[17] Methods used to monitor ventilation include visual monitoring for chest wall movement, listening for breath sounds with a precordial stethoscope, determination of respiratory rate, and capnography. Capnography is considered the gold standard for monitoring ventilatory status and will reveal respiratory compromise within 15 seconds.

The capnography monitor (Fig. 14-16, *A*), detects both the presence and the quality of ventilation by analyzing the concentration of carbon dioxide in the exhaled gasses through differential infrared absorption. The end-tidal carbon dioxide concentration is the concentration of carbon dioxide measured at the terminal portion of the exhalation curve (Fig. 14-16, *B*).[18] The sampling line is placed either in the nostril or in close approximation to the nose or mouth and allows for suctioning of a sample of exhaled air into the unit. There are limitations to the accuracy of readings that must be kept in mind, especially when the device is used in children. Head movement, mouth breathing, crying, and tube blockage by mucous all result in inaccurate readings. Technology is being developed to overcome these obstacles. In the future, capnography will become the most important monitoring instrument when patient sedation is used.

The availability of appropriately trained personnel to evaluate the patient and interpret monitoring results is just as important as using the correct monitoring devices. In addition to the operating practitioner, an individual trained to monitor appropriate physiologic parameters must be present during conscious sedation. Both individuals must be certified in basic life-support techniques and must be familiar with the office emergency cart or kit.

POSTOPERATIVE MONITORING

Before any patient receiving conscious sedation is discharged, all vital signs must be stable. The child must be reasonably alert, able to talk, ambulating with minimal assistance, and sitting unaided. For the very young or disabled patient who might be incapable of the usually expected responses, a level of awareness that is as close to the usual state for that person must be achieved before discharge (see Box 14-2).

15

Hospital Dental Services for Children and the Use of General Anesthesia

JAMES A. WEDDELL

JAMES E. JONES

Dentists can provide essential services to patients within an operating room setting in addition to providing consultative and emergency services. Staff membership is necessary. National commissions such as the Joint Commission on Accreditation of Healthcare Organizations (JCAHO) issue the standards for hospital governance for all hospital services.

In recent years, with the increasing number of general practice residencies and postdoctoral specialty programs, the qualified dentist finds that hospital staff privileges are a necessity. Active involvement in hospital dentistry has added a rewarding component to the practice of many dentists. Many hospitals have incorporated not only dental specialties but also general dental services, providing a comprehensive health care facility in which to serve the community.

OBTAINING HOSPITAL STAFF PRIVILEGES

Requirements for obtaining hospital staff privileges vary among institutions. The dentist must fulfill the following three basic requirements to become a hospital staff member:

1. The applicant must have graduated from an accredited dental school.
2. The applicant must be licensed to practice dentistry in the state in which the facility is located.
3. The applicant must have high moral and ethical standards.

Additional requirements may have to be met to obtain staff privileges. Many hospitals ask staff members to sign a "Delineation of Privileges" form indicating the procedures that staff members are qualified to perform and that are accepted by the governing body of the hospital. In addition, the applicant must show proof of professional liability insurance, and membership in the American Dental Association is desirable.

In a children's hospital, dentists might be required to have adequate advanced training to treat and manage children in the hospital. The requirements may include a dental residency of 1 to 4 years in a teaching hospital in which the dentist (1) gains experience in recording and evaluating the medical history and current medical status of children; (2) receives instruction in physical examination techniques and in recognition of conditions that may influence dental treatment decisions; (3) learns to initiate appropriate medical consultations when a problem arises during treatment; (4) learns the procedure for admitting, monitoring, and discharging children; and (5) develops proficiency in operating

room protocol. A rotation in which the dental resident was actively involved in administering general anesthetics to children is highly desirable. Current certification in basic cardiopulmonary resuscitation should be maintained by all members of the hospital's professional staff, including dentists.

As active members of the hospital staff, dentists should be aware of the hospital's bylaws, rules, regulations, and meetings. A copy of the bylaws should be obtained for easy reference. Fully understanding the responsibilities of staff membership will enable dentists to treat their patients within the established protocol of the institution. Most important, dentists should endeavor to provide the highest quality care within the specialty area for which they are trained. The American Academy of Pediatric Dentistry encourages the participation of pediatric dentistry practitioners on hospital medical-dental staffs, recognizes the American Dental Association as a corporate member of the JCAHO, and encourages hospital member pediatric dentists to maintain strict adherence to the rules and regulations of the policies of the hospital medical staff.

INDICATIONS FOR GENERAL ANESTHESIA IN THE TREATMENT OF CHILDREN

The use of general anesthesia for dental care in children is sometimes necessary to provide safe, efficient, and effective care. Depending on the patient, this will be done in an ambulatory care setting or inpatient hospital setting. It should be only one component of the dentist's overall treatment regimen. Oral hygiene and preventive care must be implemented at the onset of treatment with parents or guardians and patients to eliminate the cause of the dental problem.

The safety of the patient and practitioner, as well as the need to diagnose and treat, must justify the use of general anesthesia. All available management techniques, including acceptable restraints and sedation, should be considered before the decision is made to use a general anesthetic. Crespi and Friedman cite several authors who agree in recommending that at least one or two attempts be made using conventional behavior management techniques or conscious sedation before general anesthesia is considered.[1]

Parental or guardian written consent must be obtained before the use of general anesthesia. Documentation regarding dental treatment needs, unmanageability in the dental setting, and contributory medical problems must be included in the patient's hospital record. Records must be clearly written so others are able to read and understand them. Review organizations examine dental admissions for proper documentation in the hospital chart for insurance payment and quality assurance purposes.

Patients for whom general anesthesia has been the management technique of choice include the following:

1. Patients with certain physical, mental, or medically compromising conditions
2. Patients with dental restorative or surgical needs for whom local anesthesia is ineffective because of acute infection, anatomic variations, or allergy
3. The extremely uncooperative, fearful, anxious, physically resistant, or uncommunicative child or adolescent with substantial dental needs for whom there is no expectation that the behavior will soon improve
4. Patients who have sustained extensive orofacial and/or dental trauma
5. Patients with immediate comprehensive oral or dental needs who otherwise would not receive comprehensive dental care
6. Patients requiring dental care for whom the use of general anesthesia may protect the developing psyche and/or reduce medical risks

Patients for whom general anesthesia is usually contraindicated include those with a medical contraindication to general anesthesia and healthy and cooperative patients with minimal dental needs.

PSYCHOLOGIC EFFECTS OF HOSPITALIZATION ON CHILDREN

Hospitalization is a frequent source of anxiety for children. According to King and Nielson, 20% to 50% of children demonstrate some degree of behavioral change after hospitalization.[2] Separation of the child from the parent appears to be a significant factor in posthospitalization anxiety, although other causes are also documented. Allowing the parent to stay with the child during the hospitalization, and especially to be present when the child leaves for and returns from surgery, can reduce anxiety for the child and parent alike.

According to Camm et al, postoperative behavioral changes reported by mothers in a limited sample of children who received dental treatment with general anesthesia in a hospital were similar to those observed in children who received treatment under conscious sedation in a dental clinic.[3] Mothers of children receiving dental treatment with general anesthesia in a hospital setting were found to experience more stress during the procedure. Ways to decrease these stresses include the following: providing a prior tour of the operating room facility, informing the parents of the status of the child during the procedure, and letting them know that "everything is all right." Seventy-five percent of the children receiving general anesthesia exhibited some type of behavioral change. Positive changes included less fuss about eating, fewer temper tantrums, and better appetite. Negative changes included biting the fingernails, becoming upset when left alone, being more cautious or avoiding new things, staying with the parent more, needing more attention, and being afraid of the dark. Ways to minimize negative changes include (1) involving the child in the operating room tour, (2) allowing the child to bring along a favorite doll or toy, (3) giving preinduction sedation, (4) providing a nonthreatening environment, (5) giving postprocedure sedation as needed, and (6) allowing parents to rejoin their children as early as possible in the recovery area.

To limit the severity and duration of psychologic disturbances, the dentist should strive to reduce parental apprehension concerning the operative procedure. Because children often sense apprehension in their parents, effectively reducing the parents' anxiety will put the child more at ease. Thoroughly explaining the procedure, describing the normal postanesthetic side effects, and familiarizing the child and parents with the hospital can reduce postoperative anxiety.

Peretz et al concluded that children treated for early childhood caries under general anesthesia or under conscious sedation at a very young age behaved similarly or better in a follow-up examination approximately 14 months after treatment than at their pretreatment visit, as measured by the Frankl scale and by the "sitting pattern."[4]

OUTPATIENT VERSUS INPATIENT SURGERY

During the past 25 years the popularity of outpatient anesthesia and surgery has continually increased. Currently more than 70% of all pediatric surgical and diagnostic procedures are performed on an *outpatient* basis. The criteria for and advantages of ambulatory general anesthesia procedures are well recognized. The increasing cost of inpatient hospital care, advances in anesthetic management, and quality assessment of patient care have led to changes in preoperative and postoperative management of many surgical procedures done under general anesthesia that were previously assumed to be possible only on an inpatient basis. Ambulatory care is more expeditious, better tolerated both by family and hospital teams, and less traumatic for the patient. Development of freestanding ambulatory care surgical centers (i.e., same-day surgery centers) and hospital ambulatory surgical care areas has cut health care costs for consumers and third-party providers. The advances in perioperative anesthesia care are related to the wider availability of more highly qualified anesthesia care providers (board-certified anesthesiologists with subspecialty training) and the availability of modern, safer short-acting anesthetic and adjuvant drugs and monitoring equipment. A number of studies have reported a significant decrease in anesthesia-related

SIGNATURES REQUIRED

1. If the patient is an adult (age 18 or over) – signature of patient; or, if the patient is incompetent, the guardian's signature.

2. Minor patient (under age 18) – if emancipated (providing own support and living apart from the parents) patient's signature.

   If married, signatures of patient and spouse are required.

   Otherwise, signature of parent or guardian is required.

3. In an emergency threatening the life or well-being of the patient, and if signatures as required above are not available, there should be an entry in the chart documenting the emergency nature of the procedure and the need for prompt action, attested by the signatures of two physicians. Also, the signature of the closest adult relative should be obtained, if available.

FIG. **15-1, cont'd.**

BOX 15-1 Components of the Pediatric Medical History and Physical Examination for Admission to the Hospital

A. Pediatric history
1. Identification: age, sex, racial-ethnic profile
2. Informant and estimate of reliability
3. Problem leading to admittance
4. History of present illness: date of onset, chronologic description of illness, presence or absence of previous similar episodes, treatment given prior to admittance
5. Medical survey
   a. Immunization against diphtheria, pertussis, tetanus, polio, measles, mumps, rubella
   b. Previous hospitalizations, operations, major illnesses, or injuries
   c. Allergies, including allergies to food and drugs
   d. Dietary history (under 2 years of age)
   e. Current medications
6. Developmental status
   a. Infants younger than 2 years: statement regarding motor and language development
   b. Preschool children: general statement regarding development
   c. Children in school: statement regarding school performance
7. Family history

B. Physical examination
1. Vital signs: Temperature, pulse, respiration, blood pressure if older than 12 months of age
2. Measurements: weight, height or length, head circumference if younger than 12 months of age
3. General observations: nutrition, color, distress
4. Head: description of fontanel if present
5. Eyes: pupils, extraocular movements
6. Ears: tympanic membranes
7. Nose: patency, secretions
8. Mouth: teeth, pharynx, and tonsils
9. Neck: masses
10. Lungs: auscultation
11. Cardiovascular system: heart sounds, rate, rhythm, murmurs; femoral pulses
12. Abdomen: masses, viscera
13. Genitalia
    a. Male testes
    b. Female introitus
14. Skin: eruption
15. Lymph nodes
16. Skeleton: joints, spine
17. Nervous system: state of consciousness, gait (if walking)
18. Summary list of problems on tentative diagnosis

BOX 15-2 Components of the Dental History and Intraoral Examination to be Completed Before Hospitalization

1. Past dental history
2. Head and neck physical examination
   a. General
   b. Head
   c. Neck
   d. Face
   e. Lateral facial profile
3. Intraoral examination
   a. Lips
   b. Tongue
   c. Floor of mouth
   d. Buccal mucosa
   e. Hard and soft palate
   f. Oropharynx
   g. Periodontium
4. Teeth
   a. Caries
   b. Eruption sequence
   c. Occlusion molar, cuspid, overbite, overjet, and midline
5. Oral habits
6. Behavior
7. Recommendations

INDIANA UNIVERSITY

July 7, 2003

SCHOOL OF DENTISTRY

Mr. and Mrs. Smith
75 Mulberry Lane
Indianapolis, Indiana

Dear Mr. and Mrs. Smith:

RE: William Smith

After evaluating William and discussing with you the extent of his dental
disease, it has been decided to accomplish all necessary dental care in the
hospital. A medical history and physical examination must be completed
by your physician, Dr. Charles Brown, prior to William's admission to the
hospital. It has been scheduled for him at 9:00 a.m. on August 9, 2003, at
Dr. Brown's office. You should also bring your child to the hospital at
10:00 a.m. on August 10, 2003, for admission.

You are encouraged to remain with your child overnight if possible. Your
child may bring his favorite toy or book. If any cold symptoms (runny
nose or congestion) should develop before the scheduled admission,
please contact our office immediately. It is better to postpone the
general anesthesia procedure if your child has a cold.

If you have any further questions concerning this procedure, please
contact our office.

Sincerely,

John J. Doe, D.D.S.

John J. Doe, D.D.S.

JJD/db

DEPARTMENT OF
ORAL FACIAL DEVELOPMENT

UNIVERSITY PEDIATRIC
DENTISTRY ASSOCIATES

702 Barnhill Drive
Indianapolis, Indiana
46202-5200

317-274-9604
Fax: 317-278-0760

*Located on the campus of
Indiana University
Purdue University
Indianapolis*

FIG. **15-2.** Sample letter sent to parents 2 weeks before their child's admission to the hospital.

ADMISSION TO THE HOSPITAL

If the child is to be admitted as an inpatient, the child and parents should report to the hospital the day before the surgery. If the medical history is less complex, however, the patient may be admitted for "23-hour observation." In this instance the child may come to the hospital the same day as the operative procedure and stay postoperatively until the next morning. The parents must complete the necessary forms for admission to the hospital. The dentist must write the child's admission orders, which give the nursing staff the preliminary information needed and outline the basic care procedures for the child (Fig. 15-3). The nursing staff will explain standard hospital procedures to the parents and make any recommendations needed to foster a comfortable experience for the patient.

During this time the child will be visited by the anesthesiologist involved in the anticipated procedure. The anesthesiologist will assess the child's present state of health and review the past and present hospital records, focusing on prior exposures to general anesthetics and any complications that may have occurred. The anesthesiologist will explain the procedures involved during his or her part of the procedure and answer any questions that the child or parent might have. The decision regarding how long to keep the child off solid foods and liquids before the procedure is also determined by the anesthesiologist and may vary for younger patients to prevent hypoglycemia (Fig. 15-4).

The evening before surgery the dentist should visit the child in the ward. At this time the dentist can answer any questions the parents or the child might have. The dentist should also evaluate the preoperative laboratory data so that appropriate consultations can be initiated if any abnormal values are found. The dentist should record an admitting note in the medical chart to provide the supporting staff with a concise record of the child's medical history, current medical and oral status, diagnosis, and proposed treatment (Box 15-3). Abbreviations can be used when information is recorded in the medical chart (Box 15-4).

On the morning of the procedure the dentist and the staff should be in the operating room area 30 minutes before the start of the procedure. The dentist should evaluate how the child spent the previous evening, check that preanesthetic medications have been administered, and determine that the child has been given nothing by mouth (*nil per os* [NPO]) for the recommended time. An appropriate note should be made in the medical chart. If all information is found acceptable, the child is ready to be taken to the surgical suite.

OPERATING ROOM PROTOCOL

All persons involved in the care of patients in the operating room must follow Occupational Safety and Health Administration (OSHA) guidelines. They must wear appropriate attire designed to prevent contamination of the surgical suite, hallways, and recovery room. This generally consists of a shirt, pants or skirt, and coverings for the face, head, and feet. A hood is used to cover all unshaven facial hair. Eyeglasses, goggles, or a face shield must be used to protect the surgeon's eyes, and a mask must cover the mouth and nose.

The dentist and staff should be familiar with the standard scrub technique for sterile procedures. Neither the medical nor the dental literature documents that a sterile technique is more advantageous than a modified sterile, or clean, technique for restorative dental procedures. Therefore intraoral dental procedures are generally considered clean procedures rather than sterile procedures. However, the dentist should wear sterile gloves. A sterile gown is worn at the discretion of the dentist. It is important to remember that barrier technique should be followed to prevent cross-contamination between patients in the hospital.

PROPERTIES OF INHALATION GENERAL ANESTHETICS

All inhalation anesthetic agents produce anesthesia by depressing specific areas of the brain. The magnitude of

---

1. Please admit (patient's name) to ward for comprehensive dental care under general anesthesia.
2. CBC and differential, platelet, bleeding time, PT, PTT, (if indicated)
3. UA (if indicated)
4. Lateral and PA chest films (if indicated)
5. History and physical examination by medical house officer (if not already completed)
6. Routine diet per age (special diet if indicated)
7. Weight of patient
8. Bedside privileges for parents
9. Restraints (if indicated)
10. Activity for patient (up ad lib, BRP with assistance, and so forth)
11. Continue present medications (list all normally taken, dosages, and times given), for example:

    phenytoin   50 mg   po   bid
    phenobarbital   60 mg   po   bid

12. Notify anesthesiology of admission for preoperative evaluation and medication
13. Medication for pain, infection, or sleep (if indicated)
14. Consultations (if indicated)
15. Arrange for transport to the operating room on (date) at (time)
16. Contact me if problems develop

        Answering service phone number: 555-5000
        Home phone number: 555-7886

        Signature: *John J. Doe, D.D.S.*

FIG. **15-3.** Dentist's admission orders for a patient.

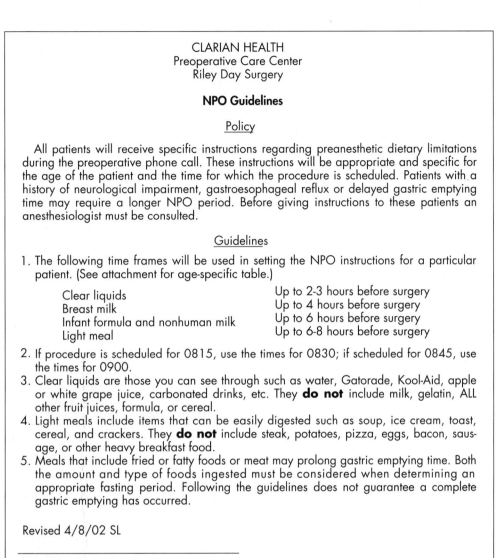

CLARIAN HEALTH
Preoperative Care Center
Riley Day Surgery

NPO Guidelines

Policy

All patients will receive specific instructions regarding preanesthetic dietary limitations during the preoperative phone call. These instructions will be appropriate and specific for the age of the patient and the time for which the procedure is scheduled. Patients with a history of neurological impairment, gastroesophageal reflux or delayed gastric emptying time may require a longer NPO period. Before giving instructions to these patients an anesthesiologist must be consulted.

Guidelines

1. The following time frames will be used in setting the NPO instructions for a particular patient. (See attachment for age-specific table.)

Clear liquids	Up to 2-3 hours before surgery
Breast milk	Up to 4 hours before surgery
Infant formula and nonhuman milk	Up to 6 hours before surgery
Light meal	Up to 6-8 hours before surgery

2. If procedure is scheduled for 0815, use the times for 0830; if scheduled for 0845, use the times for 0900.
3. Clear liquids are those you can see through such as water, Gatorade, Kool-Aid, apple or white grape juice, carbonated drinks, etc. They **do not** include milk, gelatin, ALL other fruit juices, formula, or cereal.
4. Light meals include items that can be easily digested such as soup, ice cream, toast, cereal, and crackers. They **do not** include steak, potatoes, pizza, eggs, bacon, sausage, or other heavy breakfast food.
5. Meals that include fried or fatty foods or meat may prolong gastric emptying time. Both the amount and type of foods ingested must be considered when determining an appropriate fasting period. Following the guidelines does not guarantee a complete gastric emptying has occurred.

Revised 4/8/02 SL

Gopal Krishna, MD
Director of Pediatric Anesthesia
Riley Hospital for Children

FIG. **15-4.** Nothing by mouth (*nil per os* [NPO]), times according to age.

BOX 15-3 Components of Dentist's Admitting Note on the Medical History-Physical-Progress Note Form

1. Name, age, sex, race, chief complaint, and rationale for admission
2. History of the present illness
3. Past medical history
4. Present medications (list all with dosages and times given)
5. Results of current laboratory tests
6. Documentation of informed consent and physical examination
7. Impression of case (intraoral examination, diagnosis, and prognosis)
8. Plan for treatment
9. Dentist's signature

depression is proportional to the partial pressure of the inhalation agents reaching specific sites in the central nervous system (CNS) after entering through the lungs and being distributed by the circulation to the tissues. The resulting physiologic signs of CNS depression produced by general anesthetic agents have been described by Guedel and modified by Roberts as stages of anesthesia with ether (Fig. 15-5).[10,11] Guedel's classification of the stages of anesthesia is largely of historical interest, however. The modern inhaled anesthetics are extremely potent. Induction of anesthesia occurs quickly, and passage through the stages of anesthesia is quite rapid.

Techniques of inhalation anesthesia vary with the type of equipment used (i.e., reservoir bag, directional valves), chemical absorption of expired carbon dioxide, and rebreathing of expired gases. The techniques range

BOX 15-4   Abbreviations Commonly Used in the Hospital

ac	Before meals *(ante cibos)*	MCHC	Mean corpuscular hemoglobin concentration
ad lib	At liberty or at pleasure	MCV	Mean corpuscular volume
anom	Anomalies	meds	Medication
AP	Anteroposterior	N	Normal
aq	Aqueous, water	NC	Noncontributory
B/F	Black female	neg	Negative
bid	Twice a day	N_2O	Nitrous oxide
B/M	Black male	NPO	Nothing by mouth *(nil per os)*
BP	Blood pressure	NSA	No significant abnormality
BRP	Bathroom privileges	n/v	Nausea and vomiting
BSS	Black silk sutures	OOB	Out of bed
BUN	Blood urea nitrogen	op	Operation
bx	Biopsy	OPD	Outpatient department
c	With *(cum)*	OR	Operating room
C	Celsius (formerly centigrade)	ox	Mouth *(os)*
cap	Capsule	PA	Posteroanterior
CBC	Complete blood count	pc	After meals *(post cibos)*
cc	Cubic centimeter (liquid: milliliter)	PE (or Px)	Physical examination
CC	Chief complaint	ped	Pediatric
CHD	Congenital heart disease	PH	Past history
CNS	Central nervous system	PI	Present illness
congen	Congenital	PMH	Past medical history
CP	Cerebral palsy	po	By mouth *(per os)*
CR	Cardiorespiratory	postop	Postoperative
CV	Cardiovascular	preop	Preoperative
d/c	Discontinue	prep	Prepare
Dent	Dental	prn	As required *(pro re nata)*
diff	Differential blood count	pro time	Prothrombin time
disch	Discharge	Pt	Patient
D5W	5% dextrose in water	PT	Physical therapy
Dx	Diagnosis	PTT	Partial thromboplastin time
ECG	Electrocardiogram	Px	Physical examination
El	Elixir	q	Every *(quaque)*
ER	Emergency department	qd	Every day
FH	Family history	qh	Every hour
FUO	Fever of unknown origin	qid	Four times a day *(quater in die)*
Fx	Fracture	qn	Every night
GA	General anesthesia	qod	Every other day
ging	Gingiva	qs	Sufficient quantity *(quantum sufficiat)*
gtt	Drops *(guttae)*		
h	Hour	RHD	Rheumatic heart disease
Hct	Hematocrit	RO (or R/O)	Rule out
HEENT	Head, eyes, ears, nose, and throat	ROS	Review of symptoms
Hg	Mercury	RR	Respiratory rate
hist	History	RR	Recovery room
HPI	History of present illness	RSR	Regular sinus rhythm
hs	Just before sleep *(hora somni)*	Rx	Take (or prescription) *(recipe)*
I & D	Incision and drainage	s	Without *(sine)*
IM	Intramuscular	SBE	Subacute bacterial endocarditis
I & O	Intake and output	SC	Subcutaneous
IV	Intravenous	SH	Social history
kg	Kilogram	SH	Serum hepatitis
L	Left	S/P	Status post
mand	Mandible	Stat	At once *(statim)*
max	Maxilla	r	Rectal
M	Molar, in moles	R	Right
MCH	Mean corpuscular hemoglobin		

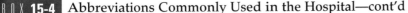

BOX 15-4 Abbreviations Commonly Used in the Hospital—cont'd

surg	Surgery		WBC	White blood count
Sx	Signs and symptoms		WD	Well developed
tbsp	Tablespoon		W/F	White female
tid	Three times a day		W/M	White male
TPR	Temperature, pulse, and respiration		WN	Well nourished
Tx	Treatment		WNL	Within normal limits
UA	Urinalysis		w/o	Without

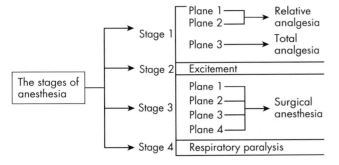

FIG. **15-5.** Stages of anesthesia observed with ether. *(Adapted from Roberts GJ: Relative analgesia in clinical practice. In Coplans MD, Green RA, editors: Anaesthesia and sedation in dentistry, vol 12, Amsterdam, 1983, Elsevier Science.)*

from insufflation to open or nonbreathing systems, semiopen systems, semiclosed systems, and closed systems. The semiclosed system is most often used in modern anesthesia. Exhaled gases mingle with fresh gas and are rebreathed after all the carbon dioxide is removed by a chemical absorber. Inhaled gases are humidified and a reservoir bag or ventilator allows assisted respiration. Reduced loss of body heat and water vapor, increased economy of flow, and decreased environmental contamination are advantages of the semiclosed system.

An anesthetic's *potency* is defined as the concentration of the agent required to inhibit response to a standard surgical stimulus. The potency is expressed in terms of the minimal alveolar concentration (MAC) value for the agent. The MAC of a given agent will abolish the response to stimulus in 50% of patients. Expressed as a number, MAC values are additive when different agents are used in combination. MAC is very useful, since it provides an estimate of the anesthetic requirement for each patient. Fine adjustment of anesthetic administration can then be made by monitoring the patient's physiologic responses (such as heart rate, blood pressure, and respiratory rate). MAC values and some other properties of inhalation anesthetics are listed in Table 15-1.

Available inhalation anesthetics include nitrous oxide, halothane, enflurane, isoflurane, desflurane, and sevoflurane. In children, because they dislike needles, anesthesia is commonly induced by inhalation of a halogenated volatile anesthetic via a face mask. For decades, halothane enjoyed widespread popularity as an induction agent in children. More recently, sevoflurane became available and in comparison to halothane has a lower blood/gas partition coefficient (producing more rapid induction and emergence) and is associated with less myocardial depression and fewer and less significant respiratory problems when used for inhalational induction. As a result, sevoflurane has become the agent of choice for inhalational induction. For maintenance of anesthesia, halothane, sevoflurane, isoflurane, and desflurane are all acceptable.

ANESTHETIC PREPARATION OF THE CHILD

After donning operating room attire, the dentist should report to the surgical suite and inform the anesthesiologist of any special requests concerning the procedure prior to induction of anesthesia. Nasotracheal intubation is preferred to ensure good access to the oral cavity. Oral tracheal intubation is not contraindicated, however, and can be used in a dental case with minimal restorative needs. The anesthesiologist should be careful to avoid complications during induction (i.e., laryngospasm, tooth avulsion or aspiration, traumatic intubation, compromised airway, malignant hyperthermia).

The anesthesiologist is responsible for starting intravenous fluids (IV), securing the necessary monitoring equipment, performing the intubation, and stabilizing the endotracheal tube. The anesthesiologist will select the type of IV fluid and calculate the estimated fluid replacement and fluid deficit volumes, and perform a physical assessment of dehydration. Since the patient is NPO, 5% dextrose lactated Ringer solution (D5LR) is initially used. The monitoring equipment should include (1) a precordial stethoscope, (2) an automatic sphygmomanometer, (3) electrocardiographic leads, (4) a temperature-monitoring device, (5) a pulse oximeter, and (6) a capnography device. The anesthesiologist must confirm that the child is in a stable condition for anesthesia and that the equipment is functioning properly (Fig. 15-6).

PIT AND FISSURE SEALANTS

In 1955 Buonocore described the technique of acid etching as a simple method of increasing the adhesion of self-curing methyl methacrylate resin materials to dental enamel.[1] He used 85% phosphoric acid to etch enamel for 30 seconds. This produces a roughened surface at a microscopic level, which allows mechanical bonding of low-viscosity resin materials.

The first materials used experimentally as sealants were based on cyanoacrylates but were not marketed. By 1965 Bowen et al had developed the bis-GMA resin, which is the chemical reaction product of bisphenol A and glycidyl methacrylate.[2] This is the base resin to most of the current commercial sealants. Urethane dimethacrylate and other dimethacrylates are alternative resins used in sealant materials.

For the chemically cured sealants, a tertiary amine (activator) in one component is mixed with another component containing benzoyl peroxide, and their reaction produces free radicals, which initiates polymerization of the sealant material.

The other sealant materials are activated by an external energy source. The early light-activated sealants were polymerized by the action of ultraviolet rays (which are no longer used) on a benzoin methyl ether or higher-alkyl benzoin ethers to activate the peroxide curing system. The visible light–curing sealants have diketones and aromatic ketones, which are sensitive to visible light in the wavelength region of 470 nm (blue region). Some sealants contain filler, usually silicon dioxide microfill or even quartz.

Sealant materials may be transparent or opaque. Opaque materials are available in tooth color or white. Transparent sealants are clear, pink, or amber. The clear and tooth-colored sealants are esthetic but are difficult to detect at recall examinations. Recent advances in sealant technology include light-activated coloring agents that allow for color change during and/or after polymerization. These compositional changes do not affect the sealant, but only offer some arguable benefit in the recognition of sealed surfaces.

The cariostatic properties of sealants are attributed to the physical obstruction of the pits and grooves. This prevents colonization of the pits and fissures with new bacteria and also prevents the penetration of fermentable carbohydrates to any bacteria remaining in the pits and fissures, so that the remaining bacteria cannot produce acid in cariogenic concentration.

CLINICAL TRIALS

Many clinical studies have reported on the success of pit and fissure sealants with respect to caries reduction. As the longevity of the sealant increases, the retention rate becomes a determinant of its effectiveness as a caries-preventive measure.

In 1983 a National Institutes of Health Consensus Panel considered the available information on pit and fissure sealants and concluded that "the placement of sealants is a highly effective means of preventing pit and fissure caries.... Expanding the use of sealants would substantially reduce the occurrence of dental caries in the population beyond that already achieved by fluorides and other preventive resources."[3]

In 1991 Simonsen reported on a random sample of participants in a sealant study recalled after 15 years.[4] He reported that, in the group with sealant, 69% of the surfaces were sound 15 years after a single sealant application, whereas 31% were carious or restored. In the group without sealant, matched by age, gender, and residence, 17% of the surfaces were sound, whereas 83% were carious or restored. He also estimated that a pit and fissure surface on a permanent first molar is 7.5 times more likely to be carious or restored after 15 years if it is not sealed with a single application of pit and fissure sealant.

The use of glass ionomer as a sealant material has the advantage of continuous fluoride release, and its preventive effect may continue with the visible loss of the material. Glass ionomer may be useful as a sealant material in deeply fissured primary molars that are difficult to isolate due to the child's precooperative behavior and in partially erupted permanent molars that the clinician believes are at risk for developing decay. In such cases, glass ionomer materials must be considered a provisional sealant to be reevaluated and probably replaced with resin-based sealants when better isolation is possible. Because questions exist regarding the strength and retention of glass ionomer, further long-term research is necessary before it is recommended as a routine pit and fissure sealant material.

A 1996 survey of Indiana dentists[5] found that 91% of them were placing sealants on permanent teeth, whereas in 1985 a similar study[6] had found that only 73.5% were placing sealants on permanent teeth. This increased use of sealants may be related to increased practitioner comfort with the materials, because a direct correlation was found between sealant usage and year of graduation from dental school. The increase may also be related to a decreased concern over the possibility of caries developing under the sealant.

Several studies have reported decreased viable bacterial counts in occlusal fissures that have been sealed. Handleman, Washburn, and Wopperer placed an ultraviolet-radiation–polymerized sealant on pits and fissures of teeth with incipient caries.[7] They reported a 2000-fold decrease in the number of cultivable microorganisms in the carious dentin samples of the sealed teeth compared with unsealed control teeth at the end of 2 years.

Going et al obtained bacteriologic samples from teeth that had been sealed with an ultraviolet-radiation—polymerized sealant for 5 years.[8] They found an apparent 89% reversal from a caries-active to a caries-free state in the sealed teeth.

Jeronimus, Till, and Sveen placed three different pit and fissure sealants on molars with incipient, moderate, and deep carious lesions.[9] Samples of carious dentin were removed immediately after and 2, 3, and 4 weeks after placement of the sealants and bacteriologic cultures were made. They reported usually positive culture results in teeth where the sealant was lost. Although their short-term study indicated that incipient carious lesions may not be of prime concern when sealants are applied, they cautioned against the use of sealants over deeper lesions because of the potential for advancement of caries when sealants over these lesions are lost. One must keep in mind that their deep-lesion group consisted of teeth with caries that had advanced pulpally greater than half the distance from the dentinoenamel junction.

Studies have shown definitively that deficient sealants are not effective in caries prevention and that loss of sealants leads to immediate risk of caries attack from undercover surfaces. Sealants require regular maintenance and repair or replacement to assure success in caries prevention over the long term.

Going declared that, given the results of many well-documented studies, practitioners' fear of sealing pits and fissures with incipient caries is not warranted.[10] He pointed out that sufficient studies of scientific merit reported negative or low bacterial concentrations after sealant had been in place for several years.

Wendt and Koch annually followed 758 sealed occlusal surfaces in first permanent molars for 1 to 10 years.[11] At the end of their study, evaluation of the surfaces that had been sealed 10 years previously revealed that only 6% showed caries or restorations. Romcke et al annually monitored 8340 sealants placed on high-risk (for caries) first permanent molars during a 10-year period.[12] Maintenance resealing was performed as indicated during the annual evaluations. One year after the sealants were placed, 6% required resealing; thereafter 2% to 4% required resealing annually. After 8 to 10 years, 85% of the sealed surfaces remained caries free.

Retrospective studies based on billing data from large third-party databases reveal that sealant use is still surprisingly low, even in populations for which sealants are a covered benefit.[13,14] In addition, these studies show that the effectiveness of sealants in preventing the need for future restorative care on the sealed surfaces declines after the first 3 years following sealant

treatment. These data argue again for the importance of vigilant recall and upkeep of sealants after placement.

Another concern is the placement of sealants immediately after topical fluoride application. Clinical and in vitro studies have shown that topical fluoride does not interfere with the bonding between sealant and enamel.[15,16]

RATIONALE FOR USE OF SEALANTS

In 1997 the ADA Councils on Access, Prevention, and Interprofessional Relations and on Scientific Affairs reconfirmed the safety and effectiveness of pit and fissure sealants as a caries-preventive measure and added that "dental sealants have proved to be highly effective in preventing pit and fissure dental caries.... Many individuals and groups stand to benefit from sealant placement. The key element is the professional judgment of the dentist, for a specific patient, at a specific time."[17]

The American Academy of Pediatric Dentistry's Pediatric Restorative Dentistry Consensus Conference[18] confirmed support for sealant use and published these recommendations:

1. Bonded resin sealants, placed by appropriately trained dental personnel, are safe, effective, and underused in preventing pit and fissure caries on at-risk surfaces. Effectiveness is increased with good technique and appropriate follow up and resealing as necessary.
2. Sealant benefit is increased by placement on surfaces judged to be at high risk or surfaces that already exhibit incipient carious lesions. Placing sealant over minimal-enamel caries has been shown to be effective at inhibiting lesion progression. Appropriate follow-up care is recommended, as with all dental treatment.
3. Presently, the best evaluation of risk is made by an experienced clinician using indicators of tooth morphology, clinical diagnostics, past caries history, past fluoride history, and present oral hygiene.
4. Caries risk, and therefore potential sealant benefit, may exist in any tooth with a pit or fissure, at any age, including primary teeth of children and permanent teeth of children and adults.
5. Sealant placement methods should include careful cleaning of the pits and fissures without removal of any appreciable enamel. Some circumstances may indicate use of a minimal-enameloplasty technique.
6. Placement of a low-viscosity, hydrophilic material-bonding layer as part of or under the actual sealant has been shown to enhance the long-term retention and effectiveness.

7. Glass ionomer materials have been shown to be ineffective as pit and fissure sealants but can be used as transitional sealants.
8. The profession must be alert to new preventive methods effective against pit and fissure caries. These may include changes in dental materials or technology.

SELECTION OF TEETH FOR SEALING

To gain the greatest benefit, the clinician should determine the caries risk; thus, the term *risk-based sealant treatment* has come into use. In risk-based sealant treatment, the practitioner takes into account prior caries experience, fluoride history, oral hygiene, and fissure anatomy in determining when sealant should be applied.

Good professional judgment should be used in the selection of teeth and patients. The use of pit and fissure sealants is contraindicated when rampant caries or interproximal lesions are present. Occlusal surfaces that are already carious with involvement of dentin require restoration.

All caries-susceptible surfaces should be carefully evaluated, because caries is unlikely in well-coalesced pits and fissures. In this case, sealants might be unnecessary or, at least, not cost effective. Finally, although sealant application is relatively simple, the meticulous technique requires patient cooperation and should be postponed for uncooperative patients until the procedures can be properly executed.

SEALANT TECHNIQUE

After selection, the tooth is washed and dried and the deep pits and fissures are reevaluated (Fig. 17-1, *A*). If caries is present, restoration or a combination of restoration and sealing may be indicated, as explained later in this chapter.

Marking centric stops with articulating paper will provide information so that excess sealant does not interfere with the occlusion. This is not necessary when the tooth has just erupted but is helpful in a well-established occlusion.

CLEANING

Adequate retention of the sealant requires that the pit and fissures be clean and free of excess moisture (Fig. 17-1, *B* and *C*). Acid etching completely removes the enamel pellicle, and a dental prophylaxis (even with a dental explorer) does not increase the retention of sealants. From a practical standpoint, in cases of poor oral hygiene, fissure cleansing with a rotating dry bristle brush may be beneficial.

Pope et al found that the use of a quarter round bur produced the greatest penetration of the sealant into etched enamel in laboratory studies.[19] The use of an aluminum oxide air abrasion system allows sealant penetration greater than that achievable by use of pumice or a dry bristle brush alone. It is not known if the increased depth of sealant penetration will result in greater sealant retention. When pumice or aluminum oxide is used, particulate matter is left in the deep recesses of the pits, the impact of which has not been determined.

Hatibovic-Kofman, Wright, and Braverman measured the microleakage of sealants placed in three groups of extracted teeth.[20] The teeth received conventional (etch), quarter round bur, or air abrasion surface preparation. Teeth prepared with the bur exhibited the least microleakage. The amount of microleakage in the conventional and air abrasion groups was about equal. No clinical studies exist to substantiate the value of using a bur to clean fissure surfaces prior to sealant placement.

The routine procedure of fissure eradication is probably not necessary. In fact, inappropriate or aggressive use of fissure opening or enameloplasty often removes the last of the enamel overlying dentin at the bottoms of fissures, which leaves the tooth more susceptible to future caries in the event of sealant loss. Good sealant methodology and proper sealant volume is probably more beneficial than enameloplasty.

ISOLATION

The tooth (or quadrant of teeth) to be sealed is first isolated. Rubber dam isolation is ideal but may not be feasible in certain circumstances. Cotton rolls, absorbent shields, and high-volume evacuation with compressed air may also be used effectively.

Eidelman, Fuks, and Chosack reported comparable retention results with the use of rubber dam and the use of cotton rolls for the isolation of teeth to be sealed.[21] Matis reported 96% retention of sealants with rubber dam isolation and 91% retention with cotton roll isolation at 12 months in young adults.[22] These values are not statistically different, however, which indicates that retention rates are probably not related to isolation technique, provided that the insertion technique is sound.

ETCHING

Microporosities in the enamel surface are created by the acid-etching technique. This permits a low-viscosity resin to be applied that penetrates the roughened surface and produces a mechanical lock of resin tags when cured.

Various phosphoric acid solutions have been evaluated for the etching procedure. Zidan and Hill tested the amount of surface loss of enamel after 60 seconds of etching with different phosphoric acid concentrations ranging from 0.5% to 80%.[23] They reported that the

18

Restorative Dentistry

RALPH E. McDONALD

DAVID R. AVERY

Advances in preventive dentistry and their application in the private dental office, the widespread acceptance of communal fluoridation, and greater emphasis on dental health education have dramatically changed the nature of dental practice. Today the dentist devotes more time to preventive procedures and less time to the routine restoration of carious teeth.

Nevertheless, the restoration of carious lesions in primary and young permanent teeth continues to be among the important services that pediatric dentists and general practitioners provide for the children in their practices. Patients and fellow practitioners often judge dentists on the effectiveness of their preventive programs and the skill with which they perform routine operative procedures.

The *Reference Manual* of the American Academy of Pediatric Dentistry (AAPD) includes a Guideline on Pediatric Restorative Dentistry (revised in 1998 and 2001) that states in part:

Restorative treatment shall be based upon the results of an appropriate clinical examination and ideally be part of a comprehensive treatment plan. The treatment plan shall take into consideration:

1. the developmental status of the dentition;
2. a caries-risk assessment based upon the caries history of the patient;
3. the patient's oral hygiene;
4. anticipated parental compliance and likelihood of timely recall;
5. the patient's ability to cooperate for treatment.

The restorative treatment plan must be prepared in conjunction with an individually tailored preventive program.
Restoration of primary teeth differs significantly from restoration of permanent teeth, due in part to the differences in tooth morphology.[1]

The AAPD, with financial assistance from the American Society of Dentistry for Children, held a pediatric restorative dentistry consensus conference on April 15-16, 2002, in San Antonio, Texas. Sixteen literature review and position papers were presented at the conference and numerous consensus statements about appropriate pediatric restorative materials and procedures were developed. All of the papers and the consensus statements may be found in *Pediatric Dentistry* 24(5), Sept/Oct 2002.

STATUS OF COMMON RESTORATIVE MATERIALS

Recent advances in the development of improved biomaterials for dental restorations have been rapid, and they continue to occur at a fast pace. This fact creates a significant challenge for dentists striving to remain at the cutting edge of dental technology. At this writing the more common restorative materials used in pediatric dentistry are composite and other resin systems, glass ionomers, silver amalgam alloys, and stainless steel alloys. Porcelain and cast metal alloy materials are also used in pediatric restorative dentistry but less frequently than those listed in the previous sentence.

Composite resins, glass ionomers, or some combination of the two are being used progressively more and silver amalgam progressively less in pediatric restorative dentistry. Many pediatric dentistry practices do not use silver amalgam at all; instead, some form of composite resin and/or glass ionomer is used. These materials have bonding capability. Glass ionomers may be considered pharmacologically therapeutic because they release fluoride over time; they also have minimal shrinkage during setting. Composite resins possess durability and superior esthetic qualities. When managed properly, both materials are capable of providing superior marginal sealing at the tooth–restorative material interface. The manufacturers of these materials have also combined them in an effort to join the primary advantages of each type of material. Berg has suggested that we think of these materials and their combinations on a continuum, with glass ionomer on the left, composite resin on the right, and the combined materials somewhere in between depending on the relative amounts of each material in the mix. Two major categories on the continuum are described as "resin-modified glass ionomer" (or "hybrid ionomer" or "light-cured glass ionomer") and "compomers" (or "polyacid-modified composite resin" or "glass ionomer–modified composite resin"). A fifth formulation has been added on the right side of the continuum in the form of "flowable composite resin." Berg points out that knowing the particular strengths and weaknesses of each type of material on the continuum will enhance the clinician's ability to make the best choices for each individual restorative situation.[2] Use of any of these restorative materials generally requires more effort and time than corresponding conventional amalgam restorations.

Despite its declining use, silver amalgam remains one of the most durable and cost-effective restorative materials. Success in using this filling material depends on adherence to certain principles of cavity preparation that do not always apply when materials on the glass ionomer–composite resin continuum are used. Some renewed interest in silver amalgam has occurred because of the development of "bonded amalgams." Bonded amalgams are silver amalgam restorations that have been condensed into etched cavity preparations lined with a dentin-bonding agent and some material on the glass ionomer–composite resin continuum. Bonded amalgams require considerable extra effort and expense to place compared with conventional amalgam restorations. The improvements in tooth support and marginal integrity gained with these restorations have been demonstrated in many studies. Some longer-term studies, however, suggest that the advantages of bonded amalgams may be transient and relatively short-lived, possibly 1 year or less.[3,4] In general, the use of bonded amalgams seems difficult to justify for the routine restoration of primary teeth because traditional silver amalgam should provide comparable quality more efficiently and cost effectively in most situations.

Stainless steel alloy is another commonly used pediatric restorative material. It is used extensively for full coronal coverage restorations of primary teeth. Stainless steel crowns have undoubtedly preserved the function of many primary teeth that otherwise would have been unrestorable. In addition, stainless steel crowns are often used to restore all posterior teeth in young patients with high caries risk who exhibit multiple proximal lesions that could otherwise be restored with silver amalgam or esthetic materials. Crowns are used instead simply because they better protect all posterior tooth surfaces from developing additional caries in the near future and because the posterior crown restoration has proven to be the most durable and cost effective in the primary dentition. Anterior stainless steel crowns may have labial resin or porcelain veneers to enhance esthetics.

MAINTENANCE OF A CLEAN FIELD

The maintenance of a clean operating field during cavity preparation and placement of the restorative material helps ensure efficient operation and development of a serviceable restoration that will maintain the tooth and the integrity of the developing occlusion.

The rubber dam aids in the maintenance of a clean field. It is generally agreed that the use of the rubber dam offers the following advantages:

1. *Saves time.* The dentist who has not routinely used the rubber dam needs only to follow the routine presented later in this chapter or a modification of it for a reasonable period to be convinced that operating time can be appreciably reduced. The time spent in placing the rubber dam is negligible, provided that the dentist works out a definite routine and uses a chairside assistant. Heise reported an average time of 1 minute, 48 seconds to isolate an average of 2.8 teeth with the rubber dam in 302 cases.[5] These applications of the rubber dam, placed with the aid of a capable dental assistant, were for routine operative dentistry procedures. The minimum time recorded for placing a rubber dam was 15 seconds (single-tooth isolation), and

the maximum time was 6 minutes. Many of the applications ranged from 25 to 50 seconds. Heise also observed that approximately 10 seconds is required to remove the rubber dam. The time required for the placement of the rubber dam will invariably be made up and additional time saved through the elimination of rinsing and spitting by the pediatric patient.

2. *Aids management.* A few explanatory words and reference to the rubber dam as a "raincoat" for the tooth or as a "Halloween mask" helps allay the child's anxiety. It has been found through experience that apprehensive or otherwise uncooperative children can often be controlled more easily with a rubber dam in place. Because the rubber dam efficiently controls the tongue and the lips, the dentist has greater freedom to complete the operative procedures.

3. *Controls saliva.* Control of saliva is an extremely important consideration when one is completing an ideal cavity preparation for primary teeth. The margin of error is appreciably reduced when a cavity is prepared in a primary tooth that has a large pulp and extensive carious involvement. Small pulp exposures may be more easily detected when the tooth is well isolated. It is equally important to observe the true extent of the exposure and the degree and type of hemorrhage from the pulp tissue. Thus the rubber dam aids the dentist in evaluating teeth that are being considered for vital pulp therapy.

4. *Provides protection.* The use of the rubber dam prevents foreign objects from coming into contact with oral structures. When filling material, debris, or medicaments are dropped into the mouth, salivary flow is stimulated and interferes with the operative or restorative procedure. A rubber dam also prevents the small child in a reclining position from swallowing or aspirating foreign objects and materials.

5. *Helps the dentist to educate parents.* Parents are always interested in the treatment that has been accomplished for their child. While the rubber dam is in place, the dentist can conveniently show parents the completed work after an operative procedure. The rubber dam creates the feeling that the dentist has complete control of the situation and that a conscientious effort has been made to provide the highest type of service.

ARMAMENTARIUM FOR RUBBER DAM PLACEMENT

The armamentarium consists of 5 × 5 inch sheets of medium latex, a rubber dam punch, clamp forceps, a selection of clamps, a flat-blade instrument, dental

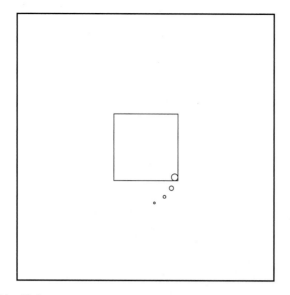

FIG. **18-1.** The corners of the square represent points where punch holes should be made for the clamp-bearing tooth.

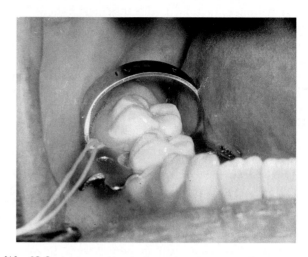

FIG. **18-2.** An Ivory No. 3 clamp has been trial-fitted to the second primary molar. The clamp will be removed and placed in the rubber dam.

floss, and a rubber dam frame. If one visualizes an approximately 1¼-inch square in the center of a sheet of rubber dam, each corner of the square indicates where the punch holes for the clamp-bearing tooth in each of the four quadrants of the mouth are to be made (Fig. 18-1). As experience is gained in applying the dam, the dentist and assistant will soon learn the proper location for punching the holes. If the holes are punched too far apart, the dam will not readily fit between the contact areas. In addition, the greater bulk of material between the teeth will greatly increase the possibility that the rubber will become a barrier to proximal surface preparation. Conversely, if the holes are punched too close together, salivary leakage will contaminate the operating field. In general, the holes should be punched the same distance apart as the holes on the cutting table of the rubber dam punch.

The large punch hole is used for the clamp-bearing tooth and for most permanent molars. The medium-sized punch hole generally is used for the premolars and primary molars. The second smallest hole is used for maxillary permanent incisors, whereas the smallest hole is adequate for the primary incisors and lower permanent incisors.

SELECTION OF A CLAMP

The operator will soon develop a personal preference for which clamps to use to secure the dam in isolating different areas in the mouth. Unless the clamp is firmly anchored to the tooth, the tension of the stretched rubber will easily dislodge it. Therefore the proper selection of a clamp is of utmost importance. It is recommended that the clamp be tried on the tooth before the rubber dam is placed to ascertain that the clamp can be securely seated

and will not be easily dislodged by the probing tongue, lip, or cheek musculature. An 18-inch length of dental floss should be doubled and securely fastened to the bow of the clamp. The floss will facilitate retrieval in the unlikely event that the clamp should slip and fall toward the pharynx (Fig. 18-2).

The following procedure is recommended for rubber dam application (Fig. 18-3). The previously selected and ligated clamp is placed in the rubber dam. The dentist grasps the clamp forceps with the clamp engaged. The assistant, seated to the left of the patient (the dentist is right-handed in this example), grasps the upper corners of the dam with the right hand and the lower left corner between the left thumb and index finger. The dam is moved toward the patient's face as the dentist carries the clamp to the tooth while holding the lower right portion of the dam. After securing the clamp on the tooth, the dentist transfers the clamp forceps to the assistant, who receives it while continuing to hold the upper corners of the dam with the right hand. The dentist then places the frame over the rubber dam. Together the assistant and dentist attach the corners of the dam to the frame. The flat blade of a plastic instrument or a right-angle explorer may be used to remove the rubber dam material from the wings of the clamp and to complete the seal around the clamped tooth. If necessary, light finger pressure may seat the clamp securely by moving it cervically on the tooth. If additional teeth are to be isolated, the rubber is stretched over them, and the excess rubber between the punched holes is placed between the contact areas with the aid of dental floss. The most anterior tooth and others if necessary are ligated to aid in the retention of the dam

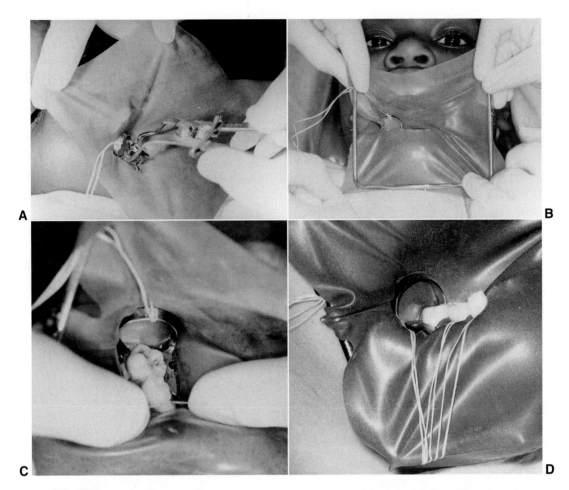

FIG. **18-3. A,** The dental assistant holds the top and lower right corners of the rubber dam as the dentist holds the lower left corner and carries the clamp to the tooth. **B,** The assistant and dentist attach the corners of the rubber dam to the frame. **C,** Dental floss is used to carry the rubber dam between the teeth. **D,** The teeth are isolated and ready for the operative procedure. **(A, B,** and **C** courtesy Dr. Richard Troyer.)

and the prevention of cervical leakage. The free ends of the floss are allowed to remain, because they may aid in the further retraction of the gingival tissue or the patient's lip during the operative procedure. At the end of the operative procedure, the length of floss will also aid in removing the ligature.

When a quadrant of restorations in the primary dentition is planned and no pulp therapy is anticipated, Croll recommends the "slit-dam method."[6] One long opening is made in the dam, and the entire quadrant is isolated without interseptal dam material between the teeth.

It is unwise to include more teeth in the rubber dam than are necessary to isolate the working area adequately. If the first or second permanent molar is the only tooth in the quadrant that is carious and if it requires only an occlusal preparation, it is often desirable to punch only one hole in the dam and to isolate the single tooth (Fig. 18-4). This procedure will require only seconds and will save many minutes.

MORPHOLOGIC CONSIDERATIONS

The crowns of the primary teeth are smaller but more bulbous than the corresponding permanent teeth, and the molars are bell-shaped, with a definite constriction in the cervical region. The characteristic sharp lingual inclination occlusally of the facial surfaces results in the formation of a distinct faciogingival ridge that ends abruptly at the cementoenamel junction. The sharp constriction at the neck of the primary molar necessitates special care in the formation of the gingival floor during class II cavity preparation. The buccal and lingual surfaces of the molars converging sharply occlusally form a narrow occlusal surface or food table; this is especially true of the first primary molar.

The pulpal outline of the primary teeth follows the dentoenamel junction more closely than that of the permanent teeth. The pulpal horns are longer and more pointed than the cusps would indicate. The dentin also has less bulk or thickness, and so the pulp is

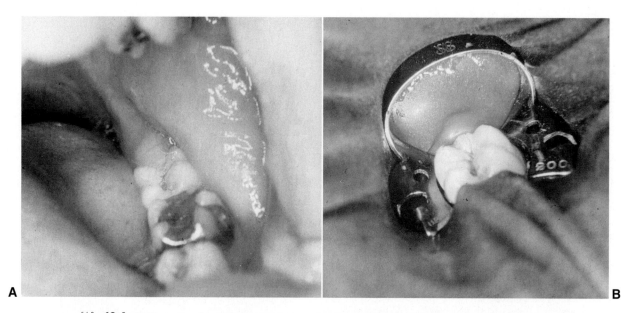

A   B

FIG. **18-4. A,** The second permanent molar requires an occlusal restoration. It is not necessary to isolate more than a single tooth. **B,** A No. 200 clamp has been selected to hold the rubber dam in place. The rubber dam has retracted the tissue that extended over the distal marginal ridge.

proportionately larger than that of the permanent teeth. The enamel of the primary teeth is thin but of uniform thickness. The enamel surface tends to be parallel to the dentinoenamel junction.

BASIC PRINCIPLES IN THE PREPARATION OF CAVITIES IN PRIMARY TEETH

Traditional cavity preparations for class I and class II lesions include areas that have carious involvement and, in addition, those areas that retain food and plaque material and may be considered areas of potential carious involvement. A flat pulpal floor is generally advocated. However, a sharp angle between the pulpal floor and the axial wall of a two-surface preparation should be avoided. Rounded angles throughout the preparation will result in less concentration of stresses and will permit better adaptation of the restorative material into the extremities of the preparation.

Although the traditional class I cavity preparation and restoration may occasionally be the most practical treatment for a tooth in certain circumstances, such treatment is currently obsolete for most class I lesions. The traditional treatment has been replaced, for the most part, by conservative caries excavation and restoration using a combination of bonding restorative and sealant materials (see Chapter 17).

Likewise, the traditional class II cavity preparation and restoration, though not yet considered obsolete, is currently used less frequently as steadily improving restorative materials with therapeutic and bonding capability are developed. In the traditional class II

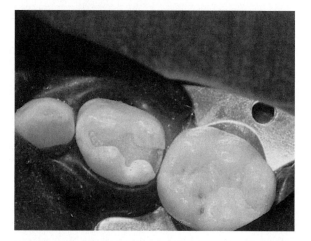

FIG. **18-5.** Conservative but adequate extension of a traditional class II cavity preparation in a mandibular first primary molar.

cavity preparation for amalgam, the buccal and lingual extensions should be carried to self-cleansing areas. The cavity design should have greater buccal and lingual extension at the cervical area of the preparation to clear contact with the adjacent tooth. This divergent pattern is necessary because of the broad, flat contact areas of the primary molars and because of the distinct buccal bulge in the gingival third. Ideally, the width of the preparation at the isthmus should be approximately one third the intercuspal dimension (Fig. 18-5). The axiopulpal line angle should be beveled or grooved to reduce the concentration of stresses and to provide greater bulk of material in this area, which is vulnerable to fracture.

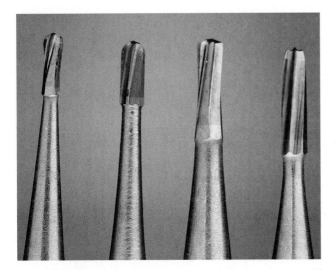

FIG. **18-6.** Rounded-end, high-speed carbide burs No. 329, No. 330, No. 245, and No. 256, which may be used for cutting cavity preparations.

Because many occlusal fractures of amalgam restorations are caused by sharp opposing cusps, it is advisable to identify these potentially damaging cusps with articulating paper before cavity preparation. The slight reduction and rounding of a sharp opposing cusp will reduce the number of such fractures.

CAVITY PREPARATION IN PRIMARY TEETH

The steps in the preparation of a cavity in a primary tooth are not difficult but do require precise operator control. Many authorities advocate the use of small, rounded-end carbide burs in the high-speed handpiece to establish the cavity outline and perform the gross preparation. For efficiency and convenience, all necessary high-speed instrumentation for a given preparation may be completed with a single bur in most situations. Therefore the dentist should select the bur that is best designed to accomplish all the high-speed cutting required for the procedure being planned. Fig. 18-6 illustrates four high-speed carbide burs designed to cut efficiently and yet allow conservative cavity preparations with rounded line angles and point angles. Alternatively, cavity preparations may be made with aluminum oxide air abrasion systems or with laser systems approved for hard-tissue procedures.

INCIPIENT CLASS I CAVITY IN A VERY YOUNG CHILD

During the routine examination of a child younger than 2 years of age, the dentist may occasionally discover a small but definite carious lesion in the central fossa of one or two first primary molars, with all other teeth being sound. Thus restorative needs are present but

minimal. Because of the child's psychologic immaturity and because it is usually impossible to establish effective communication with the child, the parent should hold the child on his or her lap in the dental chair. This will help the child feel more secure and provide a better opportunity to restrain the child's movement during the operative procedure. The small-cavity preparation may be made without the aid of a rubber dam or local anesthetic. A No. 329 or No. 330 bur is used to open the decayed area and extend the cavo-surface margin only to the extent of the carious lesion. If the patient is resistant (usually), completing the preparation with an air abrasion or laser system would be inconvenient. The preparation can be completed in just a few seconds. Restoring the tooth with amalgam or a resin-modified glass ionomer will arrest the decay and at least temporarily prevent further tooth destruction without a lengthy or involved dental appointment for the child. If the child is cooperative, a preventive resin restoration, preceded by application of a dentin-bonding agent, may be used.

PIT OR FISSURE CLASS I CAVITY

The preparation and restoration of a pit or fissure class I cavity are discussed in chapter 17 (see the section on preventive resin restoration).

DEEP-SEATED CLASS I CAVITY

If an amalgam restoration is planned, the first step in the preparation of an extensive class I cavity is to plane back the enamel that overhangs the extensive carious lesion. Then the cavity preparation should be extended throughout the remaining grooves and anatomic occlusal defects. The carious dentin should next be removed with large, round burs or spoon excavators. If a carious exposure is not encountered, the cavity walls should be paralleled and finished as previously described. With deep carious lesions and near pulp exposures, the depth of the cavity should be covered with a biocompatible base material to provide adequate thermal protection for the pulp.

If a composite resin and/or glass ionomer restoration is planned, any disease-free pits and grooves may be sealed as part of the bonded restoration. The restorative material will also provide thermal insulation to the pulp.

CLASS II CAVITY

Proximal lesions in a preschool child indicate excessive caries activity; a preventive and restorative program should be undertaken immediately.

Small Lesions. Very small incipient proximal lesions may be chemically restored with topical fluoride therapy provided by the dentist, along with the judicious use of fluoride products designed for topical

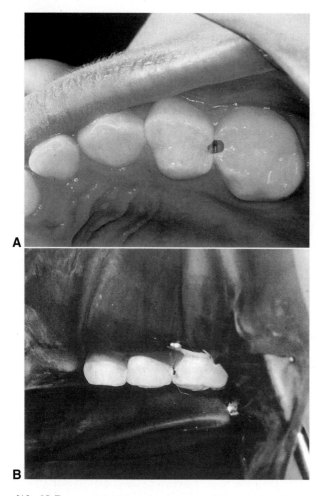

A

B

FIG. **18-7.** Approximating conservative preparations to remove small class II carious lesions in primary molars. **A,** Marginal ridge access. **B,** Facial surface access.

application at home. If this treatment regimen is accompanied by improved diet and improved oral hygiene, some incipient proximal lesions may remineralize or remain in an arrested state indefinitely. However, the parents should be informed of the incipient lesions and emphasis should be placed on the need to continue practicing the recommended procedures and to bring the child back for periodic examinations. If the parents and the patient do not follow the instructions properly, subsequent bite-wing radiographs will reveal growth of the lesion, and restorative procedures should be initiated before the defects become extensive carious lesions.

As bonded restorations have improved, especially those restorations capable of fluoride release, more conservative cavity preparation designs have also been advocated. In otherwise sound teeth free of susceptible pits and fissures, accessing small class II carious lesions via small openings in the marginal ridges or in the facial surfaces of the teeth is becoming a popular technique (Fig. 18-7). Gaining access to the lesion with openings

only large enough to allow caries excavation is the goal. Caries is removed by pendulous motions of small burs or by tilting of the air abrasion tip laterally and pulpally at the initial opening. This technique is particularly useful in cooperative patients with one or two affected primary molars who are judged to be at relatively low risk for additional caries activity.

Croll[7] as well as Vaikuntam[8] have also advocated conservative preparations and restorations with fluoride-releasing restorative materials. Our experience has shown that local anesthesia is usually unnecessary to make the preparation. When performing this short procedure in cooperative patients, rubber dam isolation is often optional, especially on maxillary teeth. Use of resin-modified glass ionomer materials results in excellent restorations for this conservative procedure (Fig. 18-8).

Marks et al[9] and also Welbury[10] et al (who also restored class I preparations) have reported very satisfactory results using conservative class II preparations and compomers to restore primary molars in studies of 36 and 42 months' duration, respectively. In a 3-year study, Hubel and Mejare reported the successful performance of conservative class II resin-modified glass ionomer restorations in primary molars.[11]

Lesions with Greater Dentin Involvement. The first step in the traditional preparation of a class II cavity in a primary tooth for an amalgam or an esthetic restoration involves opening the marginal ridge area. Extreme care must be taken when breaking through the marginal ridge to prevent damage to the adjacent proximal surface.

Amalgam. The gingival seat and proximal walls should break contact with the adjacent tooth. The angle formed by the axial wall and the buccal and lingual walls of the proximal box should approach a right angle. The buccal and lingual walls necessarily diverge toward the cervical region, following the general contour of the tooth (Fig. 18-9). The occlusal extension of the preparation should include any caries-susceptible pits and fissures. If the occlusal surface is sound and not caries susceptible, then a minimal occlusal dovetail is still often needed to enhance the cavity retention form. If carious material remains after the preparation outline is established, it should next be removed. The appropriate liner or intermediate base, if indicated, and a snug-fitting matrix should be placed before the insertion of the amalgam.

Esthetic Materials. Because of the improvements in the properties of composite resins, many dentists use them routinely for posterior restorations. More recently the use of glass ionomer restoratives (or other materials on the glass ionomer–composite resin continuum) has also been advocated. The preparation and restoration may be similar to that described earlier for amalgam

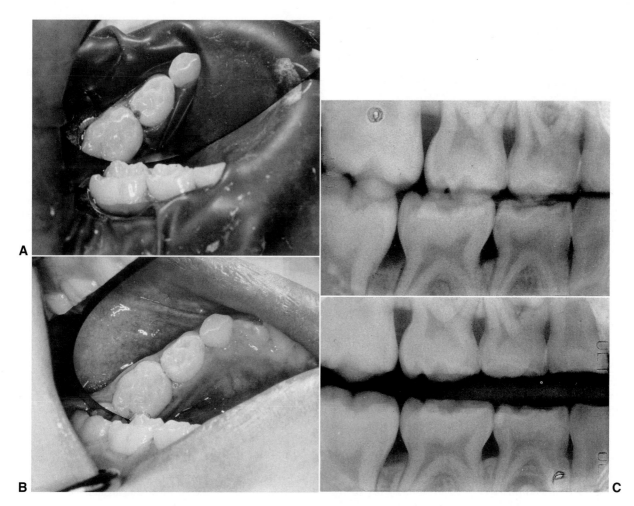

FIG. **18-8. A,** Conservative class II preparation. **B,** Resin-modified glass ionomer restoration. **C,** Preoperative radiograph *(top)* and 17-month postoperative film.

FIG. **18-9.** Traditional class II cavity preparation for a primary molar. The preparation includes diverging proximal walls and a beveled and grooved axiopulpal line angle.

when significant caries exists on both the occlusal and proximal surfaces (Fig. 18-10). However, little or no occlusal preparation may be required when the occlusal pits and fissures are caries susceptible but sound or incipient. Then the proximal restoration may be combined with application of an occlusal sealant (with or without enameloplasty). Whenever composite restorative materials are employed, enamel beveling, etching, and application of bonding agents are recommended.

Clinical trials of restoration of primary molars reported by Paquette et al[12] and by Oldenburg, Vann, and Dilley[13] revealed that traditional preparations modified only by beveling of enamel margins and restored with bonded composite resins yielded highly successful results during 12- and 24-month observation periods. Tonn and Ryge have also reported acceptable 2-year results for primary molars restored with bonded composite resins in traditional cavity preparations modified only by beveling of enamel margins.[14]

Dilley et al have demonstrated that the placement and finishing of posterior composite restorations are significantly more time consuming than those for comparable amalgam restorations.[15] In addition to increasing the cost of care, the extra time required for treatment may complicate patient management for some young patients.

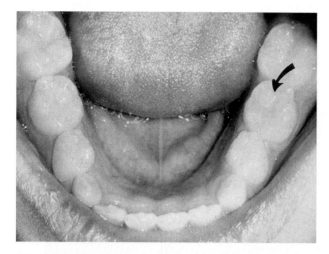

FIG. **18-10.** A distal occlusal composite resin restoration was placed in the lower left second primary molar 6 months before the photograph.

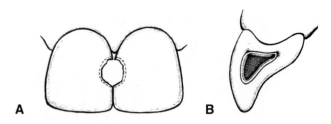

FIG. **18-11.** **A,** Schematic drawing of carious lesions on the mesial surfaces of maxillary primary central incisors that do not undermine the mesial angles of the teeth. The dotted line indicates the proposed labial outline of the class III cavity preparation. **B,** Proximal view illustrates that the class III preparation is limited to the cervical two thirds of the primary incisor. *(From Roche JR: Restorative dentistry. In Goldman HM et al, editors:* Current therapy in dentistry, *vol 4, St Louis, 1970, Mosby.)*

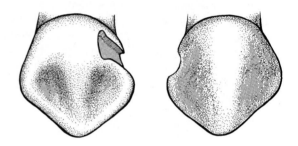

FIG. **18-12.** Lingual and labial views of a modified class III preparation for a maxillary primary canine. The dovetail improves retention form of the preparation and allows access for placing the restorative material to ensure adequate contact with the adjacent tooth.

More recently Donly et al have reported successful results for class II resin-modified glass ionomer restorations in primary molars after 3 years of observation.[16] The dentist's sound professional judgment is the key to selecting the restoration that will best serve the patient in each situation.

CLASS III CAVITY

Carious lesions on the proximal surfaces of anterior primary teeth sometimes occur in children whose teeth are in contact and in children who have evidence of arch inadequacy or crowding. Carious involvement of the anterior primary teeth, however, may be interpreted as evidence of excessive caries activity requiring a comprehensive preventive program.

If the carious lesion has not advanced appreciably into the dentin and removal of the caries will not involve or weaken the incisal angle, a small conventional class III cavity may be prepared and the tooth may be restored with the dentist's choice of bonding materials (Fig. 18-11).

Mandibular primary incisors with small proximal carious lesions may not require conventional restorations at all. Enameloplasty of the affected proximal surface (usually described as "disking") to open the proximal contact and to remove most, if not all, of the cavitation, followed by topical treatments with fluoride varnish, will often suffice until the teeth exfoliate naturally. Extraction is usually indicated when mandibular primary incisors have extensive caries.

MODIFIED CLASS III CAVITY PREPARATION

The distal surface of the primary canine is a frequent site of caries attack in patients at high risk for caries if the canine is in proximal contact with the first molar. The position of the tooth in the arch, the characteristically

broad contact between the distal surface of the canine and the mesial surface of the primary molar, and the height of the gingival tissue sometimes make it difficult to prepare a typical class III cavity and restore it adequately. The modified class III preparation uses a dovetail on the lingual or occasionally on the labial surfaces of the tooth. A lingual lock is normally considered for the maxillary canine, whereas a labial lock may be more conveniently prepared on the mandibular teeth for which the esthetic requirement is not so important (Figs. 18-12 and 18-13). The preparation allows for additional retention and access necessary to insert the restorative material properly.

RESTORATION OF PROXIMAL INCISAL CARIES IN PRIMARY ANTERIOR TEETH

PREFORMED STAINLESS STEEL BANDS

The use of preformed stainless steel bands has been advocated by McConville and Tonn for the restoration of anterior primary teeth with deep mesial or distal

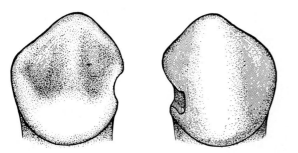

FIG. **18-13.** Lingual and labial views of a modified class III preparation for a mandibular primary canine.

caries involving the incisal angle.[17] The band is fitted before caries removal. After caries removal, the cavity and the band are filled with a creamy mix of glass ionomer cement, and the band is seated to place. After the cement has hardened, the excess cement is removed.

Although this cemented-band technique was recommended before the development of good esthetic restorative materials, it may still be the restoration of choice in the very young child with early childhood caries when the parents decide against the more time-consuming and expensive esthetic restorative procedures. If the pulps of the teeth are healthy, cemented-band restorations are preferable to extractions. With the use of accepted methods of restraining the child's movements, this procedure can be carried out quickly and yet provide a satisfactory long-term restoration. After the child has gained more maturity and has become a cooperative patient, the bands may be removed and more esthetic restorations provided, if desired.

If the carious involvement of an anterior tooth endangers the pulp, the cemented band is excellent for supporting the intermediate dressing in indirect pulp therapy. Only the gross caries is removed at the initial appointment, and the previously fitted band is cemented on the tooth to seal the cavity and arrest the caries process. A waiting period of at least 6 weeks is indicated to allow adequate reparative dentin formation before the band is taken off the tooth and the remaining caries removed. If there is no evidence of a pulp exposure, the final restorative procedure is carried out.

ESTHETIC RESIN RESTORATION

One type of preparation used for the esthetic restoration of primary incisors in which dental caries approximates or involves the incisal edge of the teeth is illustrated in Fig. 18-14. As with other operative procedures for the pediatric patient, the use of the rubber dam aids in maintenance of a dry field, provides better vision, and facilitates control of the lips and tongue.

The preparation includes a proximal reduction through the incisal angle and the carious lesion, and ends at the established cervical seat. Labial and lingual locks are then prepared in the cervical third of the tooth. The remaining caries is removed, the tooth is etched, and a bonding agent is applied.

A properly placed matrix tightly wedged at the cervical seat aids the operator in placing, shaping, and holding the composite resin during the curing process. A good matrix also simplifies the finishing procedures.

McEvoy has described a similar preparation and restoration for primary incisors, except that the retentive locking component is placed on the labial surface only in the gingival one third of the tooth.[18] The lock extends minimally across two thirds of the labial surface and may extend even farther to include decalcified enamel in the cervical area. We would also recommend slightly beveling the enamel margins before etching to further improve the marginal bonding of the restoration.

Initial shaping of the restoration may be accomplished with a flame-shaped finishing bur. The excess resin is removed, and the contour of the restoration is established. The gingival margins may be finished with a sharp scalpel blade. Final polishing may be accomplished with the rubber cup and a fine, moist abrasive material or one of the composite polishing systems (Fig. 18-15).

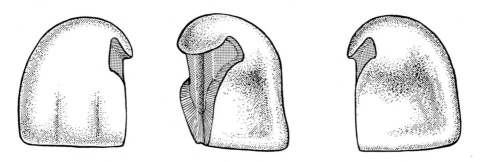

FIG. **18-14.** Labial, proximolingual, and lingual views of a preparation for an esthetic resin restoration in a primary incisor. The preparation includes a proximal reduction and the establishment of a definitive cervical seat that extends to labial and lingual locks in the cervical third of the tooth.

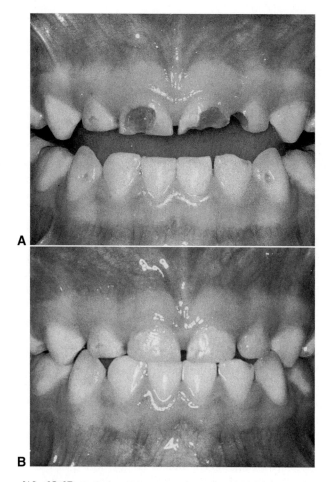

FIG. **18-15.** **A,** Extensive carious lesions of the maxillary right central, left central, and lateral incisors of a 3½-year-old patient. **B,** Postoperative view of the restored teeth. The restorations are retained with labial and lingual locks incorporated in the preparations. The maxillary lateral preparation was designed as illustrated in Fig. 18-14.

STAINLESS STEEL CROWNS

Primary incisors or canines that have extensive proximal lesions involving the incisal portion of the tooth may be restored with stainless steel crowns.

A steel crown of appropriate size is selected, contoured at the cervical margin, polished, and cemented into place. The crown technique is discussed in detail later in this chapter. Although the crown will be well retained even on teeth that require removal of extensive portions of carious tooth structure, the esthetic requirements of some children may not be met by this type of restoration.

Most of the labial metal may be cut away, leaving a labial "window" that is then restored with composite resin (Fig. 18-16). This restoration is called an *open-face stainless steel crown.*

Several brands of stainless steel crowns with esthetic facings veneered to the labial surfaces are also available

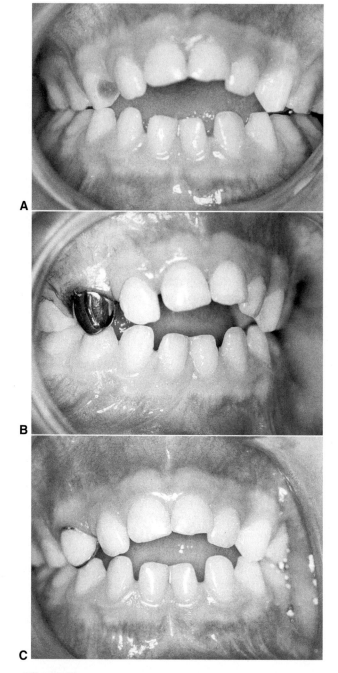

FIG. **18-16.** **A,** An extensive carious lesion is evident in the maxillary right primary canine. **B,** After the removal of caries and preparation of the tooth, a stainless steel crown was fitted to the tooth. **C,** The labial portion of the steel crown was removed and restored with resin. *(Courtesy Dr. Lionel Traubman.)*

to restore primary anterior teeth (Fig. 18-17). Such crowns are available for direct adaptation to the prepared teeth. Alternatively, the restorations may be completed in two appointments, with the labial veneers added in the laboratory after the bare steel crowns are adapted to the teeth but before final cementation.

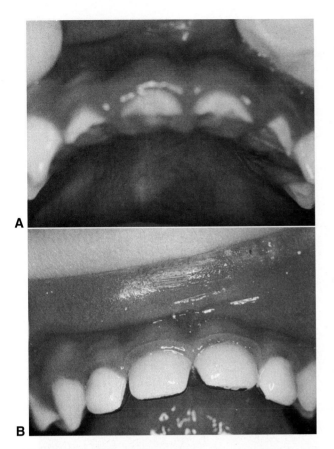

FIG. **18-17.** **A,** Extensive caries and coronal destruction of the maxillary incisors in a child 21 months of age. **B,** After pulp therapy, the teeth were restored with veneered stainless steel crowns. *(Courtesy Dr. Gary J. Hinz.)*

Croll recommends that an anterior alginate impression be made before the restorative appointment.[19] The crown preparations can then be simulated on a stone model, and most of the crown adaptation can be achieved in advance. This procedure enables the clinician to cement the crowns at the same appointment at which the preparations are made (rather than waiting for laboratory veneering of the adapted bare crowns). Croll's technique also gives the clinician a better opportunity to focus on fitting the crowns so that optimal tooth alignment will result, which further enhances the esthetic outcome.

DIRECT RESIN CROWNS

Doyle introduced a preparation design for primary incisor jacket crowns that uses an undercut area around the gingival shoulder, retains as much enamel as possible for etching, and preserves the midportion of the natural incisal edge whenever possible to improve retention.[20] After excavating the caries, protecting the exposed dentin, and etching the enamel, the dentist restores the prepared incisor with a preformed acrylic jacket crown lined with self-curing restorative resin.

Webber et al[21] have described a resin crown technique very similar to Doyle's except that the tooth is restored with composite resin using a celluloid crown form as a matrix. They did not advocate preserving a portion of the incisal edge. They point out that very little finishing of the restoration is required when the celluloid crown has been properly fitted.

Doyle's idea of preserving a portion of the tooth's natural incisal edge whenever possible seems valid.[20] Preservation of the incisal area of the tooth provides a greater surface area of etched enamel and greater length in the preparation, both of which will improve the retentive quality of the restoration.

The jacket crown technique illustrated in Fig. 18-18 incorporates the use of a celluloid crown form and composite resin as advocated by Webber et al[21] and also includes the preservation of the tooth's natural incisal edge as advocated by Doyle.[20]

Celluloid crown forms are also available for primary posterior teeth. These crown forms are useful matrices for some posterior bonded restorations. A good example of an indication for using such a crown form is to provide a bonded crown buildup to temporarily reestablish arch integrity and occlusion of an ankylosed (submerged) primary molar.

PREPARATION OF CAVITIES IN YOUNG PERMANENT TEETH

Many of the caries management procedures presented in this textbook also often apply to young permanent teeth. Entire textbooks are devoted to operative dentistry procedures, and the primary focus of these books is restoration of permanent teeth. Repeating all that information (or portions thereof) in this chapter is impractical and realistically impossible. For detailed information about the various cavity preparation designs for permanent teeth and the matrix systems to facilitate the placement and contour of restorations, please consult a standard textbook of operative dentistry listed in the references, such as those by Roberson, Heymann, and Swift[22] and by Baum, Phillips, and Lund.[23]

INTERIM RESTORATION FOR HYPOPLASTIC PERMANENT MOLARS

The dentist who routinely treats children occasionally faces a difficult restorative problem when severely hypoplastic first permanent molars erupt. Often the teeth are so defective that they require restoration at a very early stage of eruption. Many of these teeth have been saved by early restoration with stainless steel crowns as an interim procedure. However, this procedure may require sacrificing sound tooth surfaces to provide adequate space for the crown. Such full-coverage restorations are sometimes difficult to fit.

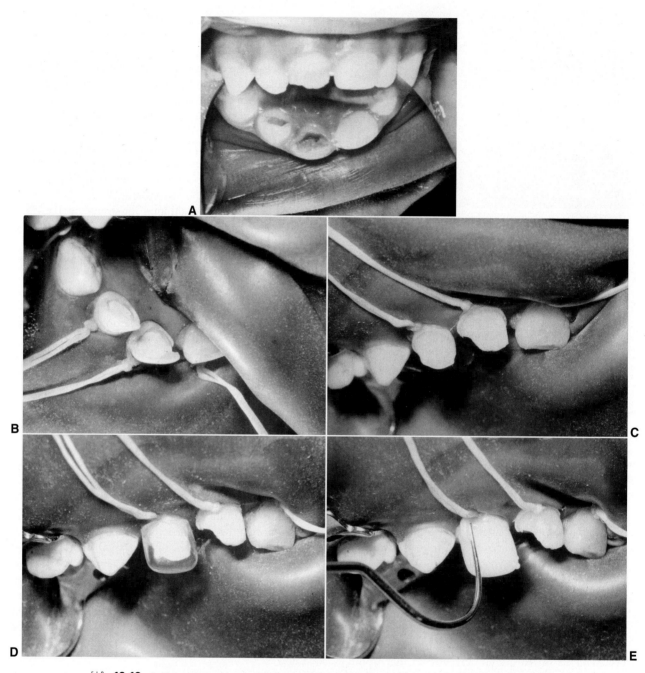

FIG. **18-18.** **A,** Extensive caries on the lingual surfaces of the maxillary right primary central and lateral incisors in a 2½-year-old patient. The caries has also severely undermined the proximal and incisal surfaces of the teeth. The maxillary left central incisor had been previously restored. **B,** The carious lesions have been excavated, and the exposed dentin has been covered with calcium hydroxide. **C,** Completed jacket preparations with cervical shoulders, slightly undercut walls at the cervical areas, and preservation of as much enamel and incisal tooth structure as possible. The enamel has been etched. **D,** Fitted celluloid crown form on the lateral incisor. The crown form should be trimmed to fit snugly and to just cover all cervical margins of the preparation. A snug fit at the cervical margin is very desirable, even if the incisal is too long, to minimize cervical finishing of the restoration. **E,** The crown form filled with composite resin has been seated, and the excess material is being carefully removed at the cervical margins with an explorer. Note excess material exuding from the vent hole placed on the mesial incisal of the crown form.

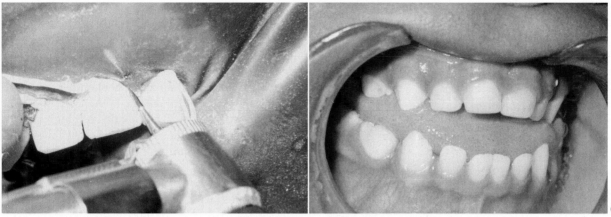

FIG. **18-18, cont'd. F,** The central incisor was restored in a similar fashion. The incisal edges of the restorations have been trimmed back to the natural tooth structure with a No. 7901 finishing bur, which is also being used to trim the cervical margins and embrasure areas before polishing. **G,** The resin jacket crown restorations 2 months postoperatively. *(Courtesy Dr. Robert Rust.)*

The composite materials have proved to be a more satisfactory interim restoration for many of these teeth. Such a bonded composite buildup restoration allows preservation of all sound tooth structure and depends on the presence of some enamel surfaces to provide bonded retention for the restorative material. Any soft defective areas are excavated, but little or no additional tooth preparation is done. Usually even undermined enamel surfaces are preserved for additional retention and support of the restorative material. In some cases gingivoplasty around the erupting tooth may first be necessary to allow adequate access to and isolation of the defective areas. Even if the restoration requires occasional repair, it still often provides a more satisfactory interim result than the stainless steel crown. Some of the newer restorative materials on the glass ionomer–composite resin continuum may also be useful interim restorations for hypoplastic teeth.

In situations in which a stainless steel crown is required to restore a young permanent molar, Radcliffe and Cullen have noted the importance of conservative tooth preparation to preserve better options for future restoration of the same tooth.[24] They advocate a preparation similar to that described in the following section.

STAINLESS STEEL CROWNS FOR POSTERIOR TEETH

Chrome steel crowns, as introduced by Humphrey in 1950, have proved to be serviceable restorations for children and adolescents and are now commonly called *stainless steel crowns.*[25] There are a number of indications for the use of stainless steel crowns in pediatric dentistry, including the following:

1. Restorations for primary or young permanent teeth with extensive and/or multiple carious lesions (Fig. 18-19)
2. Restorations for hypoplastic primary or permanent teeth that cannot be adequately restored with bonded restorations
3. Restorations for teeth with hereditary anomalies, such as dentinogenesis imperfecta or amelogenesis imperfecta
4. Restorations for pulpotomized or pulpectomized primary or young permanent teeth when there is increased danger of fracture of the remaining coronal tooth structure
5. Restorations for fractured teeth
6. Restorations for primary teeth to be used as abutments for appliances
7. Attachments for habit-breaking and orthodontic appliances

Randall published an extensive review of the literature that reports on the use of preformed metal crowns for primary and permanent molars.[26] She found five clinical studies that have compared the performance of crown restorations with that of multisurface amalgam restorations. The five studies included a total of 1210 crowns and 2201 amalgams that were followed from a minimum of 2 years to a maximum of 10 years. The findings in all five studies were in agreement that the crown restorations were superior to the amalgam restorations in the treatment of multisurface cavities in

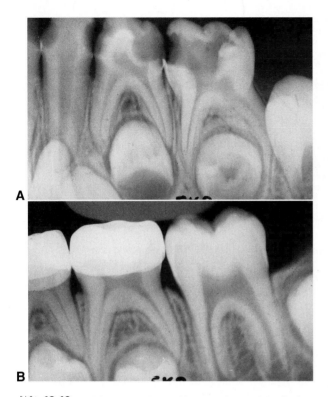

FIG. **18-19** **A,** Primary molars with extensive carious lesions. **B,** Adequately contoured steel crowns have maintained function and the relationship of the primary teeth in the arch.

primary molars. Randall's review was followed by a position paper prepared by Seale that included additional scientific evidence favoring the use of stainless steel crown restorations, especially in children at high risk for caries.[27] Seale's published abstract states in part:

> The stainless steel crown (SSC) is an extremely durable restoration.... Children with extensive decay, large lesions or multiple surface lesions in primary molars should be treated with stainless steel crowns. Because of the protection from future decay provided by their feature of full coverage and their increased durability and longevity, strong consideration should be given to the use of SSCs in children who require general anesthesia. Finally, a strong argument for the use of the SSC restoration is its cost effectiveness based on its durability and longevity.

PREPARATION OF THE TOOTH

A local anesthetic should be administered and a rubber dam placed as for other restorative procedures. The proximal surfaces are reduced using a No. 69L bur at high speed (Fig. 18-20). Care must be taken not to damage adjacent tooth surfaces during the proximal reductions. A wooden wedge may be placed tightly between the surface being reduced and the adjacent surface to provide a slight separation between the teeth for better access. Near-vertical reductions are made on

the proximal surfaces and carried gingivally until the contact with the adjacent tooth is broken and an explorer can be passed freely between the prepared tooth and the adjacent tooth. The gingival margin of the preparation on the proximal surface should be a smooth feathered edge with no ledge or shoulder present. The cusps and the occlusal portion of the tooth may then be reduced with a No. 69L bur revolving at high speed. The general contour of the occlusal surface is followed, and approximately 1 mm of clearance with the opposing teeth is required.

The No. 69L bur at high speed may also be used to remove all sharp line and point angles. It is usually not necessary to reduce the buccal or lingual surfaces; in fact, it is desirable to have an undercut on these surfaces to aid in the retention of the contoured crown. In some cases, however, it may be necessary to reduce the distinct buccal bulge, particularly on the first primary molar.

If any carious dentin remains after these steps in crown preparation are completed, it is excavated next. In the event that a vital pulp exposure is encountered, a pulpotomy procedure is usually carried out.

SELECTION OF CROWN SIZE

The smallest crown that completely covers the preparation should be chosen. Spedding has advocated adhering to two important principles that will help consistently to produce well-adapted stainless steel crowns.[28] First, the operator must establish the correct occlusogingival crown length; and second, the crown margins should be shaped circumferentially to follow the natural contours of the tooth's marginal gingivae. The crown should be reduced in height, if necessary, until it clears the occlusion and is approximately 0.5 to 1 mm beneath the free margin of the gingival tissue. The patient can force the crown over the preparation by biting an orangewood stick or a tongue depressor. After making a scratch mark on the crown at the level of the free margin of the gingival tissue, the dentist can remove the crown and determine where additional metal must be cut away with a No. 11B curved shears or a rotating stone (Fig. 18-21).

With a curved-beak pliers, the cut edges of the crown are redirected cervically and the crown is replaced on the preparation. The child is again directed to bite on an orangewood stick to forcibly seat the crown so that the gingival margins may be checked for proper extension.

The precontoured and festooned crowns currently available often require very little, if any, modification before cementation.

CONTOURING OF THE CROWN (WHEN NECESSARY)

A crown-contouring pliers with a ball-and-socket design is used at the cervical third (if loosely fitting,

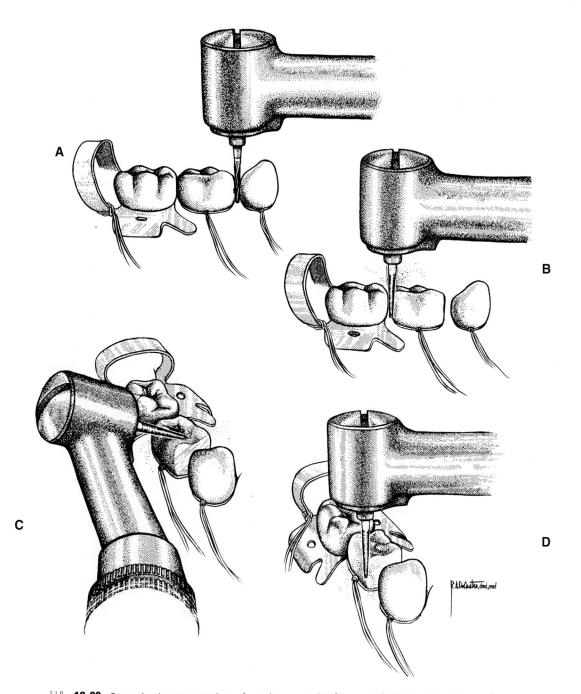

FIG. **18-20.** Steps in the preparation of a primary molar for a steel crown restoration using a No. 69L bur in the high-speed handpiece. **A,** Mesial reduction. **B,** Distal reduction. **C,** Occlusal reduction. **D,** Rounding of the line angles.

start at the middle third) of the buccal and lingual surfaces to help adapt the margins of the crown to the cervical portion of the tooth. The handles of the pliers are tipped toward the center of the crown, so that the metal is stretched and curled inward as the crown is moved toward the pliers from the opposite side. A curved-beak pliers is used to further improve the contour on the buccal and lingual surfaces (Fig. 18-22). The curved-beak pliers may also be used to contour the proximal areas of the crown and develop desirable contact with adjacent teeth. Many clinicians prefer to complete the crown contouring procedures with a crown-crimping pliers (Fig. 18-23). If necessary, solder may be added to the proximal surfaces of the crown to improve the proximal contacts and contour. Trimming and contouring are continued until the crown fits the preparation snugly and extends under the free margin of the gingival tissue.

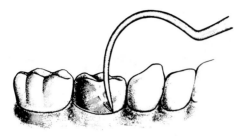

FIG. **18-21.** A scratch is made at the level of the free margin of the gingival tissue as an aid in determining where additional metal must be removed.

The crown should be replaced on the preparation after the contouring procedure to see that it snaps securely into place. The occlusion should be checked at this stage to make sure that the crown is not opening the bite or causing a shifting of the mandible into an undesirable relationship with the opposing teeth (Fig. 18-24).

The final step before cementation is to produce a beveled gingival margin that may be polished and that will be well tolerated by the gingival tissue. A rubber abrasive wheel can be used to produce the smooth margin.

On occasion the best-fitting crown may need to be modified to produce a more desirable adaptation to the prepared cervical margin. Mink and Hill have referred to methods of modifying steel crowns for primary and permanent teeth.[29] The oversized crown may be cut as illustrated in Fig. 18-25 and the cut edges overlapped. The crown is replaced on the tooth to ensure that it now fits snugly at the cervical region, and a scratch is made at the overlapped margin. The crown is removed from the tooth and the overlapped material repositioned and welded. A small amount of solder is flowed over the outside margin. The crown is finished in the previously recommended manner and cemented to the prepared tooth.

If the dentist encounters a tooth that is too large for the largest crown, a similar technique may be helpful. The crown may be cut on the buccal or lingual surface. After the crown has been adapted to the prepared tooth, an additional piece of 0.004-inch stainless steel band material may be welded into place. A small amount of solder should be added to the outer surface of the margins. The crown may then be contoured in the usual manner, polished, and cemented into place.

ALTERNATIVE RESTORATIVE TREATMENT

Alternative restorative treatment, or *ART,* has become a popular descriptive term to describe a conservative method of managing both small and large carious lesions in situations in which treating the disease by more traditional restorative procedures is impossible or impractical. This method may prevent pain and

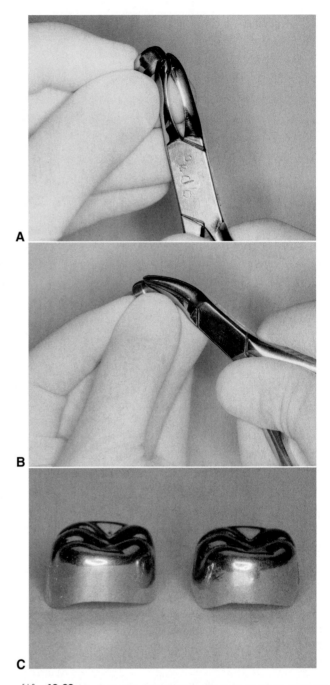

FIG. **18-22. A,** A crown-contouring pliers is used to contour the buccal and lingual surfaces of the crown. The crown is held firmly with the pliers, and pressure is exerted with the finger from the opposite side of the crown to bend the surface inward. **B,** The curved-beak pliers is "walked" completely around the cervical margins of the crown to direct all margins inward with smooth, flowing contour. **C,** The crown on the right was the same size and shape as the crown on the left before it was contoured. This illustrates the effectiveness of the contouring procedures with the pliers as described.

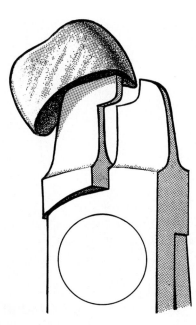

FIG. **18-23.** A crown-crimping pliers may also be used for crown contouring.

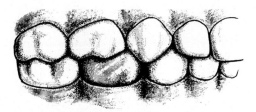

FIG. **18-24.** Final adaptation of the crown should result in good occlusion before cementation.

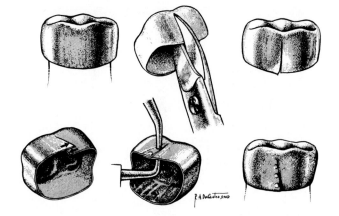

FIG. **18-25.** Technique for adapting an oversized crown to a prepared tooth.

preserve teeth in individuals who do not have access to regular and conventional oral health care. ART may be performed with only hand instruments when no other dental equipment is available, but it may be useful sometimes in the conventional dental setting as well. ART does not require the complete excavation of dentinal caries before placement of the restorative material. This is not a totally new concept in dentistry, but it has enjoyed renewed recognition as a viable restorative approach because of the development of the more durable fluoride-releasing glass ionomer and resin-modified glass ionomer restorative materials. The principles validating this technique are discussed further in Chapter 19 (in the section Treatment of the Deep Carious Lesion).

The AAPD adopted a policy on ART in 2001. The discussion and the policy statement as they appear in the AAPD *Reference Manual* (excluding references) are as follows:

Purpose

Removal of dental caries and restoration of teeth can often present unique challenges to the practitioner. Not all dental disease can be treated by "traditional" restorative techniques. Young patients, uncooperative patients, patients with special needs and situations where traditional cavity preparation and placement of traditional dental restorations is not possible, may require the use of an alternative restorative treatment.

Background

Alternative restorative treatment (ART), formerly known as atraumatic restorative treatment, is a technique used to restore defective or carious teeth with minimal cavity preparation followed by placement of a fluoride-releasing material such as glass ionomer. This technique is promoted and endorsed by the World Health Organization with the goals of preserving tooth structure, reducing infection and avoiding discomfort. The International Association for Dental Research held a symposium on ART in June 1995 recognizing the technique as a means of restoring and preventing dental caries.

The procedure does not require a traditional dental setting. Preventive measures to control the bacterial infection and the causative agents of the disease should also be utilized for optimal results following treatment.

Policy statement

The American Academy of Pediatric Dentistry recognizes ART as a useful and beneficial technique in the treatment and management of dental caries where traditional cavity preparation and placement of traditional dental restorations are not possible.[30]

COSMETIC RESTORATIVE PROCEDURES FOR YOUNG PERMANENT ANTERIOR TEETH

A common problem confronting dentists who treat children is the esthetic management of anterior teeth that are discolored, developmentally undersized or malformed, malposed, or fractured. Dentists recognize that esthetic impairments of the teeth often adversely

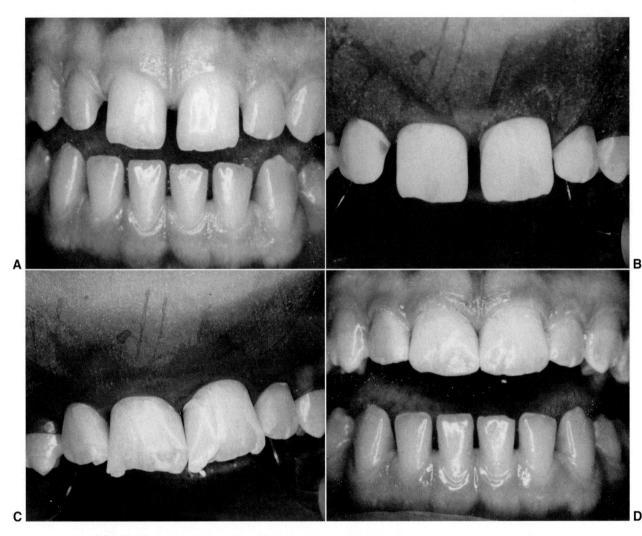

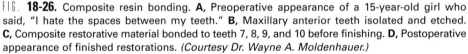

FIG. **18-26.** Composite resin bonding. **A,** Preoperative appearance of a 15-year-old girl who said, "I hate the spaces between my teeth." **B,** Maxillary anterior teeth isolated and etched. **C,** Composite restorative material bonded to teeth 7, 8, 9, and 10 before finishing. **D,** Postoperative appearance of finished restorations. *(Courtesy Dr. Wayne A. Moldenhauer.)*

affect the social and psychologic development of the growing child. Esthetic restorative systems and bonding techniques are usually employed when restorations are indicated in these situations. Although bonding procedures are also applicable to primary tooth restorations (as described earlier in this chapter), the following discussion applies primarily to permanent anterior teeth simply because few indications are encountered in the primary dentition. However, Aron has reported the successful use of porcelain laminate veneer restorations on maxillary primary incisors in one unusual case.[31]

The following discussion assumes that one understands dental bonding principles and has a working knowledge of the process. These principles and procedures are similar for sealants, restorative resins, and resin luting agents, and they are presented in Chapter 17. Some tooth preparation confined to enamel

(as much as possible) is often indicated, although not always required, before cosmetic bonding procedures are performed.

BONDED COMPOSITE VENEER RESTORATIONS (COMPOSITE RESIN BONDING)

Composite restorative resins (and bonding agents) are frequently applied directly to etched enamel. The restorative resin simply becomes a veneer to improve tooth color or contour. Restorative resin-bonding techniques are particularly useful for restoring anterior crown fractures (see Chapter 21) and for cosmetically increasing the mesial-distal widths of young permanent anterior teeth (Fig. 18-26). Bonded composite veneers are also useful for restoring small hypoplastic or discolored areas on visible tooth surfaces. Many dentists also use this type of restoration to mask intrinsic

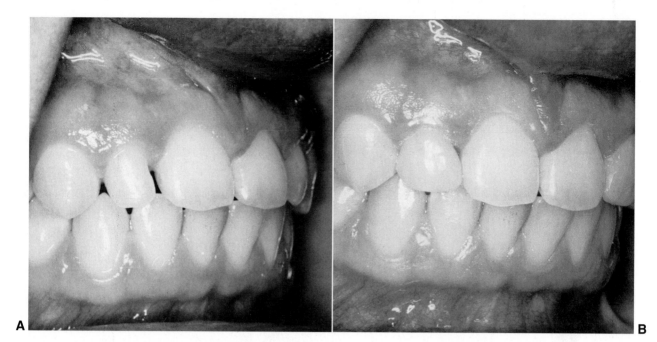

FIG. **18-27. A,** Undersized maxillary right lateral incisor in a young patient. **B,** Improved appearance of tooth after restoration with a bonded laminate veneer restoration.

discolorations by veneering the entire labial surfaces of the discolored anterior teeth. This approach may provide satisfactory cosmetic restorations for teeth with mild to moderate discolorations that will not respond to the bleaching or microabrasion procedures discussed in Chapter 7.

BONDED LAMINATE VENEER RESTORATIONS (DENTAL LAMINATES OR LAMINATE VENEERS)

The use of thin, prefitted porcelain facings (laminate veneers) that are bonded to enamel surfaces has become commonplace in cosmetic dentistry. Interest in laminate veneer restorations has grown steadily since their introduction by Faunce and Faunce.[32] Such restorations for maxillary anterior teeth are recognized as conservative, esthetically satisfactory restorations, especially in children and young adults. Laminate veneer restorations have also been used successfully on mandibular anterior teeth.

The laminate veneer technique offers esthetic improvement because the restored teeth simulate the natural hue and appearance of normal, healthy tooth structure. When properly finished, the laminate restorations are well tolerated by the gingival tissues even though their contour may be slightly excessive. Immaculate oral hygiene is essential, but experience has shown that the maintenance of gingival health around the restorations is certainly possible in cooperative patients (Fig. 18-27).

The luting materials are tooth-colored resin systems designed for use in bonding techniques. If the teeth being treated are severely discolored, tinting or opaquing agents also may be required (Fig. 18-28).

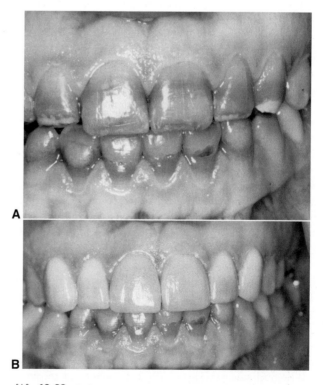

FIG. **18-28. A,** Severe intrinsic tooth discoloration in a teenager. **B,** Porcelain-bonded laminate veneer restorations have been placed onto the maxillary anterior teeth for a more natural appearance. The laminates were intentionally lengthened incisally to provide more coverage of the discolored lower incisors and to improve the patient's smile line.

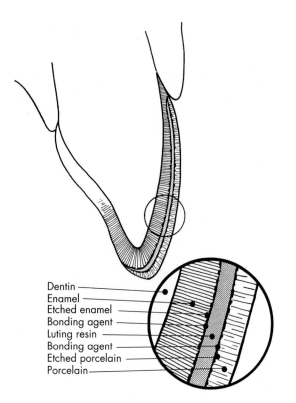

FIG. **18-29.** Cross-sectional sketch of the intraenamel preparation and the precision-fitted porcelain laminate veneer that had been fabricated in the laboratory to restore the natural tooth contours when bonded in place.

The laminate veneer procedure is not complicated, but it requires meticulous attention to detail for success.

The bonding procedure for a laminate veneer restoration requires proper preparation of the inside laminate surface and proper etching of the outer enamel surface. The inside of the porcelain laminate surface is etched with a hydrofluoric acid etchant and then coated with silane, which results in a bond with the resin luting agent similar to that achieved on etched enamel but also enhanced chemically by the silane. Excellent bond strengths to the porcelain surface have been reported by Lee et al.[33]

The intraenamel preparation includes removal of 0.5 to 1.0 mm of facial enamel, tapering to about 0.25 to 0.5 mm at the cervical margin. This margin is finished in a well-defined chamfer level with the crest of the gingival margin or not more than 0.5 mm subgingivally. The incisal margin may end just short of the incisal edge, or it may include the entire incisal edge ending on the lingual surface (Fig. 18-29). It is better not to place incisal margins where direct incising forces occur. Bonded porcelain techniques have significant value in cosmetic dental procedures (Fig. 18-30).

It is beyond the scope of this chapter to discuss in detail the many varieties of materials and techniques

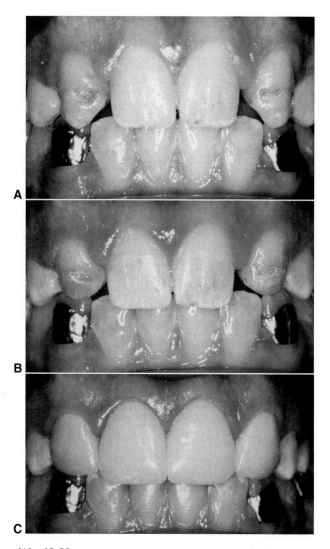

FIG. **18-30. A,** Anterior teeth of a teenaged patient immediately after the removal of bonded orthodontic appliances. Maxillary canines have been orthodontically positioned forward because of the congenital absence of the lateral incisors. Notice the interdental spaces distal to the central incisors and also the enlarged gingival tissues secondary (at least in part) to many months of orthodontic appliance therapy. The hypoplastic defects are obvious on the canines, and the central incisors are mildly affected as well. **B,** Photograph of same patient after completion of the intraenamel preparation of the canines. The central incisors received only minimal preparation so that the final restorations would provide slightly more support to the upper lip. No anesthesia was required during the tooth preparations, and no temporary restorations were necessary during the time the porcelain laminates were being fabricated in the laboratory. **C,** Bonded porcelain laminate restorations were placed several days later. The restored canines now resemble lateral incisors, and the interdental spaces are closed. Although the gingival tissues are somewhat irritated because of manipulation during the bonding procedures, some spontaneous reduction of the gingival enlargements are noticed now that better brushing and flossing have been instituted.

available for dental cosmetic procedures. Additional useful information has been published by Nixon for those interested.[34]

REFERENCES

1. American Academy of Pediatric Dentistry: Special issue: Reference manual 2002-2003, *Pediatr Dent* 24:83-85, 2002.
2. Berg JH: The continuum of restorative materials in pediatric dentistry: a review for the clinician, *Pediatr Dent* 20:93-100, 1998.
3. Bonilla E, White SN: Fatigue of resin-bonded amalgam restorations, *Oper Dent* 21:122-126, 1996.
4. Mahler DB et al: One-year clinical evaluation of bonded amalgam restorations, *J Am Dent Assoc* 127:345-349, 1996.
5. Heise AL: Time required in rubber dam placement, *J Dent Child* 38:116-117, 1971.
6. Croll TP: Restorative dentistry for preschool children, *Dent Clin North Am* 39:737-770, 1995.
7. Croll TP: Lateral-access class II restoration using resin-modified glass-ionomer or silver-cermet cement, *Quintessence Int* 26:121-126, 1995.
8. Vaikuntam J: Resin-modified glass ionomer cements (RM GICs): implications for use in pediatric dentistry, *J Dent Child* 64:131-134, 1997.
9. Marks LA et al: Dyract versus Tytin class II restorations in primary molars: 36 months evaluation, *Caries Res* 33:387-392, 1999.
10. Welbury RR et al: Clinical evaluation of paired compomer and glass ionomer restorations in primary molars: final results after 42 months, *Br Dent J* 189:93-97, 2000.
11. Hubel S, Mejare I: Conventional versus resin-modified glass-ionomer cement for class II restorations in primary molars. A 3-year clinical study, *Int J Paediatr Dent* 13:2-8, 2003.
12. Paquette DE et al: Modified cavity preparations for composite resins in primary molars, *Pediatr Dent* 5:246-251, 1983.
13. Oldenburg TR, Vann WF Jr, Dilley DC: Composite restorations for primary molars: two-year results, *Pediatr Dent* 7:96-103, 1985.
14. Tonn EM, Ryge G: Two-year clinical evaluation of light-cured composite resin restorations in primary molars, *J Am Dent Assoc* 111:44-48, 1985.
15. Dilley DC et al: Time required for placement of composite versus amalgam restorations, *J Dent Child* 57:177-183, 1990.
16. Donly KJ et al: Clinical performance and caries inhibition of resin-modified glass ionomer cement and amalgam restorations, *J Am Dent Assoc* 130:1459-1466, 1999.
17. McConville RE, Tonn EM: A method of restoring deciduous anterior teeth, *J Am Dent Assoc* 75:617-620, 1967.
18. McEvoy SA: A modified class III cavity preparation and composite resin filling technique for primary incisors, *Dent Clin North Am* 28:145-155, 1984.
19. Croll TP: Primary incisor restoration using resin-veneered stainless steel crowns, *J Dent Child* 65:89-95, 1998.
20. Doyle WA: A new preparation for primary incisor jackets, *Pediatr Dent* 1:38-40, 1979.
21. Webber DL et al: A method of restoring primary anterior teeth with the aid of a celluloid crown form and composite resins, *Pediatr Dent* 1:244-246, 1979.
22. Roberson TM, Heymann HO, Swift EJ Jr: *Sturdevant's art & science of operative dentistry*, ed 4, St Louis, 2002, Mosby.
23. Baum L, Phillips RW, Lund MR: *Textbook of operative dentistry*, ed 3, Philadelphia, 1995, WB Saunders.
24. Radcliffe RM, Cullen CL: Preservation of future options: restorative procedures on first permanent molars in children, *J Dent Child* 58:104-108, 1991.
25. Humphrey WP: Uses of chrome steel in children's dentistry, *Dent Surv* 26:945-949, 1950.
26. Randall RC: Preformed metal crowns for primary and permanent molar teeth: review of the literature, *Pediatr Dent* 24:489-500, 2002.
27. Seale NS: The use of stainless steel crowns, *Pediatr Dent* 24:501-505, 2002.
28. Spedding RH: Two principles for improving the adaptation of stainless steel crowns to primary molars, *Dent Clin North Am* 28:157-175, 1984.
29. Mink JR, Hill CJ: Modification of the stainless steel crown for primary teeth, *J Dent Child* 38:61-69, 1971.
30. American Academy of Pediatric Dentistry: Special issue: Reference manual 2002-2003, *Pediatr Dent* 24:20, 2002.
31. Aron VO: Porcelain veneers for primary incisors: a case report, *Quintessence Int* 26:455-457, 1995.
32. Faunce FR, Faunce AR: The use of laminate veneers for restoration of fractured or discolored teeth, *Tex Dent J* 93(8): 6-7, 1975.
33. Lee JG et al: Bonding strengths of etched porcelain discs and three different bonding agents, *J Dent Child* 53:409-414, 1986.
34. Nixon RL: Masking severely tetracycline-stained teeth with ceramic laminate veneers, *Pract Periodontics Aesthet Dent* 8:227-235, 1996.

The treatment of the dental pulp exposed by the caries process, by accident during cavity preparation, or even as a result of injury and fracture of the tooth has long presented a challenge in treatment. As early as 1756, Pfaff reported placing a small piece of gold over a vital exposure in an attempt to promote healing.

Although it has been established that the pulp is capable of healing, there is still much to learn regarding the control of infection and inflammation in the vital pulp. Current methods of diagnosing the extent of pulpal injury are inadequate. More effective methods of pulp therapy are still needed, and more research is necessary.

DIAGNOSTIC AIDS IN THE SELECTION OF TEETH FOR VITAL PULP THERAPY

HISTORY OF PAIN

The history of either presence or absence of pain may not be as reliable in the differential diagnosis of the condition of the exposed primary pulp as it is in permanent teeth. Degeneration of primary pulp even to the point of abscess formation without the child's recalling pain or discomfort is not uncommon. Nevertheless, the history of a toothache should be the first consideration in the selection of teeth for vital pulp therapy. A toothache coincident with or immediately after a meal may not indicate extensive pulpal inflammation. The pain may be caused by an accumulation of food within a carious lesion, by pressure, or by a chemical irritation to vital pulp protected by only a thin layer of intact dentin.

A severe toothache at night usually signals extensive degeneration of the pulp and calls for more than a conservative type of pulp therapy. A spontaneous toothache of more than momentary duration occurring at any time usually means that pulpal disease has progressed too far for treatment with even a pulpotomy.

CLINICAL SIGNS AND SYMPTOMS

A gingival abscess or a draining fistula associated with a tooth with a deep carious lesion is an obvious clinical sign of an irreversibly diseased pulp. Such infections can be resolved only by successful endodontic therapy or extraction of the tooth.

Abnormal tooth mobility is another clinical sign that may indicate a severely diseased pulp. When such a tooth is evaluated for mobility, the manipulation may elicit localized pain in the area, but this is not always the case. If pain is absent or minimal during manipulation of the diseased mobile tooth, the pulp is probably in a more advanced and chronic degenerative condition.

Pathologic mobility must be distinguished from normal mobility in primary teeth near exfoliation.

Sensitivity to percussion or pressure is a clinical symptom suggestive of at least some degree of pulpal disease, but the degenerative stage of the pulp is probably of the acute inflammatory type. Tooth mobility or sensitivity to percussion or pressure may be a clinical signal of other dental problems as well, such as a high restoration or advanced periodontal disease. However, when this clinical information is identified in a child and is associated with a tooth having a deep carious lesion, the problem is most likely to be caused by pulpal disease and possibly by inflammatory involvement of the periodontal ligament.

RADIOGRAPHIC INTERPRETATION

A recent x-ray film must be available to examine for evidence of periradicular or periapical changes, such as thickening of the periodontal ligament or rarefaction of the supporting bone. These conditions almost always rule out treatment other than an endodontic procedure or extraction of the tooth. Radiographic interpretation is more difficult in children than in adults. The permanent teeth may have incompletely formed root ends, giving an impression of periapical radiolucency, and the roots of the primary teeth undergoing even normal physiologic resorption often present a misleading picture or one suggestive of pathologic change.

The proximity of carious lesions to the pulp cannot always be determined accurately in the x-ray film. What often appears to be an intact barrier of secondary dentin protecting the pulp may actually be a perforated mass of irregularly calcified and carious material. The pulp beneath this material may have extensive inflammation (Fig. 19-1). Radiographic evidence of calcified masses within the pulp chamber is diagnostically important. If the irritation to the pulp is relatively mild and chronic, the pulp will respond with inflammation and will attempt to eliminate the irritation by blocking with irregular dentin the tubules through which the irritating factors are transmitted. If the irritation is intense and acute and if the carious lesion is developing rapidly, the defense mechanism may not have a chance to lay down the reparative dentin barrier, and the disease process may reach the pulp. In this instance the pulp may attempt to form a barrier at some distance from the exposure site. These calcified masses are sometimes evident in the pulp horn or even in the region of the pulp canal entrance. A histologic examination of these teeth shows irregular, amorphous masses of calcified material that are not like pulp stones (Fig. 19-2). The masses bear no resemblance to dentin or to a dentinal barrier. In every instance they are associated with advanced degenerative changes of the coronal pulp and inflammation of the tissue in the canal.

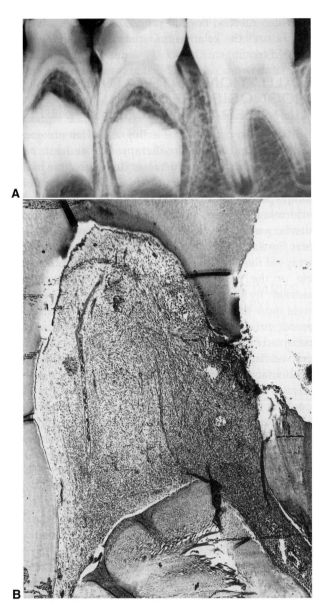

FIG. **19-1. A,** First primary molar appears to have an intact dentinal barrier beneath the carious lesion. **B,** Histologic section shows a perforation of the barrier with necrotic material at the exposure site. There is advanced inflammation of the pulp tissue, which is likely to evoke a spontaneous pain response.

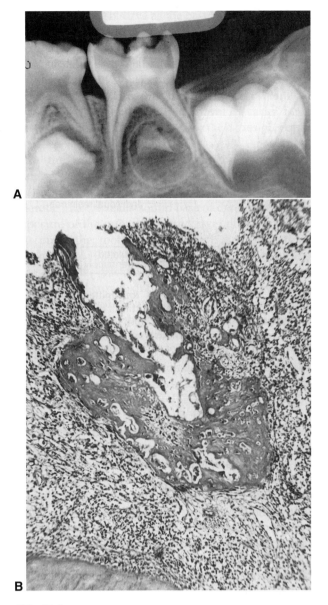

FIG. **19-2. A,** Calcified mass in the pulp chamber beneath the exposure site is associated with extensive inflammation of the pulp in the coronal area and in the pulp canals. **B,** The amorphous mass is surrounded by pulp tissue with advanced inflammation.

PULP TESTING

The value of the electric pulp test in determining the condition of the pulp of primary teeth is questionable, although it will give an indication of whether the pulp is vital. The test does not provide reliable evidence of the degree of inflammation of the pulp. A complicating factor is the occasional positive response to the test in a tooth with a necrotic pulp if the content of the canals is liquid. The reliability of the pulp test for the young child can also be questioned sometimes because of the child's apprehension associated with the test itself. Thermal

tests have reliability problems in the primary dentition, too. The lack of reliability is possibly related to the young child's inability to understand the tests.

Several methods have been developed and advocated as noninvasive techniques for recording the blood flow in human dental pulp. Two of these methods include the use of a laser Doppler flowmeter and transmitted-light photoplethysmography. As shown in the schematic in Fig. 19-3, these methods essentially work by transmitting a laser or light beam through the crown of the tooth; the signal is picked up on the other side of the

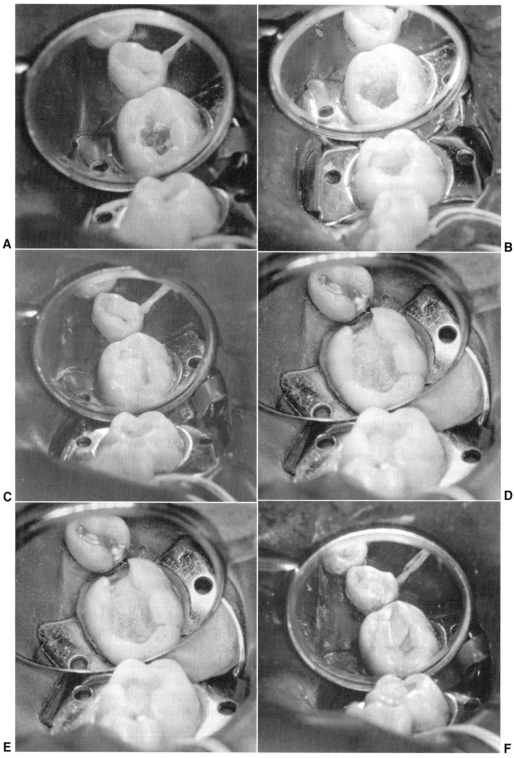

FIG. **19-5. A,** Second primary molar with deep occlusal caries. Because the tooth was free of symptoms of painful pulpitis, indirect pulp therapy was completed. **B,** The gross caries has been removed. A small amount of soft carious dentin remains at the base of the cavity. **C,** Calcium hydroxide has been placed over the remaining caries. The cavity may be sealed with a durable intermediate restorative material. **D,** After 6 to 8 weeks, the intermediate restorative material is removed. The caries in the base of the cavity appears arrested and dry. **E,** The remaining caries has been removed. **F,** After placement of a biocompatible base, the primary second molar has been restored with amalgam.

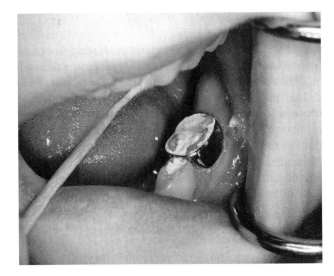

FIG. **19-6.** Preformed steel band has been cemented to the tooth to support the indirect pulp treatment material.

after the initial caries excavation. The inexperienced dentist, however, should perform the treatment in two appointments until confidence in proper case selection has been achieved.

VITAL PULP EXPOSURE

Although the routine practice of indirect pulp therapy in properly selected teeth will significantly reduce the number of direct pulp exposures encountered, all dentists who treat severe caries in children will be faced with treatment decisions related to the management of vital pulp exposures.

The appropriate procedure should be selected only after a careful evaluation of the patient's symptoms, results of diagnostic tests, and conditions at the exposure site. The health of the exposed dental pulp is sometimes difficult to determine, especially in children, and there is often lack of conformity between clinical symptoms and histopathologic condition.

SIZE OF THE EXPOSURE AND PULPAL HEMORRHAGE

The size of the exposure, the appearance of the pulp, and the amount of bleeding are valuable observations in diagnosing the condition of the primary pulp. For this reason the use of a rubber dam to isolate the tooth is extremely important; in addition, with the rubber dam the area can be kept clean and the work can be done more efficiently.

The most favorable condition for vital pulp therapy is the small pinpoint exposure surrounded by sound dentin. However, a true carious exposure, even of pinpoint size, will be accompanied by inflammation of the pulp, the degree of which is usually directly related to the size of the exposure (Fig. 19-8).

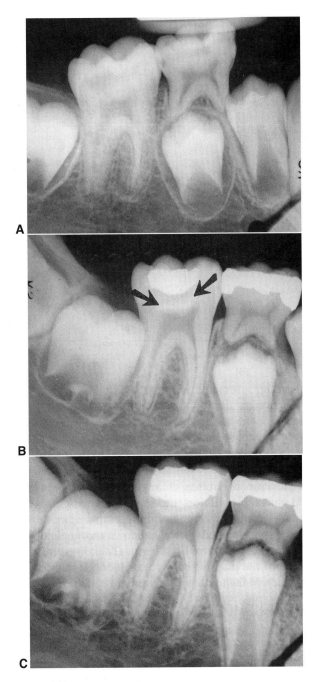

FIG. **19-7. A,** Radiograph of the first permanent molar revealed a deep carious lesion. Gross caries was removed, and calcium hydroxide was placed over the remaining caries. The tooth was restored with amalgam and was not reentered for complete caries removal for 3 months. **B,** Sclerotic dentin can be seen beneath the remaining caries and the covering of calcium hydroxide *(arrows).* **C,** The tooth was reentered, and the remaining caries was removed. A sound dentin barrier was observed at the base of the cavity. A new amalgam restoration was placed after complete caries removal.

A large exposure—the type that is encountered when a mass of leathery dentin is removed—is often associated with a watery exudate or pus at the exposure site. These conditions are indicative of advanced pulp

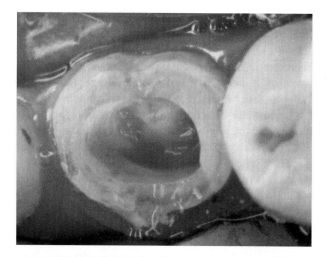

FIG. **19-10.** Cleanly excised pulpal stumps with no tags of tissue across the floor or along the walls of the chamber. The hemorrhage has been controlled. Notice also that the roof of the pulp chamber has been completely removed to provide total access to the pulp canals.

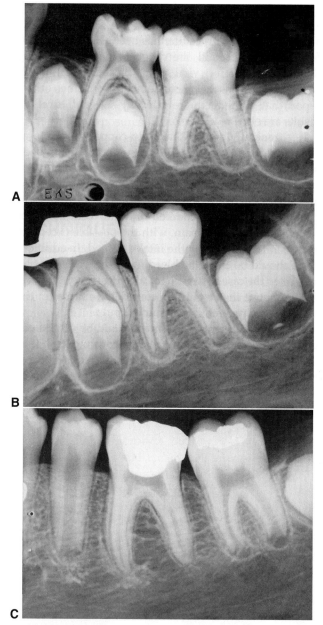

FIG. **19-11. A,** Pulp of the first permanent molar was exposed by caries. The tooth was considered a candidate for the calcium hydroxide pulpotomy technique. **B,** Calcified bridge has formed over the vital pulp in the canals. **C,** Continued root development and pulpal recession are indicative of continuing pulpal vitality. The crown should be supported with a full-coverage restoration.

the entrance of the individual root canals, may be used to amputate the coronal pulp at its entrance into the canals. The pulp stumps should be cleanly excised with no tags of tissue extending across the floor of the pulp chamber. The pulp chamber should then be irrigated with a light flow of water from the water syringe and evacuated. Cotton pellets moistened with water should be placed in the pulp chamber and allowed to remain over the pulp stumps until a clot forms (Fig. 19-10).

Laboratory and clinical observations indicate that a different technique and capping material are necessary in the treatment of primary teeth than in treatment of permanent teeth. As a result of these observations, two specific pulpotomy techniques have evolved and are in general use today.

Pulpotomy Technique for Permanent Teeth. The calcium hydroxide pulpotomy technique is recommended in the treatment of permanent teeth with carious pulp exposures when there is a pathologic change in the pulp at the exposure site. This procedure is particularly indicated for permanent teeth with immature root development but with healthy pulp tissue in the root canals. It is also indicated for a permanent tooth with a pulp exposure resulting from crown fracture when the trauma has also produced a root fracture of the same tooth. The procedure is completed during a single appointment. Only teeth free of symptoms of painful pulpitis are considered for treatment. The procedure involves the amputation of the coronal portion of the pulp as described, the control of hemorrhage, and the placement of a calcium hydroxide capping material over the pulp tissue remaining in the canals (Fig. 19-11).

A protective layer of hard-setting cement is placed over the calcium hydroxide to provide an adequate seal. The tooth is subsequently prepared for full-coverage restoration. However, if the tissue in the pulp canals appears hyperemic after the amputation of the coronal tissue, a pulpotomy should no longer be considered. Endodontic treatment is indicated if the tooth is to be saved.

After 1 year, a tooth that has been treated successfully with a pulpotomy should have a normal periodontal ligament and lamina dura, radiographic evidence of a calcified bridge if calcium hydroxide was used as the capping material, and no radiographic evidence of internal resorption or pathologic resorption. The treatment of permanent teeth by the calcium hydroxide method has resulted in a higher rate of success when the teeth are selected carefully based on existing knowledge of diagnostic techniques.

Pulpotomy Technique for Primary Teeth. The same diagnostic criteria recommended for the selection of permanent teeth for the pulpotomy procedure should be used in the selection of primary teeth for the pulpotomy procedure. The treatment is also completed during a single appointment. A surgically clean technique should be used. The coronal portion of the pulp should be amputated as described previously, the debris should be removed from the chamber, and the hemorrhage should be controlled. If there is evidence of hyperemia after the removal of the coronal pulp, which indicates that inflammation is present in the tissue beyond the coronal portion of the pulp, the technique should be abandoned in favor of the partial pulpectomy or the removal of the tooth. If the hemorrhage is controlled readily and the pulp stumps appear normal, it may be assumed that the pulp tissue in the canals is normal, and it is possible to proceed with the pulpotomy.

Although the formocresol pulpotomy technique has been recommended for many years as the principal method for treating primary teeth with carious exposures, a substantial shift away from use of this medicament has occurred because of concerns about its toxic effects. Many alternatives have been investigated to replace formocresol as the medicament of choice for a pulpotomy technique. Despite this, formocresol continues to be a very commonly used pulpotomy medicament. The pulp chamber is dried with sterile cotton pellets. Next, a pellet of cotton moistened with a 1:5 concentration of Buckley's formocresol and blotted on sterile gauze to remove the excess is placed in contact with the pulp stumps and is allowed to remain for 5 minutes. Because formocresol is caustic, care must be taken to avoid contact with the gingival tissues. The pellets are then removed, and the pulp chamber is dried with new pellets. A thick paste of hard-setting zinc oxide–eugenol is prepared and placed over the pulp stumps. The tooth is then restored with a stainless steel crown (Fig. 19-12).

Although the recommendation is that the blotted cotton pellet moistened with a 1:5 concentration of formocresol be applied to the pulp stumps for 5 minutes, it should be acknowledged that the 5-minute application time has been determined somewhat arbitrarily. Few data are available to verify the optimal application time. García-Godoy, Novakovic, and

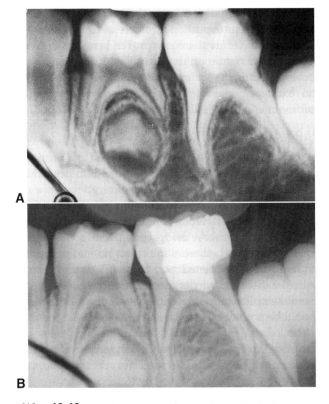

FIG. **19-12. A,** Formocresol pulpotomy technique was completed. **B,** Normal appearance of the supporting tissues is indicative of a successful treatment. The tooth should now be restored with a stainless steel crown.

Carvajal have suggested that a 1-minute application time may be adequate and perhaps superior to the recommended 5 minutes based on their limited work with pulpotomies in dogs.[11] These authors agree, however, that further studies are needed for verification.

A series of research studies by Loos and Han,[12] Loos, Straffon, and Han,[13] and Straffon and Han[14] have led to the conclusion that a dilute (1:5 concentration) of Buckley's formocresol applied to tissue achieves the desired cellular response as effectively as the full-strength formocresol agent, yet allows a faster recovery of the affected cells. The researchers suggested that the 1:5 concentration is a safer medicament that would produce equally good results with fewer postoperative problems in pulpotomy procedures. The original Buckley's formula for formocresol calls for equal parts of formaldehyde and cresol.* The 1:5 concentration of this formula is prepared by first thoroughly mixing three parts of glycerin with one part of distilled water, then adding four parts of this diluent to one part of Buckley's formocresol, and thoroughly mixing again.

Some dentists prefer to make the pulp-capping material by mixing the zinc oxide powder with equal

*Sultan Chemists, Inc., Englewood, N.J.

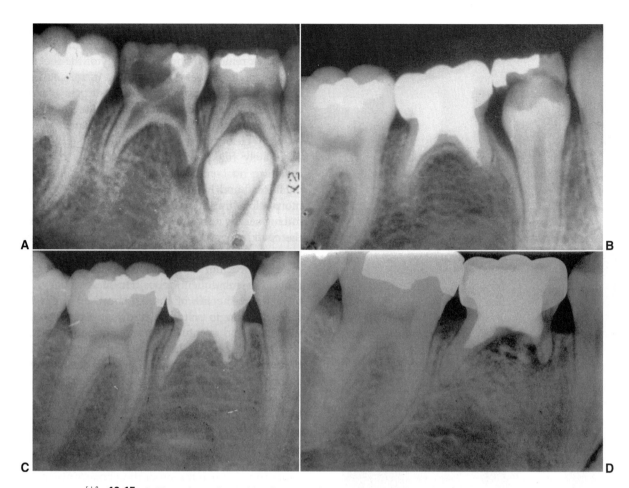

FIG. **19-15. A,** Necrotic tooth resulting from a carious exposure of the pulp of the second primary molar. Because the succedaneous second premolar was congenitally missing, a decision was made to attempt to save the tooth as a functional space maintainer through the growing years, if possible. Note the evidence of internal resorption at the floor of the pulp chamber. **B,** Radiograph made 1 year and 7 months after the pulp canals were treated and filled. The mesial canal was treated with complete pulpectomy; the distal canal was treated with partial pulpectomy. **C,** Six years and 7 months after treatment, the tooth is asymptomatic; the supporting tissues appear normal but some root resorption has occurred. **D,** Fourteen years and 6 months postoperatively, the tooth was extracted because of the development of symptoms and loss of bone support. At this time, the patient was a young adult and a fixed bridge was made.

pellet removed. If the tooth has remained asymptomatic during the interval, the remaining contents of the canals should be removed using the technique described for the partial pulpectomy. The apex of each root should be penetrated slightly with the smallest file. (The dentist should experiment with dissociated primary molars to develop a feel for the instrument as it just penetrates the apex.) A treatment pellet should again be placed in the pulp chamber and the seal completed with zinc oxide–eugenol. After another few days the treatment pellet should be removed. If the tooth has remained asymptomatic, the canals may be prepared and filled as described for the partial pulpectomy. However, if the tooth has been painful and there is evidence of moisture

in the canals when the treatment pellet is removed, the canals should again be mechanically cleansed and the treatment repeated.

Currently, pulpectomies in primary teeth are commonly completed in a single appointment (Fig. 19-16). If the tooth has painful necrosis with purulence in the canals, however, completing the pulpectomy procedure over two or three visits should improve the likelihood of success.

SUMMARY OF PULP THERAPY

The preceding discussion of various pulp therapies conforms, in principle, to the Guidelines for Pulp Therapy for Primary and Young Permanent Teeth as

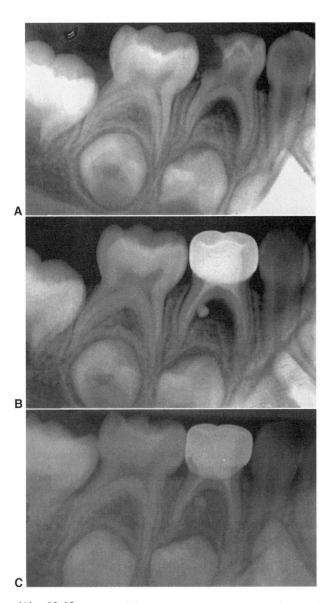

FIG. **19-16.** Successful single-appointment complete pulpectomy. Note extrusion of zinc oxide–eugenol into furcal area from distal root accessory canal, but adequate subsequent healing. **A,** Pretreatment. **B,** Immediately after treatment. **C,** 10 months after treatment.

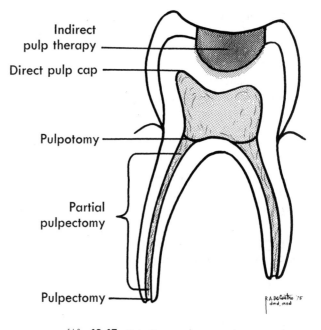

FIG. **19-17.** Pulp therapy progression.

reaffirmed by the American Academy of Pediatric Dentistry in 2002.[24]

When one encounters clinical problems that will likely require pulp therapy to return the patient to satisfactory oral health, treatment decisions are not always clear-cut. Proper diagnosis of the pulpal problem is important to allow the dentist to select the most conservative treatment procedure that offers the best chance of long-term success with the least chance of subsequent complications. The dentist should think of the possible treatment options in a progressive manner that takes into account both treatment conservatism (e.g., a pulpotomy is more conservative than a partial pulpectomy) and posttreatment problems (Fig. 19-17). The most conservative treatment possible may not always be the indicated procedure after the dentist also weighs the risks of posttreatment failure in a particular case.

RESTORATION OF THE PULPALLY INVOLVED TOOTH

It has been a common practice for some dentists to delay for weeks or months the permanent restoration of a tooth that has undergone vital pulp therapy. The purpose has been to allow time to determine whether the treatment procedure will be successful. However, failures in pulp therapy are usually not evident for many months. Rarely does a failure in pulp therapy or an endodontic procedure on a primary tooth cause the child to experience acute symptoms. Failures are usually evidenced by pathologic root resorption or rarefied areas in the bone and are discovered during regular recall appointments.

Primary and permanent molars that have been treated by the pulpotomy or pulpectomy technique have a weak, unsupported crown that is liable to fracture. Often a failure of the buccal or lingual plate occurs below the gingival attachment or even below the crest of the alveolar bone. This type of fracture makes subsequent restoration of the tooth impractical. Also, a delay in restoring the tooth with a material that will adequately seal the tooth and prevent an ingress of oral fluids is one cause for failure of pulp therapy.

The gingiva is the part of the oral mucous membrane that covers the alveolar processes and the cervical portions of the teeth. It has been divided traditionally into the free and the attached gingiva.[1] The free gingiva is the tissue coronal to the bottom of the gingival sulcus. The attached gingiva extends apically from the free gingival groove to the mucogingival junction.

The gingival tissues are normally light pink, although the color may be related to the complexion of the person, the thickness of the tissue, and the degree of keratinization. The gingival color of the young child may be more reddish due to increased vascularity and thinner epithelium. The surface of the gingiva of a child appears less stippled or smoother than that of an adult. In the healthy adult the marginal gingiva has a sharp, knifelike edge. During the period of tooth eruption in the child, however, the gingivae are thicker and have rounded margins due to the migration and cervical constriction of the primary teeth.

Delaney reports probing depths around primary teeth to be approximately 2 mm, with the facial and lingual probe sites shallower than the proximal sites.[2] Children have a wider periodontal ligament than the adult. The width of the attached gingiva is narrower in the mandible than in the maxilla, and both widths increase with the transition from the primary to permanent dentition in the child. The alveolar bone surrounding in the primary dentition demonstrates fewer trabeculae, less calcification, and larger marrow spaces.

Recent recognition that periodontal disease may have its origins in childhood has led dentists to be more aggressive in treatment. Studies confirm a high prevalence of gingival inflammation in children. Periodontal conditions that progress rapidly and result in the loss of primary and permanent teeth have been noted with increased frequency. Therefore, the American Academy of Pediatric Dentistry's Dental Health Objectives for Children for the Year 2000 includes placing greater emphasis on the prevention, early diagnosis, and treatment of gingival and periodontal disease in children.[3] By establishing excellent oral hygiene habits in children, which will carry over to adulthood, the risk of periodontal disease is lowered.

Gingivitis is an inflammation involving only the gingival tissues next to the tooth. Microscopically, it is characterized by the presence of an inflammatory exudate and edema, some destruction of collagenous gingival fibers, and ulceration and proliferation of the epithelium facing the tooth and attaching the gingiva to it. Numerous studies indicate that marginal gingivitis is the most common form of periodontal disease and starts in early childhood.

Severe gingivitis is relatively uncommon in children, although numerous surveys have shown that a large portion of the pediatric population has a mild, reversible type of gingivitis. The major etiologic factors associated with gingivitis and more significant periodontal disease are uncalcified and calcified bacterial plaque. However, gingivitis rarely progresses to periodontitis in the preschool and grade school child.

Bacterial plaque, which is composed of soft bacterial deposits that adhere firmly to the teeth, is considered to be a complex, metabolically interconnected, highly organized bacterial system consisting of dense masses of microorganisms embedded in an intermicrobial matrix. In sufficient concentration it can disturb the host-parasite relationship and cause dental caries and periodontal disease.

Eastcott and Stallard have observed that plaque begins to form within 2 hours after the teeth are brushed.[4] Coccal forms of bacteria form first on a thin fenestrated pellicle (organic bacteria-free film deposited on the tooth surface). The surface is completely covered with a smooth material 3 hours after brushing. Within 5 hours, plaque microcolonies develop, apparently by cell division. Between 6 and 12 hours, the covering material becomes thinner and is reduced to discontinuous small scattered areas. About 30% of the coccus bacteria are in various stages of division by 24 hours. Rod-shaped bacteria appear for the first time in 24-hour-old plaque. Within 48 hours the surface of the plaque is covered with a mass of rods and filaments.

Dental calculus, which is considered to be calcified dental plaque, is discussed again later in the chapter. It is classified as supragingival or subgingival, depending on its location on the tooth. Supragingival calculus occurs as hard, firmly adherent masses on the enamel of teeth. Subgingival calculus is found as a concretion on the tooth in the confines of the periodontal pocket. The surface of dental calculus is always covered by uncalcified plaque. Calculus is an important factor in the development of gingival and periodontal disease.

In a study of approximately 1700 children 9 to 14 years of age by Suomi et al, it was found that a relatively high percentage of children of all racial-ethnic groups had calculus (both supragingival and subgingival).[5] From 56% to 85% of the children in the various age, sex, and racial-ethnic groups had supragingival calculus. The findings of this study indicate that most children 9 to 14 years of age who are of low socioeconomic status would benefit from inclusion in a preventive periodontal disease program based on improvement of oral hygiene.

SIMPLE GINGIVITIS
ERUPTION GINGIVITIS

A temporary type of gingivitis is often observed in young children when the primary teeth are erupting. This gingivitis, often associated with difficult eruption, subsides after the teeth emerge into the oral cavity.

Weddell and Klein conducted a study to determine the prevalence of gingivitis in a group of children between 6 and 36 months of age.[6] The children, patients of pediatricians in the Indianapolis area, had been born in the area, which has a fluoridated water supply. Among 299 white children, gingivitis was present in 13% of those 6 to 17 months of age, 34% of those in the 18- to 23-month age group, and 39% of those in the 24- to 36-month age group. Black children were not included in the study because of the inconsistency of their gingival colors. The gingivitis observed by Weddell and Klein was for the most part eruption gingivitis.[6] Nevertheless, their findings support the view that an oral hygiene program should be initiated by parents when the child is very young.

The greatest increase in the incidence of gingivitis in children is often seen in the 6- to 7-year age group when the permanent teeth begin to erupt. This increase in gingivitis apparently occurs because the gingival margin receives no protection from the coronal contour of the tooth during the early stage of active eruption, and the continual impingement of food on the gingivae causes the inflammatory process.

Food debris, materia alba, and bacterial plaque often collect around and beneath the free tissue, partially cover the crown of the erupting tooth, and cause the development of an inflammatory process (Fig. 20-1). This inflammation is most commonly associated with the eruption of the first and second permanent molars, and the condition can be painful and can develop into a pericoronitis or a pericoronal abscess. Mild eruption gingivitis requires no treatment other than improved oral hygiene. Painful pericoronitis may be helped when the area is irrigated with a counterirritant, such as Peroxyl.* Pericoronitis accompanied by swelling and lymph node involvement should be treated with antibiotic therapy.

GINGIVITIS ASSOCIATED WITH POOR ORAL HYGIENE

The degree of dental cleanliness and the condition of the gingival tissues in children are definitely related. Horowitz et al observed significant improvements in the gingivitis scores of schoolchildren after the initiation of a supervised daily plaque removal program.[7] Children in grades 5 to 8 participated in the program, and successful results were maintained during three school years. The mean gingivitis scores were reduced 40% among girls and 17% among boys during the program period, whereas the children in the control group maintained essentially the same gingivitis scores for the period of the study. Adequate mouth hygiene and cleanliness of the teeth are related to frequency of brushing and the thoroughness with which bacterial plaque is removed from the teeth. Favorable occlusion and the chewing of coarse, detergent-type foods, such as raw carrots, celery, and apples, have a beneficial effect on oral cleanliness.

In a study of 2876 children residing in a naturally fluoridated area, Murray confirmed the high prevalence of gingivitis in the young population.[8] He observed that inflammation of one or more papillae or margins associated with the incisor and canine teeth occurred in 90% of children 8 to 18 years of age. He, too, pointed to the importance of a good standard of oral cleanliness in reducing gingivitis and, ideally, preventing the progression of the disease in later life.

Gingivitis associated with poor oral hygiene is usually classified as early (slight), moderate, or advanced. Early gingivitis is quickly reversible and can be treated with a good oral prophylactic treatment and instruction in good toothbrushing and flossing techniques to keep the teeth free of bacterial plaque (Figs. 20-2 and 20-3). Gingivitis is generally less severe in children than in adults with similar plaque levels.

ALLERGY AND GINGIVAL INFLAMMATION

Matsson and Moller studied the degree of seasonal variation of gingival inflammation in children with allergies to birch pollen.[9] Thirty-four allergic children were examined during two successive spring seasons and the one intervening fall. Age- and sex-matched

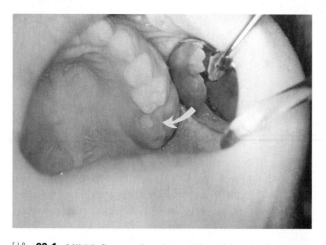

FIG. **20-1.** Mild inflammation *(arrow)* is evident in the tissue partially covering the crown of the erupting first permanent molar.

*Colgate-Palmolive Co., New York, NY.

controls were also examined in the fall. Gingival inflammation and the presence or absence of plaque were recorded, and a bleeding/plaque ratio was calculated for each subject. The results indicated an enhanced gingival inflammatory reaction in the allergic children during the pollen seasons. Although the authors acknowledge that the significance of gingival reaction during short allergic seasons is difficult to assess, they speculate that patients with complex allergies who have symptoms for longer periods may be at higher risk for more significant adverse periodontal changes.

ACUTE GINGIVAL DISEASE
HERPES SIMPLEX VIRUS INFECTION

Herpesvirus causes one of the most widespread viral infections. The primary infection usually occurs in a child under 6 years of age who has had no contact with the type 1 herpes simplex virus (HSV-1) and who therefore has no neutralizing antibodies. It is believed that 99% of all primary infections are of the subclinical type. The infection may also occur in susceptible adults who have not had a primary infection (Fig. 20-4).

In some preschool children the primary infection may be characterized by only one or two mild sores on the oral mucous membranes, which may be of little concern to the child or may go unnoticed by the parents. In other children the primary infection may be manifested by acute symptoms (*acute herpetic gingivostomatitis*). The active symptoms of the acute disease can occur in children with clean mouths and healthy oral tissues. In fact, these children seem to be as susceptible as those with poor oral hygiene. The symptoms of the disease develop suddenly and include, in addition to the fiery red gingival tissues, malaise, irritability, headache, and pain associated with the intake of food and liquids of acid content. A characteristic oral finding in the acute primary disease is the presence of yellow or white liquid-filled vesicles. In a few days the vesicles rupture

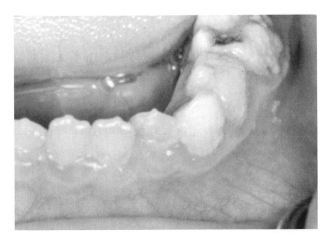

FIG. **20-2.** Gingivitis resulting from poor oral hygiene and reduced function in the area. A painful second primary molar has interfered with normal function on this side of the mouth.

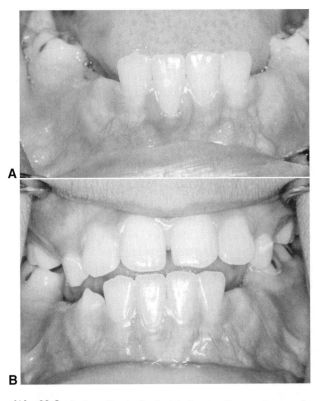

FIG. **20-3. A,** Localized gingival inflammation and recession associated with minimal plaque accumulation on mandibular right central incisor. **B,** Gingival health was greatly improved after a thorough plaque removal regimen was initiated at home.

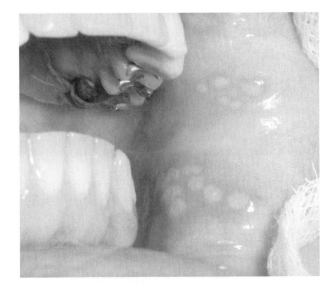

FIG. **20-4.** Ulcerated stage of primary herpes in a young adult. Notice the circumscribed confluent areas of inflammation.

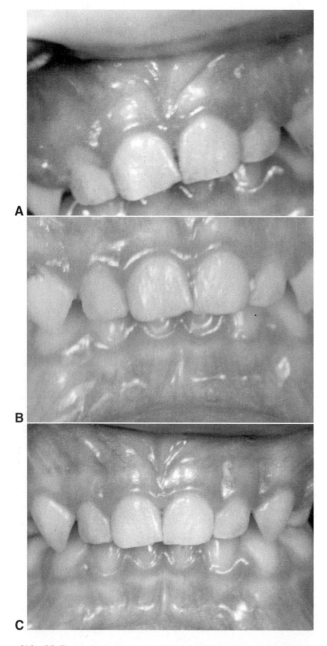

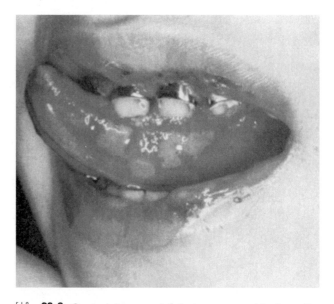

FIG. **20-6.** Several large, painful ulcers are evident on the tongue of a preschool child with acute herpetic gingivostomatitis.

FIG. **20-5.** **A,** Acute herpetic gingivostomatitis in an 18-month-old child. The fiery red gingival tissues and the presence of ulcers on the mucous membrane are characteristic findings. **B,** Considerable improvement is evident within a week after the occurrence of the acute symptoms. **C,** Symptoms of the disease have subsided in 2 weeks. Mild inflammation of isolated gingival papillae is still evident.

and form painful ulcers, 1 to 3 mm in diameter, which are covered with a whitish gray membrane and have a circumscribed area of inflammation (Figs. 20-5 and 20-6). The ulcers may be observed on any area of the mucous membrane, including buccal mucosa, tongue, lips, hard and soft palate, and the tonsillar areas. Large ulcerated lesions may occasionally be observed on the palate or gingival tissues or in the

region of the mucobuccal fold. This distribution makes the differential diagnosis more difficult. An additional diagnostic criterion is a fourfold rise of serum antibodies to HSV-1. The lesion culture will also show positive results for HSV-1.

Treatment of acute herpetic gingivostomatitis in children, which runs a course of 10 to 14 days, should include specific antiviral medication as well as provision for the relief of the acute symptoms so that fluid and nutritional intake can be maintained. The application of a mild topical anesthetic, such as dyclonine hydrochloride (0.5%) (Dyclone) before mealtime will temporarily relieve the pain and allow the child to take in soft food. Another topical anesthetic, lidocaine (Xylocaine Viscous), can be prescribed for the child who can hold 1 teaspoon of the anesthetic in the mouth for 2 to 3 minutes and then expectorate the solution. Schaaf recommends as an alternative to the anesthetic a mixture of equal parts of diphenhydramine (Benadryl) elixir and Kaopectate.[10] This material can be compounded by the pharmacist or mixed by the parent. The diphenhydramine has mild analgesic and anti-inflammatory properties, whereas the kaolin-pectin compound coats the lesions. Because fruit juices are usually irritating to the ulcerated area, ingestion of a vitamin supplement during the course of the disease is indicated.

Although the treatments just described may prove useful at certain times, they are only palliative. The mainstay of definitive therapy is regular doses of specific systemic antiviral medication combined with systemic analgesics (acetaminophen or ibuprofen) during the course of the disease.[11] The antiviral medications currently available are acyclovir, famciclovir, and valacyclovir. These medications inhibit viral replication in cells infected with the virus. Acyclovir (Zovirax*) should be administered in 5 daily doses to equal 1000 mg per day for 10 days. Acyclovir is available in capsules or suspension. Acyclovir therapy has been successfully used in infants and children. Famciclovir (Famvir[†]) and valacyclovir (Valtrex[‡]) are newer and possibly more effective antiviral agents, but their use in pediatric populations has not yet been studied. If the newer antivirals are prescribed for teenagers, the course of treatment is also 10 days but daily doses are less frequent and usually fewer milligrams daily than acyclovir. Valacyclovir should not be prescribed for immunocompromised patients.

Bed rest and isolation from other children in the family are also recommended. Hale et al reported an outbreak of herpes simplex infection in a group of 13 children occupying one floor in an orphanage.[12] The children ranged in age from 11 to 35 months. In three of the children a mild fever of brief duration and small oral lesions were the only signs of infection, and these might easily have been unobserved in a situation different from that of an institutional study. The remaining children had symptoms of acute infection.

After the initial primary attack during early childhood, the herpes simplex virus becomes inactive and resides in sensory nerve ganglia. The virus will often reappear later as the familiar cold sore or fever blister, usually on the outside of the lips (Fig. 20-7). Thus the disease has been commonly referred to as *recurrent herpes labialis* (RHL). However, approximately 5% of recurrences are intraoral. With the recurring attacks, the sores develop in essentially the same area. Kleinman, Swango, and Pindborg published the results of a national survey of 39,206 schoolchildren aged 5 to 17 years.[13] A history of RHL was reported by 33% of the children.

The recurrence of the disease has often been related to conditions of emotional stress and lowered tissue resistance resulting from various types of trauma. Excessive exposure to sunlight may be responsible for the appearance of the recurrent herpetic lesions on the lip. Use of sunscreen can prevent sun-induced recurrences. Lesions on the lip may also appear after dental treatment and may be related to irritation from rubber dam material or even routine daily procedures.

The most effective treatment for these recurrences is the use of the specific systemic antiviral medications already discussed in connection with the treatment of the primary herpetic infection (acyclovir, famciclovir,

FIG. **20-7.** Recurrent herpes labialis. **A,** Early vesicular lesions. **B,** Mature vesicular lesion. **C,** Appearance of herpes labialis after rupture of vesicles and crusting of the lesion. *(A, B, and C Courtesy Dr. Susan L. Zunt.)*

and valacyclovir).[11] The medication should be taken immediately after the prodromal symptom of recurrence. The daily dosages are the same as those for the primary infection, but the course of treatment is usually 5 days instead of 10. One-day therapy for recurrent herpes labialis is a total of 4 g valacyclovir given in a divided dose; 2 g initially with the prodrome, followed 12 hours later with another 2 g. This regimen has been approved for children 12 years of age and older. Another topical antiviral agent, penciclovir cream (Denavir*), may be applied to perioral lesions but

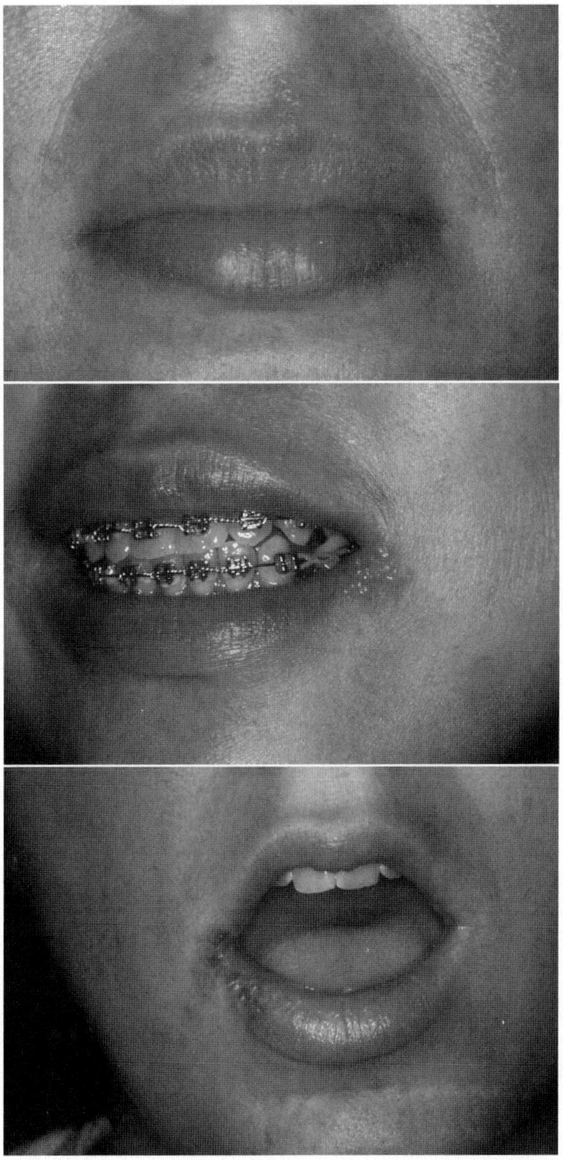

*GlaxoSmithKline, Inc., Research Triangle Park, NC.
†Novartis Pharmaceuticals Corporation, East Hanover, NJ.
‡GlaxoSmithKline, Inc., Research Triangle Park, NC.

*Novartis Consumer Health, Inc., Parsippany, NJ.

should not be applied to intraoral lesions. The penciclovir cream and systemic antivirals should not be prescribed for concurrent use. The cream can be applied every 2 hours while awake for 4 days, and it is approved for use in children 12 years of age and older. Topical 5% acyclovir cream may be prescribed for use 5 times daily for 4 days in children 12 years of age and older.

Other remedies for herpes simplex infection also include the amino acid lysine. The oral therapy is based on lysine's antagonistic effect on another amino acid, arginine. Griffith, Norins, and Kagan conducted an initial study in which 250 patients were given daily lysine doses of 1000 mg and were told to avoid eating arginine-rich foods, such as chocolate and nuts.[14] The lysine therapy was continued until the patients had been lesion free for 6 months. L-Lysine monohydrochloride is available commercially in capsule form or tablets containing 100 or 312 mg of L-Lysine.* The patients reported that pain disappeared overnight in virtually every instance. New vesicles failed to appear, and a majority considered the resolution of the lesions to be more rapid than in the past. There was also a reduction in frequency of occurrences. Griffith, Norins, and Kagan conclude that improper food selection may make adequate lysine intake precarious for some persons.[14] Ingestion of cereals, seeds, nuts, and chocolate would produce a high arginine/lysine ratio and favor the development of herpetic lesions. Similar results are obtained when arginine is added to the medium in the laboratory to induce herpes proliferation. The avoidance of these foods, coupled with the selection of foods with adequate lysine, such as dairy products and yeast, should discourage herpes infection. These authors postulate that this may explain the low incidence of herpes in infants before they are weaned from a predominantly milk diet. Prophylactic lysine is apparently useful in managing selected cases of RHL if serum lysine is maintained at adequate concentrations.

Brooks et al have reported that dentists are frequently exposed to HSV-1.[15] They evaluated the risk of infection with the virus by assessing disease experience, comparing the individual's history with the results of a complement fixation or antibody titration test or both. Their study group consisted of 525 dental students, 94 dental faculty members, and 23 staff members. Although almost all of those with a history of herpetic infection showed antibodies to HSV-1, only 57% of those lacking such a history had neutralizing antibody titers of 1:10 or higher. This finding suggests that a significant portion of practicing dentists risk primary herpetic infection. Consequently, dentists and dental auxiliaries without a history of herpetic lesions might benefit from serologic testing. Considering the occupational disability that

often accompanies HSV-1 infection of the finger or eye, effective barrier protection for health professionals is important.

Primary herpetic infection has been observed on the dorsal surface of the thumb of a pediatric patient (Fig. 20-8). The child was a thumb sucker, and the acute primary infection was present in the mouth. The dorsal surface of the thumb, which rested on the lower incisor teeth, apparently became irritated, and an inoculation of the virus took place. The oral condition and the lesions on the thumb subsided in 2 weeks.

RECURRENT APHTHOUS ULCER (CANKER SORE)

The *recurrent aphthous ulcer (RAU)*—also referred to as *recurrent aphthous stomatitis (RAS)*—is a painful ulceration on the unattached mucous membrane that occurs in school-aged children and adults. The peak age for RAU is between 10 and 19 years of age. It has been reported to be the most common mucosal disorder in people of all ages and races in the world. This disorder, according to definitions adopted in the epidemiologic literature, is characterized by recurrent ulcerations on the moist mucous membranes of the mouth, in which both discrete and confluent lesions form rapidly in certain sites and feature a round to oval crateriform base, raised reddened margins, and pain. They may appear as attacks of minor or single, major or multiple, or herpetiform lesions. They may or may not be associated with ulcerative lesions elsewhere.

In the national survey reported by Kleinman, Swango, and Pindborg mentioned earlier, a history of RAU was reported by 37% of the schoolchildren.[13] Ship et al reported the prevalence estimates of RAU to range between 2% to 50% with most estimates between 5% and 25% (among medical and dental students, estimated prevalence is between 50% and 60%).[16] Lesions persist for 4 to 12 days and heal uneventfully, leaving scars only rarely and only in cases of unusually large

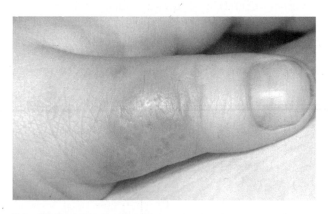

FIG. **20-8.** Primary herpetic infection involving the dorsal surface of the thumb of a 3-year-old child. An acute primary infection was present in the mouth.

*General Nutrition Corp., Pittsburgh, Pa.

lesions. The description of RAU frequently includes the term *canker sores* (Fig. 20-9). The major form (RAS) is less common and has been referred to as periadenitis mucosa necrotica recurrens and Sutton disease. RAS has been associated with other systemic diseases: PFAPA (periodic fever, aphthous stomatitis, pharyngitis, adenitis), Behçet disease, Crohn disease, ulcerative colitis, celiac disease, neutropenia, immunodeficiency syndromes, Reiter syndrome, systemic lupus erythematosus, and MAGIC (mouth and genital ulcers with inflamed cartilage) syndrome.

The cause of RAU is unknown. Local and systemic conditions and genetic, immunologic, and infectious microbial factors have been identified as potential causes. The condition may be caused by a delayed hypersensitivity to the L form of *Streptococcus sanguis*, which is a common constituent of the normal oral microbiota of humans. It is also possible that the lesions are caused by an autoimmune reaction of the oral epithelium. Epidemiologic studies by Ship et al have

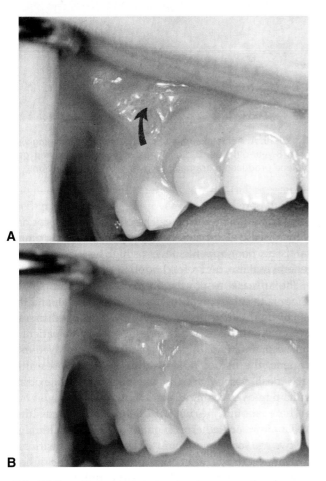

FIG. **20-9. A,** Evidence of the development of a recurrent aphthous ulcer in the mucobuccal fold above the primary canine. An area of inflammation and vesicle formation is apparent *(arrow).* **B,** Five days later the lesion is a well-developed ulcer with a circumscribed area of inflammation.

provided evidence for this hypothesis.[16] These data indicate that both RHL and RAU may be produced by the same mechanism, despite the known infectious agent of RHL and the absence of any known virus for RAU. Graykowski, Barile, and Stanley have isolated the L form of bacteria from patients with aphthous lesions.[17] Cultures of blood from patients with lesions in the acute stage tested positive for the organisms, whereas blood examined during quiescence was sterile.

Local factors include trauma, allergy to toothpaste constituents (sodium lauryl sulfate), and salivary gland dysfunction. In a review of the clinical problem, Antoon and Miller suggested that minor trauma is a common precipitating factor accounting for as many as 75% of the episodes.[18] Injuries caused by cheek biting and minor facial irritations are probably the most common precipitating factors. Nutritional deficiencies are found in 20% of persons with aphthous ulcers. The clinically detectable deficiencies include deficiencies of iron, vitamin B_{12}, and folic acid. While screening patients with aphthous ulcers, Wray et al observed a history of unusually high incidence of gastrointestinal disorders.[19] Stress may prove to be an important precipitating factor, particularly in stress-prone groups, such as students in professional schools and military personnel.

According to Greenspan et al, either nonspecific factors (trauma, food allergy) or specific factors (bacterial or viral infection) may trigger a temporary imbalance in various cell subpopulations.[20] This imbalance could then upset immune regulation and result in local destruction of the oral epithelium and thus ulceration. Ship et al also suggested herpes simplex virus, human herpesvirus type 6, cytomegalovirus, Epstein-Barr virus, and varicella-zoster virus as possible causes of RAS.[16]

Current treatment is focused on promoting ulcer healing, reducing ulcer duration and patient pain, maintaining the patient's nutritional intake, and preventing or reducing the frequency of recurrence of the disease.

A variety of treatments have been recommended for RAU, but a completely successful therapy has not been found. Topical antiinflammatory and analgesic medicines and/or systemic immunomodulating and immunosuppression agents have been used for RAU. The primary line of treatment uses topical gels, creams, and ointments as antiinflammatory agents. Currently, a topical corticosteroid (e.g., 0.5% fluocinonide, 0.025% triamcinolone, 0.5% clobetasol) is applied to the area with a mucosal adherent (e.g., isobutyl cyanoacrylate, Orabase). For example, the application of triamcinolone acetonide (Kenalog in Orabase) to the surface of the lesions before meals and before sleeping may also be helpful. Binnie et al report that an antiinflammatory and antiallergic medication in the form of a topical paste is effective in reducing pain and accelerating healing of RAU ulcers.[21]

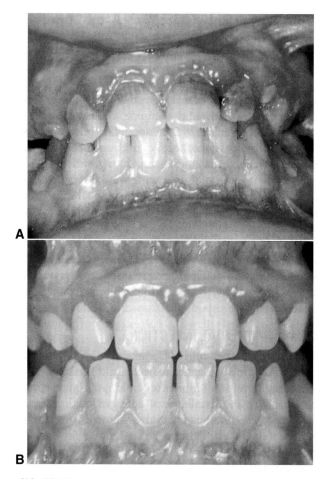

FIG. **20-12.** **A,** Chronic nonspecific gingivitis. The cause of this type of gingivitis is complex, and it often persists for prolonged periods without significant improvement. **B,** After 9 months of treatment, hyperplastic gingival tissue is still evident in the anterior maxillary region.

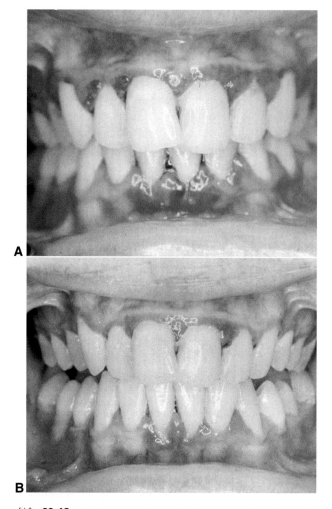

FIG. **20-13.** **A,** Fiery red gingival lesions essentially limited to the anterior labial tissues. Only minimum local deposits were evident. The gingivitis was classified as the chronic nonspecific type. **B,** Limited improvement was evident after 6 months of local treatment. A hormonal imbalance and vitamin deficiency were suspected as contributing etiologic factors.

prophylactic treatment. The age of the patients involved and the prevalence of the disease in girls suggested a hormonal imbalance as a possible factor. Histologic examination of tissue sections and the use of special stains ruled out a bacterial infection. Inadequate oral hygiene, which allows food impaction and the accumulation of materia alba and bacterial plaque, is undoubtedly the major cause of this chronic type of gingivitis.

Kaslick, West, and Chasens studied 238 young adults and looked for a correlation between their periodontal status and their ABO blood type.[28] They discovered that the chronic gingivitis group had a larger percentage of AB blood types and a smaller percentage of O blood type than the control group.

The cause of gingivitis is complex and is considered to be based on a multitude of local and systemic factors. Because dietary inadequacies are often found in the preteenage and teenage groups, the 7-day diet survey described in Chapter 10 is an important diagnostic aid. Insufficient quantities of fruits and vegetables in the diet, leading to a subclinical vitamin deficiency, may be an important predisposing factor. An improved dietary intake of vitamins and the use of multiple-vitamin supplements will improve the gingival condition in many children.

Malocclusion, which prevents adequate function, and crowded teeth, which make oral hygiene and plaque removal more difficult, are also important predisposing factors in gingivitis. Carious lesions with irritating sharp margins, as well as faulty restorations with overhanging margins (both of which cause food accumulation), also favor the development of the chronic type of gingivitis.

A wide variety of local irritants can produce a hyperplastic type of gingivitis in children and young adults. The irritation to the gingival tissue produced by mouth breathing is often responsible for the development of the chronic hyperplastic form of gingivitis, particularly in the maxillary arch. All these factors should be considered contributory to chronic nonspecific gingivitis and should be corrected in the treatment of the condition. The importance of thorough daily oral hygiene must be emphasized repeatedly to the patients.

CHLORHEXIDINE AS A THERAPEUTIC PLAQUE CONTROL AGENT

Chlorhexidine (CH) is a chlorophenyl biguanide with broad antimicrobial activity. It has been used commonly as an antiseptic skin and wound cleanser for presurgical preparation of the patient and as a hand wash and surgical scrub for health care personnel. It has also been added as a preservative to ophthalmic products and has been used internally in very dilute concentrations in the peritoneal cavity and urinary bladder.

In dentistry, CH has been studied for control of smooth surface caries, for use as a denture disinfectant, and as a plaque control agent. Its use in controlling dental plaque accumulations has received the most attention in dental research. Mouthrinses containing CH have been very popular as therapeutic agents in several countries for some time, and in 1986 CH was approved for use in the United States. As of this writing, two products under the trade names Peridex* and PerioGard† have received Food and Drug Administration approval as prescription agents. This mouthrinse contains 0.12% CH gluconate as the active ingredient.

Widespread use of CH mouthrinses over many years, especially in Europe, has had an excellent safety record. Few adverse side effects have been reported with CH mouthrinses, but their use has been linked to mouth dryness and burning sensations in some persons. Poorly defined desquamative lesions have been observed in others after the mouthrinse was used. Allergic reactions to CH are rare. If the rinse is inadvertently swallowed, it has essentially little systemic effect due to poor absorption in the gastrointestinal system.

Löe and Schiött reported highly significant inhibition of plaque formation and the prevention of gingivitis with use of an aqueous solution of 0.2% CH digluconate as a mouthrinse twice daily with swishing for 1 minute.[29] Studies by Grossman et al compared the 0.12% CH gluconate mouthrinse with a placebo over 3 and 6 months.[30] The study included 430 subjects who rinsed twice daily for 30 seconds with 15 ml of mouthrinse solution. At both the 3-month and 6-month evaluations, the CH group had significantly less gingivitis, gingival bleeding, and plaque accumulation. However, the accumulation of dental calculus and extrinsic dental stain increased in the CH group. Yankell et al have shown that dental stain from CH mouthrinse can be significantly reduced with regular use of a tartar-control dentifrice.[31]

It is important to recognize that the beneficial use of CH as a therapeutic mouthrinse should be considered adjunctive to the practice of sound conventional plaque control measures as presented in Chapter 11 and elsewhere in this text. Its adjunctive use would also seem most appropriate for therapy in cases in which attaining adequate plaque control is more difficult, such as during illness or convalescence after serious injuries.

GINGIVAL DISEASES MODIFIED BY SYSTEMIC FACTORS

GINGIVAL DISEASES ASSOCIATED WITH THE ENDOCRINE SYSTEM

Puberty gingivitis is a distinctive type of gingivitis that occasionally develops in children in the prepubertal and pubertal period. Cohen, in a study of 270 boys and girls in the 11- to 14-year age group, observed that gingival enlargement in the anterior segment occurred with regularity in the prepubertal and premenarcheal period, as well as in pubescence.[32] The gingival enlargement was marginal in distribution and, in the presence of local irritants, was characterized by prominent bulbous interproximal papillae far greater than gingival enlargements associated with local factors.

Sutcliffe's survey of a group of children between 11 and 17 years of age revealed an initial high prevalence of gingivitis that tended to decline with age.[33] In both sexes the prevalence of gingivitis tended to decrease with age. Initially, 89% of 11-year-olds and 92% of 12-year-olds were affected. It should be recalled, however, that with increasing age there is increased evidence of more adequate brushing. Girls tended to reach their maximum gingivitis experience earlier than boys did.

The enlargement of the gingival tissues in puberty gingivitis is confined to the anterior segment and may be present in only one arch. The lingual gingival tissue generally remains unaffected (Fig. 20-14). Treatment of puberty gingivitis should be directed toward improved oral hygiene, removal of all local irritants, restoration of carious teeth, and dietary changes necessary to ensure an adequate nutritional status. Cohen observed a sharp improvement in gingival inflammation and enlargement after the oral administration of 500 mg of ascorbic acid.[34] However, the improvement did not occur until the vitamin had been taken for approximately 4 weeks.

Severe cases of hyperplastic gingivitis that do not respond to local or systemic therapy should be treated by gingivoplasty. Surgical removal of the thickened fibrotic marginal and interproximal tissue has been

*Zila Pharmaceuticals, Phoenix, Ariz.
†Colgate-Palmolive Co., New York, NY.

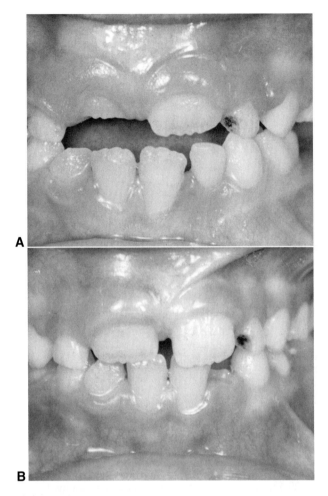

FIG. **20-19. A,** Mild gingivitis caused by a vitamin C deficiency. The marginal tissue and papillae were painfully enlarged. A dietary history revealed that the child's diet was grossly deficient in fruits and vegetables. **B,** Improvement in diet and greater emphasis on oral hygiene resulted in a great improvement in the oral health.

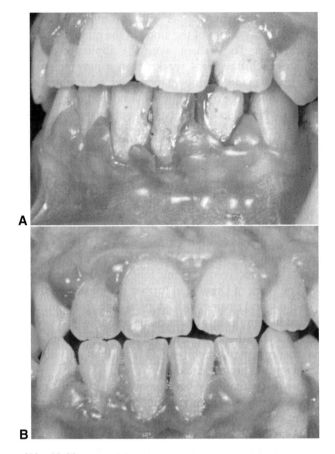

FIG. **20-20. A,** Scorbutic gingivitis in a 13-year-old girl. The diet was almost entirely lacking in foods containing vitamin C. **B,** An improved diet, supplemental amounts of fresh fruit juices, and toothbrushing instruction resulted in an improved gingival condition in 2 weeks.

Distances between 2 and 3 mm can be defined as questionable bone loss and distances greater than 3 mm indicate definite bone loss.

According to Delaney, in preschool children with periodontitis, recession, gingival erythema, and edema are not usually found unless the child is neutropenic.[2] Periodontal probing for attachment loss and bite-wing radiography are often used to clinically confirm the diagnosis. Bone loss is usually between the primary first and second molars. Bimstein, Delaney, and Sweeney demonstrated abnormal alveolar bone resorption in 7.6% of 4-year-old children and in 5.9% of 5-year-old children of primarily Hispanic origin with high caries.[56]

In its classification of periodontitis, the American Academy of Periodontology has categorized the early-onset form under Aggressive Periodontitis.[57,58]

EARLY-ONSET PERIODONTITIS

Albandar et al proposed the term *early-onset periodontitis (EOP).*[59] EOP is used as a generic term to describe a heterogeneous group of periodontal disease occurring in young individuals who are otherwise healthy. EOP can be viewed as three categories of periodontitis that may have overlapping etiologies and clinical presentations: (1) a localized form (localized juvenile periodontitis [LJP]), (2) a generalized form (generalized juvenile periodontitis [GJP]), and (3) a prepubertal category that is thought to have both localized and generalized forms (localized and generalized prepubertal periodontitis). Albandar, Brown, and Löe, using data from a 1986-87 survey, estimated the prevalence of EOP in adolescent schoolchildren in the United States to be 10% in blacks, 5% in Hispanics, and 1.3% in whites.[60]

Löe and Brown have reported observations from a periodontal assessment of 1107 adolescents aged 14 to 17 years.[61] Approximately 0.53% were estimated to have LJP, 0.13% to have GJP, and 1.61% to have incidental loss of attachment. Boys were more likely to have GJP than girls (ratio of 4.3:1).

Page et al believe that there are four different forms of periodontitis: prepubertal, juvenile, rapidly progressing, and adult.[62] As mentioned earlier, a new classification of periodontal disease has been published which recommends that EOP be recategorized as aggressive periodontitis and that its subclassifications be discarded. The old categorization has been retained because the new classification is not as widely used.

PREPUBERTAL PERIODONTITIS

Prepubertal periodontitis of the primary dentition can occur in a localized form but usually is seen in the generalized form. *Localized prepubertal periodontitis (LPP)* is localized attachment loss and alveolar bone loss only in the primary dentition in an otherwise healthy child. The exact time of onset is unknown, but it appears to arise around or before 4 years of age, when the bone loss is usually seen on radiographs around the primary molars and/or incisors. Abnormal probing depths with minor gingival inflammation, rapid bone loss, and minimal to varying amounts of plaque have been demonstrated at the affected sites of the child's dentition. Abnormalities in host defenses (e.g., leukocyte chemotaxis), extensive proximal caries facilitating plaque retention and bone loss, and a family history of periodontitis have been associated with LPP in children. As the disease progresses, the child's periodontium shows signs of gingival inflammation with gingival clefts and localized ulceration of the gingival margin.

The onset of *generalized prepubertal periodontitis (GPP)* is during or soon after the eruption of the primary teeth. It results in severe gingival inflammation and generalized attachment loss, tooth mobility, and rapid alveolar bone loss with premature exfoliation of the teeth (Fig. 20-21). The gingival tissue may initially demonstrate only minor inflammation with a minimum of plaque material. Chronic cases display the presence of clefting and pronounced recession with associated acute inflammation. Testing may reveal a high prevalence of leukocyte adherence abnormalities and an impaired host response against bacterial infections. Alveolar bone destruction proceeds rapidly, and the primary teeth may be lost by 3 years of age. Microorganisms predominating in the gingival pockets include *Actinobacillus actinomycetemcomitans* (Aa), *Porphyromonas* (Bacteroides) *gingivalis, Bacteroides melaninogenicus, Prevotella intermedia, Capnocytophaga sputigena,* and *Fusobacterium nucleatum.* Recent findings of Asikainen et al suggest that the major periodontal pathogens are transmitted among family members.[63] Often the past medical history of the child reveals a history of recurrent infections. (e.g., otitis media, skin infections, upper respiratory tract infections).

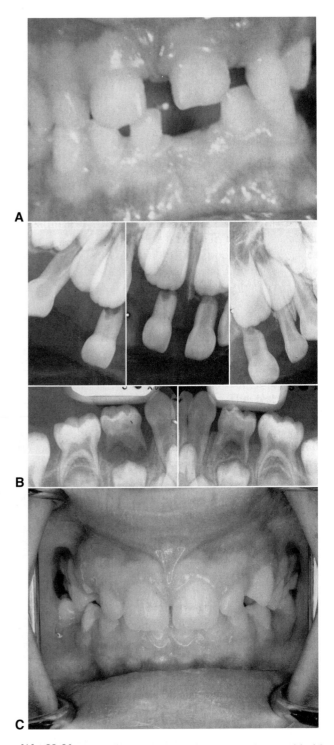

FIG. **20-21. A,** Prepubertal periodontitis in a 4½-year-old girl. Loosening, migration, and spontaneous loss of the primary teeth occurred. **B,** A generalized loss of alveolar bone can be seen in the radiographs. **C,** Eight years after the initial observation of an involvement of the supporting tissues, there is evidence of normal gingival tissues. It is believed that dietary counseling and excellent oral hygiene contributed to the success of the treatment. *Continued*

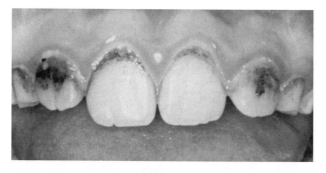

FIG. **20-39.** Dark green stain is evident on maxillary anterior teeth. Papillary and marginal gingivitis is also present. The patient had poor oral hygiene and was a mouth breather.

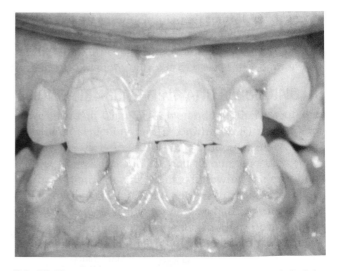

FIG. **20-40.** Orange stain is evident in the gingival third of the mandibular anterior teeth.

believed to be the result of the action of chromogenic bacteria on the enamel cuticle. The color of the stain varies from dark green to light yellowish green. The deposit is seen most often in the gingival third of the labial surface of the maxillary anterior teeth. The stain collects more readily on the labial surface of the maxillary anterior teeth in mouth breathers. It tends to recur even after careful and complete removal. The enamel beneath the stain may be roughened or may have undergone initial demineralization. The roughening of the surface is believed to be related to the frequency of recurrence of the stain (Fig. 20-39).

ORANGE STAIN

The cause of orange stain is likewise unknown. Orange stain occurs less frequently and is more easily removed than green stain. The stain is most often seen in the gingival third of the tooth and is associated with poor oral hygiene (Fig. 20-40).

BLACK STAIN

A black stain occasionally develops on the primary or permanent teeth of children, but it is much less common than the orange or green type (Fig. 20-41). The stain may be seen as a line following the gingival contour or it may be apparent in a more generalized pattern on the clinical crown, particularly if there are roughened or pitted areas. The black type of stain is difficult to remove, especially if it collects in pitted areas. Many children who have black stain are relatively free from dental caries.

REMOVAL OF EXTRINSIC STAINS

Extrinsic stains can be removed by polishing with a rubber cup and flour pumice. If the stain is resistant and difficult to remove, the excess water should be blotted from the pumice and the teeth should be dried before the polishing procedure is performed. Because stains

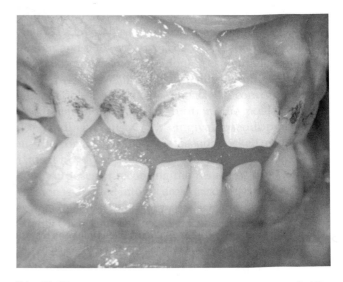

FIG. **20-41.** Black stain is evident on the primary teeth. The stain is difficult to remove, particularly when it collects in roughened areas of the tooth.

are most often seen in a mouth in which there is poor oral hygiene, improving the oral hygiene will minimize the recurrence of the stain.

PIGMENTATION CAUSED BY STANNOUS FLUORIDE APPLICATION

During the first clinical trials involving the topical application of an 8% stannous fluoride solution, certain areas of the tooth became discolored. A characteristic pigmentation of both carious and precarious lesions has been found to be associated with exposure to stannous fluoride (Fig. 20-42).

CALCULUS

Calculus is not often seen in preschool children, and even in children of grade school age it occurs with much lower frequency than in adult patients. A low caries incidence is related to high calculus incidence.

Bhat has reported findings in 14- to 17-year-old children who participated in the 1986-1987 National Survey of Oral Health.[83] Supragingival calculus was observed in nearly 34% of the children and subgingival calculus in approximately 23%. Both types show a predilection for molars in the maxilla and incisors and canines in the mandible.

Children with mental retardation often have accumulations of calculus on their teeth. This accumulation may be related to abnormal muscular function, a soft diet, poor oral hygiene, and stagnation of saliva.

The observations of Turesky, Renstrup, and Glickman regarding early calculus formation in children and adults substantiate those of others and indicate that calculus begins as a soft, adherent, bacteria-laden plaque that undergoes progressive calcification.[84] They observed calculus formation on cellulose acetate strips that were fixed in children's mouths. Plaque material that accumulated on the strips underwent progressive hardening. A soft plaque material consisted for the most part of bacteria appearing as a dense meshwork of diffusely distributed gram-negative cocci with occasional rod forms. Filamentous or thread-shaped organisms were scarce. Leukocytes and epithelial cells were also scattered within the amorphous matrix.

Gross accumulations of calculus are occasionally seen in teenaged and preteenaged children (Figs. 20-43 and 20-44). Traiger reported on a 14-year-old girl who had excessive deposits of supragingival and subgingival calculus.[85] The calculus covered the labial surfaces of the anterior teeth, extended into the mucobuccal fold, and covered the attached gingiva.

Supragingival deposits of calculus occur most frequently and in greater quantity on the buccal surfaces of the maxillary molars and the lingual surfaces of the mandibular anterior teeth. These areas are near the openings of the major salivary glands. Local factors are unquestionably important in the initiation of calculus formation.

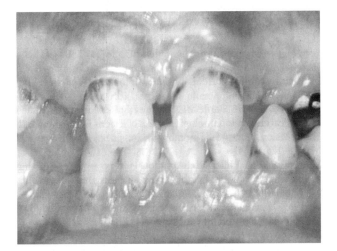

FIG. **20-42.** Pigmentation of carious and precarious enamel. The color ranges from light brown to black, the darker pigmentation being evident in the area of greatest caries involvement. The pigmentation is evidence of caries arrest following stannous fluoride application.

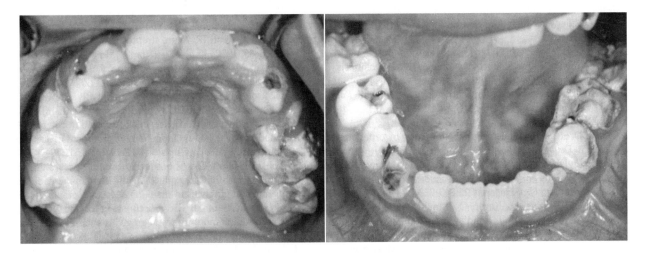

FIG. **20-43.** Gross accumulations of calculus are seen on the clinical crowns of the posterior teeth on the left side of the mouth. The fact that the child chewed mostly on his right side accounts partially for the greater cleanliness on that side.

A trauma with accompanying fracture of a permanent incisor is a tragic experience for the young patient and is a problem whose management requires experience, judgment, and skill perhaps unequaled by any other portion of the dentist's practice. The dentist whose counsel and treatment are sought after a trauma is obligated either to treat the patient with all possible means or to immediately refer the patient to a specialist. The oral and emotional health of the young patient is involved, and the child's appearance, marred by an unsightly oral injury, must be restored to normal as soon as possible to relieve the consciousness of being different from other children. Slack and Jones observed that the progress of children in school and their behavior elsewhere, as well as their psychologic well-being, can be adversely influenced by an injury to the teeth that causes an unsightly fracture.[1] In addition, the short- and long-term costs associated with managing trauma to the oral and perioral structures can be large. Borum and Andreasen estimate that the yearly cost from traumatic dental injuries in Denmark ranges from US $2 million to US $5 million per 1 million inhabitants per year.[2]

Injuries to the teeth of children or adults present unique problems in diagnosis and treatment. The diagnosis of the extent of the injury after a blow to a tooth, regardless of loss of tooth structure, is difficult and often inconclusive. Trauma to a tooth is invariably followed by pulpal hyperemia, the extent of which cannot always be determined by available diagnostic methods. Congestion and alteration in the blood flow in the pulp may be sufficient to initiate irreversible degenerative changes, which over time can cause pulpal necrosis. In addition, the apical vessels may have been severed or damaged enough to interfere with the normal reparative process. Treatment of injuries causing pulp exposure or tooth displacement are particularly challenging, because the prognosis of the involved tooth is often uncertain.

The treatment of fractured teeth, particularly in young patients, is further complicated by the often difficult but extremely important restorative procedure. Although the dentist may prefer to delay the restoration because of a questionable prognosis for the pulp, often a malocclusion can develop within a matter of days as a result of a break in the normal proximal contact with adjacent teeth. Adjacent teeth may tip into the area created by the loss of tooth structure (Fig. 21-1). This loss of space will create a problem when the final restoration is contemplated. There must often be a compromise of an ideal esthetic appearance, at least in the initial restoration, because the prognosis is questionable or because the tooth is young and has a large pulp or is still in the stage of active eruption.

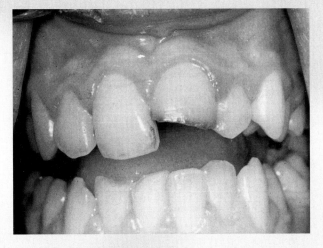

FIG. **21-1.** Loss of the incisal third of the maxillary left central incisor has allowed the right central incisor to tip into the area. Satisfactory restoration of the fractured tooth cannot be accomplished until the space is regained. Orthodontic treatment will be required.

Often the likelihood of success depends on the rapidity with which the tooth is treated after the injury, regardless of whether the procedure involves protecting a large area of exposed dentin or treating a vital pulp exposure. Several factors can be considered common to all types of injury to the anterior teeth. These important considerations should become a checklist invariably used by the dentist in the diagnosis of and treatment planning for traumatic injuries.

The International Association of Dental Traumatology reports that one out of every two children sustains a dental injury, most often between the ages of 8 and 12. They suggest that in most cases of dental trauma a rapid and appropriate treatment can lessen its impact from both an oral and an esthetic standpoint. To that end the association has developed guidelines for the evaluation and management of traumatic dental injuries, which is available at the following web site: http://www.iadtdentaltrauma.org/Trauma/dental_trauma.htm.

HISTORY AND EXAMINATION

The routine use of a clinical evaluation sheet for injured anterior teeth is helpful during the initial examination and subsequent examinations of an injured tooth (Fig. 21-2). The form, which becomes a part of the patient's record, serves as a checklist of important questions that must be asked and observations that must be made by the dentist and the auxiliary personnel during the examination of the child.

HISTORY OF THE INJURY

The time of the injury should first be established. Unfortunately, many patients do not seek professional advice and treatment immediately after an injury. Occasionally the accident is so severe that dental

ASSESSMENT OF ACUTE TRAUMATIC INJURIES	PATIENT NAME:_____ DATE OF BIRTH:_____
DATE: **TIME:**	**REFERRED BY:**

HISTORY	MEDICAL HISTORY:
	ALLERGIES:
	DATE OF LAST TETANUS INNOCULATON:
	DATE AND TIME OF INJURY:
	TIME LAPSED SINCE INJURY:
	WHERE INJURY OCCURRED:
	HOW INJURY OCCURRED:

	Check if present and describe	**MANAGEMENT PRIOR TO EXAM** By whom: Describe:
HISTORY	Nondental injuries	
	Loss of consciousness	
	Altered orientation/mental status	
	Hemorrhage from nose/ears	
	Headache/nausea/vomiting	
	Neck pain	
	Spontaneous dental pain	
	Pain on mastication	
	Reaction to thermal changes	
	Previous dental trauma	
	Other complaints	

	Check if present and describe	**OTHER FINDINGS/COMMENTS:**
EXTRAORAL EXAM	Facial fractures	
	Lacerations	
	Contusions	
	Swelling	
	Abrasions	
	Hemorrhage/drainage	
	Foreign bodies	
	TMJ deviation/asymmetry	

	Check if injured and describe	**DIAGRAM OF INJURIES**
INTRAORAL EXAMINATION	Lips	
	Frenae	
	Buccal mucosa	
	Gingivae	
	Palate	
	Tongue	
	Floor of mouth	
	Occlusion	
	Molar classification R___ L___	
	Canine classification R___ L___	
	Overbite (%)_____	
	Overjet (mm)_____	
	Crossbite Y N	
	Midline deviation Y N	
	Interferences Y N	

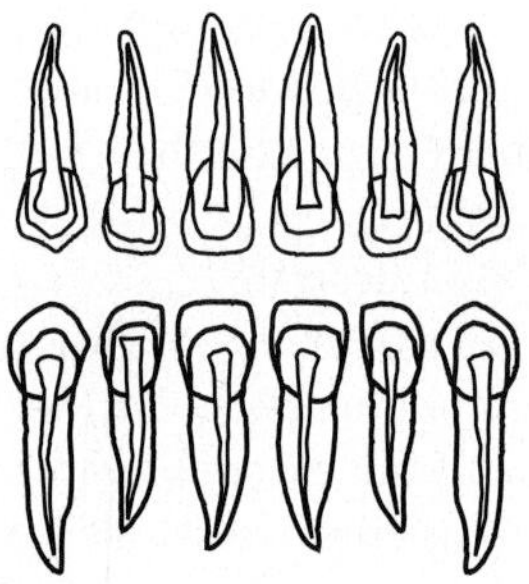

FIG. **21-2.** Clinical evaluation sheet for injured anterior teeth. *(Adapted from American Academy of Pediatric Dentistry: Pediatr Dent 24(7 suppl):95-96, 2002.)*

	TOOTH NUMBER					
DENTAL INJURIES	AVULSION — Extraoral time					
	Storage medium					
	INFRACTION					
	CROWN FRACTURE					
	PULP EXPOSURE — Size					
	Appearance					
	COLOR					
	MOBILITY (mm)					
	PERCUSSION					
	LUXATION — Direction					
	Extent					
	PULP TESTING — Electric					
	Thermal					
	CARIES/PREVIOUS RESTORATIONS					
RADIOGRAPHS	PULP SIZE					
	ROOT DEVELOPMENT					
	ROOT FRACTURE					
	PERIODONTAL LIGAMENT SPACE					
	PERIAPICAL PATHOLOGY					
	ALVEOLAR FRACTURE					
	FOREIGN BODY					
	DEVELOPMENTAL ANOMALY					
	OTHER					

TREATMENT

Check if performed and describe
- Soft tissue management
- Medication
- Pulp therapy
- Repositioning
- Stabilization
- Restoration
- Extraction
- Prescription
- Referral
- Other

SUMMARY

INSTRUCTIONS AND DISPOSITION

Check if discussed
- Diet
- Hygiene
- Pain
- Swelling
- Infection
- Prescription
- Complications:
  - Damage to developing teeth
  - Abnormal position/ankylosis
  - Tooth loss
  - Pulp damage to injured teeth
- Other:
- Follow-up:
- Other

Subsequent visit No. 1   Date_____

                7 8   9 10
1. Pulpal response   ☐☐ ☐☐
2. Radiographic exam ☐☐ ☐☐
                  2625 2423
3. Treatment and comments:_____
_____

                         Date_____
Subsequent visit No. 2

                7 8   9 10
1. Pulpal response   ☐☐ ☐☐
2. Radiographic exam ☐☐ ☐☐
                  2625 2423
3. Treatment and comments:_____

Subsequent visit No. 3   Date_____

                7 8   9 10
1. Pulpal response   ☐☐ ☐☐
2. Radiographic exam ☐☐ ☐☐
                  2625 2423
3. Treatment and comments:_____
_____

                         Date_____
Subsequent visit No. 4

                7 8   9 10
1. Pulpal response   ☐☐ ☐☐
2. Radiographic exam ☐☐ ☐☐
                  2625 2423
3. Treatment and comments:_____

FIG. **21-2, cont'd**. See legend on opposite page.

treatment cannot be started immediately because other injuries have higher priority. Davis and Vogel emphasized that a force strong enough to fracture, intrude, or avulse a tooth is also strong enough to result in cervical spine or intracranial injury. The dentist must be particularly alert to such potential problems, be prepared ahead of time to make a neurologic assessment, and make appropriate medical referral when indicated without delay.[3] The patient should be assessed for nausea, vomiting, drowsiness, or possible cerebral spinal fluid leakage from the nose and ears, which would be indicative of a skull fracture. In addition, the patient should be evaluated for lacerations and facial bone fractures, and even such things as baseline temperature, pulse, blood pressure, and respiratory rate could be considered as information to be gathered prior to addressing the dental needs of the patient. Finally, Davis[4] recommends a quick cranial nerve evaluation involving the following four areas:

Extraocular muscles are intact and functioning appropriately; that is, the patient can track a finger moving vertically and horizontally through the visual field with the eyes remaining in tandem.

Pupils are equal, round, and reactive to light with accommodation.

Sensory function is normal as measured through light contact to various areas of the face.

Symmetry of motor function is present, as assessed by having the patient frown, smile, move the tongue, and perform several voluntary muscular movements.

The prognosis of an injured tooth depends logically, often to a great extent, on the time that has elapsed between the occurrence of the accident and the initiation of emergency treatment. This is particularly true in cases of pulp exposure, for which pulp capping or pulpotomy would be the procedure of choice. Rusmah treated 123 traumatized permanent incisors and monitored them over a 24-month period. His findings suggest that the interval between trauma and emergency treatment is directly related to the severity of the injury and the dental awareness of the patients.[5] Furthermore, the prognosis of the injured teeth maintaining pulpal vitality diminished when treatment was delayed. The loss of vitality of some injured teeth occurred as early as 3 months and as late as 24 months after the injury, which justifies a long follow-up period after injury.

For practical and especially economic reasons, Andreasen et al have attempted to classify pulpal and periodontal healing of traumatic dental injuries based on the effect of treatment delay.[6] They developed three major categories of treatment timing: acute treatment (i.e., within a few hours), subacute treatment (i.e., within the first 24 hours), and delayed treatment (i.e., after the

first 24 hours). Unfortunately, they lament that we presently have a rather limited knowledge of the effect of treatment delay on wound healing, with very little data available in the literature.

Taking a complete dental history can help the dentist learn of previous injuries to the teeth in the area. Repeated injuries to the teeth are not uncommon in children with protruding anterior teeth and in those who are active in athletics. In these patients the prognosis may be less favorable. The dentist must rule out the possibility of a degenerative pulp or adverse reaction of the supporting tissues as a result of previous trauma.

The patient's complaints and experiences after the injury are often valuable in determining the extent of the injury and in estimating the ability of the injured pulp and supporting tissues to overcome the effects of the injury. Pain caused by thermal change is indicative of significant pulpal inflammation. Pain occurring when the teeth are brought into normal occlusion may indicate that the tooth has been displaced. Such pain could likewise indicate an injury to the periodontal and supporting tissues. The likelihood of eventual pulpal necrosis increases if the tooth is mobile at the time of the first examination; the greater the mobility, the greater the chance of pulp death.

Trauma to the supporting tissues may cause sufficient inflammation to initiate external root resorption. In instances of severe injury, teeth can be lost as a result of pathologic root resorption and pulpal degeneration.

CLINICAL EXAMINATION

The clinical examination should be conducted after the teeth in the area of injury have been carefully cleaned of debris. When the injury has resulted in a fracture of the crown, the dentist should observe the amount of tooth structure that has been lost and should look for evidence of a pulp exposure. With the aid of a good light, the clinical crown should be examined carefully for cracks and craze lines, the presence of which could influence the type of permanent restoration used for the tooth. With light transmitted through the teeth in the area, the color of the injured tooth should be carefully compared with that of adjacent uninjured teeth. Severely traumatized teeth often appear darker and reddish, although not actually discolored, which indicates pulpal hyperemia (Fig. 21-3). This appearance suggests that at some later time the pulp may undergo degenerative change terminating in pulpal necrosis.

The Ellis and Davey classification of crown fractures is useful in recording the extent of damage to the crown.[7] The following is a modification of their classification (Fig. 21-4):

Class I—Simple fracture of the crown involving little or no dentin

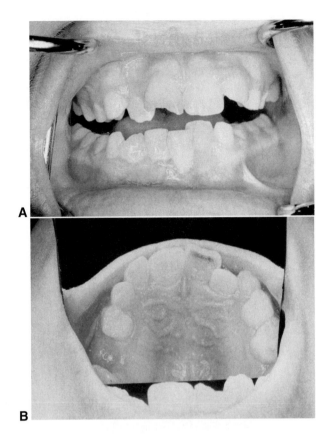

A

B

FIG. **21-3. A,** Fractured central incisor appeared darker than the adjacent teeth 3 days after the injury. The pulp was not exposed, but it was in a state of shock and did not respond to pulp tests. **B,** The reddish appearance of the dentin is evidence of severe hyperemia within the pulp tissue. The prognosis for retaining vitality of the pulp is poor.

Class II—Extensive fracture of the crown involving considerable dentin but not the dental pulp

Class III—Extensive fracture of the crown with an exposure of the dental pulp

Class IV—Loss of the entire crown

A vitality test of the injured tooth should be performed, and the teeth in the immediate area, as well as those in the opposing arch, should be tested. The best prediction of continued vitality of the pulp of a damaged or traumatized tooth is the vital response to electric pulp testing at the time of the initial examination. A negative response, however, is not reliable evidence of pulp death because some teeth that give such a response soon after the injury may recover vitality after a time. When the electric pulp tester is used, the dentist should first determine the normal reading by testing an uninjured tooth on the opposite side of the mouth and recording the lowest number at which the tooth responds. If the injured tooth requires more current than does a normal tooth, the pulp may be undergoing degenerative change. If less current is

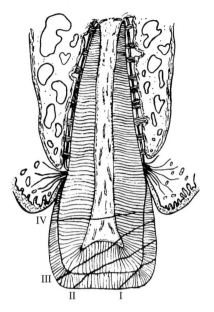

FIG. **21-4.** Classification of crown fractures of anterior teeth.

needed to elicit a response from a traumatized tooth, pulpal inflammation is usually indicated.

Many practitioners question the need for the electric vitality test immediately after the injury. Because the electrical stimulus has been shown to produce negligible additional pulpal irritation, its use is not contraindicated on this basis. However, the patient's measured responses to the test may be almost meaningless. The reliability of the electric pulp test depends on eliciting valid responses from the patient. The mere presence of this new, unknown instrument may create anxiety in children that hampers their ability to respond accurately to the test. Because an unscheduled emergency appointment for treatment of an injury is a new experience, it seems reasonable to introduce the child to the instrument during the first emergency visit when the child does not know what to expect. This gives the dentist an opportunity to allay the child's anxiety about the instrument during a time when the responses are not as important as they will be on subsequent visits. It should also be remembered that the electric pulp test is frequently unreliable even on normal teeth when apices are incompletely formed.

The thermal test is also somewhat helpful in determining the degree of pulpal damage after trauma. Although there are difficulties with the thermal test, it is probably more reliable in testing primary incisors in young children than the electric pulp test. Failure of a tooth to respond to heat is indicative of pulpal necrosis. The response of a tooth to a lower degree of heat than is necessary to elicit a response in adjacent teeth is an indication of inflammation. Pain occurring when ice is applied to a normal tooth will subside when the ice is removed. A more painful and often lingering reaction to cold indicates a pathologic change within the pulp, the nature of which can be determined when the reaction is correlated with other clinical observations.

Failure of a recently traumatized tooth to respond to the pulp test is not uncommon and may indicate a previous injury with a resulting necrotic pulp. However, the traumatized tooth may be in a state of shock and as a result may fail to respond to the accepted methods of determining pulp vitality. The failure of a pulp to respond immediately after an accident is not an indication for endodontic therapy. Instead, emergency treatment should be completed, and the tooth should be retested at the next follow-up visit.

Laser Doppler flowmetry has been reported to be a significant aid in determining vascular vitality of traumatized teeth by Olgart, Gazelius, and Lindh-Stromberg[8] and more recently by Mesaros and Trope.[9] Although this technology is not yet affordably priced for dental offices, it may be in the future.

RADIOGRAPHIC EXAMINATION

The examination of traumatized teeth cannot be considered complete without a radiograph of the injured tooth, the adjacent teeth, and sometimes the teeth in the opposing arch. It may even be necessary to obtain a radiograph of the soft tissue surrounding the injury site in search of a fractured tooth fragment (Fig. 21-5). The relative size of the pulp chamber and canal should be carefully examined. Irregularities or an inconsistency in the size of the chamber or canal compared with that of adjacent teeth may be evidence of a previous injury. This observation is important in determining the immediate course of treatment. In young patients the stage of apical development often indicates the type of treatment, just as the size of the coronal pulp and its proximity to the area of fracture influence the type of restoration that can be used. A root fracture as a result of the injury or one previously sustained can be detected by a careful examination of the radiograph. However, the presence of a root fracture may not influence the course of treatment, particularly if the fracture line is in the region of the apical third. Teeth with root fractures in this area rarely need stabilization, and a fibrous or calcified union will usually result. If teeth have been discernibly dislocated, with or without root fracture, two or three radiographs of the area at different angles may be needed to clearly define the defect and aid the dentist in deciding on a course of treatment.

Another value of the radiograph is that it provides a record of the tooth immediately after the injury. Frequent, periodic radiographs reveal evidence of continued pulp vitality or adverse changes that take place within the pulp or the supporting tissues. In young teeth in which the pulp recovers from the initial trauma, the pulp chamber and canal will decrease in

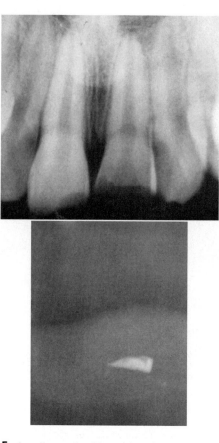

FIG. 21-5. A radiograph with a reduced exposure time (25% of the usual time) was useful in detecting where this fractured tooth fragment was located within the patient's lip.

size coincident with the normal formation of secondary dentin. After a period of time, an inconsistency in the true size or contour of the pulp chamber or canal compared with that of adjacent teeth may indicate a developing pathologic condition.

In cases in which more complex facial injuries have occurred or jaw fractures are suspected, extraoral films may also be necessary to help identify the extent and location of all injury sequelae. Oblique lateral jaw radiographs and panoramic films are often useful adjuncts to this diagnostic process.

EMERGENCY TREATMENT OF SOFT TISSUE INJURY

Injury to the teeth of children is often accompanied by open wounds of the oral tissues, abrasion of the facial tissues, or even puncture wounds. The dentist must recognize the possibility of the development of tetanus after the injury and must carry out adequate first-aid measures.

Children with up-to-date active immunization are protected by the level of antibodies in their circulation produced by a series of injections of tetanus toxoid.

Primary immunization is usually a part of medical care during the first 2 years of life. However, primary immunization cannot be assumed but must be confirmed by examining the child's medical record.

When the child who has had the primary immunization receives an injury from an object that is likely to have been contaminated, the antibody-forming mechanism may be activated with a booster injection of toxoid. An unimmunized child can be protected through passive immunization or serotherapy with tetanus antitoxin (tetanus immune globulin, or TIG).

The dentist examining the child after an injury should determine the child's immunization status, carry out adequate débridement of the wound, and, when indicated, refer the child to the family physician. Tetanus is often fatal, and preventive measures must be taken if there is a possibility that an injured child is not adequately immunized.

Débridement, suturing, and/or hemorrhage control of open soft tissue wounds should be carried out as indicated. Working with an oral and maxillofacial surgeon or a plastic surgeon may also be indicated.

EMERGENCY TREATMENT AND TEMPORARY RESTORATION OF FRACTURED TEETH WITHOUT PULP EXPOSURE

A trauma to a tooth that causes a loss of only a small portion of enamel should be treated as carefully as one in which greater tooth structure is lost. The emergency treatment of minor injuries in which only the enamel is fractured may consist of no more than smoothing the rough, jagged tooth structure. However, without exception a thorough examination should be conducted as previously described. The patient should be reexamined at 2 weeks and again at 1 month after the injury. If the tooth appears to have recovered at that time, continued observation at the patient's regular recall appointments should be the rule.

Sudden injuries with a resultant extensive loss of tooth structure and exposed dentin require an immediate temporary restoration or protective covering, in addition to the complete diagnostic procedure. In this type of injury, initial pulpal hyperemia and the possibility of further trauma to the pulp by pressure or by thermal or chemical irritants must be reduced. In addition, if normal contact with adjacent or opposing teeth has been lost, the temporary restoration or protective covering can be designed to maintain the integrity of the arch. Because providing an adequate permanent restoration may depend on maintaining the normal alignment and position of teeth in the area, this part of the treatment is as important as maintaining the vitality of the teeth. Several restorations that will satisfy these requirements can easily be fabricated.

FRAGMENT RESTORATION (REATTACHMENT OF TOOTH FRAGMENT)

Occasionally the dentist may have the opportunity to reattach the fragment of a fractured tooth using resin and bonding techniques. Tennery reported the successful reattachment of tooth fragments for eight teeth in five patients.[10] One reattached fragment was subsequently lost as the result of a second traumatic episode. Starkey reported successful reattachment of one tooth fragment on a lower central incisor 2 days after the injury.[11]

This procedure is atraumatic and seems to be the ideal method of restoring the fractured crown. Sealing the injured tooth and esthetically restoring its natural contour and color are accomplished simply and constitute an excellent service to the patient. The procedure provides an essentially perfect temporary restoration that may be retained a long time in some cases.

It is not often that the fractured tooth fragment remains intact and is recovered after an injury, but when this happens, the dentist may consider the reattachment procedure. The tooth requires no mechanical preparation because retention is provided by enamel etching and bonding techniques. If little or no dentin is exposed, the fragment and the fractured tooth enamel are etched and reattached with bonding agents and materials. Farik et al have tested the use of the new single-bottle dentin adhesives with and without unfilled resins in the fragment-bonding technique.[12] Their hypothesis was that the amount of resin in single-bottle dentin adhesives might not be sufficient to secure an adequate fragment bond. The results of their study showed that all but one of the seven dentin adhesive systems that they tested should be used with an additional unfilled resin when fractured teeth are restored by reattachment.

For cases in which considerable dentin is exposed or a direct pulp cap is indicated, some controversy currently exists about the best treatment to enhance the likelihood of maintaining pulpal vitality. Some believe that the meticulous use of bonding agents and materials to directly cap the exposed dentin and the pulp (if exposed) is best, whereas others believe that calcium hydroxide should be applied to the exposed dentin and pulp before completing the bonding procedure. The former method has been called the total-etch technique.

Fig. 21-6 illustrates the successful management of a class II fracture of the maxillary left central incisor in a 15-year-old boy who was treated approximately 2 hours after the injury. This reattached fragment has been a successful restoration for more than 7 years. The fragment has been reattached twice during this time, and each failure resulted from an additional direct blow to the tooth. The natural labial position of the tooth made it more susceptible to injury, especially in this very

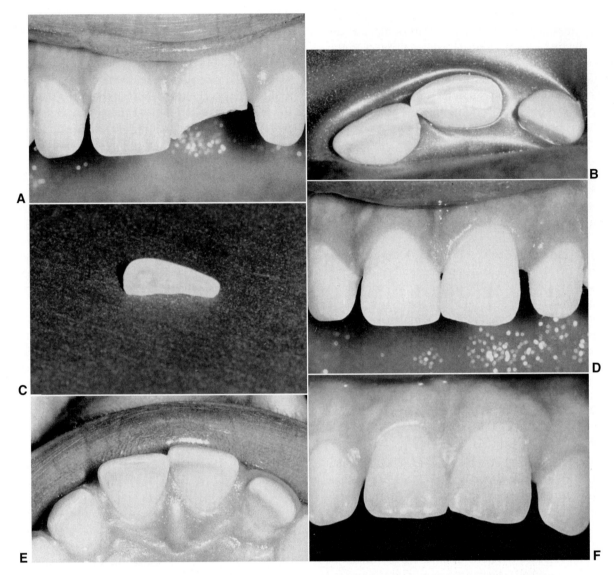

FIG. **21-6. A,** Class II fracture of the crown of a maxillary left central incisor. **B,** The exposed dentin of the tooth is covered with hard-setting calcium hydroxide; all fractured enamel remains exposed. **C,** Part of the dentin is removed from the tooth fragment; the enamel is not disturbed. **D,** Fragment restoration immediately after removal of the rubber dam. **E,** Incisal view of the restored tooth illustrates the tooth's natural susceptibility to fracture because of its labial position. **F,** Restored tooth 22 months after injury.

athletically active patient. After the fragment was trial-seated to confirm a precise fit, the exposed dentin of the fractured tooth was covered with a thin layer of hard-setting calcium hydroxide that was allowed to remain as a sedative dressing between the tooth and the restored fragment. A portion of the dentin in the fragment was removed to provide space for the calcium hydroxide dressing. The fragment was then soaked in etchant, and the fractured area of the tooth was also etched well beyond the fracture site. After thorough rinsing and drying of all etched enamel, the fragment and the etched portion of the tooth were painted with a light-curing sealant material. Although no bonding

agent was used here, its use is currently recommended. The selected shade of composite resin was used to fill the prepared void in the fragment, and it was then carefully seated into its correct position and held firmly while the material was cured with the light. A small amount of external enamel had been lost, which left a defect about 1 mm in diameter on the labial surface. This defect was also filled with the composite resin, and a second layer of sealant was painted over all margins and cured. Subsequent radiographs and vitality tests indicated that the tooth had probably responded favorably. Croll has reported successfully using light-hardened glass ionomer material for reattaching

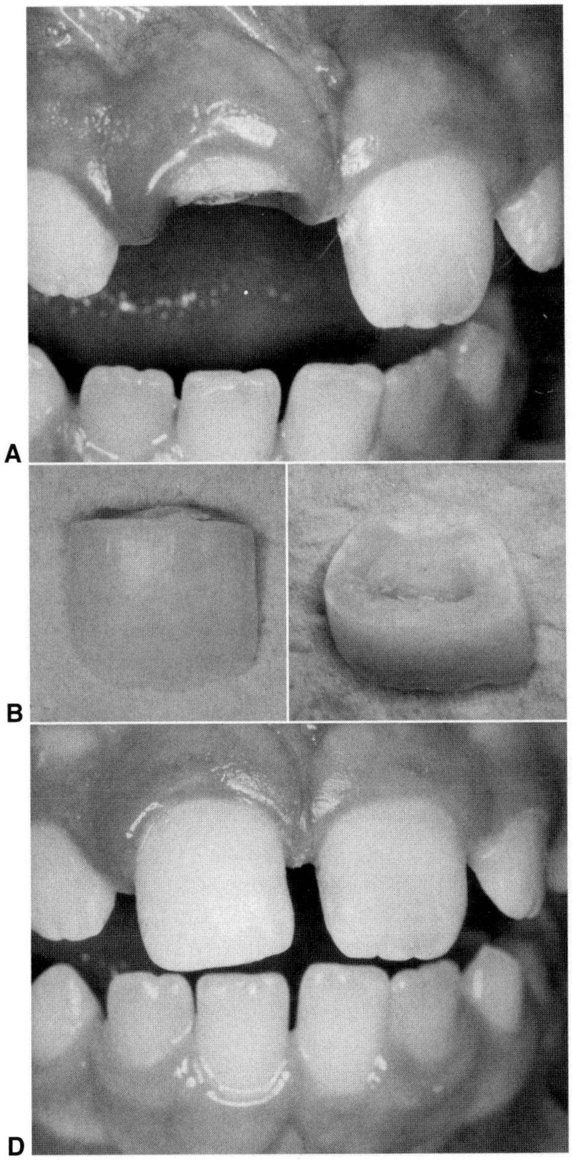

FIG. **21-7.** **A,** Clinical appearance of the anterior teeth of a young boy after a sledding accident that resulted in a mesial-incisal class II crown fracture of the maxillary left central incisor and a class IV fracture of the maxillary right central incisor. The right incisor has been treated by calcium hydroxide pulpotomy. **B** and **C,** Labial and cervical views, respectively, of the coronal fragment of the right central incisor; **C** also illustrates the cavity preparation of the crown made by enlargement of the pulp chamber. **D,** Clinical appearance of the right central incisor after the fragment restoration procedure, which used the mechanical retention of composite resin placed in the pulp canal and pulp chamber preparations along with enamel bonding and cure into a single unit. This fragment restoration served for 7 years 2 months before the tooth was finally restored with a root canal filling, post and core, and crown. During the time the fragment restoration was in place, the patient underwent 2 years of comprehensive orthodontic therapy in which a bonded bracket was attached to the fragment. The fragment broke off and was reattached, but in each instance, failure occurred as a result of new traumatic episodes (once while a protective mouth guard was being

fragments.[13] Kanca reported reattachment of a fragment that successfully capped the pulp using the total-etch technique.[14] The restoration was more than 5 years old (replaced once) and was still in place at the time of the report.

Ludlow and LaTurno have reported the success of a fragment restoration for a 13-year-old patient in which essentially the entire clinical crown of a maxillary incisor was fractured away (Class IV fracture).[15] The remaining tooth was first treated with a root canal filling, and then the pulp canal of the tooth and the enlarged pulp chamber in the fragment crown were used as retentive internal cavities to strengthen the reattached crown. One of the authors (Avery) has performed a similar crown restoration for a younger patient who required a pulpotomy (Fig. 21-7 and also Fig. 21-12).

TEMPORARY BONDED RESIN RESTORATION

The excellent marginal seal and retention derived from applying esthetic restorative materials to etched enamel surfaces have revolutionized the approach to restoring fractured anterior teeth. These bonding techniques are highly successful and versatile in many situations involving anterior trauma.

It may not be advisable to restore an extensive crown fracture with a finished esthetic resin restoration on the day of the injury, because it is usually best not to manipulate the tooth more than is absolutely necessary to make a diagnosis and provide emergency treatment. Also, such emergencies are usually treated at unscheduled appointments, and this treatment should be carried out as efficiently as possible to prevent significant disruption of the dentist's scheduled appointments. A temporary restorative resin restoration can be placed in an efficient manner and is often the treatment of choice.

The restorative resin material is applied as a protective covering at the fracture site using conventional bonding procedures. As a short-term temporary restoration, it requires little or no finishing and does not need to restore the tooth to normal contour. However, the restoration should cover the fractured surfaces and maintain any natural proximal contacts the patient may have had before the injury (Fig. 21-8). After an adequate recovery period, an esthetic resin restoration may be completed, often without removing all the temporary resin material. However, the outer surfaces of the temporary restoration should be removed superficially

worn). Despite the occasional need to reattach the crown, we believe that overall it was the best and most convenient restoration for the patient during his young and accident-prone growing years.

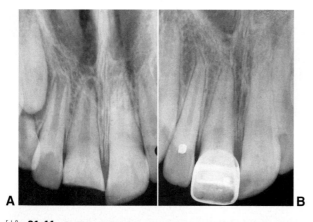

FIG. **21-11.** **A,** The pulp of a permanent central incisor has been exposed as a result of trauma. The pulp was capped with calcium hydroxide. **B,** A successful pulp capping has been accomplished. Continued root end development indicates pulp vitality. The tooth was restored with an esthetic resin-faced steel crown, but a bonded resin restoration is currently recommended.

providing this treatment. The pulp will remain functional and reparative, and dentin will develop and allow the tooth to be restored without loss of normal pulp vitality.

PULPOTOMY

If the pulp exposure in a traumatized, immature permanent (open apex) tooth is large, if even a small pulp exposure exists and the patient did not seek treatment until several hours or days after the injury, or if there is insufficient crown remaining to hold a temporary restoration, the immediate treatment of choice is a shallow pulpotomy or a conventional pulpotomy (Fig. 21-12). A shallow or partial pulpotomy is preferable if coronal pulp inflammation is not widespread and if a deeper access opening is not needed to help retain the coronal restoration.[16] This treatment is also indicated for immature permanent teeth if necrotic pulp tissue is evident at the exposure site with inflammation of the underlying coronal tissue, but a conventional or cervical pulpotomy would be required. Yet another indication is trauma to a mature permanent (closed apex) tooth that has caused both a pulp exposure and a root fracture.

The exposure site should be conservatively enlarged, and 1 to 2 mm of coronal pulp tissue should be removed for the shallow pulpotomy or all pulp tissue in the pulp chamber removed for the conventional pulpotomy. When pulp amputation has been completed to the desired level, the pulp chamber should be thoroughly cleaned with copious irrigation. No visible dentin chips or pulp tissue tags should remain. If the remaining pulp is healthy, hemorrhage will be easy to control with a pledget of moist cotton lightly compressed against the tissue. The pulp should also have a bright reddish pink

color and a concave contour (meniscus). A deeper amputation may be necessary if the health of the pulp is questionable. A dressing of calcium hydroxide is gently applied to the vital pulp tissue so that it is in passive contact with the pulp. The remaining access opening is filled with a hard-setting, biocompatible material with excellent marginal sealing capability. Then the crown may be restored with a separate bonding procedure.

Some experts on pulp therapy recommend conventional pulpectomy and root canal fillings for all teeth treated with calcium hydroxide pulpotomies soon after the root apices close. They view the calcium hydroxide pulpotomy as an interim procedure performed solely to achieve normal root development and apical closure. They justify the pulpectomy and root canal filling after apical closure as necessary to prevent an exaggerated calcific response that may result in total obliteration of the root canal (calcific metamorphosis or calcific degeneration).

We have observed this calcific degenerative response and agree that it should be intercepted with root canal therapy if possible after apical closure (Fig. 21-13). However, long-term successes after calcium hydroxide pulpotomy in which no calcific metamorphosis has been observed can be documented. We have followed such successful cases for more than 10 years without seeing any adverse results. McCormick has reported one case of a tooth successfully treated with a calcium hydroxide pulpotomy that was observed for more than 19 years and never required further pulp therapy.[17]

If healthy pulp tissue remains in the root canal, if the coronal pulp tissue is cleanly excised without excessive tissue laceration and tearing, if the calcium hydroxide is placed gently on the pulp tissue at the amputation site without undue pressure, and if the tooth is adequately sealed, there is a high probability that long-term success can be achieved without follow-up root canal therapy.

PULPECTOMY WITH ENDODONTIC TREATMENT

One of the most challenging endodontic procedures is the treatment and subsequent filling of the root canal of a tooth with an open or funnel-shaped apex. The lumen of the root canal of such an immature tooth is largest at the apex and smallest in the cervical area and is often referred to as a blunderbuss canal. Hermetic sealing of the apex with conventional endodontic techniques is usually impossible without apical surgery. This surgical procedure is traumatic for the young child and should be avoided if possible.

In instances of class III or class IV fractures of young permanent teeth with incomplete root growth and a vital pulp, the pulpotomy technique (as just described) is the procedure of choice. The successful pulpotomy allows the pulp in the root canal to maintain its vitality and also allows the apical portion to continue to

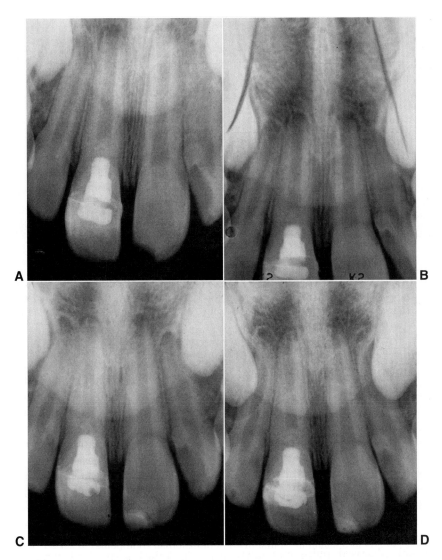

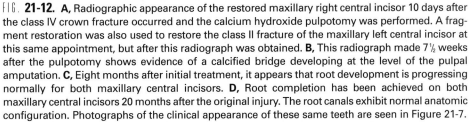

FIG. **21-12.** **A,** Radiographic appearance of the restored maxillary right central incisor 10 days after the class IV crown fracture occurred and the calcium hydroxide pulpotomy was performed. A fragment restoration was also used to restore the class II fracture of the maxillary left central incisor at this same appointment, but after this radiograph was obtained. **B,** This radiograph made 7½ weeks after the pulpotomy shows evidence of a calcified bridge developing at the level of the pulpal amputation. **C,** Eight months after initial treatment, it appears that root development is progressing normally for both maxillary central incisors. **D,** Root completion has been achieved on both maxillary central incisors 20 months after the original injury. The root canals exhibit normal anatomic configuration. Photographs of the clinical appearance of these same teeth are seen in Figure 21-7.

develop (apexogenesis). For class IV fractures the eventual restoration may require a post in the root canal. Before this type of restoration is completed, the dentinal bridge that has formed after the pulpotomy can be perforated and routine endodontic procedures can be undertaken in a now completely developed root canal.

Occasionally a patient has an acute periapical abscess associated with a traumatized tooth. The trauma may have caused a very small pulp exposure that was overlooked, or the pulp may have been devitalized as a result of injury or actual severing of the apical vessels.

A loss of pulp vitality may have caused interrupted growth of the root canal, and the dentist is faced with the task of treating a canal with an open apex.

If an abscess is present, it must be treated first. If there is acute pain and evidence of swelling of the soft tissues, drainage through the pulp canal will give the child almost immediate relief. A conventional endodontic access opening should be made into the pulp chamber. If pain is caused by the pressure required to make the opening into the pulp, the tooth should be supported by the dentist's fingers. Antibiotic therapy is also generally indicated.

of infection seem to be controlled after two or three appointments, the dentist may elect to proceed with the calcium hydroxide paste treatment.

As a general rule the treatment paste is allowed to remain 6 months. The root canal is then reopened to determine if the tooth is ready for a conventional gutta-percha filling as determined by the presence of a "positive stop" when the apical area is probed with a file. Often there is also radiographic evidence of apical closure. Frank has described four successful results of apexification treatment[18]: (1) continued closure of the canal and apex to a normal appearance, (2) a dome-shaped apical closure with the canal retaining a blunderbuss appearance, (3) no apparent radiographic change but a positive stop in the apical area, and (4) a positive stop and radiographic evidence of a barrier coronal to the anatomic apex of the tooth.

If apical closure has not occurred in 6 months, the root canal is retreated with the calcium hydroxide paste. If weeping in the canal was not controlled before filling, retreatment is recommended 2 or 3 months after the first treatment.

Although apical closure often occurs in a 6-month period, one of the authors (Avery) has monitored retreatment for more than 2½ years before favorable results were achieved. Retreatment of the canal at 3- to 6-month intervals for an extended period seems justified as long as the patient remains free of adverse signs and symptoms, because apical closure is likely to occur eventually.

Ideally the postoperative radiographs should demonstrate continued apical growth and closure as in a normal tooth. However, any of the other three previously described results are considered successful. When closure has been achieved, the canal is obliterated in the conventional manner with gutta-percha.

Currently there seems to be a trend away from incorporating antibacterial agents, such as CMCP, in the calcium hydroxide treatment paste. It is generally agreed that calcium hydroxide is the major ingredient responsible for stimulating the desired calcific closure of the apical area. Calcium hydroxide is also an antibacterial agent. It may be that CMCP does not enhance the repair; on the other hand, its use as described here has not been shown to be detrimental. Certainly more than one treatment paste has been employed with success. Giulinani et al have demonstrated the use of mineral trioxide aggregate (MTA) to form an apical plug for apexification in three clinical cases.[20] The root canals of central incisors that had suffered premature interruption of root development as a consequence of trauma were rinsed with 5% sodium hypochloride. Calcium hydroxide was then placed in the canals for 1 week. Following this, the apical portion of the canal (4 mm) was filled with MTA, and the remaining portion of the root canals were closed with thermoplastic gutta-percha. At 6-month and 1-year follow-up periods the clinical and radiographic appearance of the teeth showed resolution of the periapical lesions. These researchers suggest that MTA is a valid option for apexification. They also suggest that long-term outcome studies are needed to test whether this treatment modality will be successful in a large group of teeth.

Trairatvorakul reported on a most interesting and unusual case in which a maxillary primary central incisor successfully responded to apexification therapy.[21] A 14-month-old child experienced early childhood caries to the extent that one maxillary central incisor was necrotic and the root of the tooth was not fully formed. The tooth was treated in a manner similar to that just described. The tooth was retreated with calcium hydroxide 3 months later and restored with composite resin. An additional 3 months later (6 months after initial treatment) an apical stop was present when the area was probed from the root canal access opening. The root canal was then filled with zinc oxide–eugenol paste. The tooth remained functional and radiographically and clinically successful until its normal exfoliation 6 years after initial treatment.

It should be recognized that teeth treated by the apexification method are susceptible to fracture because of the brittleness that results from nonvitality and from the relatively thin dentinal walls of the roots. In addition, another important problem with the calcium hydroxide apexification technique is the duration of therapy, which often lasts many months.

REACTION OF THE TOOTH TO TRAUMA

PULPAL HYPEREMIA

The dentist must be cognizant of the inadequacies of present methods of determining the initial pulpal reaction to an injury and of the difficulty in predicting the long-range reaction of the pulp and supporting tissues to the insult. A trauma of even a so-called minor nature is immediately followed by a condition of pulpal hyperemia.

Congestion of blood within the pulp chamber a short time after the injury can often be detected in the clinical examination. If a strong light is directed to the labial surface of the injured tooth and the lingual surface is viewed in a mirror, the coronal portion of the tooth will often appear reddish compared with the adjacent teeth. The color change may be evident for several weeks after the accident and is often indicative of a poor prognosis.

INTERNAL HEMORRHAGE

The dentist will occasionally observe temporary discoloration of a tooth after injury. Hyperemia and increased pressure may cause the rupture of capillaries and the

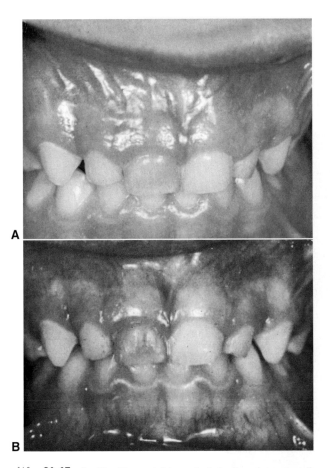

FIG. **21-15.** **A,** Maxillary right central incisor became discolored within 2 weeks after trauma. A pulp test indicated that the pulp was vital. **B,** Six months after the injury, the tooth responded to the vitality test and there was less discoloration of the crown.

escape of red blood cells, with subsequent breakdown and pigment formation. The extravasated blood may be reabsorbed before gaining access to the dentinal tubules, in which case little if any color change will be noticeable and what appears will be temporary (Fig. 21-15). In more severe cases there is pigment formation in the dentinal tubules. The change in color is evident within 2 to 3 weeks after the injury, and although the reaction is reversible to a degree, the crown of the injured tooth retains some of the discoloration for an indefinite period. In cases of this type there is some chance that the pulp will retain its vitality, although the likelihood of vitality is apparently low in primary teeth with dark gray discoloration. Croll, Pascon, and Langeland found that 33 of 51 traumatized teeth (65%) with gray-black discoloration were necrotic.[22] Holan and Fuks conducted a retrospective study of 88 pulpectomized primary incisors, of which 48 met their 9 clinical and radiographic criteria for further investigation.[23] Briefly, their criteria included dark-gray coronal discoloration as the primary diagnostic

sign before pulpectomy. The remaining criteria were indicative of normal conditions or conditions only somewhat suggestive of a pulpal problem. They found that 47 (98%) of the teeth included in the study were either necrotic (37, or 77%) or partially necrotic (10, or 21%). Because all of these teeth were previously determined to need pulpectomy, the 98% confirmation is not so surprising. However, the fact remains that all the teeth exhibited dark-gray discoloration and few, if any, other minor signs or symptoms of a problem.

Discoloration that becomes evident for the first time months or years after an accident, however, is evidence of a necrotic pulp.

CALCIFIC METAMORPHOSIS OF THE DENTAL PULP (PROGRESSIVE CANAL CALCIFICATION OR DYSTROPHIC CALCIFICATION)

A frequently observed reaction to trauma is the partial or complete obliteration of the pulp chamber and canal (Fig. 21-16). Although the radiograph may give the illusion of complete obliteration, an extremely fine root canal and remnants of the pulp will persist.

The crowns of teeth that have undergone this reaction may have a yellowish, opaque color. Primary teeth demonstrating calcific metamorphosis will usually undergo normal root resorption, although Peterson, Taylor, and Marley have reported observing one patient who exhibited calcific metamorphosis of a maxillary primary central incisor that subsequently showed evidence of significant internal resorption in the root.[24] They emphasize the need for careful monitoring of traumatized teeth that have undergone calcific metamorphosis.

Permanent teeth will often be retained indefinitely. However, a permanent tooth showing signs of calcific changes as a result of trauma should be regarded as a potential focus of infection. A small percentage demonstrate pathologic change many years after the injury (Fig. 21-17).

INTERNAL RESORPTION

Internal resorption is a destructive process generally believed to be caused by odontoclastic action. It may be observed radiographically in the pulp chamber or canal within a few weeks or months after an injury. The destructive process may progress slowly or rapidly. If progression is rapid, it may cause a perforation of the crown or root within a few weeks (Fig. 21-18). Mummery described this condition as "pink spot" because when the crown is affected, the vascular tissue of the pulp shines through the remaining thin shell of the tooth.[25] He referred to the occurrence of a perforation as "perforating hyperplasia of the pulp."

If evidence of internal resorption is detected early, before it becomes extensive with resulting perforation,

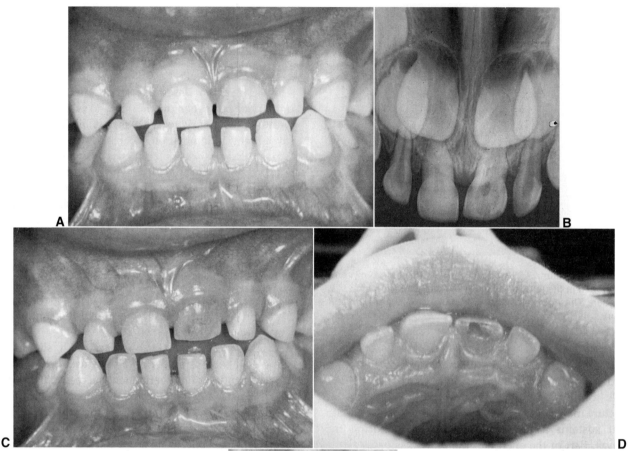

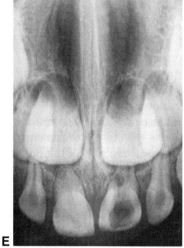

FIG. **21-18.** Internal resorption in a traumatized maxillary left primary incisor. **A,** The tooth 6 months after the injury. The crown had a slightly pinkish color. **B,** The radiograph shows internal resorption in the pulp chamber and canal and some evidence of attempted repair. **C,** There was subsequent deep discoloration of the crown as the destructive process continued, accompanied by proliferation of the pulp tissue. **D,** A perforation can be seen on the lingual surface of the primary incisor. **E,** The radiograph shows the degree of the resorption. The tooth was extracted.

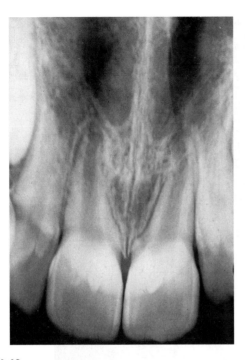

FIG. **21-19.** Radiographic evidence of peripheral root resorption. In these teeth the pulpal vitality was retained, and root resorption did not continue.

ESTHETIC BONDED COMPOSITE RESIN RESTORATION

The feathered-edge restorative technique without mechanical tooth preparation is appropriate in some situations, but it requires excessive contour in the restoration. It offers the advantage of creating less irritation to the pulp, because little or no enamel modification is required. In some cases the excess contour is relatively insignificant, but it may be more significant if the restoration is large (50% or more of the crown) or the fracture extends near or below gingival tissue. Excessive contour on the lingual surface of a maxillary anterior tooth may interfere with normal occlusion.

A beveled preparation affords the dentist the opportunity to reduce the amount of overcontouring of larger restorations and also reduces contour in areas where the occlusion prohibits overcontouring. The dentist may elect the feathered-edge technique (no preparation) on the labial tooth surface and the beveled preparation on the proximal or lingual surfaces or both. Both techniques are described in the following discussion.

When a beveled preparation is desired, the bevel is made in the enamel around the entire circumference or the selected part of the fracture (Figs. 21-23 and 21-24). The bevel should be about 1 to 2 mm incisocervically and about halfway (or more) through the thickness of the enamel at the fracture margins. The labial enamel margin should be irregular to provide a better esthetic blending of the resin with the tooth structure. It should

be mentioned that this sequence may be altered if the practitioner uses some of the latest-generation bonding adhesive systems.

The exposed dentin from a recent injury may be covered with a calcium hydroxide liner. Dilute phosphoric acid (etchant or tooth conditioner) is applied to the enamel surface of the preparation for about 20 seconds (longer for primary teeth). The tooth is then thoroughly flushed with water, and excess moisture is removed with air. The etched area should appear frosty and opaque. Alternatively, the total-etch technique may be employed. In either case a bonding agent is applied to all etched tooth structure. Again, this sequence may be altered with the use of some of the latest bonding adhesive systems.

A celluloid matrix strip may be placed interproximally and wedged for close adaptation at the gingival margin. In large restorations a custom-cut celluloid crown form matrix may be used to help contour the restoration.

Often, little or no mechanical preparation of the fractured incisor is necessary with the feathered-edge technique. Instead, the resin margins are allowed to overlap the fractured edges to become feathered-edge margins on the etched sound enamel cervical to the fracture (Figs. 21-25 to 21-29). As already mentioned, this procedure requires a slightly overcontoured restoration and therefore has limitations. The dentist should be alert to resultant potential undesirable changes in gingival health or the creation of traumatic occlusion. Slight beveling of the fractured enamel margins is usually recommended with the feathered-edge technique to remove loose enamel rods and ensure a fresh surface for etching. The exposed dentin may be protected with a layer of hard-setting calcium hydroxide, and etching should extend 2 or 3 mm beyond the fracture to allow an adequate surface for feather-edging the resin restorative materials. Most manufacturers supply a kit, which usually includes an etchant, a bonding agent, the restorative materials, and a shade guide. The bonding agent is applied to the etched surfaces.

The light-polymerized materials offer the advantage of allowing the clinician to build or sculpt the restoration in small increments and minimize finishing time. Clinical studies have confirmed that excellent and durable restorations may be obtained. Finishing disks and large, round finishing burs or diamonds may be used to contour the labial and lingual surfaces. A sharp, curved scalpel blade (No. 12) may be used to remove flash from the proximal margins of the restoration.

REACTION OF PERMANENT TOOTH BUDS TO INJURY

The dentist who provides emergency care for a child after an injury to the anterior primary teeth must be

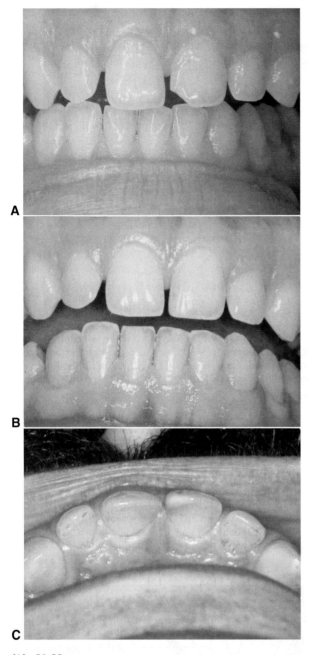

FIG. **21-26.** **A,** Fractured central incisor for which a feathered-edge bonded resin restoration is indicated. **B** and **C,** One-year postoperative photographs of the restoration. The incisal view exhibits the amount of overcontouring that naturally occurs with this technique. In this situation the overcontouring does not adversely affect esthetic appearance, occlusion, or gingival health.

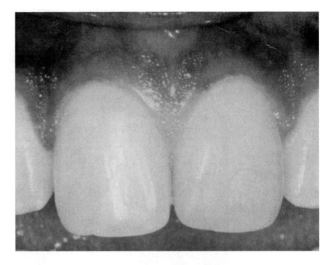

FIG. **21-27.** Mesial-incisal composite restoration on the maxillary left central incisor is more than 6 years old. No additional treatment or repair has been required since the restoration was placed.

human teeth as a result of trauma, infection, or both.[27] He observed small areas that showed destruction of the ameloblasts and a pitted area where a thin enamel layer had been laid down before the injury. In other teeth there was evidence of destruction of the ameloblasts before any enamel had been laid down, resulting in hypoplasia that clinically appeared as deep pitting.

Erupted permanent teeth in the human may show a variety of these defects, including gross malformations of the crown (Figs. 21-32 and 21-33). The presence of a small, pigmented hypoplastic area has been referred to as Turner tooth. Small hypoplastic defects may be restored by the resin-bonding technique.

REPARATIVE DENTIN PRODUCTION

In cases in which the injury to the developing permanent tooth is severe enough to remove the thin covering of developing enamel or cause destruction of the ameloblasts, the subjacent odontoblasts have been observed to produce a reparative type of dentin. The irregular dentin bridges the gap where there is no enamel covering to aid in protecting the pulp from further injury.

DILACERATION

The condition referred to as dilaceration occasionally occurs after the intrusion or displacement of an anterior primary tooth. The developed portion of the tooth is twisted or bent on itself, and in this new position growth of the tooth progresses. Cases have been observed in which the crown of a permanent tooth or a portion of it develops at an acute angle to the remainder to the tooth (Fig. 21-34). Kilpatrick, Hardman, and Welbury reported a dilacerated root of a primary central incisor

not appear to have caused any dental injuries initially, but the problem may be noticed several months or years later (Fig. 21-31).

HYPOCALCIFICATION AND HYPOPLASIA

Cutright's experiments with miniature pigs have shown many lesions similar to those seen in permanent

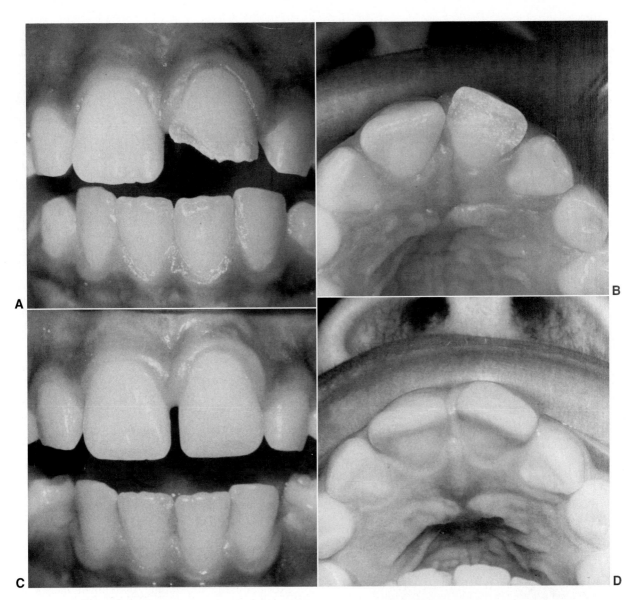

FIG. **21-28. A,** Class II crown fracture involving the entire incisal edge of the maxillary left central incisor. **B,** Incisal view illustrates rotation and labial position of the tooth, which makes it more susceptible to trauma. **C** and **D,** Six-month postoperative views of the tooth restored with an esthetic bonded composite resin restoration using the feathered-edge technique. Incisal view illustrates how an illusion of better tooth alignment was achieved when the mesial half of the labial surface was deliberately undercontoured during finishing.

in a 6-year-old boy.[28] The tooth was necrotic, the root had not resorbed, and the apex of the root was exposed in the labial sulcus and was associated with a draining sinus. No specific history of trauma could be confirmed, but the child was prone to accidents. The authors speculate that this unusual dilaceration may have been due to injury soon after initial eruption of the tooth.

Rushton reported that an injury during development may cause the subsequent appearance of an additional cusp, crown, or denticle.[29] Partial duplication of the affected teeth may occur, with the appearance of gemination in the part of the tooth formed after the injury.

DISPLACEMENT OF PRIMARY AND PERMANENT ANTERIOR TEETH (LUXATION)

INTRUSION AND EXTRUSION OF TEETH

The displacement of anterior primary and permanent teeth presents a challenge in diagnosis and treatment for the dentist (Figs. 21-35 to 21-37). Relatively few studies have been reported that can be used as a guide in treating injuries of this type.

Primary Teeth. The intrusion by forceful impaction of maxillary anterior primary teeth is a common occurrence in children during the first 3 years of life. Frequent

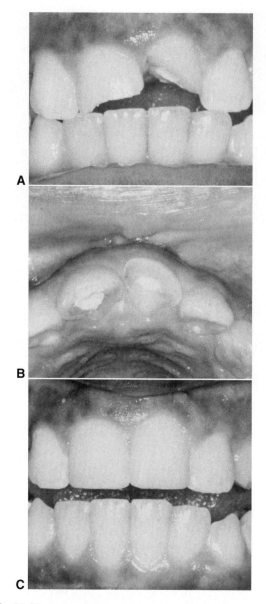

A

B

C

FIG. **21-29.** **A** and **B,** Extensive crown fractures caused pulp exposures of both maxillary central incisors. The entire lingual plate of enamel was lost on the right central incisor. Pulpotomies have been completed. **C,** The occlusion permitted restorations using the feathered-edge technique. The teeth were restored with esthetic bonded composite resin restorations. Additional retention was gained by placement of restorative material in the pulp chambers; no pins or posts were used.

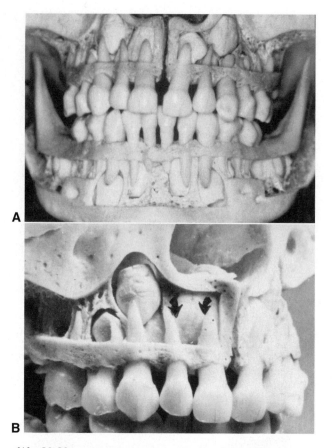

A

B

FIG. **21-30.** **A,** Skull of a 5-year-old child, revealing the relationship between primary and permanent teeth. **B,** Both the central and lateral primary incisors are in close relationship to the permanent incisors *(arrows). (From Andreasen JO, Sundström B, Ravn JJ: Scand J Dent Res 79:219-283, 1971.)*

falls and striking of the teeth on hard objects may force the teeth into the alveolar process to the extent that the entire clinical crown becomes buried in bone and soft tissue. Although there is a difference of opinion regarding treatment of injuries of this type, it is generally agreed that immediate attention should be given to soft tissue damage. Intruded primary teeth should be observed; with few exceptions, no attempt should be made to reposition them after the accident. Most injuries of this type occur at an age when it would be

difficult to construct a splint or a retaining appliance to stabilize the repositioned teeth.

Normally the developing permanent incisor tooth buds lie lingual to the roots of the primary central incisors. Therefore, when an intrusive displacement occurs, the primary tooth usually remains labial to the developing permanent tooth (Fig. 21-38). If the intruded primary tooth is found to be in a lingual or encroaching relationship to the developing permanent tooth, it should be removed. Such a relationship may be confirmed from a lateral radiograph of the anterior segment.

The examination should be carried out as previously described, and radiographs should be made to detect evidence of root fracture, fracture of the alveolar bone, and damage to permanent teeth. However, predicting whether the permanent successors will show evidence of interrupted growth and development is impossible unless actual encroachment of their space can be seen radiographically.

Primary anterior teeth intruded as a result of a blow may often reerupt within 3 to 4 weeks after the injury.

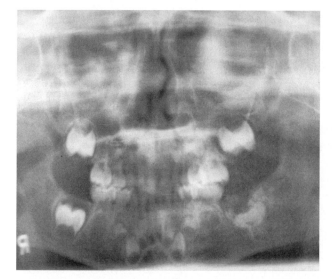

FIG. **21-31.** This radiograph of a 4-year-old child reveals improper formation of the mandibular left first permanent molar. At 18 months, the child had been viciously attacked by a dog. There had been a severe puncture wound of the lower left jaw from the dog's canines, although it was not known then that the injury involved the permanent molar tooth bud. The calcified lesion was removed and microscopically diagnosed as a developing tooth with displaced enamel matrix into follicular tissue. Early removal enhances the potential of the normally developing second permanent molar to eventually acquire an acceptable first permanent molar position.

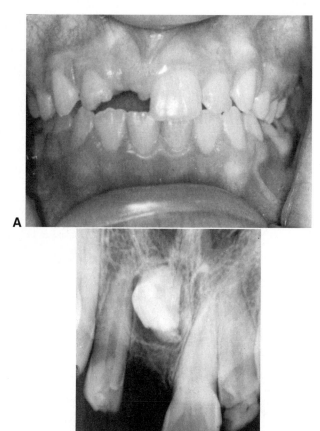

FIG. **21-33.** **A,** Hypoplastic areas on the permanent lateral incisors. The right central incisor has not erupted. **B,** Malformed central incisor. This condition can be traced to a severe trauma to the primary teeth.

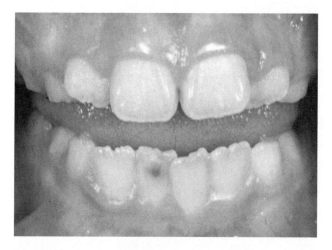

FIG. **21-32.** Isolated hypoplastic area on the labial surface of the mandibular right permanent central incisor. There was a history of a trauma to the primary tooth when the child was younger than 2 years old.

In a study of the results of 248 traumatic episodes to primary incisors, Ravn reported 88 cases of intrusion.[30] Of these teeth, four were extracted within 2 weeks because of infection and four did not reerupt and were extracted several months later, but the remaining 80 teeth fully reerupted within 6 months. Incipient reeruption was observed 14 days after the injury in a few instances. These teeth may even retain their vitality and later undergo normal resorption and be replaced on schedule by their permanent successors. During the first 6 months after the injury, however, the dentist often observes one or more of the reactions of the pulp and supporting tissues that have been mentioned previously in this chapter, the most common of which is pulpal necrosis. Even after reeruption a necrotic pulp can be treated if the tooth is sound in the alveolus and no pathologic root resorption is evident.

Primary teeth that are displaced but not intruded should be repositioned by the dentist or parent as soon as possible after the accident to prevent interference with occlusion. The prognosis for severely loosened primary teeth is poor. Frequently the teeth remain mobile and undergo rapid root resorption.

Skieller observed 60 children treated for looseness of one or more young teeth.[31] Loosened teeth were divided into three groups: simple looseness, dislocation with impaction, and dislocation with extrusion. He concluded

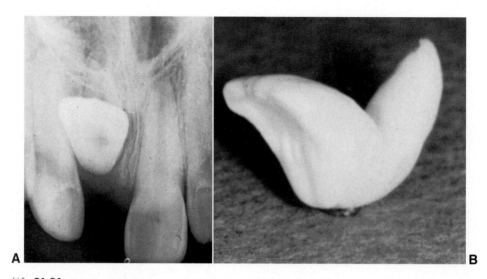

FIG. **21-34.** **A,** Dilacerated unerupted permanent central incisor. There was a history of a trauma at the age of 3 years. **B,** Dilacerated tooth after its surgical removal.

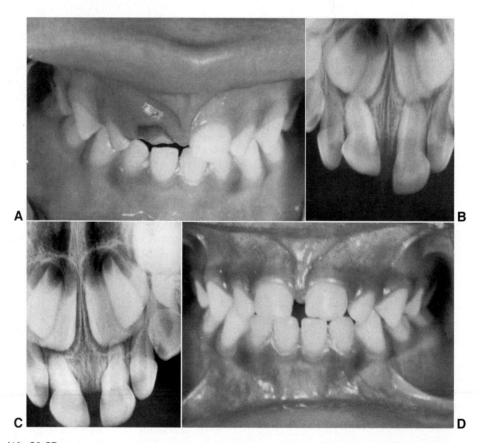

FIG. **21-35.** **A,** Intrusion of the maxillary right primary central incisor. **B,** The degree of intrusion of the primary tooth. Damage to the permanent teeth often results from an injury of this type. **C,** A radiograph taken 8 months after the injury shows that the injured tooth has reerupted. The pulp has retained its vitality, although there is evidence of partial obliteration of the pulp canal. External root resorption has occurred on the adjacent central incisor. **D,** The injured central incisor has assumed its normal place in the arch and probably will be retained until its normal exfoliation time.

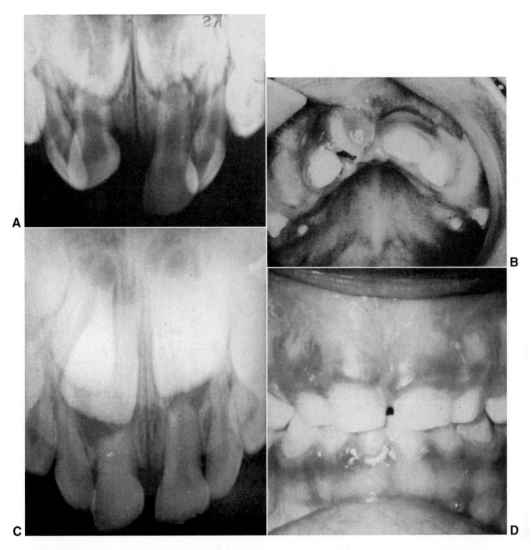

FIG. **21-36.** **A,** Radiograph made shortly after the total intrusion of the maxillary right primary central incisor of a child 22 months of age. The tooth was rotated approximately 90 degrees. **B,** Appearance of tooth and healing soft tissues 2 weeks after the initial injury. No definitive treatment of the tooth was rendered. **C** and **D,** The same patient at 6 years, 5 months of age (4 years, 7 months after injury). The intruded tooth has undergone advanced root resorption and calcific metamorphosis, but the area is asymptomatic and the soft tissues appear healthy. The improved position of the tooth occurred spontaneously as the tooth reerupted. One year after this photograph was made, the tooth exfoliated normally.

that the immediate and future prognosis for the pulp was more favorable if root formation was still incomplete at the time of the accident. Root resorption, which was observed in all three groups of loosened teeth, was most common in impaction cases. Teeth with complete root formation seemed to undergo resorption more frequently than those with incomplete root formation. However, when resorption did occur, it was more extensive and progressed more rapidly in teeth with incomplete root development.

Permanent Teeth. Intruded permanent teeth apparently have a poorer prognosis than similarly injured primary teeth. The tendency for the injury to be followed

by rapid root resorption, pulpal necrosis, or ankylosis is greater. The treatment for a permanent tooth with a closed root end consists in gradually repositioning the tooth orthodontically over a 2- or 3-week period and then continuing to stabilize the tooth for 2 to 4 weeks. The pulp should be extirpated 2 weeks after the injury, and calcium hydroxide should be placed in the root canal as an interim dressing. This treatment approach is recommended by Malmgren, Malmgren, and Goldson[32] and also by Trope, Chivian, and Sigurdsson.[33]

These same authors recommend that intruded immature permanent teeth be left to reerupt spontaneously, unless the intrusion is severe. If the immature tooth does

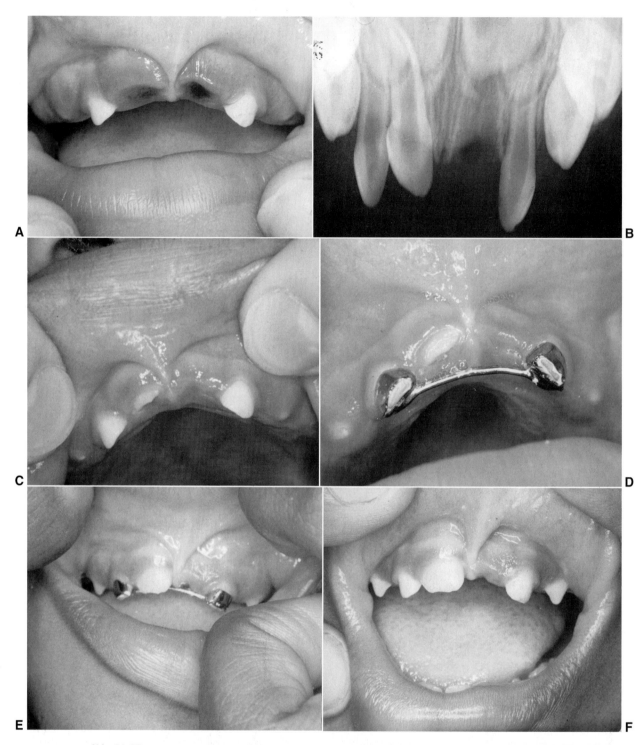

FIG. **21-37.** **A,** A partially intruded maxillary right primary lateral incisor, a totally intruded right central incisor, an avulsed left central incisor, and a loosened left lateral incisor in a 14-month-old child. **B,** Radiograph of injured area made the same day as the trauma. **C,** Area 2 weeks after injury; the right central incisor shows evidence of reeruption. Space loss was a special concern, since the canines were actively erupting. **D,** Cemented space maintainer in position. **E,** Eruption of right central incisor is continuing 2 months after the injury. **F,** Four months after the injury the response is favorable. The space maintainer should be recemented and should remain in place at least until the canines and the central incisor are fully erupted. A more esthetically pleasing space maintainer may be considered later.

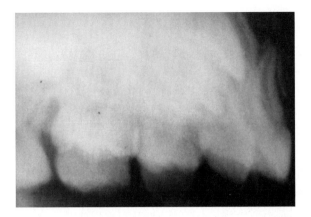

FIG. **21-38.** Radiograph of intruded primary central incisor with its root apex lying labial to the permanent central incisor.

not show early evidence of spontaneous reeruption (after 1 to 2 weeks) or if the intrusion is severe, orthodontic repositioning should be initiated. The clinician may elect to reposition the tooth orthodontically but delay endodontic therapy in the absence of unfavorable signs or symptoms. Endodontic therapy is often required, however, and the tooth should be monitored closely while a decision on endodontic therapy is pending.

Tronstad et al have reported on the management of severely intruded mature maxillary central incisors in an 11-year-old patient in whom spontaneous reeruption occurred.[34] Rather than repositioning the teeth to gain endodontic access, they performed a palatal gingivectomy and endodontic treatment 10 days after the injury while the teeth remained in their intruded position. Eight weeks after the injury the teeth had reerupted naturally and were judged to be near their original position. Similar management of severely intruded immature central incisors has been reported by Shapira, Regev, and Liebfeld.[35] In these cases the palatal gingivectomies and endodontic treatment were performed 8 to 10 weeks after injury when periapical rarefactions and root resorption were noted radiographically. They noted accelerated spontaneous reeruption of all treated teeth soon after the gingivectomies and calcium hydroxide endodontic treatments were performed. Complete reeruption of the teeth and apparent periapical and periodontal healing had occurred 2 to 3 months after the surgical intervention.

It seems that both treatment approaches to treatment of severely intruded permanent teeth (early repositioning or waiting for spontaneous reeruption) have demonstrated reasonably successful results. However, the affected teeth seem to benefit by early calcium hydroxide endodontic therapy with either treatment approach. The decision to reposition mechanically or hope for spontaneous reeruption of intruded permanent teeth remains a matter of clinical judgment that may be based on several conditions associated with the particular case.

The extrusive luxation of a permanent tooth usually results in pulpal necrosis. The immediate treatment involves the careful repositioning of the tooth and stabilization following the technique described later in this chapter. If mature repositioned teeth do not respond to pulp vitality tests within 2 to 3 weeks after repositioning, endodontic treatment should be undertaken before there is evidence of root resorption, which often occurs after severe injuries of this type. The need for endodontic intervention is virtually certain in cases of significant extrusion (more than 2 mm) of mature teeth (Fig. 21-39). With extruded immature teeth, the clinician should monitor the situation frequently and be prepared to intervene with endodontic therapy, as described later, if conditions warrant.

AVULSION AND REPLANTATION

Replantation is the technique in which a tooth, usually one in the anterior region, is reinserted into the alveolus after its loss or displacement by accidental means. There are few reports in the literature of this technique's proving successful for indefinite periods of time. For example, Barry reports on functioning teeth that were replanted 42 years earlier.[36] However, slow or even rapid root resorption often occurs with even the most precise and careful technique. Replantation of permanent teeth continues to be practiced and recommended, however, because prolonged retention is also achieved in many cases, especially when replantation occurs soon after the accident. The replanted tooth serves as a space maintainer and often guides adjacent teeth into their proper position in the arch, a function that is important during the transitional dentition period. The replantation procedure also has psychologic value. It gives the unfortunate child and parents hope for success; even though they are told of the possibility of eventual loss of the tooth, the early result often appears favorable and softens the emotional blow of the accident (Fig. 21-40).

The success of the replantation procedure is undoubtedly related to the length of time that elapses between the loss of the tooth and its replacement in the socket. The condition of the tooth, and particularly the condition of the periodontal ligament tissue remaining on the root surface, are also important factors that influence the success of replantation. There have been reports that immediate replacement of a permanent tooth occasionally results in maintenance of vitality and indefinite retention. However, replantation should generally be viewed as a temporary measure. Under favorable conditions, many replanted teeth are retained for 5 or 10 years and a few for a lifetime. Others, however, fail soon after replantation.

Camp reports that the tooth most commonly avulsed in both the primary and the permanent dentition is a maxillary central incisor.[37] Most often an avulsion injury involves only a single tooth. Avulsion injuries are three

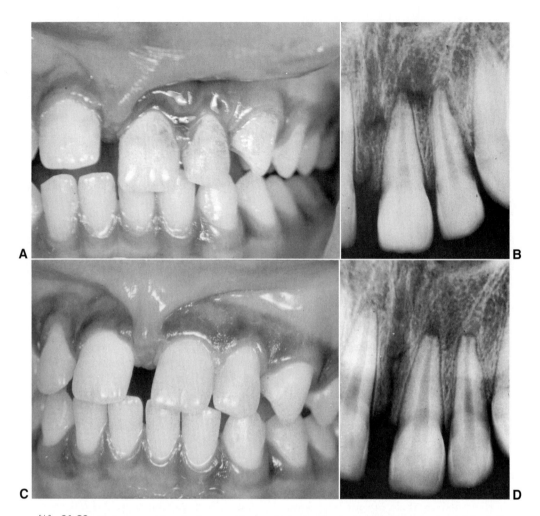

FIG. **21-39.** **A,** A severe blow to the maxillary anterior teeth resulted in the extrusion of the left central and lateral incisors. **B,** A radiograph demonstrates a fracture of alveolar bone. **C,** One month after the repositioning and stabilization of the teeth, they are firmly attached and the gingival tissues appear normal. **D,** A radiograph demonstrates healing of the fractured alveolar bone, but there is evidence of apical root resorption. Endodontic treatment was recommended.

times more frequent in boys than in girls and occur most commonly in children 7 to 9 years of age when permanent incisors are erupting. Andreasen suggests that the loosely structured periodontal ligament surrounding the erupting teeth favors complete avulsion.[38]

The sooner a tooth can be replanted in its socket after avulsion, the better the prognosis will be for retention without root resorption (Figs. 21-41 and 21-42). Andreasen and Hjørting-Hansen reported a follow-up study of 110 replanted teeth. Of those replanted within 30 minutes, 90% showed no discernible evidence of resorption 2 or more years later.[39] However, 95% of the teeth replanted more than 2 hours after the injury showed root resorption. If the tooth has been out of the mouth for less than 30 minutes, the prognosis is therefore more favorable. Also, if the apical end of the tooth is incompletely developed at the time of the injury, there is a greater chance of regaining pulp vitality after

replantation. If the apex is closed, the dentist should proceed with a pulpectomy a few days after the replantation, even if the extraoral time for the tooth was brief.

If a parent calls to report that a tooth has been avulsed and it can be determined that the injury is without other oral, neurologic, or higher-priority physical complications, the dentist may instruct the parent to replace it in the socket immediately and to hold it in place with light finger pressure while the patient is brought to the dental office. If the avulsion occurred in a clean environment, nothing should be done to the tooth before the parent replants it. If the tooth is dirty, an attempt should be made to clean the root surface, but it is very important to preserve any remnants of the periodontal ligament that are still attached to the root. Therefore the parent would then be instructed to keep the tooth immersed in a suitable storage medium and bring the child and the tooth for immediate care.

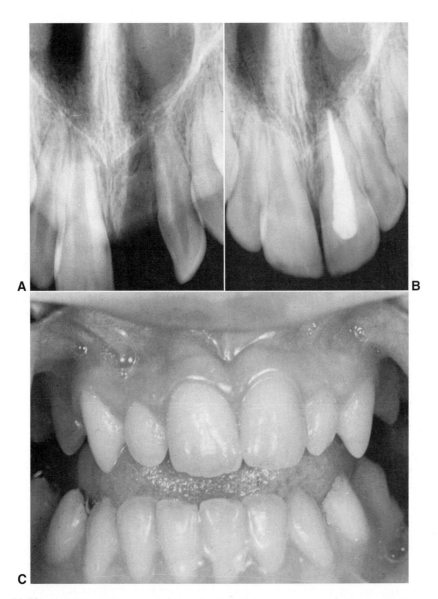

FIG. **21-40. A,** Radiograph of a patient who lost a central incisor as the result of trauma. Replantation was performed. **B,** After the replantation procedure, peripheral root resorption is evident along the mesial surface. **C,** The relationship of the replanted tooth in the arch; the gingival tissue is normal.

Milk has been shown to be a suitable storage medium that is also often readily available (skim or low-fat milk, if available, is preferred). Isotonic saline is another excellent solution to use for this purpose if it is available. A commercial product designed specifically for storing avulsed teeth is the Emergency Medical Treatment Toothsaver (EMT Toothsaver).* The system includes an appropriate container for storage and transport of the tooth while immersed in a pH-balanced cell culture fluid (similar to Hanks balanced salt solution). This product has a 2-year shelf-life without refrigeration.

*SmartPractice, Phoenix, Ariz.

The tooth must be kept moist during the trip to the dental office if the parent cannot or will not replant it. Allowing the avulsed tooth to dehydrate before replantation is damaging to a favorable prognosis. Many studies, including that by Blomlöf, Otteskog, and Hammarström, have compared various storage solutions for avulsed teeth.[40] A compilation of this information indicates that Hanks buffered saline, isotonic saline, and pasteurized bovine milk may be the most favorable known storage media. If none of these solutions is readily available, human saliva is an acceptable short-term substitute storage liquid. Presumably, the patient's saliva (and perhaps blood) would be readily available to collect in a small container (or a

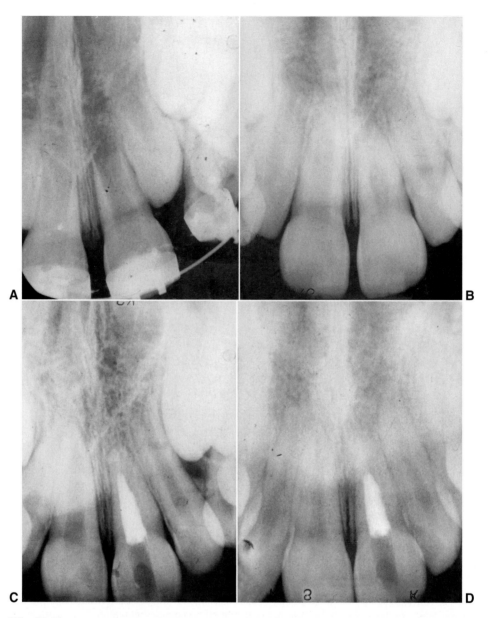

FIG. **21-41. A,** An immature permanent left central incisor soon after replantation and stabilization. The tooth was replanted by the mother within 15 minutes after avulsion. The dentist instructed her by phone before the child was brought to the dental office. The tooth had erupted only about 3 mm when it was avulsed. **B,** Replanted tooth 11 months after injury shows continued but blunted root development and thickened apical calcification. The tooth was then treated with a paste of calcium hydroxide and camphorated mono-parachlorophenol for several months. **C,** Two years after the injury, soon after the root canal was obliterated with gutta-percha. **D,** A favorable response can be seen 11½ years after the injury. The crown was restored with a full-coverage restoration approximately 25 years after the avulsion. *(Courtesy Dr. Guthrie Carr.)*

cupped hand) in which to keep the tooth moist while transporting it to the dental office. Although tap water has been a commonly recommended storage solution (and its use would be preferable to allowing dehydration of the tooth), saliva is a better storage medium. Neither water nor saliva is as good as milk or saline, if the tooth must be stored for a long period (more than 30 minutes before replantation). Because water is hypotonic, its use leads to rapid cell lysis and increased inflammation on replantation.

The patient should receive immediate attention after arriving at the dental office. If the tooth has not already been replanted, the dentist should make every effort to minimize the additional time that the tooth is out of the

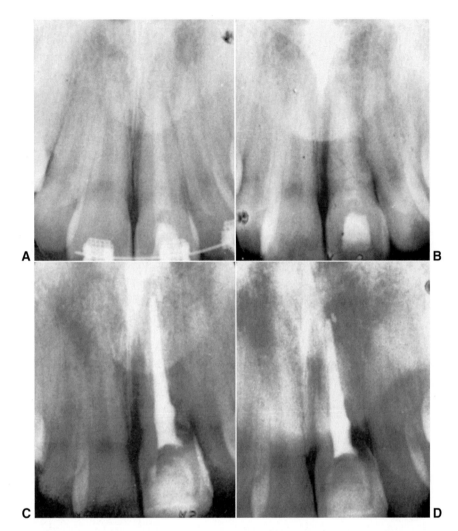

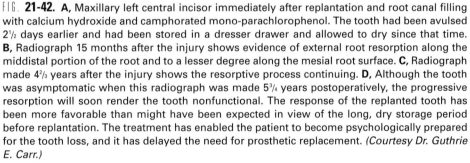

FIG. **21-42.** **A,** Maxillary left central incisor immediately after replantation and root canal filling with calcium hydroxide and camphorated mono-parachlorophenol. The tooth had been avulsed 2½ days earlier and had been stored in a dresser drawer and allowed to dry since that time. **B,** Radiograph 15 months after the injury shows evidence of external root resorption along the middistal portion of the root and to a lesser degree along the mesial root surface. **C,** Radiograph made 4⅔ years after the injury shows the resorptive process continuing. **D,** Although the tooth was asymptomatic when this radiograph was made 5¾ years postoperatively, the progressive resorption will soon render the tooth nonfunctional. The response of the replanted tooth has been more favorable than might have been expected in view of the long, dry storage period before replantation. The treatment has enabled the patient to become psychologically prepared for the tooth loss, and it has delayed the need for prosthetic replacement. *(Courtesy Dr. Guthrie E. Carr.)*

socket. The patient's general status should be quickly assessed to confirm that there are no higher-priority injuries.

If an evaluation of the socket area shows no evidence of alveolar fracture or severe soft tissue injury, the tooth is intact, and only a few minutes have elapsed since the injury, the dentist should replant the tooth immediately. Under the conditions just described, every effort should be directed toward preserving a viable periodontal ligament. Trope correctly asserts that treatment is directed at avoiding or minimizing the resultant inflammation, which occurs as a direct result of the two main consequences of tooth avulsion: attachment damage and pulpal infection.[41] If the tooth was cleanly avulsed, it can probably be replanted without local anesthetic, and obtaining the initial radiograph can also be delayed until the tooth is replaced in the socket and held with finger pressure. The minutes saved may contribute to a more successful replantation. If a clot is present in the socket, it will be displaced as the tooth is repositioned; the socket walls should not be scraped with an instrument. If the tooth does not slip back into position with

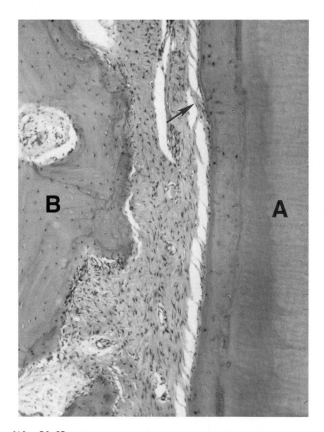

FIG. **21-43.** Microscopic section of a tooth replanted with the periodontal ligament intact. The reattachment of the periodontal fibers is illustrated by their crossing the tear in the periodontal ligament. A, Tooth; B, alveolar bone. (Courtesy Dr. Philip Sherman, Jr.)

relative ease when finger pressure is used, local anesthesia and a radiographic evaluation are indicated. Local anesthetic should also be administered when fractured and displaced alveolar bone must be repositioned before the tooth is replanted. Soft tissue suturing may be delayed until the tooth has been replaced in the socket; however, the suturing should be performed to control hemorrhage before the tooth is stabilized with a bonded splint. Splinting techniques are discussed in the next section of this chapter.

Sherman studied the mechanism by which the replanted tooth becomes secured in the alveolus.[42] Intentional replantation was performed on 25 incisors in dogs and monkeys. The root canals were hermetically sealed with gutta-percha, and the teeth were splinted for 1 month. Subsequent microscopic examination under fluorescent and incandescent light revealed deposition of secondary cementum and new alveolar bone, which entrapped the periodontal fibers (Fig. 21-43).

The preservation of an intact and viable periodontal ligament is the most important factor in achieving healing without root resorption. Delicate handling of the tooth, storage in an appropriate moist environment,

quick replantation, and appropriate stabilization are all important in preserving the periodontal ligament. Undesirable periodontal ligament reactions may result in replacement resorption (ankylosis) or inflammatory resorption of the root. Either reaction may cause eventual loss of the tooth unless the resorption can be controlled. Use of an enamel matrix derivative (Emdogain*) has been shown to increase the incidence of healed periodontal ligament when this gel is applied to the root surface of the avulsed tooth and/or inserted directly into the alveolar socket prior to implantation. It appears to aid in preventing or retarding resorption and ankylosis.

In the past, few attempts were made to replant avulsed primary teeth; however, there have been a few reports of success with this procedure. Andreasen and Andreasen have stated that replantation of primary teeth is contraindicated because of the poor prognosis for success and the additional risk of further injury to the succedaneous tooth.[43] We agree that, even under the most ideal conditions, replanting a primary tooth has higher risk and poorer prognosis despite the remote chance for a favorable outcome.

Stabilization of Replanted Teeth. After replantation of a tooth that has been avulsed, a splint is required to stabilize it during at least the first week of healing. Camp[37] has stated that an acceptable splint should meet the following criteria:

1. It should be easy to fabricate directly in the mouth without lengthy laboratory procedures.
2. It should be able to be placed passively without causing forces on the teeth.
3. It should not touch the gingival tissues, causing gingival irritation.
4. It should not interfere with normal occlusion.
5. It should be easily cleaned and allow for proper oral hygiene.
6. It should not traumatize the teeth or gingiva during application.
7. It should allow an approach for endodontic therapy.
8. It should be easily removed.

The splint should also allow mobility of the replanted tooth that is comparable with the normal mobility of a tooth. Rigid stabilization seems to stimulate replacement resorption of the root. Hurst has demonstrated that rigid stabilization of a replanted tooth is detrimental to proper healing of the periodontal ligament.[44]

The bonded resin and wire splint satisfies all the criteria just described. It can be used in most situations requiring the stabilization of one or more teeth if

*Biora, Chicago, Ill., and Malmö Sweden.

sufficient sound teeth remain for anchorage (see Fig. 21-48). Rectangular or round orthodontic wire is bent to approximate the arch configuration along the midportion of the labial surfaces of the teeth to be incorporated in the splint. At least one sound tooth on each side of the tooth to be stabilized is included. The size of the wire is not too critical, but rectangular wire should be at least 0.016 × 0.022 inch and round wire at least 0.018 inch. If three or four teeth must be stabilized, a stiffer wire (such as 0.028-inch round wire) is required. If round wire is used, a right-angle bend should be made near each end of the wire to prevent rotation of the wire in the resin. A 20- to 30-pound-test monofilament nylon line is an acceptable substitute for wire in the splint.

If the labial enamel surfaces to be etched are not plaque free, they should be cleaned with a pumice slurry, rinsed, thoroughly dried, and isolated with cotton rolls. The enamel surfaces are etched with a phosphoric acid etchant; the gel form is convenient. The enamel surfaces are thoroughly washed and dried again. The wire is then attached to the abutment teeth by placing increments of the resin material over the wire and onto the etched enamel. The resin should completely surround a segment of the wire, but it should not encroach on the proximal contacts or embrasures. The replanted tooth is then held in position while resin is used to bond it to the wire. The resin may be lightly finished if necessary after polymerization. The splint is easily removed (usually 7 to 14 days later) by cutting through the resin with a bur to uncover the wire. The remaining resin may then be removed with conventional finishing instruments. If the splint is used to stabilize lower teeth, it may be necessary to affix the wire to the lingual surfaces if placing it on the labial surfaces will interfere with natural occlusion. Because lingual surfaces are more likely to be contaminated with saliva during the procedure, however, labial placement is preferred whenever possible.

Direct-bonded orthodontic brackets may also be placed on the teeth, and a light labial archwire bent to accurately conform to the natural curvature of the arch is then ligated to the brackets. The brackets are properly aligned on the archwire and bonded to the abutment teeth first. Then the avulsed tooth is ideally positioned and additional bonding material is placed, if necessary, to fill any remaining small space between the tooth and the bracket before bonding it to the splint. If performed properly, this technique results in an excellent splint (Fig. 21-44). However, it requires much more accurate and precise wire bending than the bonded resin and wire technique (without brackets) to achieve a passive appliance.

If the patient is mentally disabled or has immature behavior and does not tolerate foreign objects in the mouth well, or if there are insufficient abutment teeth

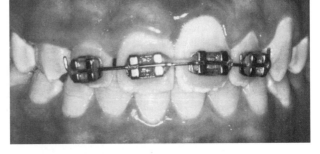

FIG. **21-44.** Bonded brackets and archwire splint.

available for the bonded resin and wire splint, the suture and bonded resin splint advocated by Camp[37] may be an acceptable alternative (Fig. 21-45). Examples of other types of splint are shown in Fig. 21-46. The titanium trauma splint has been developed by von Arx, Filippi, and Buser to ease the application and removal of the splint and to increase comfort for the patient.[45]

In general, stabilization for replanted teeth without other complications is required for 7 to 14 days. The periodontal ligament fibers should have healed sufficiently after the first week to remove the splint. However, the patient should be advised not to bite directly on the replanted tooth for 3 to 4 weeks after the injury and then gradually to begin to return to normal use of the tooth. During this time, food may be cut into bite-size pieces and chewed carefully with unaffected teeth. The patient should maintain good oral hygiene by brushing and flossing normally and using chlorhexidine mouthrinses.

We recommend that systemic antibiotic therapy begin immediately and continue for at least a week following replantation. If the apex is closed, extending the antibiotic therapy until the pulp is extirpated seems to be a good way to determine the duration of antibiotic coverage. Research by Sae-Lim, Wang, and Trope has shown that antibiotic therapy is effective in preventing the development of external inflammatory root resorption of replanted teeth in which the pulps were not extirpated.[46] This finding suggests that antibiotic therapy may also be helpful in those cases in which the pulps of immature replanted teeth are allowed to remain while hoping for revitalization. Additional studies in this area are indicated. In fact, research in this area is ongoing to find better storage and soaking media. Various antibiotics, fluoride liquids and gels, glucocorticoids, and a liver transport medium are being investigated. Krasner and Rankow have published detailed recommendations for replanting a tooth based on its status as judged by the clinician's determination of the physiologic condition of the root periodontal ligament cells, the development of the root apex, and the length of extraoral time.[47] Their recommendations recognize 10 different

and the surrounding viable tissue becomes more apparent. The necrotic tissue, known as *eschar*, becomes charred or crusty in appearance and begins to separate from the surrounding viable tissue (Fig. 21-50). The eschar sloughs off 1 to 3 weeks after the burn incident. Healing occurs by secondary intention as granulation tissue proliferates and matures. Two or 3 months after the accident the wound becomes indurated as a result of fibrous tissue formation. For an additional 6 months the immature scar tissue may bind the lips, alveolar ridges, and other involved structures. If it is not treated, contraction of the fibrotic scar tissue results in unesthetic and functionally debilitating microstomia. The scar tissue softens as it matures, and by 9 months to 1 year after the injury the potential for tissue contraction is greatly decreased. The duration of the healing process and the selected course of treatment depend on the extent and severity of tissue destruction. Because of the variable nature of burn injuries, surgery or appliance therapy may be used or no treatment may be needed.

TREATMENT

Assessing the general physical status of a patient who has sustained an electrical burn to the mouth is the first priority. Subsequently, the extent of the burn is carefully evaluated and local measures are initiated, such as control of minor hemorrhage or conservative débridement of nonviable tissue.

The immunization status of the patient must be ascertained, and tetanus toxoid or depot triple antigen (diphtheria-pertussis-tetanus vaccine) administered when appropriate. Many physicians prescribe a broad-spectrum antibiotic as prophylaxis. However, it may not be necessary or prudent to prescribe antibiotics in the absence of infection.

The parents should be informed of the possibility of spontaneous arterial hemorrhage during the first 3 weeks. They should be instructed to place firm pressure, with gauze, to the bleeding area for 10 minutes. If bleeding persists, they should take the child to the emergency department. Usually, hemorrhage is not a significant problem and does not warrant prophylactic hospitalization except for the most severe and extensive injuries.

The surgical management of burn injuries to the mouth, especially with regard to the time when such surgery should be performed, is controversial. Initially, no surgical intervention is generally warranted. Instead, the treatment of choice is the use of a prosthetic appliance. The primary functions of such an appliance are to prevent contracture of healing tissue and to serve as a framework on which a more normal-appearing commissure may be created and preserved after completion of the healing process. Many patients at James Whitcomb Riley Hospital for Children have been successfully treated with these appliances. Moreover, surgical procedures have not been needed in cases with good patient compliance in appliance use.

The major components of the burn appliance are illustrated in Fig. 21-51. The appliance is removed when the patient eats, when the teeth and appliance are cleaned, or when modifications of the wings are

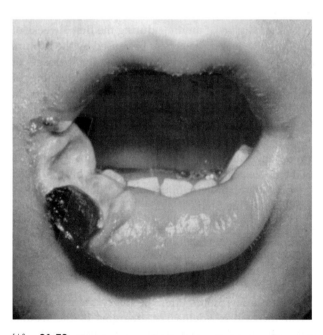

FIG. **21-50.** Appearance of injury to the lower lip and commissure 10 days after electrical burn. The dark lesion on the lower lip is an eschar. *(Courtesy Dr. Theodore R. Lynch.)*

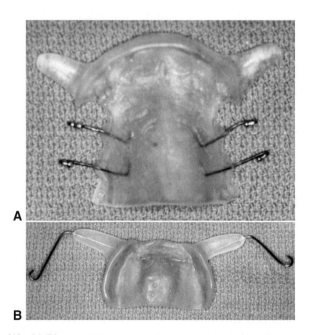

A

B

FIG. **21-51. A,** Example of a burn appliance designed for intraoral retention. **B,** Example of a burn appliance designed for intraoral and extraoral retention in combination with headgear. **(A** *courtesy Dr. David K. Hennon;* **B** *courtesy Dr. John D. Hiester.)*

necessary. The appliance is a static base with wings extending laterally to provide contact with both commissures. If symmetry relative to the midline is to be maintained during the healing process, the wings must contact the commissures equidistant from the midline and must exert essentially equal pressure at these points.

The shape and location of the wings are important, not only in preventing contracture or cohesion of the lips during healing but also in shaping the affected commissure to duplicate the unaffected side. The wing is contoured so that it is thickest in its occlusocervical dimension on the labial aspect. It is tapered as thinly as possible at the point of contact with the commissure (Fig. 21-52). The wings should be large enough just to maintain the correct shape of the commissure. Wings of the proper size will look more pleasing during wear and will enhance acceptance and compliance by the child and parent.

If compliance is a problem with an acrylic appliance, a modified fixed appliance can be constructed and ligated in the mouth. Bands are adapted on the upper second primary molars, and an impression is made. Headgear tubes are welded on the bands, and a Nance appliance is constructed from 0.036- or 0.040-inch wire. If the Nance button is not used, the wire is contoured along the gingival portion of the teeth (Fig. 21-53, *A*). For even more rigidity, an additional wire can be contoured and soldered transpalatally from molar to molar.

After the stabilizing framework is made, the outer portion of the appliance is formed. Using 0.045-inch wire, the anterior arch form is established. Horizontal loops are placed in the area approximating the location of the commissures, as determined by clinical measurements. The wire is continued posteriorly, and omega loops are placed mesial to the headgear tubes. Fig. 21-53, *B*, illustrates the completed outer portion of the appliance. Adjustments are made in the acrylic in one or both of the omega loops to achieve the correct fit. With the omega loops used as tiebacks, the appliance is ligated in the mouth. The patient should be evaluated as often as needed during the first month to make any necessary adjustments. Then the patient should be seen at least once a month.

Ideally the patient with an electrical burn to the mouth should be seen by the dentist between the fifth and tenth days after the accident. The initial appointment is probably the most crucial to the success or failure of treatment with the burn appliance. Parental apprehension and feelings of guilt are often high, and the trust and confidence of both the parents and the child must be acquired as soon as possible. They should be told in detail what they can expect from the dental services offered and what is expected of them. The parents and the child should be shown pictures from previous cases. This not only demonstrates the appearance and purpose of the appliance but also emphasizes that they are not the only ones who have experienced the physical and psychologic trauma associated with such an accident. Pictures of patients who did not have an appliance or who did not wear their appliance as instructed are also shown. The impact of such illustrative materials is dramatic.

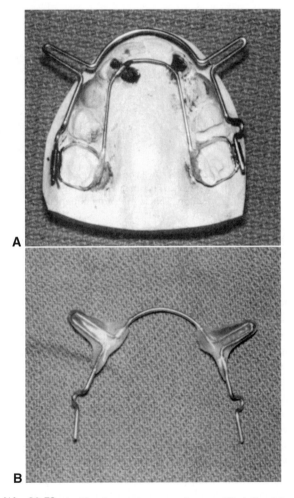

FIG. **21-53. A**, Metal components of a modified fixed burn appliance on the working model. **B**, Finished outer portion of the appliance ready to insert and ligate to the cemented lingual arch. *(Courtesy Dr. Stephanie M. Litz.)*

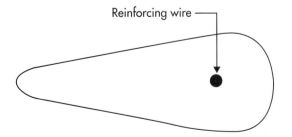

Reinforcing wire

FIG. **21-52.** Cross-sectional view of the commissure wing of the burn appliance.

predominant in dentistry for children. We strive to prevent dental caries, periodontal disease, malocclusion, and anxiety about dental care. If disease is present, our treatment becomes part of an overall prevention plan designed to halt the progress of disease and prevent its recurrence. The success of the prevention plan, provided that there is parent and patient cooperation, is reasonably predictable.

Unfortunately, our ability to prevent injuries to oral structures is limited. Living and growing carry a high risk of trauma. A child will not learn to walk without falling, and few children reach 4 years of age without having received a blow to the mouth. We cannot totally prevent trauma. Moreover, the results of treatment of trauma are often less predictable than those of other types of dental treatment.

On the brighter side, there are preventive measures that have been proved to reduce the prevalence of traumatic episodes in certain environmental situations. For example, because the prevalence of fractured incisors is higher among those with protrusive anterior teeth, many dentists are recommending early reduction of excessive protrusion to reduce the susceptibility of such teeth to injury. The use of car safety seats and restraining belts has prevented many injuries to infants and young children. The protective mouth guard described in Chapter 22 has prevented or reduced the severity of countless injuries to the teeth of youngsters participating in organized athletic activities; active youngsters should be encouraged to wear their mouth guards during high-risk unsupervised athletic activities as well.

Parents should be reminded that accessible "live" electric cords are potentially dangerous, especially to small children who still use their mouths to evaluate their environment. In addition, anticipatory guidance and education are necessary to advise our patients regarding the negative health effects of intraoral and perioral body piercing (see Fig. 7-48). Possible problems that can occur include scar tissue formation, fracture of the dentition, allergic reactions, and bacterial endocarditis in susceptible patients. When we have the opportunity to save a child from pain and suffering, an ounce of prevention is worth a pound of cure.

REFERENCES

1. Slack GL, Jones JM: Psychological effect of fractured incisors, *Br Dent J* 99:386-388, 1955.
2. Borum MK, Andreasen JO: Therapeutic and economic implications of traumatic dental injuries in Denmark: an estimate based on 7549 patients treated at a major trauma center, *Int J Paediatr Dent* 11(4):249-258, 2001.
3. Davis MJ, Vogel L: Neurological assessment of the child with head trauma, *J Dent Child* 62:93-96, 1995.
4. Davis MJ: Orofacial trauma management. Patient assessment and documentation, *N Y State Dent J* 61(7):42-46, 1995.
5. Rusmah M: Traumatized anterior teeth in children: a 24-month follow-up study, *Aust Dent J* 35:430-433, 1990.
6. Andreasen JO et al: Effect of treatment delay upon pulp and periodontal healing of traumatic dental injuries—a review article, *Dent Traumatol* 18(3):116-128, 2002.
7. Ellis RG, Davey KW: *The classification and treatment of injuries to the teeth of children,* ed 5, Chicago, 1970, Mosby.
8. Olgart L, Gazelius B, Lindh-Stromberg U: Laser Doppler flowmetry in assessing vitality in luxated permanent teeth, *Int Endod J* 21:300-306, 1988.
9. Mesaros SV, Trope M: Revascularization of traumatized teeth assessed by laser Doppler flowmetry: case report, *Endod Dent Traumatol* 13:24-30, 1997.
10. Tennery TN: The fractured tooth reunited using the acid-etch bonding technique, *Tex Dent J* 96:16-17, 1978.
11. Starkey PE: Reattachment of a fractured fragment to a tooth, *J Indiana Dent Assoc* 58(5):37-38, 1979.
12. Farik B, Munksgaard EC, Andreasen JO, et al: Fractured teeth bonded with dentin adhesives with and without unfilled resin, *Dent Traumatol* 18:66-69, 2002.
13. Croll TP: Rapid reattachment of fractured crown segment: an update, *J Esthet Dent* 2:1-5, 1990.
14. Kanca J: Replacement of a fractured incisor fragment over pulpal exposure: a long-term case report, *Quintessence Int* 27:829-832, 1996.
15. Ludlow JB, LaTurno SA: Traumatic fracture—one-visit endodontic treatment and dentinal bonding reattachment of coronal fragment: report of a case, *J Am Dent Assoc* 110:341-343, 1985.
16. Cvek M: A clinical report on partial pulpotomy and capping with calcium hydroxide in permanent incisors with complicated crown fractures, *J Endod* 4:232-237, 1978.
17. McCormick FE: Calcium-hydroxide pulpotomy: report of a case observed for nineteen years, *J Dent Child* 48:222-225, 1981.
18. Frank AL: Therapy for the divergent pulpless tooth by continued apical formation, *J Am Dent Assoc* 72:87-93, 1966.
19. Weine FS: *Endodontic therapy,* ed 6, St Louis, 2004, Mosby.
20. Giuliani V et al: The use of MTA in teeth with necrotic pulps and open apices, *Dent Traumatol* 18:217-221, 2002.
21. Trairatvorakul C: Apexification of a primary central incisor: 6-year follow up, *Pediatr Dent* 20:425-427, 1998.
22. Croll TP, Pascon EA, Langeland K: Traumatically injured primary incisors: a clinical and histological study, *J Dent Child* 54:401-422, 1987.
23. Holan G, Fuks AB: The diagnostic value of coronal dark-gray discoloration in primary teeth following traumatic injures, *Pediatr Dent* 18:224-227, 1996.
24. Peterson DS, Taylor MH, Marley JF: Calcific metamorphosis with internal resorption, *Oral Surg* 60:231-233, 1985.
25. Mummery JH: Some further cases of chronic perforating hyperplasia of the pulp, the so-called "pink spot," *Br Dent J* 47:801-811, 1926.
26. Andreasen JO, Sundström B, Ravn JJ: The effect of traumatic injuries to the primary teeth on their permanent successors, *Scand J Dent Res* 79:219-283, 1971.
27. Cutright DE: The reaction of permanent tooth buds to injury, *Oral Surg* 32:832-839, 1971.
28. Kilpatrick NM, Hardman PJ, Welbury RR: Dilaceration of a primary tooth, *Int J Paediatr Dent* 1:151-153, 1991.
29. Rushton MA: Partial duplication following injury to developing incisors, *Br Dent J* 104:12, 1958.

30. Ravn JJ: Sequelae of acute mechanical traumata in the primary dentition, *J Dent Child* 35:281-289, 1968.

31. Skieller V: The prognosis for young teeth loosened after mechanical injuries, *Acta Odontol Scand* 18:171-181, 1960.

32. Malmgren O, Malmgren B, Goldson L: Orthodontic management of the traumatized dentition. In Andreasen JO, Andreasen FM, editors: *Textbook and color atlas of traumatic injuries to the teeth,* ed 3, St Louis, 1994, Mosby.

33. Trope M, Chivian N, Sigurdsson A: Traumatic injuries. In Cohen S, Burns RC, editors: *Pathways of the pulp,* ed 7, St Louis, 1998, Mosby.

34. Tronstad L et al: Surgical access for endodontic treatment of intruded teeth, *Endod Dent Traumatol* 2:75-78, 1986.

35. Shapira J, Regev L, Liebfeld H: Reeruption of completely intruded immature permanent incisors, *Endod Dent Traumatol* 2:113-116, 1986.

36. Barry GN: Replanted teeth still functioning after 42 years: report of a case, *J Am Dent Assoc* 92:412-413, 1976.

37. Camp JH: Replantation of teeth following trauma. In McDonald RE et al, editors: *Current therapy in dentistry,* vol 7, St Louis, 1980, Mosby.

38. Andreasen JO: Effect of extra-alveolar period and storage media upon periodontal and pulpal healing after replantation of mature permanent incisors in monkeys, *Int J Oral Surg* 1:43-53, 1981.

39. Andreasen JO, Hjørting-Hansen E: Replantation of teeth. I. Radiographic and clinical study of 110 human teeth replanted after accidental loss, *Acta Odontol Scand* 24: 263-286, 1966.

40. Blomlöf L, Otteskog P, Hammarström L: Effect of storage in media with different ion strengths and osmolalities on human periodontal ligament cells, *Scand J Dent Res* 89: 180-187, 1981.

41. Trope M: Clinical management of the avulsed tooth: present strategies and future directions, *Int Endod J* 18:1-11, 2002.

42. Sherman P Jr: A histologic study of intentional replantation of teeth in dogs and monkeys, master's thesis, Indianapolis, 1967, Indiana University School of Dentistry.

43. Andreasen JO, Andreasen FM, editors: *Textbook and color atlas of traumatic injuries to the teeth,* ed 3, St Louis, 1994, Mosby.

44. Hurst RV: Regeneration of periodontal and transseptal fibers after autografts in rhesus monkeys: a qualitative approach, *J Dent Res* 51:1183-1192, 1972.

45. von Arx T, Filippi A, Buser D: Splinting of traumatized teeth with a new device: TTS (titanium trauma splint), *Dent Traumatol* 17:180-184, 2001.

46. Sae-Lim V, Wang CY, Trope M: Effect of systemic tetracycline and amoxicillin on inflammatory root resorption of replanted dogs' teeth, *Endod Dent Traumatol* 14:216-220, 1998.

47. Krasner P, Rankow HJ: New philosophy for the treatment of avulsed teeth, *Oral Surg Oral Med Oral Pathol Oral Radiol Endod* 9:616-623, 1995.

48. Fountain SB, Camp JH: Traumatic injuries. In Cohen S, Burns RC, editors: *Pathways of the pulp,* ed 6, St Louis, 1994, Mosby.

49. Cvek M, Andreasen JO, Borum MK: Healing of 208 intraalveolar root fractures in patients age 7-17 years, *Dent Traumatol* 17:53-62, 2001.

50. Cvek M, Mejare I, Andreasen JO: Healing and prognosis of teeth with intraalveolar fractures involving the cervical part of the root, *Dent Traumatol* 18:27-65, 2002.

SUGGESTED READINGS

Aeinehchi M, Eslami B, Ghanbariha M, et al: Mineral trioxide aggregate (MTA) and calcium hydroxide as pulp-capping agents in human teeth: a preliminary report, *Int Endod J* 36(3):225-31, 2003.

American Academy of Pediatric Dentistry: Special Issue: Reference Manual 2002-2003, *Pediatr Dent* 24(7 suppl):91-96, 2002.

Flores MT: Traumatic injuries in the primary dentition, *Dent Traumatol* 18:287-298, 2002.

Garcia-Godoy F, Pulver F: Treatment of trauma to the primary and young permanent dentitions, *Pediatr Dent* 44(3):597-631, 2000.

Hammarström L et al: Replantation of teeth and antibiotic treatment, *Endod Dent Traumatol* 2:51-57, 1986.

Iqbal MK, Bamaas NS: Effect of enamel matrix derivative (EMDOGAIN®) upon periodontal healing after replantation of permanent incisors in Beagle dogs, *Dent Traumatol* 17:36-45, 2001.

Kenny DJ, Barrett EJ: Recent developments in dental traumatology, *Pediatr Dent* 23(6):464-468, 2001.

Lee JY, Vann WF, Sigurdsson A: Management of avulsed permanent incisors: a decision analysis based on changing concepts, *Pediatr Dent* 23(4):357-360, 2001.

Linsuwanont P: MTA apexification combined with conventional root canal retreatment, *Aust Endod J* 29(1):45-49, 2003.

Rock WP et al: The relationship between trauma and pulp death in incisor teeth, *Br Dent J* 136:236-239, 1974.

Taylor LB, Walker J: A review of selected microstomia prevention appliances, *Pediatr Dent* 19(6):413-418, 1997.

Scientific advancements in the areas of preventive dentistry, access to and use of dental services, water fluoridation, topical application of fluorides, and new commercial preventive dentistry products have led to substantial reductions in dental disease in developed countries. However, Caplan and Weintraub determined that adolescents are still affected by caries, particularly those who are minorities, rural inhabitants, have minimal fluoride exposure, and are from less educated and less affluent families.[1] Results of a recent health and nutrition survey reported by Vargas, Crall, and Schneider also supports a higher caries prevalence among lower-income children and minorities.[2] Assessments of periodontal health by Barmes and Leous[3] and by Bader et al[4] show a decrease in severity but indicate that some adolescents are still affected.

Dental trauma continues to be a significant problem among adolescents as supported by Gift and Bhat's assessment of orofacial injury[5]; Bader, Martin, and Shugars' estimates of the incidence and consequences of tooth fracture[6]; and Haug, Prather, and Indresano's epidemiologic study of facial fractures and concomitant injuries.[7] Pilo et al indicate that congenital anomalies continue to result in missing or malformed teeth.[8] In addition, bulimia, anorexia, and dietary habits have led to an increase in the erosion of tooth structure among teenagers, particularly in girls.

Some of the esthetic treatment needs resulting from these conditions can be managed with resin-bonding procedures and porcelain laminate veneers, and whenever possible these should be considered as the treatments of first choice. When these procedures have not been able to provide a satisfactory result or when teeth are missing, then prosthodontics such as single crowns, fixed partial dentures, implant prostheses, or removable prostheses are indicated.

Because adolescents are often affected psychologically by the unacceptable appearance of diseased, damaged, or missing teeth, one should not allow chronologic age to preclude performance of whatever treatment is necessary to provide proper function and esthetics. If the teeth involved are fully erupted, have achieved complete root formation, and may be prepared without causing irreversible damage to the pulp, successful prosthodontic treatment can often be provided for patients as young as 12 to 14 years of age. Patient cooperation, however, is mandatory during and after treatment. Adolescent patients must be able to tolerate long appointments and remain still for extended periods while teeth are being prepared and impression materials are setting. Also, they must be able to achieve and maintain good oral hygiene around both the provisional and definitive restorations, as well as in

the rest of the mouth. All these conditions make it highly desirable to perform the necessary treatment as expeditiously as possible. Finally, it must be understood that an adolescent is more likely to sustain trauma to the oral structures than is an adult and thus there is greater risk of damage to restorations and prostheses than in an adult patient.

Prosthodontic treatment of the adolescent patient often requires highly intricate procedures that go beyond the scope of this chapter. The goal of this chapter is to offer the reader an opportunity to develop a better appreciation of the achievable and available solutions for the young patient with a prosthodontic need. The interested reader should consult the prosthodontic literature and current textbooks on fixed, removable, and implant prosthodontics for more detailed information in this area of dentistry.

RESTORATION OF SINGLE MALFORMED, DISCOLORED, OR FRACTURED TEETH

ALL-CERAMIC AND METAL-CERAMIC CROWNS

All-ceramic crowns are the most esthetic complete-coverage restorations currently available in dentistry. The achievement of optimal longevity with all-ceramic crowns requires normal tooth preparation form because the prepared tooth must provide support for the restoration. Therefore, if a large portion of tooth structure is missing because of trauma or caries, or if previous restorations become dislodged during tooth reduction, then a separate restoration that is well retained in remaining tooth structure should be placed to establish an ideal preparation form (Fig. 22-1). Also, the fracture resistance of all-ceramic crowns is enhanced when other characteristics are present. Occlusal forces should be average or below-average. The centric occlusal contacts should ideally be located over the concave lingual portion of the prepared tooth and not cervical to the cingulum where fracture of the crown is more likely to occur. The prepared tooth should possess average or greater incisocervical length and should not be short, round, or overtapered in form.

The tooth preparation for an all-ceramic crown (Fig. 22-2) should possess a well-defined, smooth finish line that is 0.8 mm deep around the entire tooth, with the axial surfaces reduced to a depth of 0.8 mm. The lingual reduction for occlusal clearance should be 1.0 mm. An incisal edge reduction of 1.5 to 2.0 mm is required and is biologically acceptable even in the presence of large pulps. The use of resin cement and associated dentin bonding is recommended because crown strength is significantly improved. Both chamfer and shoulder finish lines can be used in conjunction with resin cement without compromising restoration

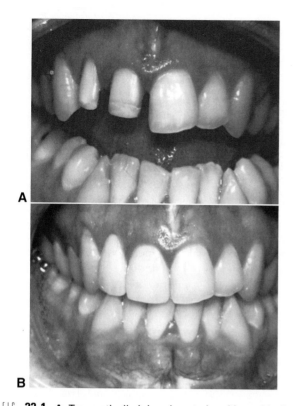

A

B

FIG. **22-1.** **A**, Traumatically injured central and lateral incisors that have been restored with bonded resins and then prepared to receive all-ceramic crowns. **B**, All-ceramic crowns have been cemented.

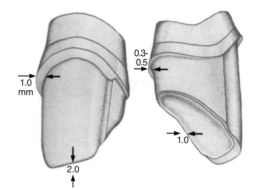

FIG. **22-3.** Two views of metal-ceramic crown preparation showing minimal facial reduction and shoulder finish line, minimal incisal reduction, lingual axial reduction depth and chamfer finish line, and lingual reduction for occlusal clearance.

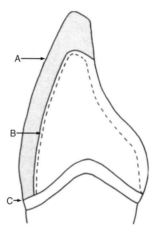

FIG. **22-4.** Collarless metal-ceramic framework design that eliminates visible cervical metal. *A* indicates porcelain; *B* indicates underlying metal framework that does not cover shoulder finish line; *C* is margin where porcelain contacts only prepared tooth.

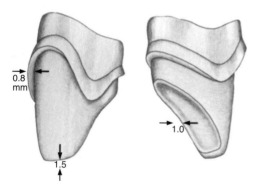

FIG. **22-2.** Two views of all-ceramic (porcelain jacket crown) preparation showing recommended reduction depths and shoulder finish line.

strength. If zinc phosphate or glass ionomer cement is used, however, then a shoulder finish line should be used to optimize crown strength.

When the ideal tooth preparation form is seriously compromised or the magnitude of occlusal forces contraindicates restoration with an all-ceramic crown, use of the stronger metal-ceramic crown is indicated. The tooth preparation design and reduction depths for a metal-ceramic crown are shown in Fig. 22-3. When

cervical esthetics must be optimized in a metal-ceramic restoration, one can employ a collarless design that eliminates facial cervical metal and uses a porcelain facial margin (Figs. 22-4 and 22-5).

Whenever possible, cervical margins should not be extended into the gingival sulcus of an adolescent patient. If oral hygiene is inadequate, subgingival margins may produce accelerated gingival recession or interfere with the normal cervical relocation of the gingival tissues as the patient matures. Both occurrences produce an esthetic liability (Figs. 22-6 and 22-7).

In addition to the conventional all-ceramic crowns, several computer-aided design and computer-aided manufacturing (CAD-CAM) systems for fabricating

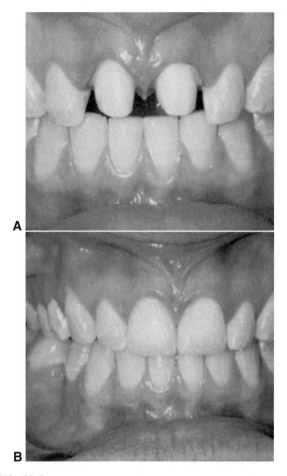

A

B

FIG. **22-5. A,** Injured vital central incisors prepared for metal-ceramic restoration in a young patient. **B,** Maxillary central incisors restored with collarless metal-ceramic crowns.

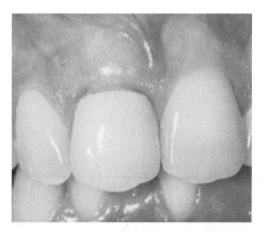

FIG. **22-6.** Gingival contour in 25-year-old patient resulting from placement of subgingival crown on maxillary right central incisor at 8 years of age. The gingival crest is not positioned as far apically on the restored central incisor, and its form is rounded and thick rather than the normal form of the gingival margin, which is thinner and sharper.

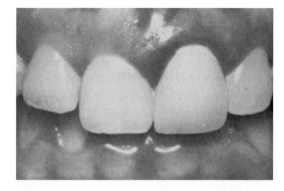

FIG. **22-7.** Accelerated gingival recession around maxillary left central incisor resulting from metal-ceramic crown with subgingival margins placed at a young age. The gingiva is edematous and red, and the gingival margin is rounded and thick.

all-ceramic crowns are now available. The CAD-CAM systems are generally designed to help streamline the fabrication and placement of esthetic crowns. Some of these systems are intended to allow preparation and placement at the same appointment. The AllCeram and CEREC systems are among the popular CAD-CAM systems.

The Procera AllCeram system (Nobel Biocare AB, Göteburg, Sweden) uses CAD-CAM technology to fabricate a densely sintered aluminum oxide coping. The coping is then veneered with dental porcelain by a dental laboratory technician. Oden et al, during a 5-year clinical trial, noted that 3 of 97 Procera AllCeram crowns had fractures involving both the veneering porcelain and the aluminum oxide coping.[9] They also reported that 2 of the 97 crowns experienced fractures in the veneering porcelain only. In their review of the Procera AllCeram system, Ottl et al described its use in fabricating implant-supported single crowns.[10]

Boening et al evaluated the clinical fit of 80 Procera AllCeram crowns.[11] They reported marginal gap widths of 80 to 95 μm for anterior teeth, and 90 to 145 μm for posterior teeth. May et al found mean marginal openings of less than 63 μm in an in vitro study.[12] Boening's study concluded that the accuracy of fit of the Procera AllCeram system was within the range of clinical acceptance.[11]

The CEREC CAD-CAM system (Sirona, Bensheim, Germany) is designed to fabricate all-ceramic restorations (crown, inlays, and onlays) at the chairside. This one-appointment approach, without the need for a provisional restoration, is its principal potential advantage. The CEREC CAD-CAM system incorporates an optical scanning of the prepared tooth and adjacent teeth. The CAD-CAM instrumentation is then used to mill internal and external surfaces of the restoration.

Mou et al noted criticisms of the marginal fit and adaptation of these restorations. Their in vitro study found average internal gaps ranging from 100 to 200 μm.[13] They found little differences in internal fit when the tooth preparations had a convergence angle of 12 to 20 degrees and a total tooth preparation height of 6 mm or less, occlusal cervically.

Reiss and Walther, using the Kaplan-Meier method of analysis, reported the probability of survival of CEREC restorations to be 90% at 10 years.[14] Restorations of premolars were rated better than those of molars, and restorations of vital teeth better than those of nonvital teeth. The most frequent reasons for failure were ceramic and tooth fractures.

TEETH WITH PULPAL INVOLVEMENT

When tooth fracture or caries involves the pulp and root development is complete, a routine pulpectomy and gutta-percha root canal filling should be completed. Because posts and cores do not strengthen endodontically treated teeth, their use is indicated only when remaining coronal tooth structure does not provide adequate retention for the definitive restoration.[15] Restorations that do not employ a post should be used whenever possible to replace missing tooth structure and serve as a retentive foundation. It is particularly important that teeth in the mouths of accident-prone adolescents or those in whom athletic trauma has previously occurred be restored without using a post, if possible. This practice helps to avoid irreparable damage in the form of root fracture should the restored tooth once again be subjected to trauma. Even though trauma may result in restoration dislodgement or perhaps even fracture of the tooth, the tooth will have survived at least one more traumatic experience.

In the case of pulpal involvement when the root is incompletely formed, a pulpotomy followed by placement of an appropriate restoration is indicated. Subsequently, when root formation is completed, a pulpectomy is performed, followed by placement of the definitive restoration or crown, if needed.

FIXED PARTIAL DENTURES

Although preventive procedures have reduced the number of teeth lost, fixed partial dentures continue to be needed in adolescent patients because of trauma or congenital lack of tooth formation, and occasionally for reasons such as extensive caries and periodontal disease. When a tooth is lost, space maintenance should be provided immediately after extraction to prevent tipping, tilting, or rotation of the abutment teeth or eruption of the opposing teeth. Space maintenance should be continued until the fixed prosthesis is completed. If the abutment teeth are malaligned

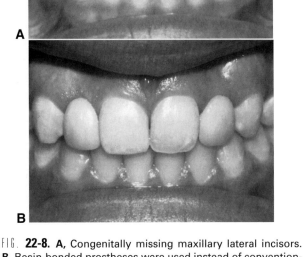

FIG. 22-8. A, Congenitally missing maxillary lateral incisors. B, Resin-bonded prostheses were used instead of conventionally cemented prostheses to preserve as much tooth structure as possible on the central incisor and canine abutments.

and pulp size does not permit the amount of tooth reduction necessary to align the preparations, orthodontic repositioning of the abutment teeth should be initiated.

RESIN-BONDED RETAINERS

For reasons of pulpal and periodontal health and conservation of tooth structure, resin-bonded retainers should be the first choice whenever possible (Fig. 22-8). Retention and resistance form is achieved through tooth preparations, terminating in enamel, coupled with acid etching of the enamel and fixation with resin cement. The conservative approach of using resin-bonded retainers does, however, require that the abutment teeth be intact or minimally restored, with substantial enamel present for bonding procedures. To produce an adequate area for resin bonding, the existing crown should be of average or greater length. A maximal amount of the nonvisible portions of the lingual and proximal surfaces should be covered by the retainers, because Pegoraro and Barrack have determined that bond strength increases with the area of enamel covered.[16] The existing crown form, color, and axial alignment must be satisfactory, because this prosthesis

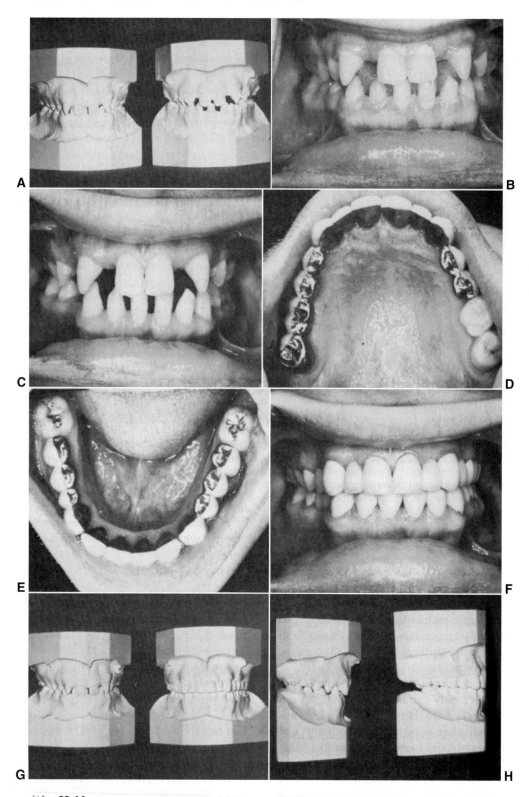

FIG. **22-14. A,** Casts of patient exhibiting incomplete dental manifestation of hereditary ectodermal dysplasia. *Left,* Casts before orthodontic treatment. *Right,* Progress casts near completion of orthodontic treatment. **B,** Dentition of the patient shown in **A** after orthodontic treatment. Notice vertical overbite correction and space adjustment to facilitate prosthetic treatment. Additional illustration of the treatment may be seen in **C** through **H. C,** After periodontal treatment, gingivoplasty was performed to gain crown length and improve tissue contours. **D,** Mirror view of maxillary arch after prosthetic treatment. **E,** Mirror view of mandibular arch after prosthetic treatment. **F,** Anterior view in occlusion after prosthetic treatment. Metal-ceramic fixed partial dentures were employed to correct abnormal tooth form, replace congenitally missing teeth, and restore occlusion. **G** and **H,** Anterior and right lateral views of casts before and after treatment.

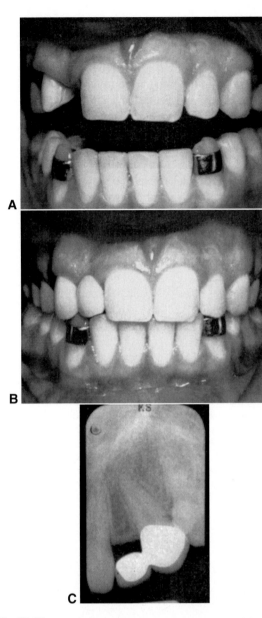

FIG. 22-15. A, Maxillary canine has been prepared for metal-ceramic cantilevered prosthesis. Notice discrepancy in path of insertion with central incisor, which necessitated cantilever design. B, Facial view of cemented prosthesis. C, Postinsertion periapical radiograph showing malalignment of canine and central incisor roots.

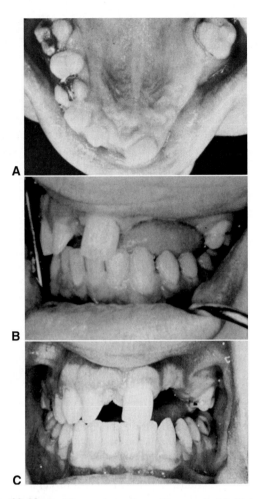

FIG. 22-16. A, Mirror view of maxillary arch. Multiple teeth have been lost in this young adult as a result of a gunshot accident. B, Left lateral view in centric occlusion. C, Anterior view in centric occlusion.

The development of proper speech can be ensured if the parts of the partial denture are given correct form, dimension, and position in their relationships to the tongue, cheek, and lips.

The restoration of esthetics is often the most important personal consideration for adolescent patients. Artificial teeth of compatible color, size, and form, naturally arranged and positioned, enhance dental esthetics. In addition, the form and size of the base of a partial denture must be correct to ensure the restoration of normal facial contours.

The preservation of the remaining teeth and their supportive tissues is the most important objective of all but will not be achieved without adequate mouth preparation, correct partial denture design, accurate fabrication of that design, periodic professional follow-up care, and continued proper home care by the patient.

Additional dental procedures may be required to create an oral environment that will furnish proper support and retention for the removable partial denture and that will prevent the development of forces or processes that are harmful to the remaining teeth and their supportive tissues. These preparatory procedures may involve all phases or branches of dentistry. Adolescents may require periodontal procedures, particularly to increase crown length for crown or fixed

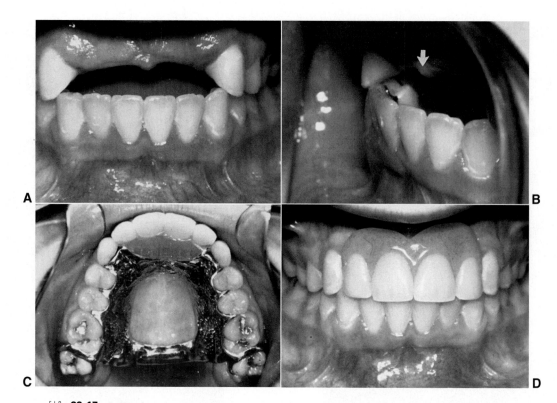

FIG. **22-17. A,** The four maxillary incisors have been lost as a result of traumatic injury. Note the long span, short clinical crowns, and facial flare to the canines, which make retention and resistance form difficult to achieve for a conventional fixed partial denture. **B,** Lateral view showing the relationship of the mandibular incisors to the residual alveolar ridge. The trauma caused substantial bone loss, and the ridge is located lingual to the mandibular incisors (the *arrow* indicates the position of the incisive papilla on the crest of the residual alveolar ridge), which necessitates use of a removable partial denture base for lip support and proper esthetics. **C,** Occlusal view of maxillary removable partial denture. **D,** Facial view of completed prosthesis.

partial denture retention or to improve tissue contours so that more ideal results can be achieved.

Orthodontic procedures can be used to reposition severely malpositioned teeth that would otherwise require extraction. Orthodontic procedures are particularly indicated for malpositioned teeth that are vital to an adequate plan of treatment (Fig. 22-18).

OVERDENTURES

Occasionally, congenital abnormalities or trauma result in the loss of multiple teeth and the resulting interarch relationship does not allow a conventional removable partial denture to reestablish proper occlusion with opposing teeth. This situation may necessitate fabrication of a prosthesis that overlays all or part of the remaining teeth so that proper function and facial esthetics are established (Fig. 22-19).[35]

IMPLANT PROSTHESES

The routine successful use of osseointegrated dental implants in total or partial support of prostheses in

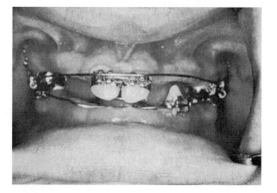

FIG. **22-18.** Orthodontic treatment is in progress to erupt the molars, depress the mandibular left canine, and close the maxillary central incisor diastema.

adults has heightened interest in their use in younger patients. Adolescents who have congenital anomalies, have undergone ablative surgical procedures, or have experienced traumatic tooth loss are frequently seen, and the use of dental implants would greatly assist

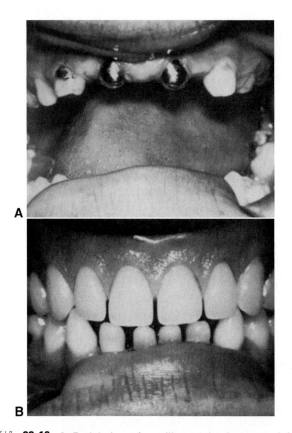

A

B

FIG. **22-19.** **A,** Facial view of maxillary arch where remaining primary and permanent teeth were improperly spaced and lacked adequate bone support for a fixed prosthesis. Lip support, facial esthetics, and proper occlusal interdigitation with the opposing mandibular teeth could be achieved only by use of an overdenture. Central incisors required endodontic treatment and have been restored with cast posts and cores. **B,** Facial view of overdenture.

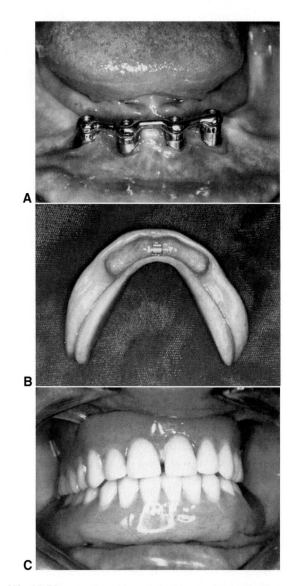

A

B

C

FIG. **22-20.** **A,** Prepubertal periodontitis resulted in extensive and aggressive bone changes and loss of the teeth. Four implants were placed at age 12. This treatment greatly enhances prosthesis stability and will help preserve the remaining mandibular anterior bone. Because the mandibular symphysis fuses at birth or shortly thereafter, early implant placement in this area is less affected by future growth. **B,** Mandibular overdenture prosthesis that will be supported by the four implants and bar. **C,** Facial view of the completed prostheses.

prosthesis support (Figs. 22-20 and 22-21). Replacement of congenitally missing teeth with implants can often be accomplished in an esthetic manner that preserves the integrity of adjacent teeth (Fig. 22-22). However, dental and skeletal growth is a major confounding variable related to the use of dental implants in adolescent patients.

There are two primary concerns related to the placement of implants before growth is completed: (1) the effect of growth on the long-term relative position of the dental implant, and (2) the effect of the implant-supported prosthesis on future dental and skeletal growth.

An understanding of dental development and craniofacial growth are certainly a prerequisite for anyone anticipating the use of dental implants in growing patients.[36] Growth and development in the maxilla and mandible are essentially quite different, as are growth and development in the specific areas of each arch.[37-40]

In the maxilla, growth is intimately associated with the growth of the cranial base in early childhood, whereas later growth primarily occurs by enlargement of the maxilla. This growth is extremely variable and can be observed as vertical growth, transverse growth, and anteroposterior growth. Transverse growth occurs primarily at the midpalatal suture of the maxilla. The sutural growth site is extremely important and poses a

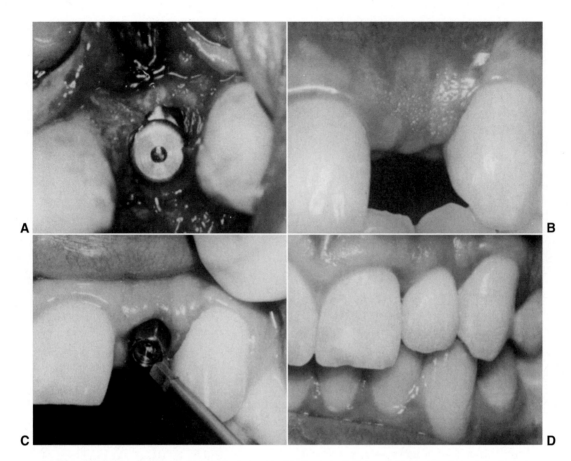

FIG. **22-21.** **A,** A 16-year-old boy traumatically fractured the maxillary left lateral incisor, rendering it nonrestorable. An implant is being placed in the socket immediately after extraction. **B,** Edentulous ridge following implant placement. **C,** Abutment being connected to implant with screwdriver. **D,** Completed metal-ceramic restoration.

risk to the placement of an implant-supported prosthesis that crosses this suture and could limit its growth potential. The maxilla also grows vertically by passive displacement as well as by alveolar appositional growth. It is the vertical component of maxillary growth that causes the most concern in the long-term positional stability of the individual implant and its effect on restorative function and esthetics.

Mandibular growth differs greatly from the complex growth in the maxilla. Not closely associated with major cranial passive growth, mandibular growth is primarily downward and forward, mediated by appositional condylar growth. This growth is not purely linear but can be rotational secondary to the precise direction of condylar growth patterns. The appositional growth is also refined by certain areas of resorption, primarily seen on the anterior aspect of the ramus. As the mandible increases in length, it also increases in width, secondary to the flaring of posterior growth direction. Anterior stabilization is accomplished by the early closure of the mandibular synthesis. Although less

dynamic than maxillary growth, mandibular growth can create many complexities that could place dental implants at positional risk, especially in the posterior mandible, secondary to vertical changes and resorptive processes.

In addition to understanding growth and development, the clinician must also comprehend the dynamics of the positional relationship between the dental implant and its biologic environment in the growing patient. A wealth of dental literature using in vivo evidence-based studies attests to the long-term success of dental implants and their associated prostheses in adults. Such a wealth of knowledge does not exist, however, for the growing patient. The behavior of an osseointegrated dental implant essentially resembles that of an ankylosed tooth and the latter therefore provides an accurate model of the behavior of an implant in a growing patient. Two facets of the relationship of ankylotic teeth to their actively growing environment must be understood. *First,* the ankylotic tooth, lacking the adaptive mechanisms of a healthy

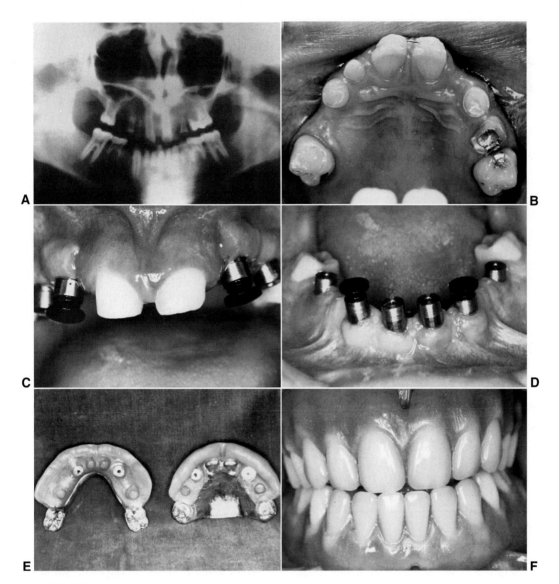

FIG. 22-22. A, Panoramic radiograph of a 12-year-old with partial anodontia of unknown origin. B, Occlusal view of maxillary arch showing primary teeth that will be extracted. C, Four maxillary implants have been placed and the mouth prepared for an impression. D, Six mandibular implants have been placed to provide prosthesis stability and preserve bone. E, Maxillary and mandibular overdentures using magnets to augment stability and retention. F, Facial view of completed overdentures.

tooth, does not erupt normally and becomes buried. *Second,* failing to participate in vertical growth, it often creates severe malocclusions secondary to tipping and associated growth changes in normal teeth adjacent to the affected ankylotic tooth. It seems logical that an osseointegrated implant placed prematurely could elicit the same negative growth effects.

An understanding of growth and development and its variability in the male and female adolescent population raises serious concern about the premature placement of implants. The reader is referred to Chapter 25 for a more in-depth discussion of this topic.

IMPLANT USAGE BEFORE GROWTH COMPLETION

Although it is best to wait until maxillary and mandibular growth is completed before placing osseointegrated implants, dentists are constantly faced with apparent indications for implant treatment. The clinician must understand the disadvantages of early placement and weigh those factors against the functional and esthetic advantages afforded by implants. If a determination is made that implants are needed before growth completion, it is more predictable to restore larger edentulous areas with implants than to place a single

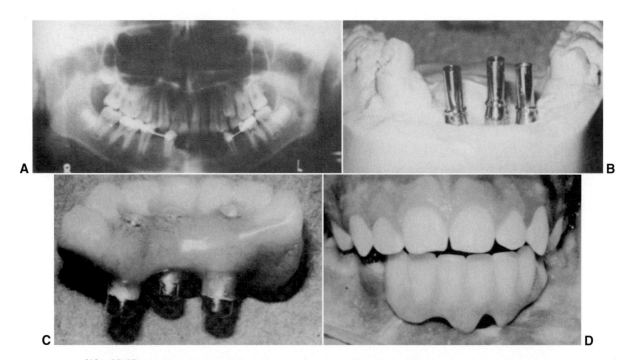

FIG. **22-23. A,** Panoramic radiograph of a 13-year-old patient after removal of a giant cell granuloma from the anterior mandible. **B,** Working cast showing ridge defect and the location of the three implants. **C,** Fixed prosthesis that will be attached to the three implants. **D,** Prosthesis in place.

implant-supported crown in a growing patient (Fig. 22-23). The successful use of implant-assisted prostheses in patients with multiple missing teeth has been reported.[41-43] Implants have been placed in the anterior mandible in patients as young as 5 years of age (Fig. 22-24). Often, the placement of implants in this area will diminish the residual alveolar resorption anticipated from many years of removable prosthesis wear. Unfortunately, one of the most frequently encountered implant indications is treatment of the traumatic loss or congenital absence of a single anterior maxillary tooth. The placement of dental implants in this area should not be attempted until the accelerated phase of peripubertal growth is close to complete.

IMPLANTS FOR ORTHODONTIC ANCHORAGE

Osseointegrated implants have been used as valuable adjuncts to orthodontic treatment when there is a need for anchorage but no conventional tooth anchorage is available.[44] Because the implants act as ankylosed teeth and are incapable of being moved by orthodontic or orthopedic forces, they serve as ideal anchorage units.[45] Their use has produced tooth movements that otherwise would not be possible, particularly in cases in which a large number of teeth are missing as a

result of trauma or congenital anomalies. Implants are especially valuable when their postorthodontic positioning permits them to be used to support a future prosthesis.

RECARE PROGRAM

The prosthodontic treatment of an adolescent does not end with the placement of the prosthesis. Periodic recare appointments for inspection, maintenance, repair, or replacement are a necessity. For patients who have removable partial dentures, relining or rebasing should be performed when indicated. When all-ceramic crowns or metal-ceramic restorations are used in an adolescent patient, replacement may be needed periodically as the gingival tissue assumes its adult position. Patients with fixed partial dentures should be examined periodically for soft tissue health, evidence of occlusal wear, and response of the supportive tissues to the added stress loads. Patients with implant-assisted restorations should be evaluated frequently to ensure the health of the osseointegrated implant and its surrounding tissue, as well as to assess the effect of the implant-supported prosthesis on the overall growth and development of the patient. The use of dental implants to assist in the support of a prosthesis necessitates an extremely vigilant recare program.

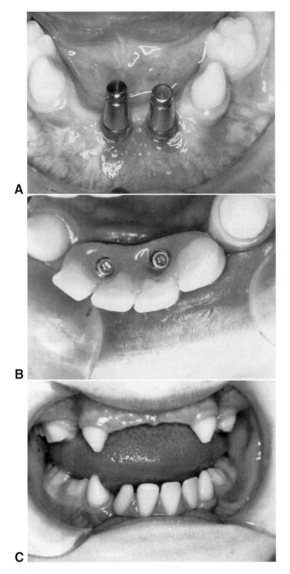

FIG. **22-24.** **A,** Two implants placed at age 5 in a young patient with partial anodontia resulting from ectodermal dysplasia. Impression copings have been attached for the impression procedure. Because of the early fusion of the mandibular symphysis, future bone growth will have minimal impact. **B,** Incisal view of the retrievable prosthesis showing two lingually located screws. A retrievable design permits the prosthetic teeth to be replaced when the surrounding teeth change positions from growth. **C,** Facial view of completed prosthesis.

Every adolescent patient must be taught proper oral hygiene and home care for his or her prosthodontic restorations and must be motivated until adequate performance is routinely achieved. Each patient with fixed or implant-supported prostheses should be taught the use of aids such as the floss threader and interproximal brush to enhance oral hygiene efforts.

Only with regular recare programs can maximum longevity of service can be realized.

PROTECTIVE MOUTH GUARDS

Although this chapter is concerned with the prosthodontic treatment of adolescents, emphasis should always be placed on the prevention of oral disease and injury. The number and severity of injuries to the teeth and jaws can be significantly reduced through the faithful use of protective mouth guards by athletes who are engaged in contact sports.[46]

Effective and relatively inexpensive prefabricated mouth guards are available at sporting goods stores. A custom-made guard may be fabricated, however, by vacuum-molding a sheet of thick, clear material over a stone cast of the maxillary arch. Seals and Dorrough have reviewed the advantages of custom-made mouth protectors.[47]

Studies comparing custom-made (laboratory) mouth guards with standard (manufactured) or intraorally formed mouth guards have shown that the custom-made mouth guards provide better fit and comfort, are less likely to adversely affect the player's speech, and are less likely to come loose.[48] In a study reported by Bass and Williams, the majority of athletes felt that they were more likely to wear their mouth guards if they fit better and were comfortable.[49]

Several materials have been suggested for use in mouth guards, including poly (vinyl acetate-ethylene) copolymer thermoplastic, polyurethane, and laminated thermoplastic. Chaconas, Caputo, and Bakke demonstrated that the laminated thermoplastic underwent significantly less dimensional change than other materials.[50]

Because a custom-made mouth guard accurately fits individual tooth and arch form, it affords maximal resistance to dislodgement. The technique of fabrication involves placing the mouth guard material (Fig. 22-25, *A*) in a molding machine, which softens the material by heat (Fig. 22-25, *B*) and closely adapts it to a dry stone cast by vacuum (Fig. 22-25, *C*). After the adapted material has cooled, the guard is removed from the cast and the excess peripheral material is trimmed off with scissors (Fig. 22-25, *D*). The borders are rounded by trimming the material with a resin-trimming bur and flaming with a torch or polishing with wet pumice on a rag wheel (Fig. 22-25, *E*).

Maximum retention is obtained when the entire hard palate is covered. If the guard interferes with speech, however, a portion of the palatal area of the guard can be removed.

The successful use of mouth guards by many young athletes has proven that they can be worn with comfort and serve as effective safeguards against injuries to the teeth.

23

Dental Problems of Children with Disabilities

JAMES A. WEDDELL

BRIAN J. SANDERS

JAMES E. JONES

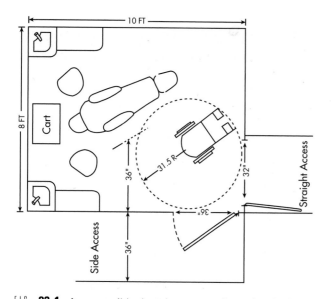

FIG. **23-1.** An accessible dental operatory floor plan designed for either a straight or side access doorway. *(From Bill D, Weddell JA: Spec Care Dentist 7:246–252, 1987.)*

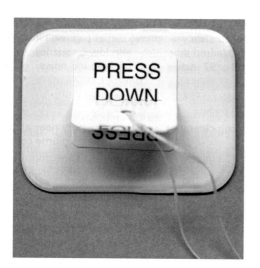

FIG. **23-2.** Bite-wing radiographic film secured with floss.

PREVENTIVE DENTISTRY

Preventing oral disease before it starts is the most desirable way of ensuring good dental health for any dental patient. An effective preventive dentistry program is important for a child with disabilities because of the predisposing factors that make restorative dental care harder to obtain when it is necessary. After the diagnosis the dentist should determine the patient's needs, assume the responsibility for formulating an individual program for the child, and adequately communicate to the parents and patient how such a program can be effected. A clear perception of the situation by everyone involved is essential for a successful preventive program; adequate communication is vital.

HOME DENTAL CARE

The parents (or the guardian) are initially responsible for establishing good oral hygiene in the home. Reinforcement of good home dental care is provided through mass media (e.g., newspapers, radio, and television), communication with other people, and school activities (e.g., health classes, parent-teacher association meetings, and observation of National Dental Health Month). This supplementary support relieves the dentist having sole responsibility for explaining the need for home dental care and reinforces the receptivity of the parent and child to such a program. The dentist or the hygienist is responsible for consulting with the caregiver of the child with disabilities (i.e., parent, guardian, or nursing home attendant) in those cases in which continued oral hygiene problems appear. Follow-up observation is essential for effective implementation of the preventive dental treatment plan.

Home dental care should begin in infancy; the dentist should teach the parents to gently cleanse the incisors daily with a soft cloth or an infant toothbrush. For older children who are unwilling or physically unable to cooperate, the dentist should teach the parent or guardian correct toothbrushing techniques that safely restrain the child when necessary. Fig. 23-4 shows several positions for toothbrushing that permit firm control and support of the child, adequate visibility, and convenient positioning of the adult, with reasonable comfort for both adult and child (also see Fig. 11-16). Some of the positions most commonly used for children requiring oral care assistance are as follows:

- The standing or sitting child is placed in front of the adult so that the adult can cradle the child's head with one hand while using the other hand to brush the teeth.
- The child reclines on a sofa or bed with the head angled backward on the parent's lap. Again, the child's head is stabilized with one hand while the teeth are brushed with the other hand.
- The parents face each other with their knees touching. The child's buttocks are placed on one parent's lap, with the child facing that parent, while the child's head and shoulders lie on the other parent's knees; this allows the first parent to brush the teeth.
- The extremely difficult patient is isolated in an open area and reclined in the brusher's lap. The patient is then immobilized by an extra attendant while the brusher institutes proper oral care. If a child cannot be adequately immobilized by one person, then both parents and perhaps siblings may be required to complete the home dental care procedures.
- The standing and resistive child is placed in front of the caregiver so that the adult can wrap his or her

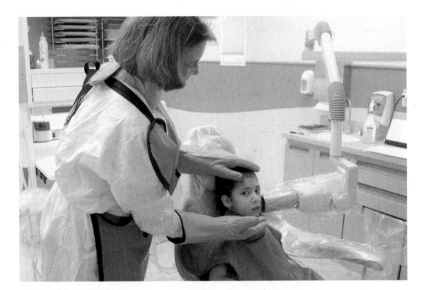

FIG. **23-3.** Extra assistance in holding the patient's head steady to prevent movement while a radiograph is being made.

legs around the child to support the torso while using the hands to support the head and brush the teeth.

If a child is institutionalized, the staff should be instructed in the proper dental care regimen for the child. Wrapped tongue blades may be of benefit in helping to keep a child's mouth open while plaque is being removed. Stabilization of the child's head will prevent the occurrence of any unnecessary trauma from sudden movements. Follow-up observation is carried out by the dentist or the hygienist, and it is appropriate to offer in-service training sessions and to check with the staff periodically to identify and solve the problems associated with an oral hygiene program in the institution.

Some parents and health centers have encouraged children with disabilities to assume the responsibility for their own oral hygiene, but the results are usually poor. Although independent brushing is not contraindicated, parents and staff should be aware that, without their follow-up, unsupervised oral hygiene procedures in children with disabilities can have serious dental consequences. The amount of supervision and assistance provided by the parents or staff should depend on the child's willingness to cooperate and ability to maintain good oral hygiene.

A plaque control program is essential in monitoring oral hygiene in the child with disabilities and determining the level of success achieved by each patient. The brushing technique for patients with disabilities who have fine or gross motor deficiencies limiting their ability to brush should be effective and yet simple for the person performing the brushing. One technique often recommended is the horizontal scrub method because it is easy to perform and can yield good results. This technique consists of performing gentle horizontal strokes on cheek, tongue, and biting surfaces of all teeth and gums. Other patients without such motor problems can use age-appropriate techniques previously discussed in Chapter 11. A soft, multitufted nylon brush should be used.

Fig. 23-5 illustrates some modifications that may be made to a toothbrush to help persons with poor fine motor skills improve their brushing techniques. Although many types of grips are available, using the patient's hand to custom-design a handle has often had good results (Fig. 23-6). Electric toothbrushes have also been used effectively by children with disabilities. The vibration and noise tend to desensitize the patient for future dental appointments if followed by positive reinforcement.

DIET AND NUTRITION

Diet and nutrition influence dental caries by affecting the type and virulence of the microorganisms in dental plaque, the resistance of teeth and supporting structures, and the properties of saliva in the oral cavity. A proper diet, as outlined in Chapter 12, is essential to a good preventive program for a child with disabilities. As discussed in Chapter 10, one should assess the diet by reviewing answers on a diet survey with the parent, realizing that allowances must be made for certain conditions for which dietary modifications are required. For example, conditions associated with difficulty in swallowing, such as severe cerebral palsy, may require that the patient be on a pureed diet. Patients with certain metabolic disturbances or syndromes, such as phenylketonuria, diabetes, or Prader-Willi syndrome,

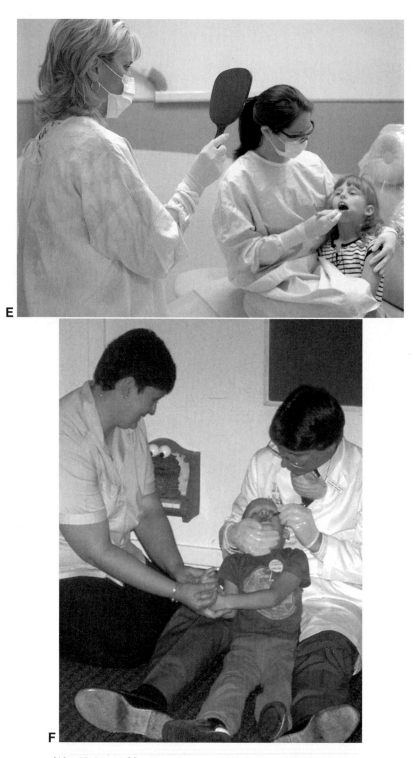

FIG. **23-4, cont'd. E,** "Leg-lock" position. **F,** Reclining on floor.

Association–accepted dentifrice containing a therapeutic fluoride compound should also be used daily. Some clinicians treating patients with disabilities who have chronically poor oral hygiene and high decay rates suggest a daily regimen of rinsing with 0.05% sodium fluoride solution. Nightly application of a 0.4% stannous fluoride brush-on gel has also been successfully used to decrease caries in children.

PREVENTIVE RESTORATIONS

Pit and fissure sealants have been shown to reduce occlusal caries effectively. Sealants are appropriate in

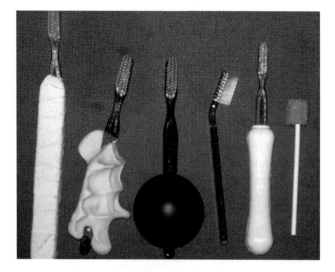

FIG. **23-5.** Various toothbrush handle modifications.

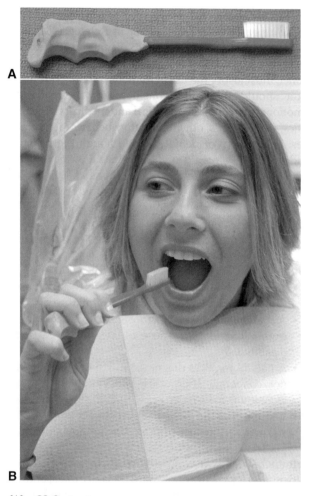

FIG. **23-6. A,** Custom-designed acrylic handle. **B,** Patient using the custom-handle toothbrush.

patients with disabilities. For a patient who requires dental work under general anesthesia, deep occlusal pits and fissures should be restored with amalgam or long-wearing composites to prevent further breakdown and decay. Patients with severe bruxism and interproximal decay may need their teeth restored with stainless steel crowns to increase the longevity of the restorations.

REGULAR PROFESSIONAL SUPERVISION

Close observation of caries-susceptible patients and regular dental examinations are important in the treatment of patients with disabilities. Although most patients are seen semiannually for professional prophylaxis, examination, and topical fluoride application, certain patients can benefit from recall examinations every 2, 3, or 4 months. This is particularly true of patients who are confined to institutions in which dental health programs are inadequate.

MANAGEMENT OF A CHILD WITH DISABILITIES DURING DENTAL TREATMENT

The principles of behavior management discussed in Chapter 3 are even more important in treating a child with disabilities. Because hospital visits or previous appointments with a physician frequently result in the development of apprehension in the patient, additional time must be spent with the parent and the child to establish rapport and dispel the child's anxiety. If patient cooperation cannot be obtained, the dentist must consider alternatives such as treatment immobilization and conscious sedation to allow performance of the necessary dental procedures.

TREATMENT IMMOBILIZATION

Partial or complete immobilization of the patient is sometimes a necessary and effective way to diagnose and

deliver dental care to patients who need help controlling their extremities, such as infants or patients with certain neuromuscular disorders. Immobilization is also useful for managing combative, resistant patients, so that the patient, practitioner, and/or dental staff may be protected from injury while care is being provided. Treatment immobilization can be performed by the dentist, staff, or parent, with or without the aid of an immobilization device.

The parents, guardian, or patient (if an adult) must be informed and must give consent, and the consent must be documented, before immobilization is used. These individuals should have a clear understanding of the type of immobilization to be used, the rationale, and the duration of use. In many cases this information should be included in the explanation of the overall management approach for the child during the initial examination and conference with the parents.

In October 1990 the Omnibus Budget Reconciliation Act of 1987 became effective. It provided recommended guidelines to reduce the risk of injury and death from the use of patient restraints.

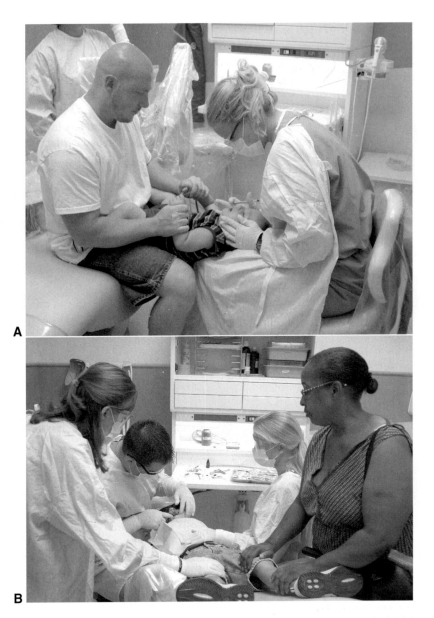

FIG. **23-8.** Assistance for immobilization. **A,** Parental aid during an examination. **B,** Additional assistance during the dental procedure.

The child's arms and legs can be immobilized with help from the parent or the dental assistant, with Posey straps,* or with a towel and adhesive tape (Fig. 23-11). If movement of the extremities is the only problem, having a dental assistant restrain the child is very helpful. Posey straps fasten to the arms of the dental chair and allow limited movement of the patient's forearm and hand. This limited movement frequently prevents overaction by resistant or combative patients. Wrapping a towel wrapped around the patient's forearms and fastening it with adhesive tape (without impeding circulation) is often helpful for an athetoid-spastic cerebral

palsy patient who tries desperately, but without success, to control body movements. Immobilization actually encourages relaxation and prevents undesired reflexes by keeping the patient's arms in the midline of the body.

A patient's head position can usually be successfully maintained through the use of forearm-body pressure by the dentist. Other options include presence of an additional assistant to stabilize the child's head or use of a Papoose Board head positioner or a plastic bowl (doggie bowl) to provide position guidance (Fig. 23-12).

An explanation of the benefits of this management should be presented by the dentist before use if communication with the patient is possible. The mouth prop

*J.T. Posey Co., Arcadia, Calif.

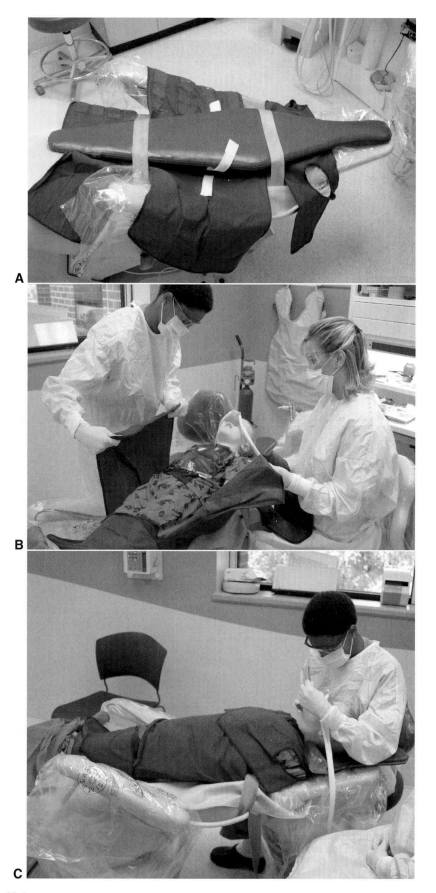

FIG. **23-9.** **A,** The Olympic Papoose Board secured to a dental chair. **B,** Patient being placed in Papoose Board. **C,** Papoose Board in use.

unmanageable patient. In addition, patients who have unintelligible speech, uncontrollable jaw movements, and spastic tongue are often erroneously assumed to be intellectually delayed. A clinician who is not knowledgeable about cerebral palsy and other physically and mentally disabling conditions may feel uncomfortable about treating such patients and may refuse to do so.

In providing treatment for children with cerebral palsy, it is imperative that a dentist evaluate each patient thoroughly in terms of personal characteristics, symptoms, and behavior and then proceed as conditions and needs dictate.

The dentist should never make assumptions about the degree of a child's physical or mental impairments without first acquiring the facts. Taking a thorough medical and dental history is very important, and the parent or guardian should be interviewed before the initiation of any treatment. It may also be beneficial to consult the patient's physician regarding the patient's medical status.

A patient with cerebral palsy who has involuntary head movements may be cognizant of the need to minimize these movements while receiving dental care. Paradoxically, the patient's own endeavors to control these movements may only exacerbate the problem. Therefore it is imperative that all dental personnel be empathic about the fears and frustrations that such a person experiences. The importance of maintaining a calm, friendly, and professional atmosphere cannot be overemphasized.

The following suggestions are offered to the clinician as being of practical significance in treating a patient with cerebral palsy:

1. Consider treating a patient who uses a wheelchair in the wheelchair. Many patients express such a preference, and it is frequently more practical for the dentist. For a young patient, the wheelchair may be tipped back into the dentist's lap.
2. If a patient is to be transferred to the dental chair, ask about a preference for the mode of transfer. If the patient has no preference, the two-person lift is recommended.
3. Make an effort to stabilize the patient's head throughout all phases of dental treatment.
4. Try to place and maintain the patient in the midline of the dental chair, with arms and legs as close to the body as feasible.
5. Keep the patient's back slightly elevated to minimize difficulties in swallowing. (It is advisable not to have the patient in a completely supine position.)
6. On placing the patient in the dental chair, determine the patient's degree of comfort and assess the position of the extremities. Do not force the limbs into unnatural positions. Consider the use of pillows, towels, and other measures for trunk and limb support.

7. Use immobilization judiciously to control flailing movements of the extremities.
8. For control of involuntary jaw movements, choose from a variety of mouth props and finger splints. Patient preference should weigh heavily, since a patient with cerebral palsy may be very apprehensive about the ability to control swallowing. Such appliances may also trigger the strong gag reflex that many of these patients possess.
9. To minimize startle reflex reactions, avoid presenting stimuli such as abrupt movements, noises, and lights without forewarning the patient.
10. Introduce intraoral stimuli slowly to avoid eliciting a gag reflex or to make it less severe.
11. Consider the use of the rubber dam, a highly recommended technique, for restorative procedures.
12. Work efficiently and minimize patient time in the chair to decrease fatigue of the involved muscles.

SPINA BIFIDA AND LATEX ALLERGY

Although the etiology of spina bifida is unknown, it is thought to be the result of a genetic predisposition whose manifestation is triggered by the environment. There are two common forms of this neural tube defect, spina bifida occulta and myelomeningocele. Spina bifida occulta (i.e., closed) presents with skin covering an area where tissue protrudes through a bony cleft in the vertebral column. These children may develop foot weakness or bowel and bladder sphincter disturbances. Myelomeningocele (spina bifida aperta, i.e., open) is the most severe because the spinal cord, spinal fluid, and membranes protrude in a sac through the defect. These children can suffer from hydrocephalus, paralysis, orthopedic deformities, and genitourinary abnormalities. Taking folic acid during the first 6 weeks of pregnancy can prevent over 50% of neural tube defects.

Children with neural tube defects are at higher risk for caries secondary to poor hygiene, poor nutritional intake, and long-term drug therapy. They are also at higher risk for latex allergy because they are frequently exposed to latex as a result of undergoing procedures in which latex products are used. Therefore, Nettis et al[7] recommend that all patients be screened for conditions such as spina bifida and exposure to recurrent surgical procedures, and for a history of atopy, cross-reactive food allergies (i.e., allergies to banana, avocado, kiwi, and chestnuts, which may sensitize allergic patients to latex exposure), and previous reactions to natural rubber latex.

For all patients with a latex allergy or latex allergy risk factors, all equipment that comes in intimate contact with the patient should be made of nonlatex substitutes. Nettis et al[6] suggest avoiding handling of nonlatex products while wearing latex gloves or with unwashed hands to prevent the transfer of latex allergens to nonlatex products. They suggest that the ideal time to schedule dental appointments for such individuals is at the beginning of a working session, such as in the morning or after a vacation when the office has been closed. This will allow for settling of airborne latex particles. Another good scheduling time is after the office has been professionally vacuumed and cleaned to remove latex-tainted cornstarch. Mild irritant reactions to latex can be managed with immediate removal of the rubber object and administration of an antihistamine. However, systemic reactions may require immediate treatment with drugs such as adrenaline and may necessitate emergency resuscitation.

RESPIRATORY DISEASES

ASTHMA (REACTIVE AIRWAY DISEASE)

Asthma is a very common childhood disease, affecting 1 in 10 children. Although often thought of as acute respiratory distress brought on by environmental factors, asthma is a chronic airway disease characterized by inflammation and bronchial constriction.

Asthma is a diffuse obstructive disease of the airway caused by edema of the mucous membranes, increased mucous secretions, and spasm of smooth muscle. It is twice as common in prepubertal boys but affects both sexes equally during adolescence and adulthood. The etiology includes biochemical, immunologic, infectious, endocrine, and psychologic factors. The typical symptoms of asthma are coughing, wheezing, chest tightness, and dyspnea. The clinical onset of an episode may occur over minutes (acute) or hours and days. An acute attack is associated with exposure to irritants such as cold air, fumes, or dust, and it may develop in minutes. An attack developing over days is usually precipitated by a viral respiratory infection. Severe bronchial obstruction results in labored breathing, wheezing, tachypnea, profuse perspiration, cyanosis, hyperventilation, tachycardia, and sometimes chest pain. A dental procedure constitutes an acute irritant to the airways of the asthmatic child and may precipitate an attack.

Fortunately, three fourths of childhood asthma is mild, with minimal daily symptoms and short-lived exacerbations. Before initiating dental treatment, the dentist should know what are the frequency and severity of the attacks, what are the triggering agents, when the patient was hospitalized and/or in the emergency department, when the last attack occurred, what medications the patient takes, and what limitations on activity the patient may have. Patients taking systemic corticosteroids and those who were hospitalized or in the emergency department in the past year should be treated with caution because they are at higher risk of morbidity and mortality. Sometimes, deferring the dental visit until the patient's asthma is controlled is the best approach.

Patients who use bronchodilators should take a dose before their appointment, and they should bring their inhalers or nebulizers into the dental office in case trouble arises. Acute symptoms may be prevented by the use of the child's bronchodilator (inhaled β_2 receptor agonist such as albuterol or terbutaline sulfate). Behavioral methods are employed to reduce anxiety, and the use of nitrous oxide–oxygen analgesia may be helpful. Hydroxyzine hydrochloride (Vistaril) and diazepam (Valium) have been successful in alleviating anxiety. Barbiturates and narcotics are not indicated because of their potential for histamine release leading to a bronchospasm. Aspirin compounds and nonsteroidal antiinflammatory agents are contraindicated because about 4% of patients experience wheezing after taking these drugs. Acetaminophen is recommended. Positioning a child with mild asthmatic symptoms in an upright or semiupright position for the dental procedure may be beneficial.

Oral findings of children with moderate to severe asthma include higher caries rate, decreased salivary rate, increased prevalence of oral mucosal change characteristic of chronic mouth breathers, and increased levels of gingivitis. Increased incidence of orofacial abnormalities such as high palatal vault, more posterior crossbites, greater overjets, and increased facial height is also seen.

Dental goals are similar to those for other patients, with care taken to avoid the potential for dental materials and products to exacerbate the asthma. The patient's pulmonary function, propensity for developing an attack, immune status, and adrenal status should be evaluated prior to dental treatment. Emergency treatment for a person with asthma who is in respiratory distress requires discontinuing the dental procedure, reassuring the patient, and opening the airway. Administer 100% oxygen while placing the patient in an upright or comfortable position. Keeping the airway open, administer the patient's β_2 agonist with an inhaler or nebulizer. If there is no improvement, administer subcutaneous epinephrine (0.01 mg/kg of 1:1000 solution) and obtain medical assistance immediately.

BRONCHOPULMONARY DYSPLASIA

Bronchopulmonary dysplasia is a chronic lung disease usually resulting from the occurrence during infancy of respiratory distress syndrome that requires prolonged ventilation with a high concentration of inspired oxygen. Chronic lung changes are more likely to occur in the premature infant. The incidence is 80% to 90% in infants weighing less than 1000 g at birth. With the increased survival of low-birth-weight infants, the prevalence of bronchopulmonary dysplasia has increased. The lung pathology of children with bronchopulmonary dysplasia shows evidence of bronchial ulceration, necrosis with plugging of bronchiolar lumina, and inflammatory cells. This bronchiolar injury compromises further lung development. Inflammatory changes and bronchiolar fibrosis lead to increased airway resistance and contribute to the hypoxemia seen in infants with bronchopulmonary dysplasia. Some children with bronchopulmonary dysplasia develop right ventricular hypertrophy (cor pulmonale). Other significant pulmonary complications include tracheal stenosis, upper airway obstruction secondary to subglottic cysts, and hoarseness because of partial or complete vocal cord paralysis. About 20% of infants with bronchopulmonary dysplasia die within the first year of life. The major causes of death are cor pulmonale, respiratory infections, and sudden death.

An increased oxygen supply must be provided to prevent hypoxic pulmonary vasoconstriction and to decrease the work of breathing. The nasal cannula provides continuous oxygen delivery, which results in fewer fluctuations in oxygen tension. Weaning off oxygen is possible with improved lung function and lung size. Children who develop cor pulmonale may require diuretic therapy to prevent congestive heart failure.

Dental care for children with bronchopulmonary dysplasia requires more chair time than usual. These children often spend a significant part of their early lives in the hospital and exhibit significant oral defensiveness.

After the initial dental evaluation, consultation with a pulmonologist is beneficial to plan safe dental treatment for the patient. If the dental patient is taking oxygen continuously via a nasal cannula, short appointments with frequent breaks are necessary to prevent the development of pulmonary vasoconstriction. Parents of children with bronchopulmonary dysplasia may need to provide additional oral hygiene for their children when these children are required to eat frequent small meals to maintain the proper caloric intake. Any non-emergent dental care should be avoided when the patient is not doing well medically.

CYSTIC FIBROSIS

Cystic fibrosis is an autosomal recessive disorder occurring in 1 of every 2000 births. It is the most common lethal genetic disorder affecting whites. The genetically altered protein affects exocrine gland function. The defective exocrine gland function leads to microobstruction of the pancreas, which results in cystic degeneration of the pancreas and ultimately a digestive enzyme deficiency producing malabsorption of nutrients.

The defective gene products cause abnormal water and electrolyte transport across epithelial cells, which results in a chronic disease of the respiratory and gastrointestinal system, elevated levels of electrolytes in sweat, and impaired reproductive function.

In the lungs, retention of mucus occurs, which causes obstructive lung disease and increased frequency of infections. As the progressive lung disease develops, there is an increase in chest diameter, clubbing of the fingers and toes, decreased exercise tolerance, and a chronic productive cough. Before advances in antibiotic therapy, physical therapy, and nutritional supplementation, these individuals rarely survived childhood. The median life expectancy has been increased to 31 years. Death is most frequently the result of pneumonia and anoxia after a long period of respiratory insufficiency. Cystic fibrosis–related diabetes is becoming more common as patients live longer.

Children with cystic fibrosis have a high incidence of tooth discoloration when systemic tetracyclines are taken during tooth formation. With the advent of alternative antibiotics the incidence of tooth discoloration is decreasing. The incidence of dental caries in children with cystic fibrosis is low secondary to long-term antibiotic therapy, buffering capacity of excess calcium in the saliva, and pancreatic enzyme replacement therapy. There is a high incidence of mouth breathing and open-bite malocclusion associated with chronic nasal and sinus obstruction. Patients with cystic fibrosis may prefer to be treated in a more upright position to allow them to clear secretions more easily. The use of sedative agents that interfere with pulmonary function should be avoided, and the patient's physician should be contacted before using nitrous oxide–oxygen sedation in a patient exhibiting evidence of severe emphysema.

HEARING LOSS

Hearing loss (deafness) is a disability that is often overlooked because it is not obvious. Total hearing loss affects 1.8 million people, and there are 14 million hearing-impaired individuals in the United States. About 1 in 600 neonates has a congenital hearing loss. During the neonatal period, many more acquire hearing loss from other associated conditions. Almost inevitably, speech is affected. If an impairment is severe enough that dentist and child cannot communicate verbally, the dentist must use sight, taste, and touch to communicate and to allow the child to learn about dental experiences. Table 23-3 shows how speech and psychologic problems relate to various degrees of hearing loss. Many times, mild hearing losses are not diagnosed, which leads to management problems because of the child's misunderstanding of instructions; children with more severe hearing losses already have psychologic and social disturbances that make dental behavior management more complex. Parents may suspect profound hearing loss if their infant does not respond to ordinary sounds or voices. Early identification and correction of hearing loss is essential for normal

TABLE 23-3	Implications of Auditory Disability Relative to International Standards Organization (ISO) Reference Levels*

ISO (DB)	DISABILITY	SPEECH COMPREHENSION	PSYCHOLOGIC PROBLEMS IN CHILDREN
0	Insignificant	Little or no difficulty	None.
>25	Slight	Difficulty with faint speech; language and speech development within normal limits	Child may show a slight verbal deficit.
>40	Mild-moderate	Frequent difficulty with normal speech at 3 feet (91.4 cm); language skills are mildly affected	Psychologic problems can be recognized.
>55	Marked	Frequent difficulty with loud speech at 3 feet (91.4 cm); difficulty understanding with hearing aid in school situation	Child is likely to be educationally retarded, with more pronounced emotional and social problems than in children with normal hearing.
>70	Severe	May understand only shouts or amplified speech at 1 foot (30.5 cm) from ear	The prelingually deaf show pronounced educational retardation and evident emotional and social problems.
>90	Extreme	Usually no understanding of speech even when amplified; child does not rely on hearing for communication	The prelingually deaf usually show severe educational retardation and emotional underdevelopment.

Adapted from Goetzinger CP: The psychology of hearing impairment. In Katz J, editor: *Handbook of clinical audiology,* ed 2, Baltimore, 1978, Williams & Wilkins.

*Reference levels are in decibels relative to threshold in young patients with normal hearing.

development of communication skills. No abnormal dental findings are associated with hearing loss.

The following are known causes of hearing loss:

Prenatal factors

Viral infections, such as rubella and influenza
Ototoxic drugs, such as aspirin, streptomycin, neomycin, kanamycin
Congenital syphilis
Heredity disorders (e.g., Alport, Arnold-Chiari, Crouzon, Hunter, Klippel-Feil, Stickler, Treacher Collins, and Waardenburg syndromes)

Perinatal factors

Toxemia late in pregnancy
Prematurity
Birth injury
Anoxia
Erythroblastosis fetalis

Postnatal factors

Viral infections, such as mumps, measles, chickenpox, influenza, poliomyelitis, meningitis
Injuries
Ototoxic drugs, such as aspirin, streptomycin, neomycin, kanamycin

The following should be considered when treating a hearing-impaired patient:

1. Prepare the patient and parent before the first visit with a welcome letter that states what is to be done and include a medical history form.

2. Let the patient and parent determine during the initial appointment how the patient desires to communicate (i.e., interpreter, lipreading, sign language, note writing, or a combination of these). Look for ways to improve communication. It is useful to learn some basic sign language. Face the patient and speak slowly at a natural pace and directly to the patient without shouting. Exaggeration of facial expressions and the use of slang make lipreading difficult. Even the best lip-readers comprehend only 30% to 40% of what is said.

3. Assess speech, language ability, and degree of hearing impairment when taking the patient's complete medical history. Identify the age of onset, type, degree, and cause of hearing loss, and determine whether any other family members are affected.

4. Enhance visibility for communication. Watch the patient's expression. Make sure the patient understands what the dental equipment is, what is going to happen, and how it will feel. Have the patient use hand gestures if a problem arises. Write out and display information.

5. Reassure the patient with physical contact; hold the patient's hand initially, or place a hand reassuringly on the patient's shoulder while the patient maintains visual contact. Without visual contact the child may be startled. Explain to the patient if you must leave the room.

6. Employ the tell-show-feel-do approach. Use visual aids and allow the patient to see the instruments,

and demonstrate how they work. Hearing-impaired children may be very sensitive to vibration.

7. Display confidence; use smiles and reassuring gestures to build up confidence and reduce anxiety. Allow extra time for all appointments.

8. Avoid blocking the patient's visual field, especially with a rubber dam.

9. Adjust the hearing aid (if the patient has one) before the handpiece is in operation, because a hearing aid amplifies all sounds. Many times the patient will prefer to have it turned off.

10. Make sure the parent or patient understands explanations of diagnosis, treatment, and payment. Deaf persons have different levels of skill with English. Use of an interpreter is extremely helpful.

VISUAL IMPAIRMENT

Total visual impairment (blindness) affects more than 30 million people. The list that follows gives some of the known causes of visual impairment; however, in more than 35% of those affected the cause is either unknown or unreported. Blindness is not an all-or-nothing phenomenon; a person is considered to be affected by blindness if the visual acuity does not exceed 20/200 in the better eye with corrective lenses or if the acuity is greater than 20/200 but is accompanied by a visual field of no greater than 20 degrees.

The following are known causes of visual impairment:

Prenatal causes
Optic atrophy
Microphthalmos
Cataracts
Colobomas
Dermoid and other tumors
Toxoplasmosis
Cytomegalic inclusion disease
Syphilis
Rubella
Tuberculous meningitis
Developmental abnormalities of the orbit

Postnatal causes
Trauma
Retrolental fibroplasia
Hypertension
Premature birth
Polycythemia vera
Hemorrhagic disorders
Leukemia
Diabetes mellitus
Glaucoma

Visual impairment may be only one aspect of a child's disability. For example, a patient with congenital rubella may have deafness, mental retardation, congenital heart disease, and dental defects, as well as blindness resulting from congenital cataracts. Total visual impairment is one disorder that may result in frequent hospitalizations, separation from family, and slow social development. Because the capabilities of a child with blindness are difficult to assess, the child may be considered developmentally delayed.

Consideration must be given to every developmental aspect of a child with blindness. Early in development the parents may experience guilt and either overprotect or reject the child; this can result in a lack of development of self-help skills and delayed development in general, which is often misinterpreted as mental retardation. Assessment of parental attitudes is of primary importance in behavioral management. In addition, children with blindness may exhibit self-stimulating activities, such as eye pressing, finger flicking, rocking, and head banging. Therefore assessment of the child's socialization is useful in the management of dental behavior.

A distinction should be made between children who at one time had sight and those who have not and thus do not form visual concepts. More explanation is needed for children in the latter category to help them perceive the dental environment. Dentists should realize that congenitally visually impaired children need a greater display of affection and love early in life and that they differ intellectually from children who are not congenitally visually impaired. Although explanation is accomplished through touching and hearing, reinforcement takes place through smelling and tasting. The modalities of listening, touching, tasting, and smelling are extremely important for these children in helping to learn coping behavior. Reports indicate that, once speech is developed, the other senses assume heightened importance and other development can occur that is comparable to that in children with sight.

Reports also reveal that motor activity affects the development of language and perception. Visually impaired children tend to have more accidents than other children during the early years while they are acquiring motor skills.

Hypoplastic teeth and trauma to the anterior teeth have been reported to occur with greater than average frequency in visually impaired children. Such children are also more likely to have gingival inflammation because of their inability to see and remove plaque. Other dental abnormalities occur with the same frequency as in the general population.

Before initiating dental treatment for a visually impaired child, the dentist should keep the following points in mind:

1. Determine the degree of visual impairment (e.g., can the patient tell light from dark?).

2. If the patient is accompanied by a companion, find out if the companion is an interpreter. If he or she is not, address the patient.

3. Establish rapport; afterward offer verbal and physical reassurance. Avoid expressions of pity or references to visual impairment as an affliction.

4. In guiding the patient to the operatory, ask if the patient desires assistance. Do not grab, move, or stop the patient without verbal warning. Encourage the parent to accompany the child.

5. Paint a picture in the mind of the visually impaired child by describing the office setting and treatment. Always give the patient adequate descriptions before performing treatment procedures. It is important to use the same office setting for each dental visit to allay the patient's anxiety.

6. Introduce other office personnel very informally.

7. When making physical contact, do so reassuringly. Holding the patient's hand often promotes relaxation.

8. Allow the patient to ask questions about the course of treatment and answer them, keeping in mind that the patient is highly individual, sensitive, and responsive.

9. Allow a patient who wears eyeglasses to keep them on for protection and security.

10. Rather than using the tell-show-feel-do approach, invite the patient to touch, taste, or smell, recognizing that these senses are acute. Avoid sight references.

11. Describe in detail instruments and objects to be placed in the patient's mouth. Demonstrate a rubber cup on the patient's fingernail.

12. Because strong tastes may be rejected, use smaller quantities of dental materials with such characteristics.

13. Some patients may be photophobic. Ask parents about light sensitivity and allow these patients to wear sunglasses.

14. Explain the procedures of oral hygiene and then place the patient's hand over yours as you slowly but deliberately guide the toothbrush.

15. Use audiocassette tapes and braille dental pamphlets explaining specific dental procedures to supplement information and decrease chair time.

16. Announce exits from and entrances to the dental operatory cheerfully. Keep distractions to a minimum, and avoid unexpected loud noises.

17. Limit providers of the patient's dental care to one dentist whenever possible.

18. Maintain a relaxed atmosphere. Remember that your patient cannot see your smile.

The provision of dental care to a visually impaired child is facilitated by an in-depth understanding of the patient's background. A team approach by all health professionals involved in the care of the child is ideal. Disease prevention and continuity of care are of utmost importance.

HEART DISEASE

Heart disease can be divided into two general types: congenital and acquired. Because individuals with heart disease require special precautions during dental treatment (such as antibiotic coverage for prevention of bacterial endocarditis), a dentist should closely evaluate the medical histories of all patients to ascertain their cardiovascular status.

CONGENITAL HEART DISEASE

The incidence of congenital heart disease is approximately 9 in 1000 births. The following is the relative incidence of congenital heart defects (Toronto Heart Registry):

Defect	Percent
Ventricular septal defect	22
Patent ductus arteriosus	17
Tetralogy of Fallot	11
Transposition of the great vessels	8
Atrial septal defect	7
Pulmonary stenosis	7
Coarctation of the aorta	6
Aortic stenosis	5
Tricuspid atresia	3
All others	14

The cause of a congenital heart defect is obscure. Generally it is a result of aberrant embryonic development of a normal structure or the failure of a structure to progress beyond an early stage of embryonic development. Only rarely can a causal factor be identified in congenital heart disease. Maternal rubella and chronic maternal alcohol abuse are known to interfere with normal cardiogenesis. If a parent or a sibling has a congenital heart defect, the chances that a child will be born with a heart defect are about 5 to 10 times greater than average. Congenital heart disease can be classified into two groups: acyanotic and cyanotic.

Acyanotic Congenital Heart Disease. Acyanotic congenital heart disease is characterized by minimal or no cyanosis and is commonly divided into two major groups. The first group consists of defects that cause left-to-right shunting of blood within the heart. This group includes ventricular septal defect and atrial septal defect. Clinical manifestations of these defects can include congestive heart failure, pulmonary congestion, heart murmur, labored breathing, and cardiomegaly.

The second major group consists of defects that cause obstruction (e.g., aortic stenosis and coarctation of the aorta). The clinical manifestations can include labored breathing and congestive heart failure.

Kanner L: *Childhood psychosis: initial studies and new insights,* Washington, DC, 1973, VH Winston & Sons.

Kisby L: Understanding the blind child, *J Pedod* 2:67-72, 1977.

Leslie ND, Sperling MA: Relation of metabolic control to complications in diabetes mellitus, *J Pediatr* 108:491-497, 1986.

Ligh RQ: The visually handicapped patient in dental practice, *J Dent Handicap* 4:38-40, 1979.

McCrindle BW et al: An evaluation of parental concerns and misconceptions about heart murmurs, *Clin Pediatr* 34:25-31, 1995.

Morsey SL: Communicating with and treating the blind child, *Dent Hyg* 65:288-290, 1980.

Nowak AJ: *Dentistry for the handicapped patient,* St Louis, 1976, Mosby.

Phillips S, Liebert RM, Poulos RW: Employing paraprofessional teachers in a group language training program for severely and profoundly retarded children, unpublished manuscript, 1972, State University of New York at Stony Brook.

Pope JEC, Curzon MEJ: The dental status of cerebral palsied children, *Pediatr Dent* 13(3):156-162, 1991.

Posnick WR, Feigal RJ: Cystic fibrosis and its dental implications, *J Dent Handicap* 5:21-23, 1980.

Rituo ER, Freeman BJ: National society of autistic children definition of the syndrome of autism, *J Pediatr Psychol* 2:146, 1977.

Rosenberg DJ et al: Estimating treatment and treatment times for special and nonspecial patients in hospital ambulatory dental clinics, *J Dent Educ* 50:665-672, 1986.

Rosenstein SN: *Dentistry in cerebral palsy and related handicapping conditions,* Springfield, Ill, 1978, Charles C Thomas.

Sanders BJ, Weddell JA, Dodge NN: Managing patients who have seizure disorders: dental and medical issues, *J Am Dent Assoc* 126:1641-1647, 1995.

Shapira J et al: Oral health status and dental needs of an autistic population of children and young adults, *Spec Care Dentist* 9:38-41, 1989.

Simko A et al: Fragile X: recognition in young children, *Pediatrics* 83:547-551, 1989.

Steinbacher DM, Glick M: The dental patient with asthma: an update and oral health consideration, *J Am Dent Assoc* 132:1229-1239, 2001.

Storhaug K, Hallonsten AL, Nielsen LA: Dentistry with handicapped children. In Koch G et al, editors: *Pedodontics: a clinical approach,* Munksgaard, 1991, Schmidt, Vojens.

Swallow JN, Swallow BG: Dentistry for physically handicapped children in the International Year of the Child, *Int Dent J* 30:1-5, 1980.

Tarnopol L: Delinquency and minimal brain dysfunction, *J Learn Disabil* 3:200-207, 1970.

Tesini DA, Fenton SJ: Oral health needs of persons with physical or mental disabilities, *Dent Clin North Am* 38:483-498, 1994.

Tunis W, Dixter C: Dentistry and the hearing impaired child, *J Pedod* 3:321-334, 1979.

Waldman BH: Fetal alcohol syndrome and the realities of our time, *J Dent Child* 56:435-437, 1989.

Waldman BH: Almost eleven million special people, *J Dent Child* 58:237-240, 1991.

Waldman BH, Swerdloff M, Perlman S: Children with mental retardation and epilepsy: demographics and general concerns, *J Dent Child* 67:268-274, 2000.

Wandera A, Conry JP: Aspiration and ingestion of a foreign body during dental examination by a patient with spastic quadriparesis: case report, *Pediatr Dent* 15:362-363, 1993.

Williams BJ: Practical oral hygiene for handicapped children, *J Dent Child* 46:408-409, 1979.

Zhu J et al: Dental management of children with asthma, *Pediatr Dent* 18:363-370, 1996.

24

Management of the Medically Compromised Patient: Hematologic Disorders, Cancer, Hepatitis, and AIDS

BRIAN J. SANDERS

AMY D. SHAPIRO

RANDY A. HOCK

JAMES A. WEDDELL

CHRISTOPHER EDWARD BELCHER

CHAPTER OUTLINE

To achieve optimal oral health for the medically compromised patient, the dentist and physician must establish a close working relationship. Because of the complexity of many of these medical conditions additional treatment time may be needed to provide these services. To minimize the risk of possible complications that may affect the physical health of medically compromised patients, an aggressive prevention-oriented program is needed for such individuals. Each patient presents a unique set of challenges to the dentist, but achieving a successful outcome can be a rewarding experience. This chapter discusses major medical conditions and their dental management.

HEMOPHILIA
DISORDERS OF HEMOSTASIS

The hemophilias are disorders of hemostasis resulting from a deficiency of a procoagulant. Hemophilia is an inherited bleeding disorder affecting approximately 1 in 7500 males.

Hemophilia A, or classic hemophilia, is a deficiency of factor VIII, also known as *antihemophilic factor*. Factor VIII deficiency is the most common of the hemophilias and is inherited as an X-linked recessive trait. Therefore males are affected, females are carriers, and there is no male-to-male transmission. If a normal male has children with a carrier of hemophilia, there is a 50% chance that hemophilia will occur in each male offspring and a 50% chance that each female offspring will be a carrier. If a male hemophilic has children with a normal female, all male offspring will be normal, and all female offspring will be carriers.

Hemophilia B, or Christmas disease, is caused by a deficiency of factor IX (plasma thromboplastin component) and is also inherited as an X-linked recessive trait. Factor IX deficiency is one fourth as prevalent as factor VIII deficiency.

Factor XI (plasma thromboplastin antecedent) deficiency is inherited as an autosomal recessive trait, with male and female offspring equally affected. This disorder is most frequently observed in those of Ashkenazi Jewish descent.

Other factor deficiencies, such as those of factors II, V, and XIII (one case per 1 million) and factor VII (one case per 500,000) are rare and are also inherited as autosomal recessive traits.

Von Willebrand disease is a hereditary bleeding disorder resulting from an abnormality of the von Willebrand factor (VWF) that is found in the plasma, platelets, megakaryocytes, and endothelial cells. VWF circulates in conjunction with factor VIII and is important in platelet adhesion to the subendothelium via collagen and therefore in the formation of the primary platelet plug. In von Willebrand disease, the VWF may have a quantitative or qualitative abnormality. The VWF is composed of subunits called *multimers*. Von Willebrand disease is divided into subtypes based on the platelet and plasma multimeric structure of the VWF. Treatment of this disorder is dependent on the subtype.

Impaired formation of the platelet plug may result in bleeding from the skin and mucosa, bruising, epistaxis, prolonged bleeding after surgical procedures, and menorrhagia. This is in contrast to hemophilia involving deficiencies of factors VIII and IX, in which bleeding tends to involve muscles and joints.

PROCOAGULANT CLASSIFICATION

Hemophilia A (factor VIII deficiency) and hemophilia B (factor IX deficiency) are classified into the following three groups based on the level of the procoagulant present (normal levels range from 55% to 100%):

- Severe deficiency: levels less than 1%
- Moderate deficiency: levels between 1% and 5%
- Mild deficiency: levels greater than or equal to 5%

Patients with severe deficiency may experience frequent bleeding episodes, occurring two to four times per month. Bleeding episodes are often spontaneous, without a specific history of trauma. The common sites of bleeding include joints, muscles, and skin. Hemarthroses (joint hemorrhages) are common, and symptoms include pain, stiffness, and limited motion. Repeated episodes of hemarthroses or muscle hemorrhage result in chronic musculoskeletal problems. Individuals with hemophilia may develop debilitating painful arthritis. Commonly affected joints include knees, elbows, ankles, hips, and shoulders.

Pseudotumors (hemorrhagic pseudocysts) may occur in several locations including the jaw, in which case curettage is indicated.

Patients with moderate deficiency experience less frequent bleeding episodes (approximately four to six times per year). However, if a patient with moderate deficiency develops a target joint (a joint with repeated episodes of bleeding), spontaneous bleeding may occur.

Patients with mild deficiency bleed infrequently and only in association with surgery or injury. The diagnosis of a mild deficiency may be when an abnormality is found during presurgical evaluation or when bleeding occurs in association with surgery or trauma.

Mouth lacerations are a common cause of bleeding in children with all severities of hemophilia. Sonis and Musselman evaluated 132 patients with factor VIII–deficient hemophilia and noted that "persistent oral bleeding resulted in the diagnosis of 13.6% of all cases of hemophilia."[1] About 29% of the cases of mild hemophilia observed were discovered as a result of bleeding from the oral cavity. Of the cases diagnosed secondary to oral bleeding, 78% were the result of bleeding from the maxillary frenum, and 22% resulted from tongue bleeds. Thus initial diagnosis of hemophilia, especially in moderate or mild disease, may directly involve the dentist.

TREATMENT

The mainstay of therapy for hemophilia is replacement of the deficient coagulation factor, by the use of either purified concentrate made from pooled plasma or factor produced through recombinant technology. In the past, whole blood, plasma, or cryoprecipitate was used for replacement therapy. Factor concentrates are advantageous because they are generally accessible, easy to handle and store, and virally inactivated, and lead to more consistent hemostatic results. The dosage, frequency of administration, and duration of therapy depend on the activity level needed, the half-life of the procoagulant, and the location and severity of the bleeding episode. The half-life of factor VIII is approximately 12 hours, whereas that for factor IX is approximately 24 hours.

Hemophilia A. Factor VIII concentrate is used for treatment of hemophilia A. Vials of factor concentrate are labeled with the number of units of activity contained, where 1 U is the amount of activity of the procoagulant present in 1 ml of normal plasma. For routine hemorrhagic episodes, such as early joint, soft tissue, and oral bleeds, a one-time correction of the procoagulant to approximately a level of 40% will achieve hemostasis and resolution of the bleeding episode. For mild factor VIII–deficient hemophilia, DDAVP* (1-deamino-8-D-arginine vasopressin) may be used for minor hemorrhagic episodes to achieve hemostasis. DDAVP is a synthetic analogue of vasopressin (antidiuretic hormone). This drug, when given intravenously, subcutaneously, or intranasally Stimate (desmopressin)[†] causes a rise in factor VIII activity and in VWF, often to the hemostatic range. An appropriate rise in factor VIII activity to hemostatic levels should be document for a given patient before the therapeutic use of DDAVP, since response may vary across individuals. Peak levels are obtained approximately 1 hour after administration. Repeated administration of DDAVP may result in tachyphylaxis. Use of DDAVP to treat hemorrhagic disorders may also be associated with water retention, hyponatremia, and, rarely, seizures.

Hemophilia B. Factor IX–deficient hemophilia is treated with purified coagulation factor IX concentrate (monoclonal and recombinant). In the past less pure

products in the class of prothrombin complex concentrate (PCC) were used. PCCs contained several other coagulation factors in addition to factor IX. Individuals who require high doses or repeated infusions of PCC are at risk for development of disseminated intravascular coagulation and thrombosis. The level necessary for hemostasis is the same for factor IX as for factor VIII (40%). However, the number of units needed to achieve that level is different because the volume of distribution of plasma-derived factor IX (1.0) is greater than that for factor VIII (0.5). The volume of distribution of recombinant factor IX is greater than that of plasma-derived factor IX (estimated minimum volume of 1.2 compared to 1, respectively).

von Willebrand Disease. Patients with von Willebrand disease should undergo subtyping to determine optimal therapy. DDAVP may be used to achieve hemostasis in type I von Willebrand disease. Type I von Willebrand disease is a quantitative deficiency of VWF with all multimers present. When DDAVP is used, a test dose should be administered to document adequate response. For patients who have less common subtypes of von Willebrand disease, patients who do not respond to DDAVP or for whom it is inappropriate, or bleeding events for which DDAVP should not be used, other therapeutic modalities may be needed, and interventions should be discussed with a hemophilia comprehensive center.

COMPLICATIONS

Inhibitors are antibodies that may develop in approximately 28% of patients with severe factor VIII deficiency and in 3% to 5% of patients with severe factor IX deficiency. The key to successful treatment of patients with inhibitors is accurate knowledge of the classification and level of the inhibitor. Patients with inhibitors are divided into two general groups, high responders and low responders, based on the past peak anamnestic response.

Patients in the low-response group may continue to be treated with factor concentrate, whereas those in the high-response group must be given bypassing products (either PCC or activated PCC and recombinant factor VIIa). Hemophilic patients with inhibitors pose a challenging treatment problem and should be managed only in conjunction with a hemophilia comprehensive center, since hemostasis may be difficult to achieve.

Other complications of hemophilia include arthritis and degenerative joint disease secondary to recurrent bleeding, and bloodborne viral infections that may have been transmitted via the necessary blood or blood products used for therapy. Therefore hepatitis (either B or C) and resultant liver disease have been a significant source of morbidity and mortality in this patient population. The human immunodeficiency virus (HIV)

---

*Aventis Pharmaceuticals Products Inc., Bridgewater, N.J.
†Aventis Behring, King of Prussia, Penn.

has also been a major source of morbidity and mortality since approximately 1979. Before 1985, there was no antibody test for HIV and no consistent method of inactivation of this virus in the manufacture of factor concentrates. Therefore between 1979 and 1985, factor concentrates and blood products may have been contaminated with HIV. Approximately 90% of hemophilic patients with severe factor VIII deficiency and 30% of those with severe factor IX deficiency who received factor concentrate during these risk years may have become infected with HIV. HIV infection is a sensitive issue to these individuals, who may now bear the burden of two chronic conditions. Present-day treatment of factor concentrate and recombinant technology have effectively eliminated new transmission of HIV by this mode. Nevertheless, universal precautions should be followed in treating all hemophilic patients with a history of receiving either factor VIII or factor IX concentrate.

RISKS TO DENTAL STAFF

The risk of acquiring hepatitis B virus infection following an accidental stick with a needle used by a hepatitis B virus carrier ranges from 6% to 30%, far higher than the risk of HIV infection (less than 1%) following a stick with a needle used by a patient infected with HIV. Moreover, although HIV antibodies have been isolated in saliva and other body fluids, there is no evidence to suggest that the disease is easily transmitted through saliva alone.

A study by Klein et al demonstrated a less than 0.5% occupational risk of HIV infection among dental professionals despite their infrequent compliance with recommended infection control precautions, frequent occupational exposure to persons at increased risk for HIV infection, and frequent accidental parenteral inoculations with sharp instruments.[2]

DEVELOPMENT OF A TREATMENT PLAN

With recent advances in treatment, most hemophilic patients can receive outpatient dental care routinely. With a thorough understanding of the patient's coagulopathy, the dentist, in conjunction with the hematologist, can make appropriate decisions regarding treatment.

The dentist must be fully aware of the procedures that can be safely performed and those in which complications may arise. The dentist should confer with the patient's physician and hematologist to formulate an appropriate treatment plan. The dentist should know the specific type of bleeding disorder, the severity of the disorder, the frequency and treatment of bleeding episodes, and the patient's inhibitor status. Many individuals with hemophilia self-administer the infusion products at home. The dentist should be prepared to discuss with the hematologist the type of anesthetic anticipated to be administered, the invasiveness of the dental procedure, the amount of bleeding anticipated, and the time involved in oral wound healing to help establish an appropriate treatment plan.

USE OF ANTIFIBRINOLYTICS

Antifibrinolytics are adjunctive therapeutic agents for dental management of patients with bleeding disorders to help control oral bleeding. These agents include ε-aminocaproic acid (Amicar*) and tranexamic acid (Cyklokapron†). Hemophilic patients form loose, friable clots that may be readily dislodged or quickly dissolved. Antifibrinolytics prevent lysis of clots within the oral cavity. They are used as an adjunct to factor concentrate replacement to prevent or control oral bleeding. For some dental procedures in which minimal bleeding is anticipated, they may be used alone without factor replacement.

Dosages. In children, ε-aminocaproic acid is given immediately before dental treatment in an initial loading dose of 100 to 200 mg/kg by mouth up to a total dose of 10 g. Subsequently, 50 to 100 mg/kg per dose up to a total dose of 5 g of ε-aminocaproic acid is administered orally every 6 hours for 5 to 7 days. Alternatively, for patients of approximately adult size, a regimen of 3 g by mouth four times daily without a loading dose may also be used. The advantage of ε-aminocaproic acid for children is that it is available in both tablet and liquid form.

Adults require a 10 g initial loading dose and 5 g every 6 hours for 5 to 7 days.

The adult and pediatric dosage of tranexamic acid is 25 mg/kg given immediately before dental treatment. The same dose is continued every 8 hours for 5 to 7 days.

Side Effects. The common side effects associated with the use of antifibrinolytics include headache, nausea, and dry mouth. These side effects are usually tolerable and, unless severe, do not require discontinuation of the medication. To avoid thrombosis, antifibrinolytics should not be used when renal or urinary tract bleeding is present or when there is any evidence of disseminated intravascular coagulation. Repeated use of PCC or bypassing products (activated PCC) in patients with inhibitors should also be avoided during a course of antifibrinolytic therapy because they may predispose the patient to thrombotic episodes.

PAIN CONTROL

Analgesia. If patient apprehension is significant, sedation or nitrous oxide–oxygen inhalation analgesia may be considered. Hypnosis has also proved beneficial for some individuals. Intramuscular injections of

*Lederle Laboratories, Pearl River, N.Y.
†Upjohn Co., Kalamazoo, Mich.

For simple extractions of single-rooted primary teeth (i.e., incisors and canines), one must evaluate the amount of root development present to determine whether factor replacement therapy is required. If there is complete root development, factor replacement therapy may be necessary. If there is only partial root formation, antifibrinolytic therapy along with local hemostatic agents may be all that is required.

The normal exfoliation of primary teeth does not usually require factor replacement, and bleeding can usually be controlled with direct finger and gauze pressure maintained for several minutes. The direct topical application of hemostatic agents may also help with local hemostasis. If there is continuous slow bleeding, antifibrinolytic therapy may be started.

Surgical Complications. Despite all precautions, bleeding may occur 3 to 4 days postoperatively when the clot begins to break down. Both systemic and local treatment must be used for control of hemorrhage. Sufficient replacement factor should be administered to control any recurrent bleeding.

It is not prudent to protect a loose clot. The typical clot in this situation is characterized as a "liver clot." It is dark red and usually protrudes from the surgical site, often covering the surfaces of several teeth. Following adequate replacement with factor concentrate, usually to achieve a 30% to 40% activity level, the clot should be removed and the area cleansed to help isolate the source of bleeding. The socket should then be repacked.

Antibiotic Prophylaxis. Total joint replacement, usually of the hip or knee, may be performed in patients with hemophilia to restore function and alleviate the pain associated with degenerative arthritis that has developed after multiple hemarthroses. Antibiotic prophylaxis is required for patients with artificial joints before invasive dental procedures. The American Heart Association recommendations for subacute bacterial endocarditis prophylaxis, as revised in 1997, are usually followed. If the patient is immunocompromised because of HIV infection, intravenous antibiotic prophylaxis may be considered.

Orthodontic Treatment. Early recognition of an orthodontic problem is important, because selective guidance can diminish or eliminate complex orthodontic problems. Both interceptive and full-banded orthodontics may be performed. Care must be taken in the adaptation and placement of bands to avoid lacerating the oral mucosa and to avoid leaving protruding sharp edges and wires. Bleeding caused by an accidental scratch or minor laceration of the gingiva usually responds to applied pressure for 5 minutes. The use of preformed orthodontic bands and brackets, which can be bonded directly to the teeth, almost totally eliminates contact of orthodontic appliances with the gingiva during placement. Longer-acting wires and springs require less frequent adjustment of orthodontic appliances. Oral hygiene is particularly important to avoid inflamed, edematous, and hemorrhagic gingival tissues. A water-irrigating device may be helpful for good home dental care.

Dental Emergencies. Oral trauma is a common occurrence during childhood. Management of bleeding injuries, including hematomas, in the oral cavity of the patient with hemophilia may require a combination of factor replacement and antifibrinolytic therapy, and treatment with local hemostatic agents.

VIRAL HEPATITIS

Viral hepatitis is an infection that produces inflammation of liver cells, which may lead to necrosis or cirrhosis of the liver. Acute hepatitis classically presents with lethargy, loss of appetite, nausea, vomiting, abdominal pain, and ultimately jaundice.

Acute viral hepatitis may be caused by any of the following: hepatitis A virus (HAV), hepatitis B virus (HBV), hepatitis delta virus (HDV), and two forms of non-A, non-B hepatitis virus (NANB)—parenterally transmitted NANB or hepatitis C virus (HCV), and enterically transmitted NANB or hepatitis E virus.

Infection with hepatitis A virus results in an acute febrile illness with jaundice, anorexia, nausea, and malaise. Most HAV infections in infants and children cause mild, nonspecific symptoms without jaundice. HAV is spread by the fecal-oral route and is endemic in developing areas. Spread occurs readily in households and day-care centers, where symptomatic illness occurs primarily among adult contacts of children. No HAV carrier state exists, and the presence of immunoglobulin G–anti-HAV indicates past infection and lifelong immunity to HAV.

Hepatitis B transmission is of major concern to the dentist. Members of the dental profession assume a risk of acquiring HBV that is at least three times higher than that in the general population. An additional concern, beyond that of acquiring HBV, is the potential of becoming an asymptomatic yet infectious carrier of HBV and of having the capability of transmitting the disease to patients and dental staff members and family.

HBV is transmitted from person to person by parenteral, percutaneous, or mucous membrane inoculation. It can be transmitted by the percutaneous introduction of blood, administration of certain blood products, or direct contact with secretions contaminated with blood containing HBV. Infection may also result from inoculation of mucous membranes, including sexual transmission. Wound exudate contains HBV, and open-wound–to–open-wound contact can transmit infection. There can also be vertical transmission from an infected mother to her baby, and this almost always leads to chronic infection.

A medical history is unreliable in identifying patients who have actually had HBV infection, because approximately 80% of all HBV infections are undiagnosed. However, the medical history is useful in indicating groups of patients who are at higher risk of being undiagnosed carriers. Among populations at high risk for HBV infection are patients undergoing hemodialysis, patients requiring frequent large-volume blood transfusions or administration of clotting factor concentrates, residents of institutions for the mentally disabled, and users of illicit injectable drugs.

In 2001, an estimated 78,000 people in the United States became infected with HBV, and an estimated 1.25 million chronically infected people live in America. Overall, chronic liver disease from hepatitis B claims 5000 lives a year in the United States.

Chronic active hepatitis develops in more than 25% of carriers and often progresses to cirrhosis. Furthermore, HBV carriers have a risk of developing primary liver cancer that is between 12 and 300 times higher than that of uninfected individuals.

For detection of acute or chronic HBV infection, the serologic test for hepatitis B surface antigen (HepBsAg) is most commonly used. The antibody to surface antigen (HepBsAb or anti-HepBsAg) is protective and indicates a resolved natural infection or successful vaccination. Antibody to the core antigen (HepBcAb or anti-HepBc) indicates exposure to natural hepatitis B virus but can be present in either resolved or chronic infection. The hepatitis Be antigen (HepBeAg) is a useful marker for infectivity. Patients who test positive for HepBeAb and HepBsAg are most likely to transmit the disease. If the patient still shows a positive test result for HepBsAg 6 months after an acute HBV infection, the patient is considered to be chronically infected.

The availability of a safe, effective hepatitis B vaccine affords the dentist and staff additional protection against acquiring HBV infection. HBV vaccine is recommended for all health care personnel. The vaccine is derived from recombinant DNA and therefore does not have the potential to transmit the disease. When administered in a three-dose injection regimen (0, 1, 6 months), the recombinant DNA vaccine has induced protective antibody production (anti-HepBs) in 95% to 100% of adults.

A fulminant type of hepatitis occurs with infection by HDV but only with coexisting or simultaneous infection with HBV. HDV is defective in that it requires HBV for outer coat proteins (HepBsAg), as well as requiring HBV for replication. Transmission is similar to that of HBV, by parenteral, percutaneous, or mucous membrane inoculation.

According to Cottone, HDV infection occurs in two primary modes:

The first is simultaneous infection with HBV and HDV. When simultaneous infection occurs, the acute clinical course of hepatitis often is limited with resolution of both hepatitis B and HDV infections. The second mode of transmission, acute delta super-infection, involves those with chronic Hepatitis B infection. In this situation, the patient already has a high titer of circulating HepBsAg; thus HDV can rapidly replicate. These patients are more likely to have a serious and possibly acute fulminant form of hepatitis that more often leads to chronic HDV.[3]

Hepatitis C (formally known as parentally transmitted NANB hepatitis) is of great concern to the dentist, because it can be transmitted by needle stick (risk of about 1.8% with a range of 0% to 10%) and no immunization is available. Patients at risk of hepatitis C include those who received blood transfusions or organ transplants before 1992, those who received clotting factors before 1987, those who have experimented with illicit intravenous drugs regardless of how many times or how long ago, and those on chronic dialysis. Of those infected, 70% to 85% develop chronic infection, and about 70% develop chronic liver disease. Although only 3% of infected people die from liver failure, hepatitis C is the leading reason for liver transplantation in adults in the United States.

In 1989, parenterally transmitted NANB was identified as HCV. Subsequently, three genotypes have been identified. Diagnosis is made by detection of antibody to hepatitis C virus (anti-HCV) in the serum and can be confirmed by radiommunoblot assay. Polymerase chain reaction testing (PCR) can be done in a qualitative fashion to confirm diagnosis or in a quantitative fashion to assess response to treatment. Treatment, when indicated, includes administration of interferon or pegylated interferon with or without ribavirin. Response rates vary from 50% for type 1 infection to 80% for types 2 and 3.

In 2001, the Centers for Disease Control and Prevention estimated that there were 25,000 new cases of infection with hepatitis C in the United States.[4] There are 2.7 million carriers of hepatitis C in America, and chronic liver disease in these patients results in 8000 to 10,000 deaths per year. The number of new cases per year in the United States dropped from a high of 291,000 in 1989 to 25,000 in 2001. Infection associated with drug use accounts for 60% of the new cases in the United States.

As noted earlier, of concern to dentists and staff is the present unavailability of immunization against HCV. Antibodies formed in patients with HCV are not protective antibodies. However, the use of universal precautions should provide adequate protection.

Enterically transmitted NANB has now been identified as the hepatitis E virus. Transmission is by the fecal-oral route. Large, well-documented outbreaks have been seen in India, the former Soviet Union, North America, Mexico, and Southeast Asia. There appears to be a 6- to 8-week incubation period and a low incidence of carrier state after infection. However, a high fatality rate (10% to 20%) is seen in women in their third trimester of pregnancy who contract this virus. There is no immunization presently available against this pathogen.

SICKLE CELL ANEMIA

Patients with sickle cell anemia have an autosomal recessive hemolytic disorder that occurs predominantly in persons of African descent but is also found among Italian, Arabian, Greek, and Indian people.

Patients with sickle cell anemia produce hemoglobin S instead of the normal hemoglobin A. Hemoglobin S has a decreased oxygen-carrying capacity. Decreased oxygen tension causes the sickling of cells. These patients are susceptible to recurrent acute infections, which result in an "aplastic crisis" caused by decreased red blood cell production and in subsequent joint and abdominal pain with fever. Over time there is a progressive deterioration of cardiac, pulmonary, and renal function.

Many factors can precipitate a sickle cell crisis, including acidosis, hypoxia, hypothermia, hypotension, stress, hypovolemia, dehydration, fever, and infection.

Radiographic changes are associated with sickle cell anemia. There is a generalized radiolucency and loss of trabeculae with prominent lamina dura, caused by increased erythropoietic demands that result in expansion of the marrow spaces. Bone growth may be decreased in the mandible, resulting in retrusion, and the teeth may be hypomineralized. Occasionally, patients with sickle cell anemia have infarcts in the jaw, which may be mistaken for a toothache or osteomyelitis. The patients experience dental pain with absence of pathology.

Dental appointments should be short to reduce potential stress on the patient. The importance of an aggressive preventive program cannot be understated, and such a program should have the goal of maintaining excellent oral health and decreasing the possibility of oral infection. Dental treatment should not be initiated during a sickle cell crisis. If emergency treatment is necessary during a crisis, only treatment that will make the patient more comfortable should be provided. Patients with sickle cell anemia may have skeletal changes that make orthodontic treatment beneficial. Special care must be taken to avoid tissue irritation, which may induce bacteremias, and the disease process may compromise the proposed treatment. Careful monitoring is a necessity when proposing elective orthodontic treatment in patients with sickle cell anemia.

Many patients with sickle cell anemia have defective spleen function or undergo a splenectomy, which leaves them more vulnerable to infection because immunoglobulin production is decreased and phagocytosis of foreign antigens is thus impaired. Most patients with sickle cell anemia are taking low-dose daily prophylactic antibiotics, and the need for additional antibiotics for dental procedures is debatable. Some authors have recommended the use of antibiotics for all dental procedures, whereas others recommend the administration of additional antibiotics when there is obvious dental or periodontal infection. The selection of an antibiotic is usually similar to that in cases of heart defect.

The use of local anesthetics with a vasoconstrictor is not contraindicated in patients with sickle cell anemia. Some textbooks do recommend against the use of vasoconstrictors, although there is no evidence to support this practice. Similarly, the use of nitrous oxide is not contraindicated in these patients. Care must be taken in treating patients with sickle cell anemia to avoid diffusion hypoxia at the completion of the dental procedure.

The restoration of teeth, including pulpotomies, is preferable to extraction. Pulpectomy in a nonvital tooth is reasonable if the practitioner is fairly confident that the tooth can remain noninfected. If the tooth is likely to persist as a focus of infection, then extraction is indicated.

The use of general anesthesia for dental procedures must be approached cautiously in consultation with the hematologist and anesthesiologist. Previously, the standard protocol was to perform a direct transfusion (immediate introduction of whole blood or blood components) or an exchange transfusion (repetitive withdrawal of small amounts of blood and replacement with donor blood until a large portion of the patient blood has been exchanged) before general anesthesia. The goal of the transfusion is to increase the patient's hemoglobin level to higher than 10 g/dl and to decrease the hemoglobin S level below 40%. Transfusions do not provide complete protection against venous complications, but they may temporarily improve the patient's condition and reduce the hazards of surgery.

The current thinking is to weigh the risks associated with transfusion prior to anesthesia induction. Suggested guidelines for performing a prophylactic transfusion before general anesthesia have been proposed. Patients with a hemoglobin level of less than 7 g/dl and a hematocrit of less than 20% may require a transfusion. Pediatric patients are usually less likely to have post-transfusion complications than are adults. A high frequency of hospitalizations is indicative of a more severe anemia, and such patients may require transfusion prior to surgery. Minor surgeries may not require a transfusion.

ACQUIRED IMMUNODEFICIENCY SYNDROME

Acquired immunodeficiency syndrome (AIDS) is a clinically defined condition caused by infection with HIV type 1 or, much less commonly, type 2. Estimates are that, in the United States, about 900,000 people are infected with HIV and one quarter of them do not know they are infected. Worldwide in 2002, 38.6 million adults and 3.2 million children were HIV infected.

The incubation period from the time of infection to the appearance of symptoms of AIDS is approximately 11 years in adults. Therefore HIV-infected individuals can unknowingly spread the virus to sexual or needle-sharing partners or, in the case of infected mothers, to their children. AIDS was the fifth leading cause of death in the United States in 2001 among people from 25 to 44 years of age.

HIV infects cells of the immune system, specifically lymphocytes and macrophages. These white blood cells contain the greatest number of CD4 cell surface receptors (glycoproteins), which permit attachment with viral surface proteins (GP120) and enhance host-cell invasion and infection. Under the control of the HIV "POL" gene, the virus produces the enzyme reverse transcriptase, which is essential for incorporating viral RNA into host nuclear DNA. The viral genome is integrated into the host-cell genome and leads to progressive and eventually irreversible immunosuppression by producing more virus and further killing the CD4 (T_4) helper-inducer lymphocytes that are important modulators of the immune system. The subsequent immunodeficiency results in a variety of opportunistic infections, malignancies (such as Kaposi sarcoma and lymphoma), and autoimmune diseases. Diagnosis is made by screening the serum for antibodies to HIV and is confirmed by Western blot analysis. Ongoing management is guided by the patient's CD4+ cell count and viral load as measured by PCR. The former is an indication of the patient's immune status, whereas a higher viral load is associated with a more accelerated disease. The current antiretroviral drugs target the virus at several steps: (1) the fusion of the virus to the host cell (fusion inhibitors), (2) the transcription of DNA from viral RNA by reverse transcriptase (nucleoside, nonnucleoside, and nucleotide reverse transcriptase inhibitors), and (3) the cleavage of viral proteins by the viral protease enzyme (protease inhibitors). The most effective treatment strategies use a combination of several drugs to inhibit the virus at several steps.

In the United States, 60% of newly infected men acquired HIV through homosexual contact, infection from illicit drug use accounted for 25% of new cases, and 15% of infections were acquired through heterosexual contact. Among infected women in the United States, 75% acquired HIV through heterosexual contact and 25% through intravenous drug use. Almost 30% of newborns of untreated HIV-infected mothers can acquire the HIV virus through vertical transmission. However, treatment of pregnant women with antiretroviral medications, including azidothymidine (AZT), has

decreased the rate of transmission by 70%. The onset of symptoms is shortened in children who have acquired their infection prenatally and go untreated. Only 75% survive to age 5 years, and by that age 50% have severe symptoms.

Infants and children with AIDS have clinical findings similar to those in adults. Early manifestations of HIV infection include *Pneumocystis carinii* pneumonia, interstitial pneumonitis, weight loss and failure to thrive, hepatomegaly or splenomegaly, generalized lymphadenopathy, and chronic diarrhea. Unlike in adults, recurrent and severe bacterial infections are common in pediatric patients with HIV infection.

ORAL MANIFESTATIONS OF HIV INFECTION

The types of oral lesions seen in HIV infection may be caused by fungal, viral, or bacterial infections, as well as neoplastic and idiopathic processes.

Fungal Infection. Pindborg stated that the most common HIV-associated infection of the mouth is caused by the fungus *Candida albicans*.[5] Oral candidiasis is frequently present and may lead to esophageal or disseminated candidiasis. There are four major types of oral candidiasis: (1) pseudomembranous, (2) hyperplastic, (3) erythematous (atrophic), and (4) angular cheilotic.

The pseudomembranous lesion is characterized by the presence of creamy white or yellow plaques that can easily be removed from mucosa, leaving a red, bleeding surface. The most common locations for these lesions are the palate, buccal and labial mucosa, and dorsum of the tongue.

The hyperplastic lesion is characterized by white plaques that cannot easily be removed. The most common location is the buccal mucosa.

The erythematous (atrophic) lesion is characterized by a red appearance. Common locations are the palate and the dorsum of the tongue. The lesion may also appear as spotty areas on the buccal mucosa.

Angular cheilitis is characterized by fissures radiating from the commissures of the mouth, often associated with small, white plaques.

The treatment of *C. albicans* infection can be either systemic or topical. Topical therapy involves the use of nystatin (Mycostatin) rinses (100,000 U, three to five times daily) or clotrimazole (Mycelex) troches. Treatment for 1 to 2 weeks is usually effective. Systemic therapy calls for ketoconazole (Nizoral) 200 or 400 mg daily with food, or fluconazole (Diflucan), 100 mg daily. Amphotericin B or fluconazole (administered intravenously) is used when candidal infection has become systemic.

Candidal infections frequently recur. Therefore patients may remain on antifungal medication indefinitely. As an adjunctive measure, mouthrinses with

Peridex* (0.12% chlorhexidine digluconate) may be used. Chronic oral candidiasis may be a poor prognostic sign indicating a phase of more rapid decline of immune function to the terminal phase of AIDS.

Viral Infection. In the same way that fungi can cause oral disease because of the immune dysfunction induced by HIV infection, several viruses can produce lesions in the mouth following colonization or reactivation. These include herpes group viruses and papillomaviruses according to Greenspan.[6]

Oral warts may be seen in the HIV-infected patient, with human papillomavirus as the etiologic agent. Some warts have a raised, cauliflower-like appearance, whereas others are well circumscribed, have a flat surface, and almost disappear when the mucosa is stretched.

Herpes simplex virus (HSV) can produce recurrent episodes of painful ulceration. Intraorally the lesions appear most commonly on the palate. Typically these lesions present as vesicles that break open to form ulcers. However, they may also have an atypical appearance as slitlike lesions on the tongue or may mimic other diseases. Diagnosis can be made from culture or fluorescent antibody testing.

Herpetic lesions may be treated with oral acyclovir (Zovirax†). Acyclovir may also be administered intravenously (750 mg/m² in divided doses three times a day until lesions clear) in individuals with more severe oropharyngeal lesions or in those unable to swallow.

Herpes zoster (shingles) is caused by varicella-zoster virus (VZV), the chickenpox virus. VZV can produce oral ulcerations, which are usually accompanied by skin lesions generally restricted to one side of the face. These lesions are also treated with acyclovir.

Oral hairy leukoplakia (HL) is a white lesion that does not rub off, located on the lateral margins of the tongue. The surface may be smooth, corrugated, or markedly folded. HL is seen only in patients who are HIV infected. HL is a virally induced lesion caused by the Epstein-Barr virus. Treatment may include the use of high-dose acyclovir. However, the lesions usually recur.

Bacterial Infection. Bacteria causing oral lesions may include *Mycobacterium avian-intracellulare* and *Klebsiella pneumoniae*. Many of the oral lesions seen in association with HIV infection are not new entities; rather, they are known diseases that either follow an atypical course or that show an unusual response to treatment. This is frequently the case with neoplasms as well.

Neoplasms. Kaposi sarcoma is the most common malignancy seen in AIDS and occurs in 15% to 20% of AIDS patients according to Silverman.[7] Intraoral lesions may occur alone or along with skin, visceral, and lymph node lesions. Often the first lesions of Kaposi sarcoma appear in the mouth. They may be red, blue, or purple, flat or raised, and solitary or multiple. The most common oral site is the hard palate, although lesions may be found on any part of the oral mucosa. Treatment for aggressive lesions involves radiation, laser surgery, or chemotherapy. Conventional surgery may be appropriate for small lesions.

The group of malignancies whose incidence is growing the fastest among patients with AIDS is the lymphomas, most commonly the non-Hodgkin's lymphomas. The first manifestation may be a firm, painless swelling in the mouth. Biopsies of these growths are indicated to establish a diagnosis. Treatment includes multidrug chemotherapy and radiation. Less than 20% of patients survive 2 years; the mean survival time is approximately 6 months from diagnosis.

Oral squamous cell carcinomas also occur more frequently in the HIV-infected population.

Idiopathic Lesions. According to Greenspan oral ulcers of unknown etiology are being reported with increasing frequency in people with HIV infection.[6] The ulcers resemble aphthous lesions, appearing as well-circumscribed ulcers with an erythematous margin. Patients sometimes exhibit extremely large and painful necrotic ulcers that may persist for several weeks.

Salivary gland swelling has been seen in both adults and children with HIV infection. The cause of the swelling is unknown. It usually involves the parotid glands and is also accompanied by xerostomia.

HIV-infected patients may develop autoimmune disorders, including immune thrombocytopenic purpura. Oral lesions appear as small, blood-filled purpuric lesions or petechiae. Spontaneous gingival bleeding may also occur.

HIV-Associated Gingivitis and HIV-Associated Periodontitis. Progressive and premature periodontal disease is seen relatively frequently in HIV-infected individuals and may even be the first sign of HIV infection. Unlike conventional periodontal disease, these lesions do not respond effectively to standard periodontal therapy. There may be a rapid progression from mild gingivitis to advanced, painful, spontaneously bleeding periodontal disease in a few months. Treatment includes aggressive curettage, Peridex (0.12% chlorhexidine digluconate) rinses three times daily, and possibly antibiotic treatment.

LEUKEMIA

Malignancy is second only to accidents as the leading cause of death in children. Leukemias are hematopoietic malignancies in which there is a proliferation of abnormal leukocytes in the bone marrow and dissemination of these cells into the peripheral blood. The abnormal leukocytes (blast cells) replace normal cells in bone

---

*Zila Pharmaceuticals, Phoenix, Ariz.
†GlaxoSmithKline, Inc., Research Triangle Park, N.C.

marrow and accumulate in other tissues and organs of the body.

Leukemia is classified according to the morphology of the predominant abnormal white blood cells in the bone marrow (Table 24-1). These types are further categorized as acute or chronic, depending on the clinical course and the degree of differentiation, or maturation, of the predominant abnormal cells.

In the United States, about 6550 new cases of cancer are diagnosed each year in children under the age of 15. Acute leukemia is the most common malignancy in children, with about 2500 new cases diagnosed annually in the United States. Thus acute leukemia accounts for about one third of all childhood malignancies; of these, approximately 80% are lymphocytic (acute lymphocytic leukemia, or ALL). Chronic leukemia in children is rare, accounting for less than 2% of all cases.

Leukemia affects about 5 in 100,000 children in the United States. The peak incidence is between 2 and 5 years of age. Although the cause of leukemia is unknown, ionizing radiation, certain chemical agents, and genetic factors have been implicated. For example, children with chromosomal abnormalities (Down syndrome and Bloom syndrome), children with an identical twin who has leukemia, and children with immunologic disorders have an increased risk of leukemia.

The clinical manifestations of acute leukemia are caused by the infiltration of leukemia cells into tissues and organs. Infiltration and proliferation of leukemia cells in the bone marrow lead to anemia, thrombocytopenia, and granulocytopenia. Because these cytopenias develop gradually, the onset of the disease is frequently insidious. The history at presentation may reveal increased irritability, lethargy, persistent fever, vague bone pain, and easy bruising. Some of the more common findings on initial physical examination are pallor, fever, tachycardia, adenopathy, hepatosplenomegaly, petechiae, cutaneous bruises, gingival bleeding, and evidence of infection.

In approximately 90% of the cases of acute leukemia a peripheral blood smear reveals anemia and thrombocytopenia. In about 65% of cases the white blood cell count is low or normal, but it may be greater than 50,000 cells/mm^3.

When a new case of leukemia is diagnosed, the patient is hospitalized and therapy is directed toward stabilizing the patient physiologically, controlling hemorrhage, identifying and eliminating infection, evaluating renal and hepatic functions, and preparing the patient for chemotherapy.

These interventions proceed while the definitive studies to determine the exact type of leukemia are undertaken. These include obtaining bone marrow for microscopic analysis, special cytochemical staining, immunophenotyping by flow cytometry, and cytogenetic analysis.

The goal of treatment is to induce and maintain a complete remission, which is defined as resolution of the physical findings of leukemia (e.g., adenopathy, hepatosplenomegaly, petechiae) and normalization of peripheral blood counts and bone marrow (less than 5% blasts).

The basic principle of treatment of ALL is substantially different from that of acute myelogenous or nonlymphocytic leukemia (ANLL). In general, the treatment of ANLL is very intense and results in profound bone marrow hypoplasia, but the treatment duration is usually short (less than 1 year). For ALL, the treatment is less intense but more prolonged (2^1/$_2$ to 3^1/$_2$ years).

In all, the treatment regimens vary considerably depending on prognostic factors and the parameters being evaluated by the strategists' cooperative group (e.g., children's oncology group). The initial phase of treatment, induction, incorporates the use of a combination of antileukemic drugs at staggered intervals during a 4-week regimen (Table 24-2). This combination of drugs should rapidly destroy the leukemic cells, yet maintain the regenerative potential of the nonmalignant hematopoietic cells within the bone marrow. About 95% of patients with ALL will be in complete remission at day 28 of therapy.

The second phase of ALL treatment, consolidation, attempts to consolidate remission and intensify prophylactic central nervous system (CNS) treatment. Prevention of CNS relapse uses intrathecally administered chemotherapy (methotrexate with or without cytosine arabinoside and hydrocortisone) to destroy leukemic cells within the CNS. This chemotherapeutic agent is instilled directly into the lumbar spinal fluid because antileukemic drugs do not readily cross the blood-brain barrier. Intensive intrathecal chemotherapy to prevent CNS relapse has replaced cranial irradiation for patients in the good and intermediate-risk groups of ALL patients. However, both cranial irradiation and intrathecal chemotherapy are still used to prevent CNS relapse in high-risk ALL patients.

The third phase of treatment, interim maintenance, uses a combination of agents that are relatively nontoxic and require only monthly visits to the outpatient clinic. In most cases, another phase, delayed intensification, follows interim maintenance. This serves to intensify antileukemic therapy again after a short period of less intensive therapy. The addition of a late phase of intensive therapy substantially improves survival in patients with ALL. Following delayed intensification, therapy continues for 2 years for girls and 3 years for boys (maintenance phase), with chemotherapeutic agents given as in interim maintenance.

The prognosis for a child with acute leukemia has improved dramatically over the past 30 years.

ulcerations, severe pain requiring analgesia, and difficulty in or inability to swallow. Although the regimens shown are not always successful in cases of moderate or severe mucositis, consistent follow-through will minimize many signs and symptoms.

The presence of white patches (i.e., *Candida* infection) may occur. Care must be taken in obtaining culture specimens and providing specific antifungal therapy.

REMISSION PHASE

During the remission phase of post–bone marrow transplantation therapy, consistent oral hygiene should be provided by the patient or parent. For the first 90 days the dental staff should provide maintenance oral evaluations and preventive oral care reinforcement for the bone marrow transplantation patient when he or she returns for periodic hospital oncologic evaluations.

Afterward, the patient should be referred to his or her private dentist for continuity of oral health care. If the patient has no dentist, referral should be made to a dental diagnostic clinic at the patient's medical center for dental health status evaluation and dental care.

SOLID TUMORS

Solid tumors account for approximately half of the cases of childhood malignancy. The most common tumors include brain tumors, lymphoma, neuroblastoma, Wilms tumor, osteosarcoma, and rhabdomyosarcoma. Because many of the malignancies can involve bone marrow and their treatment with chemotherapy and radiation can suppress marrow function, many of the complications seen in acute leukemia are also seen with these patients. Bleeding diatheses and the propensity to infection are the most notable medical complications seen. In general, the dental management of patients with solid tumors is similar to that of patients with acute leukemia.

REFERENCES

1. Sonis AL, Musselman RJ: Oral bleeding in classic hemophilia, *Oral Surg* 53:363-366, 1982.
2. Klein RS et al: Low occupational risk of human immunodeficiency virus infection among dental professionals, *N Engl J Med* 318:89-90, 1988.
3. Cottone JA: Recent developments in hepatitis: new virus, vaccine, and dosage recommendations, *J Am Dent Assoc* 120:501-508, 1990.
4. Centers for Disease Control and Prevention: *HIV prevention strategic planning through 2005*, Atlanta, January 2001, The Centers.
5. Pindborg JJ: Oral candidiasis in HIV infection. In Robertson PB, Greenspan JS, editors: *Perspectives on oral manifestations of AIDS. Diagnosis and management of HIV-associated infections*, Littleton, Mass, 1988, PSG Publishing.
6. Greenspan D: Oral manifestations of HIV infection. In Robertson PB, Greenspan JS, editors: *Perspectives on oral manifestations of AIDS. Diagnosis and management of HIV-associated infections*, Littleton, Mass, 1988, PSG Publishing.

7. Silverman S: *AIDS, HIV infection and dentistry. Part I: epidemiology, pathogenesis and transmission. Part II: oral manifestations, diagnosis and management*, vol 7, Fairfax, Va, 1991, The California and American Dental Institutes for Continuing Education.

SUGGESTED READINGS

Aach RD: Management update: the emerging clinical significance of hepatitis C, *Hosp Pract* 27:19-22, 1992.

Alter H et al: Detection of antibody to hepatitis C virus in prospectively followed transfusion recipients with acute and chronic non-A, non-B hepatitis, *N Engl J Med* 321:1494-1500, 1989.

Alter M: Risk factors for acute non-A, non-B hepatitis in the United States and association with hepatitis C virus infection, *JAMA* 264:2231-2235, 1990.

American Academy of Pediatric Dentistry: Guidelines for the management of pediatric dental patients receiving chemotherapy, bone marrow transplantation, and/or radiation, *Pediatr Dent* 24(7 suppl):120-122, 2002 (special issue: Reference manual 2002-2003).

American Academy of Pediatrics: *Report of the committee on infectious disease*, Elk Grove Village, Ill, 1986, The Academy.

Barnett HX et al: Natural history of human immune deficiency virus disease in perinatally infected children: an analysis from the pediatric spectrum of disease project, *Pediatrics* 97:710-715, 1996.

Berkowitz RJ: Oral complications associated with bone marrow transplantation in a pediatric population, *Am J Pediatr Hematol Oncol* 5:53-57, 1983.

Carr MM: Dental management of patients with sickle cell anemia, *J Can Dent Assoc* 59:180-182, 1993.

Choo Q-L et al: Isolation of a CDNA clone derived from a blood non-A, non-B viral hepatitis genome, *Science* 244:359-362, 1989.

Conner EM et al: Reduction of maternal infant transmission of human immune deficiency virus type I with zidovudine treatment, *N Engl J Med* 331:1173-1180, 1994.

Cottone JA: Hepatitis B virus infection in the dental profession, *J Am Dent Assoc* 110:617-621, 1985.

Curtis AB: Childhood leukemias: initial oral manifestations, *J Am Dent Assoc* 83:159-164, 1971.

Curtis AB: Childhood leukemias: osseous changes in jaws on panoramic dental radiographs, *J Am Dent Assoc* 83:844-847, 1971.

da Fonseca MA: Pediatric bone marrow transplantation: oral complications and recommendations for care, *Pediatr Dent* 20(7):386-397, 1998.

DeVita VT Jr, Hellman S, Rosenberg SA: *AIDS: etiology, diagnosis, treatment and prevention*, Philadelphia, 1985, JB Lippincott.

Duggal MS et al: The dental management of children with sickle cell disease and B thalassaemia: a review, *Int J Paediatr Dent* 6:227-237, 1996.

Feinstone S: Non-A, non-B hepatitis. In Mandell G, editor: *Principle and practice of infectious diseases*, ed 3, New York, 1990, Churchill Livingstone.

Ferretti GA et al: Chlorhexidine for prophylaxis against oral infections and associated complications in patients receiving bone marrow transplants, *J Am Dent Assoc* 114:461-467, 1987.

Flemming PL et al: HIV prevalence in the United States, presented at the Ninth Conference on Retrovirus and Opportunistic Infections, Seattle, WA, February 2002.

Fox PC, Janson CC, editors: *Consensus development conference on oral complications of cancer therapies: diagnosis, prevention, and treatment,* NCI Monographs, No 9, Bethesda, Md, 1990, US Dept of Health and Human Services, Public Health Service, National Institutes of Health.

Gollin JI, Fauce AJ: *Acquired immunodeficiency syndrome (AIDS), advances in host defense mechanisms,* vol 5, New York, 1985, Raven Press.

Hsia PC, Seeff LB: Non-A, non-B hepatitis: impact of the emergence of the hepatitis C virus, *Adv Intern Med* 37:197-223, 1991.

Ketchmen L et al: Human immunodeficiency virus infection in children, *J Pediatr* 12:143-146, 1990.

Kuo G et al: An assay for circulating antibodies to a major etiologic virus of human non-A, non-B hepatitis, *Science* 244:362-364, 1989.

Lynch MA, Ship II: Initial oral manifestations of leukemia, *J Am Dent Assoc* 75:932-940, 1967.

McKown CG: Oral management of patients with bleeding disorders. Part 2: Dental considerations, *J Indiana Dent Assoc* 70:16-21, 1991.

McKown CG et al: Mouth care standards for hematology/ oncology patients undergoing bone marrow transplant, unpublished protocol, Indianapolis, 1990, Department of Hospital Dentistry, Indiana University Hospitals.

Michaud M et al: Oral manifestations of acute leukemia in children, *J Am Dent Assoc* 95:1145-1150, 1977.

Nowak AJ: Protocol for dental management of pediatric dental patients receiving radiation and/or chemotherapy, Iowa City, 1990, University of Iowa Hospitals and Clinics, Division of Pediatric Dentistry.

Peterson D, Sonis S, editors: *Oral complications of cancer chemotherapy,* The Hague, 1983, Martinus Nijhoff.

Piot P et al: The global impact of HIV/AIDS, *Nature* 410:968-973, 2001.

Pizzo PA, Poplack DG, editors: *Principles and practice of pediatric oncology,* London, 1989, JB Lippincott.

Protocol for dental management of oncology patients receiving chemotherapy and/or radiation therapy, Indianapolis, May 1990, Department of Dentistry, Indiana University Hospitals.

Raether DG: A double blind study of pediatric bone marrow transplant patients to assess the efficacy of a 0.12% chlorhexidine mouthrinse, master's thesis, Minneapolis, 1987, University of Minnesota School of Dentistry.

Recent advances in dental care for the hemophiliac. In Powell D, editor: *Proceedings of a workshop conference,* Los Angeles, 1979, Orthopaedic Hospital.

Sams DR, Thornton JB, Amamoo PA: Managing the dental patient with sickle cell anemia: a review of the literature, *Pediatr Dent* 12:316-319, 1990.

Shapiro AD, McKown CG: Oral management of patients with bleeding disorders. Part 1: Medical considerations, *J Indiana Dent Assoc* 70:28-31, 1991.

Smith HB, McDonald DK, Miller RI: Dental management of patients with sickle cell anemia, *J Am Dent Assoc* 114:85-87, 1987.

Stafford R et al: Oral pathoses as diagnostic indicators in leukemia, *Oral Surg Oral Med Oral Pathol* 50:134-139, 1980.

Steinle CJ, Dock M: *Mouthcare standards for hematology/oncology patients,* unpublished protocol, Cincinnati, Ohio, 1990, Children's Hospital Medical Center.

Taylor LB et al: Sickle cell anemia: a review of dental concerns and a retrospective study of dental and bony changes, *Spec Care Dentist* 15:38-42, 1995.

Thomas LB et al: The skeletal lesions of acute leukemia, *Cancer* 14:608-621, 1961.

Thornton JB, Sams DR: Preanesthesia transfusion and sickle cell anemia patients: case report and controversies, *Spec Care Dentist* 13:254-257, 1993.

The treatment of hemophilia, New York, 1975-1982, The National Hemophilia Foundation, Medical and Scientific Advisory Council.

White GE: Oral manifestations of leukemia in children, *Oral Surg* 29:420-427, 1970.

Wright W et al: An oral disease prevention program for patients receiving radiation and chemotherapy, *J Am Dent Assoc* 110: 43-47, 1985.

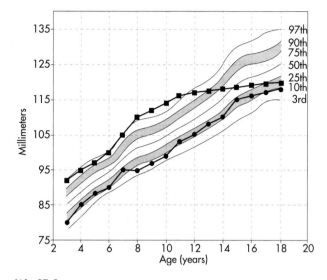

FIG. **25-6.** Cumulative growth chart for male face height (hard tissue nasion to menton), illustrating seven percentile levels. ● Relatively normal growth; ■ deviation of several percentile levels during growth, suggestive of abnormalcy. *(From Broadbent BH Sr, Broadbent BH Jr, Golden WH: Bolton standards of dentofacial developmental growth, St Louis, 1975, Mosby).*

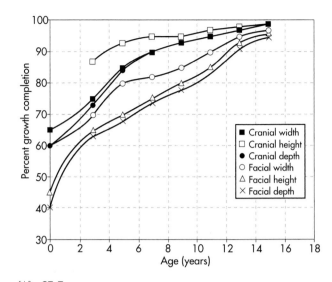

FIG. **25-7.** Cumulative growth curve for calvaria and face in width, height, and depth. *(From Scott JH: Proc R Soc Med 47:5, 1954; Meredith HV: Growth 24:215–264, 1960; and Ranley DM: A synopsis of craniofacial growth, New York, 1980, Appleton & Lange.)*

Deviations during growth of more than two percentile levels may indicate developmental problems, such as illness or disease.

Attributes (craniofacial parts) that are structurally related will also maintain a consistent relationship throughout successive stages of growth after infancy. Enlow[16] identifies the dental arches of the maxilla and mandible as an example of a structural part-counterpart relationship. An Angle class II skeletal pattern at 3 years of age will be maintained into adulthood without corrective therapy. Both dental arches in healthy individuals tend to increase in size at about the same rate. Hence, balanced or equivalent growth tends to maintain architecturally related structures of any craniofacial pattern that is present after 2 years of age.

BASIC CONCEPTS OF CRANIOFACIAL GROWTH

1. *Different parts of the craniofacial complex grow at different times.* The head takes on appearance characteristics unique to each particular growth stage. Different parts of the face experience differences in growth timing as well. The infant has a disproportionately large calvaria and forehead compared with the adult because growth of the neural tissue takes place earlier in life than facial growth.

   Size increase of the face and calvaria in the three spatial planes is a differential growth process. Scott,[19] Meredith,[20] and Ranly[21] have contributed to an understanding of this process. By birth, the cranial height dimension has attained about 70% of its adult status; cranial width, 65%; and cranial length or depth, 60% (Fig. 25-7). In contrast, only 40% of facial height and 45% of facial length (depth) has been achieved by birth. Face width (i.e., bizygomatic and bigonial), on the other hand, has attained about 60% of adult stature. Growth in face width actually falls between the classic neural and general somatic growth curves.

   After birth, a pattern in facial growth timing emerges. The anterior cranial base completes most of its growth during infancy and early childhood, but frontal and nasal bones continue outward expansion through appositional-resorptive bone growth.[22] Growth magnitude and duration are greater for the anterior maxilla than for the forehead but less than for the anterior mandible. The posterior face demonstrates the greatest incremental growth during late puberty.

2. *Differences in growth size, direction, velocity, and timing are observed among individuals.* Bergersen has also noted large variations in growth patterns among individuals and has shown that any measured attribute will demonstrate a range of expression about a central tendency.[23] Incremental growth curves for healthy males and females will demonstrate the same general disposition but may show marked differences in maturation timing (Fig. 25-8). Generally, females mature 2 years earlier than males, but Valadian and Porter have indicated that variations are so great that an early-maturing boy may mature earlier than a late-maturing girl.[3] Males tend to grow larger in size than females.

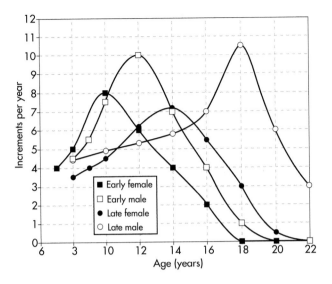

FIG. **25-8.** Incremental growth curves for early- and late-maturing males and females.

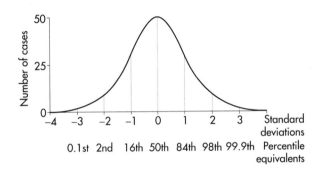

FIG. **25-9.** Normal distribution curve illustrating standard deviations and percentile equivalents.

3. *The heads and faces of no two humans are exactly the same.*
Brodie pointed out that no two humans are exactly the same.[24] This fact is no more clearly evident than when one compares, at any given age, a measured attribute shared by healthy individuals. Most attributes have a range of expression that can be graphically illustrated by a normal distribution curve (Fig. 25-9).
If the same attribute were measured in a population of individuals, the most frequently occurring value (mode), middle value in the series (median), or arithmetic average of all the measured values combined (mean) would represent the central tendency of the population. Central tendency is often referred to as *normalcy*. Another way to describe attribute distribution is by using percentile equivalents. The 50th percentile indicates the center of the distribution, the 25th percentile the lower one fourth, and so on.
A third statistical parameter often used in growth literature to indicate distribution is the standard deviation. A standard deviation (SD) of ±1 includes

about 68% of the entire population; ±2 SD and ±3 SD are equivalent to approximately 95% and 99% of the distribution, respectively. The mean values and SDs for a normative population are invaluable aids in describing a patient's condition. By comparing a patient's value to a population value for the same trait, the clinician can make statements about relative largeness or smallness. Generally, measurements beyond ±2 SD are considered clinically important because those values fall outside 95% of the population on which the normative value is based.

References will be made in the rest of this chapter to craniofacial growth principles and concepts in discussing growth of the face, occlusion, and dental arches.

CRANIOFACIAL PATTERN

In clinical assessment and treatment planning for the young patient, information about growth is often not considered to the degree that it should be. Craniofacial growth issues can be made more central to patient care concerns when a physical model is used to help visualize growth effects. For this reason, a particularly strong effort is made here to define physical craniofacial pattern.

There are two methods commonly used in dentistry to gather information about craniofacial pattern. One method is to examine the patient physically at chairside. Information collected in this fashion is based on criteria contrived and established in the practitioner's mind. The second method is to analyze dental records. Historically, cephalometric analysis has been a particularly useful tool for collecting objective information about craniofacial patterns. Generally, the patient's radiographic values measured on the cephalogram are compared with normative values derived from a population database. In this way, degrees of normalcy can be estimated by the clinician. One database is unique in its composition in that only individuals presenting with optimal or ideal craniofacial pattern were included in the study.[25] This unique conceptual approach to defining craniofacial pattern enables the practitioner to make assessments about patient optimality. Patient-measured values are compared with values from cephalograms that have relatively ideal patterns. Cephalometric analysis is discussed in Chapter 26. Darwis, Messer, and Thomas suggest that using a combination of methods, such as three-dimensional facial morphometry and Fourier analysis, can provide a more comprehensive knowledge of growth and development of craniofacial structures and thus may allow improved prediction of clinical outcomes.[26] Fourier analysis is a mathematical curve-fitting procedure that can represent boundaries so that the outlines of objects can be addressed.

IDEAL PARADIGMS FOR DENTOFACIAL PATTERN

Standards for chairside facial appraisal have been offered by Ackerman and Proffit,[27] Angle,[28] Bell, Proffit, and White,[29] Cox and van der Linden,[30] Lucker, Ribbens, and McNamara,[1] and Patterson and Powell.[31] Most of these physical appraisal models refer to the adult face. Horowitz and Hixon[32] describe idealized facial pattern as "the way things ought to be." Models available for examining the face espouse an assessment of proportion, balance, and harmony—concepts that help define overall facial attractiveness. The concept of an ideal face can be a useful clinical tool if it is used properly and its limitations are acknowledged. The first limitation is the fact that an ideal has little or no biologic basis. Biologic data can neither refute nor support the contention that the face should be ideal. Second, faces do not need to be ideal to work properly; ideal pattern, for the most part, has little connection with physiologic function. Third, an ideal model is simply a mental construct, a fiction. The words *ideal paradigm* mean "perfect example."

A perfect example can, on the other hand, be a powerful diagnostic and treatment-planning tool. The patient's facial pattern can be compared with criteria for idealness, the differences noted, and hence a problem list constructed. Criteria for an ideal face can help organize a vast array of information that is readily available to the clinician through physical observation. An ideal facial paradigm can serve as a treatment-planning tool as well. Although the concept of an ideal face is fictitious and biologically unsupported, it can serve as a guide by providing an example toward which treatment may be directed. Ideal paradigms for dental occlusion and dental arch pattern are also represented in dental literature; good examples may be found in the works of Angle,[28] Andrews,[33] and Roth.[34] The purposes served by these paradigms are the same as for ideal facial models; they are powerful diagnostic and treatment-planning aids.

GROWTH AND FACIAL PATTERN

CONSISTENCY IN PATTERN MATURATION

Following birth, the face increases in size to a greater extent than does the calvaria. Bell, Proffit, and White propose that, by adulthood, the ideal face should be equally proportioned in forehead, midface, and lower face heights.[29] Enlow has demonstrated that the facial profile flattens as the face ages. Nose and chin become more prominent and lips less pronounced.[35] (Fig. 25-10) Every healthy individual, regardless of the overall craniofacial pattern, experiences profile flattening and face height increases relative to cranium.

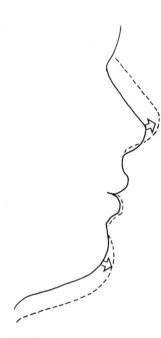

FIG. 25-10. Graphic illustration of facial profile flattening from 6 years of age *(solid line)* to 18 years of age *(broken line).*

IDEAL FRONTAL FACIAL PATTERN

Criteria for facial idealness are age dependent. Because the face elongates and the profile becomes less convex with maturity, ideal criteria appropriate for the adult face would not necessarily apply to the younger face. The ideal frontal facial pattern for a 7-year-old child might include the following criteria (Fig. 25-11):

1. Right and left face halves are symmetrical.
2. Glabella (midpoint between eyebrows) to subnasale (point where columella merges with upper lip) equals subnasale to menton (inferior aspect of chin).
3. Subnasale to lower border of upper lip represents one third the distance from subnasale to menton.
4. Upper central incisor edge is 2 mm inferior to lower border of upper lip.
5. Alar base width equals inner canthal width.

IDEAL FACIAL PROFILE PATTERN

Use of a reference plane is very helpful for evaluation of the facial profile at chairside. The Frankfort horizontal plane is an anthropometric reference line frequently used for analysis of the lateral face. It is defined by Farkas as the superior limit of the external auditory meatus and the palpated border of the infraorbital bony rim.[36] A second reference line constructed perpendicular to the Frankfort horizontal plane and through the glabella (FHP) has been used in lateral profile assessment by Legan and Burstone.[37]

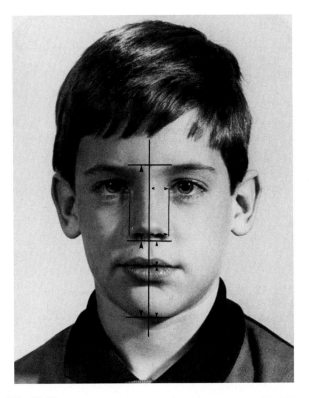

FIG. **25-11.** Ideal frontal facial pattern for a 7-year-old child.

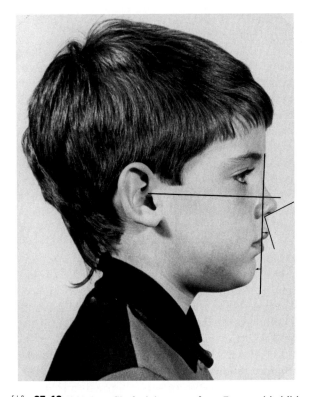

FIG. **25-12.** Ideal profile facial pattern for a 7-year-old child.

The ideal profile pattern for a 7-year-old child might include the following criteria (Fig. 25-12):

1. Chin 5 mm behind FHP
2. Most anterior aspect of lower lip on FHP
3. Most anterior aspect of upper lip 5 mm ahead of FHP
4. Nasolabial angle of 100 degrees
5. No more than 2 mm lip separation when relaxed

MAINTENANCE OF OVERALL PATTERN

The overall pattern presented by the individual at an early age will be maintained into adulthood. Although every individual experiences profile flattening and facial elongation as the face matures, Enlow et al demonstrated that the magnitude of these changes is not great enough to offset disharmonies in overall facial structure.[38] Discrepancies between the position of the maxilla and mandible persist throughout life unless clinical therapy is employed to rectify the disharmonies.

At chairside, disharmony between the maxilla and the mandible can be simply and readily identified. A list of differences can be formulated by comparing the patient's facial measurements with the criteria of an ideal face. The differences serve as a patient problem list. Adding average growth change (i.e., magnitude, direction, and velocity) to the pattern presented by the individual will give an estimate of how facial patterns will look at a later age. This growth scheme is known as a *mean-change-expansion scheme*.[32] Balbach demonstrated it to be the most useful to predict the effects of growth on facial pattern.[39] The mean-change-expansion scheme is useful for evaluation of almost all patients routinely seen in the dental office. Balanced or average growth affecting all aspects of the head and face relatively equally, however, cannot be assumed for all patients. The heads and faces of individuals who have some craniofacial congenital anomalies, hypoplastic defects, or acquired deformities that alter primary or compensatory craniofacial growth mechanisms do not grow in a typical manner. A discussion of growth in these individuals is beyond the scope of this chapter.

Because growth change in healthy children affects the face in a relatively consistent and predictable way, the key to facial diagnosis and treatment planning is the clinician's ability to identify and diagnostically describe facial pattern. Identification of balanced, proportional facial pattern, as well as recognition of facial imbalance, should be routine during patient assessment. The use of criteria related to ideal facial pattern can be helpful.

The goal in treating facial imbalance in children is to establish architectural balance in the facial pattern. If corrective measures include compensation for the effects from treatment rebound or relapse, the facial pattern established by therapy will be maintained. As the face continues to grow and increase in size, all structurally related parts of the treated face will undergo relative growth equality.

Correction of facial imbalance in the child is achieved through clinical manipulation of the means by which adaptive, compensatory facial growth occurs. Some sutures of the upper face remain patent into adolescence. Application of forces through orthopedic headgear, controlled in direction and amount, can result in an alteration of maxillary growth direction and ultimately of maxillary position. Also maxillary transverse size can be increased by judicious expansion of the palatal suture. The secondary cartilage of the mandibular condyle remains responsive to mechanical stimulation throughout life, but appositional response of this fibrocartilage decreases with age, as shown by McNamara and Carlson.[40] Facial bones respond to changes in microenvironmental stress and strain by changing form. Patterns of osseous deposition and resorption can be altered by using appliances that carefully load bone with physiologically compatible biomechanical forces.

Successful treatment of a child with facial imbalance secondary to mandibular retrognathia, for example, involves manipulation of several growth mechanisms. Mandibular anterior repositioning with a functional appliance probably affects many sites. Graber and Swain[41] believe that modification of the dentofacial complex occurs by the following means:

1. Condylar growth (secondary cartilage growth)
2. Glenoid fossa adaptation (apposition-resorption bone growth)
3. Elimination of functional retrusion
4. More favorable mandibular growth direction
5. Withholding of downward and forward maxillary arch movement (apposition-resorption bone growth)
6. Differential upward and forward eruption of lower buccal segment (apposition-resorption bone growth)
7. Orthopedic movement of maxilla and upper dentition (maxillary suture system growth)

FACIAL GROWTH EMULATES GENERAL SOMATIC GROWTH

The degree to which the facial pattern can be altered through biomechanical therapy depends on the amount of growth potential remaining. In general, the magnitude of facial pattern alteration possible is inversely proportional to age; the older the individual, the less the facial pattern can be therapeutically modified. The opportunity to alter compensatory, adaptive growth mechanisms is also greater in a rapidly growing individual. The adolescent growth spurt is characterized by increased growth velocity at about 10 to 12 years

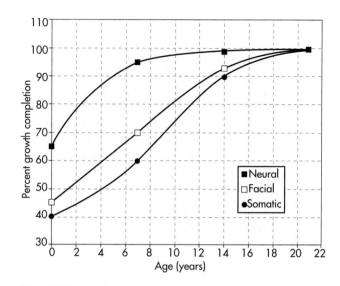

FIG. **25-13.** Cumulative growth curves for neural, facial, and general somatic tissues.

of age for girls and 12 to 14 years of age for boys. The maximum velocity or peak height velocity of growth is attained approximately 2 years after pubertal onset. Cumulative facial growth closely parallels general somatic growth (Fig. 25-13). Analysis of skeletal hand development can be helpful in estimating general skeletal maturation and, hence, facial skeletal maturation. It is relevant to evaluate a child's maturity in direct relation to the child's own pubertal growth spurt to assess whether maximum pubertal growth is imminent, has been reached, or has been passed.

GROWTH AND PATTERN OF OCCLUSION

CONSISTENCY IN PATTERN DEVELOPMENT

Usually, no teeth are clinically visible at birth. Leighton has shown that the upper anterior gum pad (intercuspid width) is typically wider than the lower anterior pad, and the upper anterior gum pad protrudes (overjet) about 5 mm relative to the lower anterior gum pad.[42] The upper anterior gum pad usually overlaps (overbite) the lower anterior pad by about 0.5 mm. In the first 6 months of postnatal life, there is marked palatal width increase, and the overjet decreases rapidly.

PRIMARY DENTITION TERMINUS

By 3 years of age, the occlusion of 20 primary teeth is usually established. The relationship of the distal terminal planes of opposing second primary molar teeth can be classified into one of three categories (Fig. 25-14). A flush terminal plane (flush terminus) means that the anterior-posterior positions of the distal surfaces of opposing primary second molars are in the same vertical

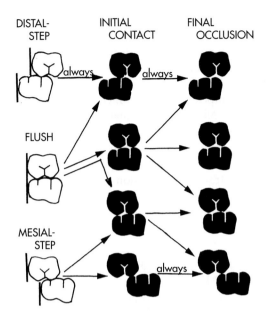

DISTAL-STEP INITIAL CONTACT FINAL OCCLUSION

always always

FLUSH

MESIAL-STEP

always

FIG. **25-14.** Graphic illustration of permanent first molar occlusion development. Outlined crown images represent three terminal plane relationships of primary second molars at about 5 years of age. Darkened images represent various permanent first molar relationships at initial occluding contact (about 6½ years of age) and at full occlusion contact (about 12 years of age). *(From Arya BS, Savara BS, Thomas DR: Am J Orthod 63:610–621, 1973; Carlsen DB, Meredith HV: Angle Orthod 30:162–173, 1960; and Moyers RA: Handbook of orthodontics, ed 3, Chicago, 1973, Mosby.)*

TABLE **25-1** Incidence of Terminal Molar Relationships at Three Stages of Occlusion Development

PRIMARY TERMINAL PLANE AT AGE 5 YEARS	INITIAL PERMANENT FIRST MOLAR OCCLUSION AT AGE 6½ YEARS	FINAL OCCLUSION AT ABOUT AGE 12 YEARS
	1% Class III	3% Class III
49% Class I (ms)	27% Class I	59% Class I
37% Flush	49% End-on	
14% Class II (ds)	23% Class II	39% Class II

From Arya BS, Savara BS, Thomas DR: *Am J Orthod* 63:610-621, 1973; Carlsen DB, Meredith HV: *Angle Orthod* 30:162–173, 1960; HEW reports: *J Clin Orthod* 12:849, 1978.
ms, Medial step; *ds*, distal step.

plane. A mesial-step terminus is defined as a lower second primary molar terminal plane that is mesial to the maxillary primary terminus. Distal-step terminal plane is descriptive of the situation in which the mandibular second primary molar terminus is distal to the upper second primary molar terminus.

Statistical studies of primary terminal plane status report that 49% of the time, the terminal plane of the lower primary second molar is mesial to the upper terminus (mesial step); the lower terminus is flush with the upper terminus 37% of the time; and the distal-step primary terminus is seen in approximately 14% of cases. These data are derived from studies reported by Arya, Savara, and Thomas[43] and by Carlsen and Meredith.[44]

OPPOSING FIRST MOLARS AT INITIAL CONTACT

The permanent first molars are clinically visible at about 6 years of age and are the first permanent teeth to emerge. The relationship of permanent first molars when initial occluding contact occurs during eruption may be represented by one of four categories (see Fig. 25-14). A class I relationship means that the mesial-buccal (m-b) cusp of the upper permanent molar contacts at or very near the buccal groove of the lower permanent first molar. This occurs approximately

55% of the time. An end-on relationship means that m-b cusps of both molars oppose one another. The incidence of this situation is about 25%. A class II relationship, occurring 19% of the time, is one in which an upper m-b cusp is anterior to the lower m-b cusp. Class III represents the situation in which an upper m-b cusp is distal to the lower buccal groove. This occurs in only 1% of the population.[44] Table 25-1 shows the incidence of medial-step, flush, and distal-step primary terminus and end-on, class I, class II, and class III permanent first molar occlusions during three stages of occlusion development.[43-45]

IDEAL STATIC OCCLUSION PATTERN

The concept of ideal occlusion development has been described by Friel[46] and by Lewis and Lehman.[47] Sanin and Savara have also shown that, to a considerable extent, ideal occlusion at a young age predisposes to an ideal adult occlusion.[48] The most desirable occlusion in the permanent dentition is a class I interdigitation, and certain features in the primary and mixed dentitions, if observed accurately, can provide clinical clues as to whether a class I relationship of the dentition will eventually develop.

The major difference between ideal adult and child occlusions is the teeth present. By 7 years of age, the primary central and lateral incisors have been or are in the process of being replaced by their permanent successors, and the permanent first molars have already erupted. The primary dentition remaining usually includes the canine and first and second molars of both arches. Criteria for ideal dental occlusion for a 7-year-old child might include the following:

1. Class I molar and canine interdigitation
2. 2-mm anterior and posterior overjet
3. 2-mm anterior overbite
4. Coincident dental midlines

The strength of the size relationships among the permanent teeth, however, is clinically important for some comparisons. Potter and Nance demonstrated that the size of an individual tooth is highly correlated with the size of the contralateral tooth in the same arch, as reflected in an *r* value of around 0.9.[57] The combined mesial-distal dimensions of contralateral quadrants of teeth show a slightly higher correlation of *r* = 0.95. Intraarch comparisons of tooth groupings, such as mesial-distal size of the lower incisors versus mesial-distal sizes of the lower canine and premolars combined, show only moderate correlation (*r* = 0.6) and therefore are not useful clinically.[58]

COMPUTATION OF TOOTH SIZE/ARCH SIZE BALANCE

The primary reason for dental arch malocclusion is imbalance between tooth size and alveolar apical size. In the transition (mixed) dentition, it is possible to accurately determine if combined mesial-distal tooth size will be balanced with alveolar arch size in later life. This process of determination is called *mixed dentition space analysis.* Many methods of mixed dentition space analysis are available. Common to all of these methods is the attempt to determine the combined mesial-distal size of the unerupted permanent canine and first and second premolars. According to Horowitz and Hixon, the lower dental arch is the focus for space analysis and the basis of orthodontic diagnosis and treatment planning.[32] The mandibular alveolar base can be modified less therapeutically than can the upper alveolus and therefore restricts treatment possibilities. The mandibular arch also undergoes less growth change than does the upper arch.

Efficacy studies by Gardner,[59] Kaplan, Smith, and Kanarek,[60] and Staley and colleagues[61-63] reveal one method to be the most accurate in predicting the combined size of the unerupted canine and premolars during the mixed dentition. This method, originally devised by Hixon and Oldfather,[58] has recently been refined by Bishara and Staley.[64] In summary, the analysis involves the following steps:

1. Measure the combined width of the lower lateral and central incisors on one side.
2. Measure directly from the radiograph the crown sizes of the unerupted 4-5 on the same side.
3. Add together the incisor and the premolar sizes.
4. Refer to the prediction chart to determine the sizes of the unerupted 3-4-5.

Techniques of mixed dentition space analysis allow estimation of the sizes of the unerupted canine and premolars on the lower arch. This size estimate must then be compared with a measurement of the arch space available between the mesial aspect of the lower molar and the distal aspect of the lateral incisor in the same quadrant. The difference between the combined width of the three unerupted permanent teeth and this arch space has been called *leeway space.*

The most favorable dental arch pattern is one in which leeway space is excessive (i.e., combined size of unerupted canine and premolars is smaller than arch space available). If leeway space is deficient, dental arch crowding will predictably result. Average growth changes in the dental arch will not be great enough to compensate for leeway deficiencies.

COMPENSATIONS IN DENTAL ARCH DEVELOPMENT

Tooth size/arch size imbalances result in dental arch conditions that are less than ideal. When combined mesial-distal tooth size exceeds alveolar arch size, compensatory adjustments occur, which results in dental arch crowding, excessive curve of Spee, or deviant axial tooth inclinations. Dental spacing results when alveolar arch size exceeds the combined mesial-distal size of the teeth.

Competent treatment planning during the mixed dentition must account not only for differences between the size of unerupted canine and premolars and the space available for them, but also for compensating dental factors. Ideal dental arch status provides a model for such planning. Each compensating factor (i.e., crowding, spacing, excess occlusal curve, or deviant axial tooth position) can be appraised relative to an ideal dental arch. Alteration of a crowded arch to an ideally aligned arch is not possible without creating extra space to resolve the crowding. Consequently, a competent dental arch treatment plan must specify the manner in which space will be clinically created. Several means are available for creating dental arch space. They include the following:

1. Move molars distally.
2. Decrease the mesial-distal dimension of the teeth present in the arch.
3. Increase the buccal-lingual axial inclination of the incisors.
4. Reduce the number of teeth in the arch by extraction.

Resolution of excessive occlusal curve also requires more space. Merrifield has indicated that generally, for each millimeter of excessive occlusal curve, 1 mm of arch length space is required.[65] To upright labially inclined incisors, arch length space is also required. In contrast, more arch length is created when retroclined incisors are proclined through therapy; the length of the arch is increased by repositioning the incisal edges from a lingual to a more labial position.

MAINTENANCE OF OVERALL PATTERN

Space analysis combined with evaluation of the impact of compensating factors on dental arch status is the means by which overall space requirements for the lower arch can be determined during the mixed dentition phase. Overall space appraisal during the mixed dentition is highly indicative of future arch status. The condition presented during the mixed dentition will, to a high degree, be maintained in the permanent dental arch. For this reason, a nonideal adult arch status can be anticipated early, and many undesirable conditions can be resolved during the transition from the primary to the permanent dental arch.

Overall space appraisal is typically expressed as millimeters of arch length space excess or deficiency. Dental arch space excess (1 to 2 mm) is a relatively ideal situation. Clinically, little intervention is usually required because mesial drifting of the permanent teeth often results in little or no crowding or residual spacing. Space excess exceeding 3 to 4 mm, however, can lead to dental arch problems. For example, congenital absence of one or more teeth can leave so much arch space that mesial drifting cannot compensate. Decisions favoring retention of primary teeth as long as possible, extraction of primary teeth and retention of space for later restorative prosthesis, or extraction followed by space closure must be made as long-term planning decisions.

Space deficiencies less than −2 mm can usually be managed with a lower lingual holding arch. Arch space deficiencies of −3 to −6 mm should be scrutinized carefully. Typically, a space-regaining lower lingual arch or arch length expansion treatment measure is indicated. Arches with deficiencies in excess of −6 mm are candidates for aggressive space-regaining techniques, dental arch expansion treatment, or one of a number of serial extraction sequences. Clinical approach to various conditions of space excess and deficiency is based on overall space appraisal (space analysis plus compensating factors) as shown in Table 25-2.

EFFECT OF ENVIRONMENTAL FACTORS ON DENTAL ARCH PATTERN

The primary determinant of dental arch malocclusion is mesial-distal tooth size/arch size imbalance. Nevertheless, secondary factors can dramatically influence the disposition of the dental arch during childhood. Dental arch status is subject to the ravaging effects of environmental factors that include early loss of primary teeth, interproximal caries, pathology, ankylosis of primary teeth, oral habits, trauma, and early eruption of permanent second molars.

The environmental factors most commonly affecting dental arch status are probably caries and premature loss of primary teeth. Early primary tooth loss and

TABLE 25-2   Clinical Disposition Guidelines for Various Dental Arch Space Conditions Resulting from Overall Mixed Dentition Space Appraisal

OVERALL APPRAISAL	mm	CLINICAL DISPOSITION
Large space excess	Greater than +3	Long-term planning
Space excess	Less than +3 to 0	No action; observation
Equivalency	0	Careful observation
Deficiency	Less than −3 to 0	Lower lingual holding arch
Moderate deficiency	−3 to −6	Space regaining or arch expansion
Large deficiency	Greater than −6	Space regaining, arch expansion, or extraction

caries can have a profound effect on dental arch status. Caries and early loss of the primary first molars (D), second molars (E), or both (D + E) result in a decrease in dental arch length. A study by Northway, Wainright, and Demirjian[50] showed the following specific details:

1. E loss had the most deleterious effect on dental arch length.
2. Early posterior primary loss resulted in 2- to 4-mm space closure per quadrant in both arches.
3. Space loss was age related in the upper but not in the lower arch.
4. Upper D loss typically resulted in blocked-out cuspids; upper E loss usually led to an impacted second permanent premolar.
5. The greatest space loss was caused by mesial molar movement.
6. More space was lost in the first year after premature tooth loss than in successive years.
7. No recovery of space was demonstrated during growth in the upper arch, and little was found in the lower arch.

SUMMARY

The goal of this chapter was to integrate basic growth principles with patient appraisal to enhance diagnostic and treatment-planning efficacy. Merging growth principles with dentofacial pattern brings to light specific growth features pertinent to clinical patient-care decision making. This chapter focused on growth events germane to a better understanding of malocclusion as it affects the face, occlusion, and dental arches. Two themes were consistent throughout the chapter.

Cephalometrics and Facial Esthetics: the Key to Complete Treatment Planning

JOHN T. KRULL

GEORGE E. KRULL

THOMAS H. LAPP

DAVID A. BUSSARD

In studying a case of malocclusion, give no thought to the methods of treatment or appliances until the case shall have been classified and all peculiarities and variations from the normal in type, occlusion, and facial lines have been thoroughly comprehended. Then the requirements and proper plan of treatment become apparent.

—Edward H. Angle

Cephalometrics, the assessment of craniofacial dimensions, particularly the ethnographic determination of cranial morphology, is an ancient skill practiced by anthropologists for centuries.

Beauty and harmony are the traditional guiding principles used to assess facial proportions, although the definition of beauty may change as civilizations change. Greek sculpture during the golden age of art (fourth century BC) shows facial proportions very similar to those found desirable today. Basic facial features of Greek male and female figures appear to be depicted identically, with most sculpture angles within 5 degrees of contemporary standards; the exceptions are a more acute mentolabial sulcus and nasofacial angle for the ancient Greek ideal.

With the advent of the twentieth century, dentistry began to include the concepts of facial harmony and balance in the theory and practice of cephalometrics. In 1922, Simon introduced this modern era with the development of gnathostatics, a photographic technique that related the teeth and their respective bony bases to each other, as well as to specific craniofacial structures. Although Racini and Carrera obtained the first x-ray films of the skull by the standard lateral view in 1926, it was not until the introduction of the cephalometer by Broadbent in 1931 that the science of cephalometrics became standardized. This sophisticated form of radiography enabled the practitioner to identify specific problem areas of craniofacial disproportion and devise detailed therapeutic interventions. Through the contributions of investigators such as Brodie, Downs, Reidel, Steiner, Tweed, and Ricketts, the clinical application of cephalometrics has developed the techniques that permit the observation of discrepancies observed in the mandible, maxilla, dental units, and soft tissue profile.

The primary aim of cephalometric analysis is to localize malocclusion within a tracing of facial bone and soft tissue structures. The analysis is performed by using standardized cephalometric landmarks to construct lines, angles, and imaginary planes, which permits linear and angular assessments of dental and facial relationships as seen on radiographic films of the head and face. These findings are compared to established normal values, and an individualized treatment protocol is developed for orthopedic, orthodontic, and orthognathic therapies.

The science of cephalometrics has often been referred to as a "numbers game" and has the reputation of being difficult to master. There appears to be a universal search for a reliable group of numbers that will ultimately lead one to an accurate diagnosis. Obviously this search is futile, because all cephalometric measurements may at times lead one to an erroneous conclusion. However, an accurate, in-depth analysis provides one with an assessment of dentofacial and craniofacial morphology. A cephalometric radiograph furnishes one with a static analysis, whereas subsequent films allow the clinician to follow the growth patterns of the adolescent patient on a longitudinal basis. In addition, comparison of serial cephalograms of the same patient may allow some developmental predictions to be made.

The use of cephalometrics serves to confirm the diagnosis and makes it possible to include the morphology of the cranium when alternative treatment modalities are considered. In patient care, cephalometrics can provide valuable data when treatment is first initiated and can serve a monitoring function during the course of orthodontic care. On completion of treatment, cephalometric radiology allows assessment of the relative degree of posttreatment stability and evaluation of treatment results produced by various mechanical and appliance selections.

Cephalometric numbers or central tendencies have been developed to serve as guidelines in evaluation of the patient. Dentists must keep in mind that they are treating individuals, not averages, and that the numbers merely help or guide in the formulation of an accurate diagnosis and treatment plan. Because of individual anatomic, biologic, and environmental variations, it is imperative that the clinician consider several factors to achieve a comprehensive case analysis. Any attempt to simplify the analysis is likely to lead to an erroneous conclusion.

The norm is commonly referred to as the mean or average. On the contrary, however, the norm, as it is applied in cephalometrics, is not a set of averages. The average patient in any given population will generally deviate from the norm, because the norm is derived from samples demonstrating ideal dental occlusions of the class I variety.

Most biologic variables are randomly distributed in the population and can be graphically illustrated by a bell-shaped curve (Fig. 26-1). Within this curve, approximately 70% of any given population lies within 1 standard deviation of the mean, whereas 95% of the group falls within 2 standard deviations. Throughout this chapter, the statistical concept of standard deviation is referred to as *clinical deviation (CD)*.

As a general rule, the goal in treatment planning is to treat in the direction of cephalometric norms.

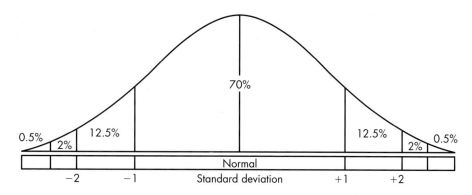

FIG. **26-1.** Bell-shaped curve illustrating the approximate distribution of biologic variables in the general population.

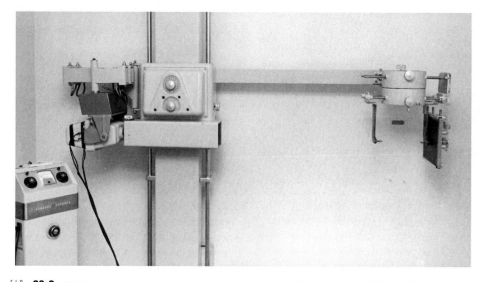

FIG. **26-2.** Wall-mounted, counterbalanced cephalometer. *(Courtesy Dr. William W. Merow.)*

The clinical advantages include the following:

1. A more favorable and predictable esthetic result
2. Greater posttreatment stability
3. Improved function and periodontal health

RADIOGRAPHIC TECHNIQUE

The technique employed in cephalometric radiology has been standardized to permit the comparison of initial and subsequent films for the same patient so that growth can be assessed and treatment progress monitored.

This standardization requires that the equipment include a headholder (cephalostat) and an x-ray tube positioned at a distance of 60 inches from the mid-sagittal plane of the subject and that the distance from the midsagittal plane of the patient to the film be approximately 7.5 inches (Fig. 26-2). The cephalostat maintains a reproducible spatial relationship with respect to the position of the patient's head, the film,

and the x-ray source. The most common device uses a counterbalanced beam with the radiographic tube on one end and the cephalostat on the other. This entire unit can be adjusted vertically to compensate for variations in patient height.

The patient is positioned in the cephalostat by means of laterally adjusted ear rods and a vertically adjusted nasal piece (Fig. 26-3). The nasal piece allows the clinician to orient the patient's head so that the Frankfort horizontal plane (a plane extending from the tragus of the ear to the inferior border of the orbital rim) is parallel to the floor. The ear posts should be centrally aligned to the source of radiation so that a transporionic axis is established.

LATERAL HEAD FILM

For a lateral head radiograph, the patient is first positioned so that the left side of the face is tangent to an 8- by 10-inch film cassette, which permits less

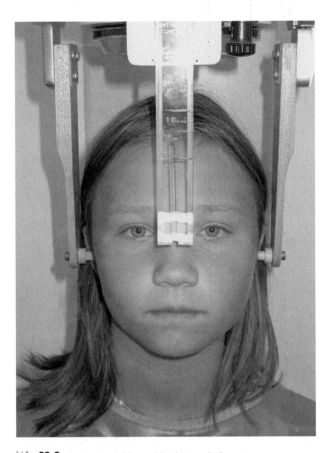

FIG. **26-3.** Patient positioned in the cephalostat.

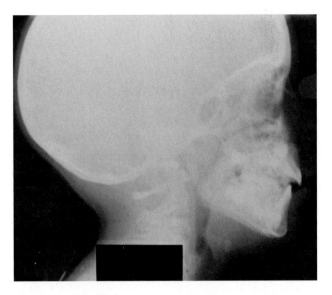

FIG. **26-4.** Lateral cephalometric film.

magnification and less distortion of the left-sided structures (Fig. 26-4).

The film cassette should be positioned as close as possible to the patient to minimize the effects of magnification, maximize resolution, and standardize the technique. The distance from the film cassette to the patient's midsagittal plane should be recorded to allow for comparison of serial films. Generally, the film is obtained with the mandible in its most retruded position and the lips in repose. Use of additional positions may be indicated. Once the patient has been positioned, the x-ray beam should enter through the ear rods perpendicular to the film.

Grids and intensifying screens are accessories used to improve the quality of the radiographic image. Rare-earth intensifying screens allow for a reduction of radiographic exposure while increasing the clarity of the radiographic image. Because the film range does not provide for sharp skeletal and soft tissue contrast, a movable aluminum screen attached to the cassette must be used over the soft tissue profile area to reduce the radiation and provide a better differential contrast between the two tissue types.

FRONTAL (POSTEROANTERIOR) FILM

Most diagnostic features related to vertical and antero-posterior (A-P) problems are evident from the lateral film, though severe maxillary transverse deficiencies or facial asymmetries may be better diagnosed by the use of a posteroanterior (P-A) film (Fig. 26-5). The patient is oriented facing the film cassette, with the ear rods and nasion piece positioning the patient so that the midsagittal and Frankfort planes are at right angles to the film cassette. After the patient's head is positioned so that the central x-ray beam passes through the head at the level of the transporionic axis and at its midpoint, the film cassette is moved into contact with the patient's nose. Because more radiation is required for this view, the milliamperage must be increased over that used in the lateral film technique.

CEPHALOMETRIC TRACING TECHNIQUE

Precise localization of the anatomic landmarks used in cephalometric analysis requires adequate knowledge of the radiographic and anatomic appearance of the facial bones and their relationships to adjacent structures. Various features are discernible: lines, shadows, the projections of bony structures, and contours of varying density. All of these make it difficult for the clinician to interpret and identify the anatomic relationships. A clear understanding of craniofacial structures and their relative spatial relationships is imperative before a lateral head film is traced.

Fig. 26-6 depicts a lateral cephalometric tracing. The lateral tracing should include the soft tissue outline, bony profile, outline of the mandible, posterior and anterior cranial base, odontoid process of the axis,

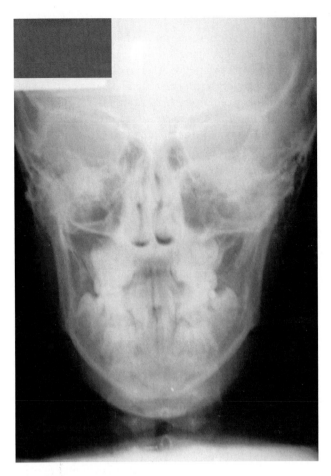

FIG. **26-5.** Frontal (posteroanterior) cephalometric film. *(Courtesy Dr. William W. Merow.)*

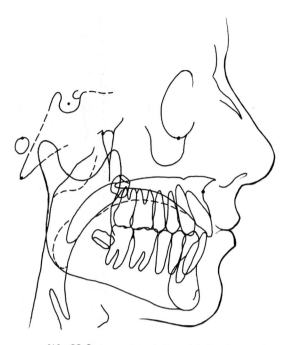

FIG. **26-6.** Lateral cephalometric tracing.

anterior lip of the foramen magnum, clivus, planum orbitale, sella turcica, orbit, pterygomaxillary fissure, floor of the nose, roof of the palate, and body of the hyoid bone. In addition to the bony tissues, at least the first permanent molars as well as the most anterior maxillary and mandibular incisors are commonly included. In certain situations it may be desirable to trace other teeth or the complete dentition as shown in Fig. 26-6.

To make the tracing, the radiograph is placed on a view box with the facial profile to the right side. Acetate tracing paper (0.003 matte) is then placed over the radiograph with the matte side up. With a sharp No. 2 or 3H drawing pencil, all the necessary structures are traced. Because all x-rays become divergent once they emanate from the collimator, magnification of the subject will result, and a double-image effect will occur along the inferior border of the mandible and the area of the posterior teeth. All paired structures will produce double images on the head films. Because left-sided structures are magnified less by the radiographic beam and are considered more accurately rendered, the outline of these structures can be traced, although some prefer to make the tracing lines bisect bilateral images.

A P-A cephalometric radiograph, as illustrated in Fig. 26-5, can be of significant diagnostic value in cases demonstrating mandibular displacement, facial asymmetry, severe posterior crossbite, or other types of bony dysplasia. Cephalometric analysis and a thorough and systematic clinical examination of these patients often reveal malocclusions accompanied by mandibular shifts when the patient is in maximum occlusion.

The P-A radiograph is traced in the same manner as the lateral film. Fig. 26-7 illustrates the important skeletal and dental structures that must be traced for an accurate and complete analysis.

REFERENCE POINTS FOR LATERAL TRACING

The ultimate diagnostic value of the cephalometric analysis is dependent on the initial accurate identification and localization of anatomic and anthropologic points (Fig. 26-8). These landmarks are used to construct the lines, angles, and planes used to make a two-dimensional assessment of the patient's craniofacial and dental relationships. Although each analysis is completed in two dimensions, when the lateral analysis and the P-A analysis for the same patient are considered together, a three-dimensional simulation emerges to contribute to the overall diagnosis and treatment plan. The following reference points are used in this chapter (see Fig. 26-8):

Sella turcica (S, or sella). The midpoint of the hypophyseal fossa. This is the ovoid area of the sphenoid bone that contains the pituitary gland.

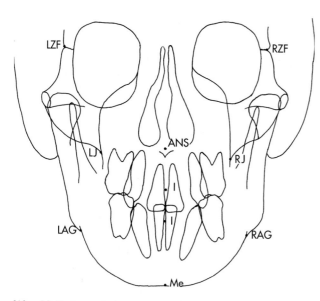

FIG. **26-7.** Frontal (posteroanterior) cephalometric tracing (see also Fig. 26-10). *ANS,* Anterior nasal spine; *I,* I (incisor) point; *LAG,* left antegonial notch; *LJ,* left jugal process of maxillary tuberosity; *LZF,* left zygomaticofrontal suture; *Me,* menton; *RAG,* right antegonial notch; *RJ,* right jugal process of maxillary tuberosity; *RZF,* right zygomaticofrontal suture.

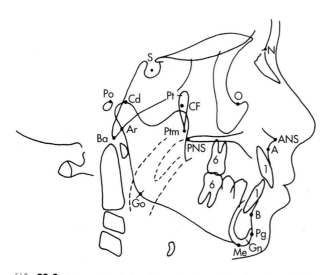

FIG. **26-8.** Lateral tracing with cephalometric reference points. *(Adapted from Dr. William W. Merow.)*

Nasion (N). The external junction of the nasofrontal suture in the median plane. If the suture is not visible, this point is located at the deepest concavity of the two bones.

Orbitale (O). The most inferior point on the external border of the orbit.

Condylion (Cd). The most superior point on the articular head of the condyle.

Anterior nasal spine (ANS). The most anterior projection of the anterior nasal spine of the maxilla in the median plane.

A point (subspinale, or A). The deepest point of the curvature of the anterior maxilla between the ANS and the alveolar crest. Although the A point may change with treatment, it represents the most forward point of the maxilla.

B point (supramentale, or B). The most posterior point on the outer curve of the mandibular alveolar process between the alveolar crest and the bony chin. The B point delineates the most anterior point of the mandible in the median plane.

Pogonion (Pg). The most anterior point on the midsagittal mandibular symphysis.

Menton (Me). The most inferior point of the mandibular symphysis.

Gnathion (Gn). A constructed point that is formed by the intersection of the facial and mandibular planes.

Gonion (Go). Another constructed point that is represented by the intersection of the lines tangent to the posterior margin of the ascending ramus and the mandibular plane.

Articulare (Ar). The point of intersection of the posterior margin of the ascending ramus and the outer margin of the cranial base.

Porion (Po). A point located at the most superior point of the external auditory meatus or the superior aspect of the metal ring that is a component of the left ear rod of the cephalostat.

Basion (Ba). The most inferior posterior point on the occipital bone that corresponds to the anterior margin of the foramen magnum.

Pterygomaxillary fissure (Ptm). A teardrop-shaped fissure of which the posterior wall is created by the anterior borders of the pterygoid plates of the sphenoid bone and the anterior wall represents the posterior border of the maxilla (maxillary tuberosity). The tip of this fissure denotes the posterior extent of the maxilla.

Posterior nasal spine (PNS). The tip of the posterior spine of the palatine bone. This landmark is usually not visible even on well-exposed lateral head films; therefore it is a constructed point that is represented by the intersection of a continuation of the anterior wall of the pterygopalatine fossa and the floor of the nose. It also denotes the posterior limit of the maxilla.

Pt point (Pt). The intersection of the inferior border of the foramen rotundum with the posterior wall of the Ptm.

CF point (center of face). The cephalometric landmark formed by the intersection of the Frankfort horizontal plane and a perpendicular line through Pt.

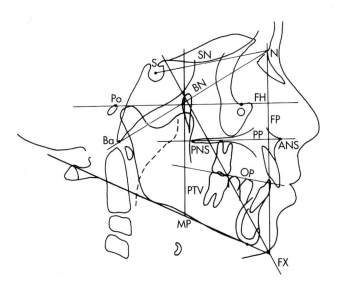

FIG. **26-9.** Cephalometric reference lines and planes. *(Adapted from Dr. William W. Merow.)*

REFERENCE LINES, ANGLES, AND PLANES

Linear assessment is derived when two reference points are connected. Angular measurements are possible when three points are used. Planes (and some lines) are actually imaginary when the cephalometric tracing is viewed because the planes are at right angles to the tracing and can be seen only as a line on the two-dimensional tracing (Fig. 26-9). In cephalometric analysis the dentist must become accustomed to thinking in three dimensions while viewing a two-dimensional representation. Therefore a point on the tracing may not only be a point but also may represent a line (or axis). A line on the tracing may actually be a line (or axis) or it may represent a plane.

Several lines or planes are used in the different cephalometric analyses, although one line or plane generally serves as the major reference on which the entire analysis is based. Two common references are the sella-nasion plane (anterior cranial base) and the Frankfort horizontal plane.

The basic units of cephalometric analysis are angles and distances (lines). Measurements may be treated as absolute values, or they may be related to one another and expressed as relative proportions. These measurements and interrelationships provide the basic framework for describing craniofacial abnormalities. The following definitions help explain the planes of reference used in this chapter (see Fig. 26-9).

Frankfort horizontal plane (FH). This plane is constructed from porion (Po) to orbitale (O) and represents the basic horizontal plane of the head.

Sella-nasion plane (SN). This plane is represented by a line connecting the sella (S) and the nasion (N).

It denotes the A-P extent of the anterior cranial base. This reference plane is of questionable diagnostic value in true mandibular prognathism.

Occlusal plane (OP). This plane separates the maxillary and mandibular permanent molars (or in younger patients the primary second molars) and passes through the contact between the most anterior maxillary and mandibular incisors. If the incisors do not contact, the line passes midway between the incisal edges. Ideally, OP is nearly parallel to both the palatal plane (PP) and the FH.

Facial plane (FP). A line constructed through the nasion (N) perpendicular to the FH represents this plane.

Mandibular plane (MP). The mandibular plane is constructed as a tangent to the inferior border of the mandible.

Pterygoid vertical plane (PTV). This plane is represented by a line perpendicular to the FH through the Pt point. Studies have shown that the intersection of FH and PTV is extremely stable, because growth has little effect on this point. An overall view of patient growth may be gained by evaluation of serial cephalometric films on which FH and PTV are superimposed. PTV represents a basic vertical reference plane.

Basion-nasion plane (BN). This plane passes through the basion (Ba) and nasion (N). The plane represents cranial base and is the dividing plane between the cranium and the face.

Facial axis (FX). This line is constructed from the Pt point through the gnathion. FX ideally crosses BN at a right angle.

Palatal plane (PP). This plane extends through the anterior nasal spine (ANS) and posterior nasal spine (PNS). The relationship of this plane to FH is useful in evaluating treatment changes occurring in the maxilla.

INTERPRETATION OF MEASUREMENTS

The objectives of cephalometric interpretation are summarized as follows:

1. To define both the skeletal and facial types
2. To evaluate the relationship between the maxillary and mandibular basal bones
3. To assess the dental relationships (the spatial relationship between the teeth, maxilla, mandible, and cranial base)
4. To locate the malocclusion within the dentofacial complex and analyze its origin (skeletal or dentoalveolar)
5. To study the facial soft tissue contours with respect to the cause of the malocclusion

6. To consider the impact of the various options for correcting the malocclusion on the facial contours as well as on the skeletal and dental components
7. To facilitate selection of a treatment plan
8. To evaluate the results of various soft tissue surgical procedures

LATERAL CEPHALOMETRIC ASSESSMENT

MAXILLARY SKELETAL

SNA: The angle between SN and N–A point
Clinical norm: 82 degrees
Clinical deviation: 2 degrees
Interpretation: Establishes horizontal location of the maxilla. Deviation in cranial base (SN, angulation, or length) or vertical maxillary excess proves that this measurement is unreliable. Therefore reduced emphasis should be given in these instances.

Maxillary depth: The angle formed by the intersection of the FH and N–A point planes
Clinical norm: 90 degrees
Clinical deviation: 3 degrees
Interpretation: Indicates horizontal position of maxilla. Class II skeletal patterns caused by a prognathic

maxilla show values exceeding 90 degrees. Chronic thumb suckers generally demonstrate large values.

Maxillary length: The measurement of the line extending from Cd to A point
Clinical norm: 85 mm female, 87 mm male
Clinical deviation: 6 mm
Interpretation: Increases 1 mm per year until adult size is attained (95 to 100 mm). This measurement determines if the class II or class III skeletal pattern is attributable to a long or short maxilla, respectively.

ANB: The difference between the SNA and SNB angles
Clinical norm: +2 degrees
Clinical deviation: 2 degrees
Interpretation: Indicates the horizontal relationship between maxilla and mandible. Positive values indicate that the maxilla is forward of the mandible, whereas negative values indicate a class III skeletal relationship.

MAXILLARY DENTAL

Maxillary incisor angulation: The angle formed by SN and the incisor long axis
Clinical norm: 102 degrees
Clinical deviation: 3 degrees

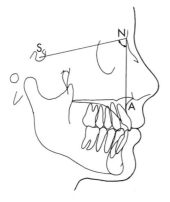

SNA

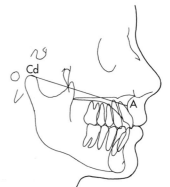

MAXILLARY LENGTH

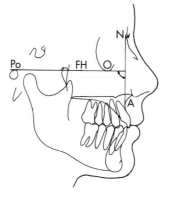

MAXILLARY DEPTH

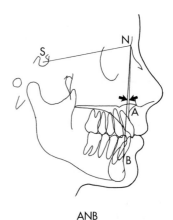

ANB

Interpretation: Relates the upper incisor angulation to the upper and middle face. Values well above 102 degrees indicate angular incisor protrusion, whereas values significantly below demonstrate angular retrusion.

Maxillary incisor A-P position: The horizontal distance from the facial surface of the maxillary central incisors to the N–A point line

Clinical norm: 4 mm

Clinical deviation: 2 mm

Interpretation: Indicates horizontal position of the maxillary incisors. Values in excess of 6 mm indicate anterior dental protrusion, whereas values 1 mm or less show dental retrusion.

Upper molar position: The horizontal distance from PTV to the distal surface of the maxillary first molar

Clinical norm: Chronologic age of the patient + 3 mm (e.g., a 10-year-old has a clinical norm of 10 + 3 = 13 mm). The growth change is approximately 1 mm per year through the years of active growth.

Clinical deviation: 3 mm

Interpretation: Determines if the dental malocclusion is caused by the A-P position of the maxillary molar. It is important in treatment planning considerations involving distal movement of the maxillary molars.

Maxillary incisor to upper lip: The vertical distance between the inferior border of the upper lip and the incisal edge of the maxillary incisor

Clinical norm: 3 mm

Clinical deviation: 1 mm

Interpretation: Gives an evaluation of the amount of upper incisor in repose. Values of 5 mm or more may be associated with vertical maxillary excess. This value must be compared with upper lip length. Obviously, patients with short upper lips will show more incisor at rest.

MANDIBULAR SKELETAL

SNB: The angle formed between the SN and N–B point planes

Clinical norm: 80 degrees

Clinical deviation: 2 degrees

Interpretation: Indicates horizontal location of the mandible. Abnormal cranial base angulation and vertical facial excess will adversely affect the reliability of this measurement.

Facial angle (depth): The angle formed between the N-Pg and FH planes

Clinical norm: 87 degrees at 9 years of age. Increases 0.33 degree per year.

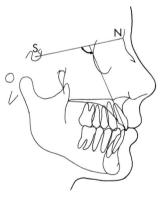

MAXILLARY INCISOR ANGULATION

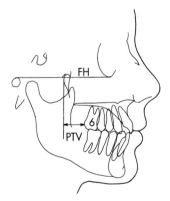

UPPER MOLAR POSITION

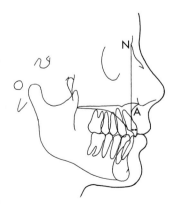

MAXILLARY INCISOR (A-P) POSITION

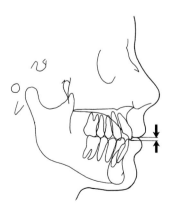

MAXILLARY INCISOR TO UPPER LIP

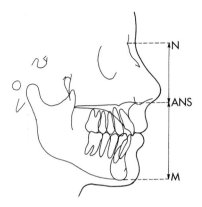

FACIAL HEIGHT

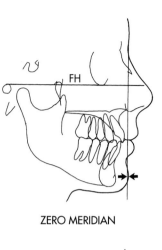

ZERO MERIDIAN

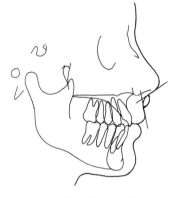

NASOLABIAL ANGLE

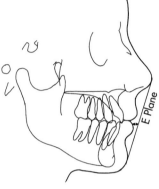

LIP PROTRUSION

Clinical norm: 90 to 110 degrees

Interpretation: Provides an assessment of the nose-to-upper-lip relationship. Values in excess of 114 degrees may indicate upper lip retrusion, whereas values of 96 degrees or less may be associated with dental protrusion.

Zero meridian: The horizontal distance from the chin to a line perpendicular to FH and tangent to the soft tissue nasion

Clinical norm: 0 mm

Clinical deviation: 2 mm

Interpretation: May be helpful in assessment of the projection of the chin relative to FH.

Interlabial distance: The vertical distance between the inferior aspect of the upper lip and the superior surface of the lower lip with the patient in repose

Clinical norm: 1.9 mm

Clinical deviation: 1.2 mm

Interpretation: High values indicate lip incompetence and are often associated with hyperactivity of the mentalis muscle. Low values may be associated with overclosure.

Lip protrusion: The horizontal distance between the lower lip and the esthetic plane (E plane). The esthetic plane is a line connecting the tip of the nose and the most anterior point on the soft tissue chin.

Clinical norm: −2 mm at 8.5 years of age; decreases 0.2 mm per year. The values tend to decrease with age until adult values of −5 mm are reached.

Clinical deviation: 2 mm

Interpretation: Indicates soft tissue balance between lips and profile (nose-chin).

FRONTAL (POSTEROANTERIOR) CEPHALOMETRIC ASSESSMENT

Frontal cephalometric points and planes are used to evaluate the overall relationships of the cranium, maxilla, mandible, and denture from a frontal view. Fig. 26-10 is a graphic representation of the points, lines, and planes used in frontal cephalometric analysis.

Dental midline: The horizontal distance between the maxillary and mandibular incisor midlines

Clinical norm: 0 mm

Clinical deviation: 1.5 mm

Interpretation: Determines dental midline asymmetry.

Maxillomandibular width: The horizontal distance between the jugal process of the maxilla and the frontal facial plane

Clinical norm: 10 mm for patient of average size at 8½ years of age. Needs to be corrected for size.

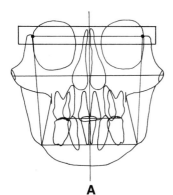 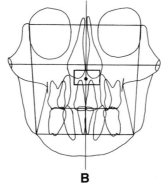 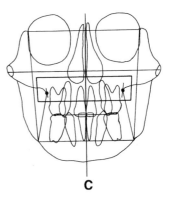

A   B   C

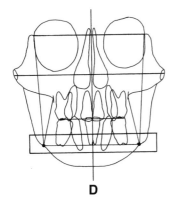 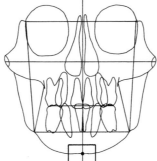 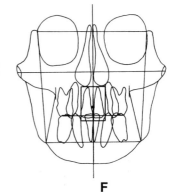

D   E   F

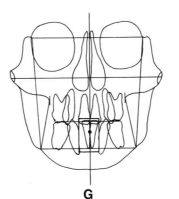

G

FIG. 26-10. Frontal reference points (see also Fig. 26-7). **A,** *LZF/RZF,* bilateral points on the medial aspect of the zygomaticofrontal sutures at the intersections of the orbits. **B,** *ANS,* tip of anterior nasal spine. **C,** *LJ/RJ,* bilateral points on the jugal processes and the intersection of the maxillary tuberosities and the zygomatic buttresses. **D,** *LAG/RAG,* points at the lateral inferior margin of the antegonial protuberances of the mandible. **E,** *Me,* menton, point of the inferior border of the mandibular symphysis directly inferior to the mental protuberance. **F,** *I point,* a point selected at the interdental papilla of the upper incisors at the junction of the crowns and gingiva. **G,** *I point,* a point selected at the interdental papilla of the lower incisors at the junction of the crowns and gingiva.

Interpretation: Determines if a crossbite is skeletal in nature. Large values are associated with skeletal lingual crossbites, whereas lesser values indicate skeletal buccal crossbites.

Maxillomandibular midline: The angle formed by the ANS-Me plane through ANS and perpendicular to the zygomatic frontal suture plane

Clinical norm: 0 mm

Clinical deviation: 2 mm

Interpretation: Determines whether facial asymmetry is attributable to total size discrepancy or a functional shift of the mandible.

Denture to jaw midlines: The horizontal distance between the midlines of the mandibular incisors and maxilla and mandible

Clinical norm: 0 mm

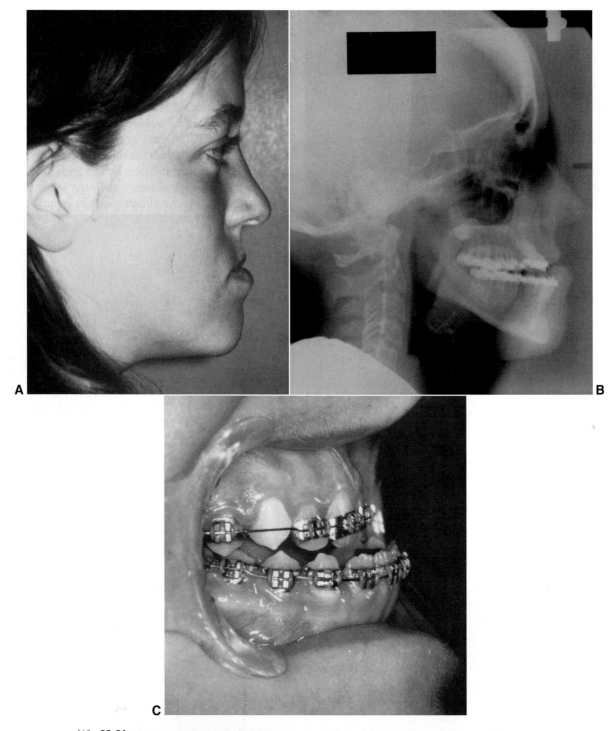

FIG. **26-21.** **A,** Mandibular prognathism (clinical appearance). **B,** Mandibular prognathism (cephalometric radiograph). **C,** Class III occlusion.

head should be positioned with the Frankfort horizontal plane parallel to the floor (Fig. 26-22). Do not ask the patient simply to "look straight ahead," because the patient will tend to place his or her head in the position the patient habitually prefers. It is also important to position the patient's occlusion in centric relation rather than centric occlusion. The patient's lips should be in repose during the examination. Patients frequently mask lip incompetence by forcing their lips together.

FRONTAL VIEW

The evaluation begins with the frontal view. This is the view people most often see of themselves. The balance

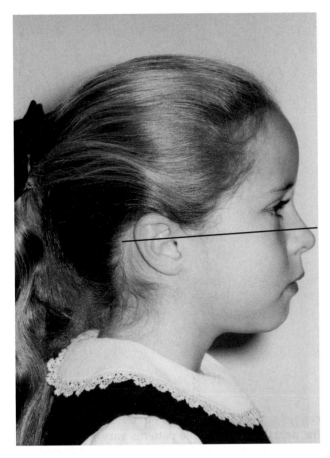

FIG. **26-22.** Patient's head positioned with the Frankfort horizontal parallel to the floor.

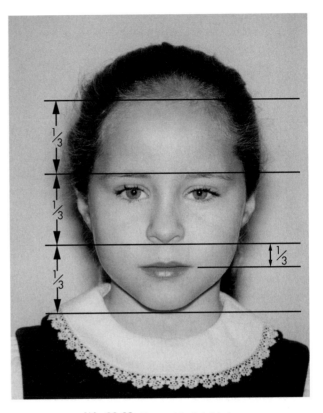

FIG. **26-23.** Frontal facial thirds.

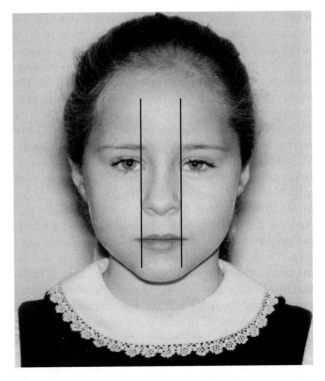

FIG. **26-24.** Comparison of the intercanthal distance and alar base width.

between the upper, middle, and lower thirds of the face is analyzed (Fig. 26-23). The upper third is bounded by the hairline (when combed back) and glabellar area. This area is least informative and is not the area to which corrections would normally be directed. More emphasis is placed on the proportions and symmetry of the middle third (from the glabellar region to subnasale) and the lower third (subnasale to menton).

In the middle third of the face, when the patient is looking straight ahead, the sclera of the eye is not seen superior or inferior to the pupil. Normal intercanthal distance is 30 to 32 mm (CD, ± 2 mm). Normal interpupillary distance is 60 to 65 mm. The inner and outer canthal tendons should fall close to a straight horizontal axis through the palpebral fissures (the fissures created when the eyelids are closed). The distance between the semilunar folds in the intercanthal area should approximate the alar base width (Fig. 26-24). Deviations from these general guidelines could indicate some deformity of the middle facial third.

Evaluation of the lower facial third is then carried out. The ratio of the middle and lower facial thirds in vertical height should be approximately 5:6. The upper

Suggested Readings

Angle EH: Classification of malocclusion, *Dent Cosmos* 41:248-264, 350-357, 1899.

Arnett GW: Facial keys to diagnosis and treatment planning—part I, *Am J Orthod Dentofacial Orthop* 103:299-312, 1993.

Arnett GW: Facial keys to diagnosis and treatment planning—part II, *Am J Orthod Dentofacial Orthop* 103:395-411, 1993.

Bell WH, Proffit WR, White RP: *Surgical correction of dentofacial deformities,* vol 1, Philadelphia, 1980, WB Saunders.

Boley JC: Serial extraction revisited: 30 years in retrospect, *Am J Orthod Dentofacial Orthop* 112:575-577, 2002.

Broadbent BH: A new x-ray technique and its application to orthodontia, *Angle Orthod* 1:45-66, 1931.

Broadbent BH: The face of the normal child, *Angle Orthod* 7:183-208, 1937.

Brodie AG and others: Cephalometric appraisal of orthodontic results: a preliminary report, *Angle Orthod* 8:261-351, 1938.

Burstone CJ: Lip posture and its significance in treatment planning, *Am J Orthod* 53:262-284, 1967.

Downs WB: Variations in facial relationships: their significance in treatment and prognosis, *Am J Orthod* 34:812-840, 1948.

Dugoni SA and others: Early mixed dentition treatment: post-treatment evaluation of stability and relapse, *Angle Orthod* 65:311-332, 1995.

James RD: A comparative study of facial profiles in extraction and nonextraction treatment, *Am J Orthod Dentofacial Orthop* 114:265-276, 1998.

Katz MI: Angle classification revisited. Is current use reliable? *Am J Orthod Dentofacial Orthop* 102:173-179, 1992.

Klocke A, Nanda RS, Kahl-Nieke B: Skeletal class II patterns in the primary dentition, *Am J Orthod Dentofacial Orthop* 112: 596-601, 2002.

Lines PA, Lines RR, Lines CA: Profilemetrics and facial esthetics, *Am J Orthod* 73:648-657, 1978.

Long RE, McNamara JA: Facial growth following pharyngeal flap surgery: skeletal assessment on serial lateral cephalometric radiographs, *Am J Orthod* 87:187-196, 1985.

McNamara JA: Influence of respiratory pattern on craniofacial growth, *Angle Orthod* 51:269-300, 1981.

Owen AH III: Diagnostic block cephalometrics, part 1, *J Clin Orthod* 18:400-422, 1984.

Owen AH III: Clinical interpretation of diagnostic block cephalometric analysis, *J Clin Orthod* 20:710-715, 1986.

Morley J: The role of cosmetic dentistry in restoring a youthful appearance, *J Am Dent Assoc* 30:1166-1172, 1999.

Reidel RA: The relation of maxillary structures to cranium in malocclusion and in normal occlusion, *Angle Orthod* 22:142-145, 1952.

Ricketts RM: Cephalometric analysis and synthesis, *Angle Orthod* 31:141-156, 1961.

Ricketts RM, Schulhof RJ, Bagha L: Orientation—sella-nasion or Frankfort horizontal, *Am J Orthod* 69:648-654, 1976.

Rody WJ Jr, Araujo EA: Extraction decision-making wigglegram, *J Clin Orthod* 36:510-519: 2002.

Sarver DM: Video cephalometric diagnosis (VCD): a new concept in treatment planning? *Am J Orthod Dentofacial Orthop* 110:128-136, 1996.

Schulhof RJ: When S-N is abnormal, *J Clin Orthod* 11:343, 1977.

Simon PW: *Fundamental principles of a systematic diagnosis of dental anomalies,* Boston, 1926, The Stratford.

Steiner C: Cephalometrics for you and me, *Am J Orthod* 39: 729-755, 1953.

Tweed CH: The Frankfort-mandibular incisor angle (FMIA) in orthodontic diagnosis, treatment planning and prognosis, *Angle Orthod* 24:121-169, 1954.

27

Management of the Developing Occlusion

JEFFREY A. DEAN

RALPH E. McDONALD

DAVID R. AVERY

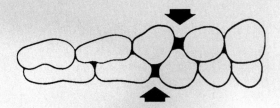

FIG. **27-1.** Primate spaces between the maxillary primary lateral incisor and primary canine and between the mandibular primary canine and mandibular first molar. *(Adapted from Baume LJ: J Dent Res 29:129, 1950.)*

The goal of every practitioner who provides dental care for children and adolescents should be to properly assess and manage the developing dental occlusion of their patients. Indeed, the following position statement is made by the American Academy of Pediatric Dentistry in the Guideline on Management of the Developing Dentition in Pediatric Dentistry[1]:

Guidance of the eruption and development of the primary and permanent dentitions is an integral part of the specialty of pediatric dentistry. Such guidance should contribute to the development of a permanent dentition that is in a harmonious, functional, and esthetically acceptable occlusion. Pediatric dentists have the responsibility to recognize, differentiate, and either appropriately manage or refer abnormalities in the developing dentition as dictated by the complexity of the problem and the individual clinician's training, knowledge, and experience. Early diagnosis and successful treatment of developing malocclusions can have both short-term and long-term benefits while achieving the goal of occlusal harmony, function, and dental facial esthetics.

The following statement was made by Ngan, Wei, and Yen[2]:

Pediatric dentistry has increasingly shifted from a conservative-restorative approach toward a concept of total pediatric patient care. Thus, all aspects of oral health care including diagnosis, prevention, oral medicine, restoration, and correction of malocclusion are increasingly the responsibility of the pediatric dentist.

With this background, it is the goal of this chapter to address management of the developing occlusion in the child and adolescent. The chapter progresses from a short review of the development of the normal occlusion to a discussion of current concepts in space maintenance for the pediatric patient. It also includes an overview of interceptive and comprehensive orthodontic care for the primary, mixed, and early permanent dentition.

DEVELOPMENT OF THE OCCLUSION

The supervision of the developing dentition and the initiation of preventive procedures, including space maintenance, require an understanding of the biogenetic course of the primary and permanent dentition. A review of the clinical studies by Baume provides this information.[3] Plaster study models of the primary dentitions of 30 children were made at various developmental stages. Two consistent morphologic arch forms of the primary dentition were found: either spaces between the teeth were present at all stages (type I) or the teeth were in proximal contact at all stages (type II). Spacing in the primary dentition is apparently congenital rather than developmental. Spaced arches frequently exhibit two

distinct diastemas: one between the mandibular canine and the first primary molar and the other between the maxillary lateral incisor and the primary canine (Fig. 27-1). Baume referred to these spaces as *primate spaces*.

Baume observed that from about 4 years of age until the eruption of the permanent molars the sagittal dimensions of the dental arches remained essentially unchanged. A slight decrease in this dimension can occur either as a result of mesial migration of the primary second molar just after eruption or after the development of dental caries on the proximal surfaces of the molar teeth. Only minor changes in the transverse dimension of the maxillary and mandibular primary arches occurred during the period from 3½ to 6 years of age.

A comparative study of models of the dentitions of 60 children before and after the eruption of the permanent molars revealed three distinct kinds of normal molar adjustment (Fig. 27-2). Any mesial shift of molars will use the leeway space. If this space is needed for the eruption of the premolars and canines, the molar shift should be prevented by a holding lingual arch.

Moyers believed that the pattern of transition involving the straight terminal plane is normal but that the occlusion forming a mesial step (distal surface of the lower second primary molar is mesial to the same surface of the maxillary molar) is more ideal.[4] Proper permanent molar occlusion was achieved by a late mesial shift of the mandibular permanent molars. A distal step (distal surface of the lower second primary molar is distal to the same surface of the maxillary molar) is abnormal and is indicative of a developing class II malocclusion.

Further evaluation of serial casts of the dentitions of 60 children were made by Baume at the time of eruption of the permanent incisors. A transverse widening of the mandibular arches occurred, representing a physiologic process to provide space for the erupting permanent incisors with their greater mesiodistal widths. This widening was brought about by lateral and frontal alveolar growth during the time of the eruption of the permanent incisors. The mean increase in intercanine

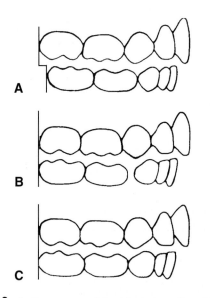

FIG. **27-2. A,** Occurrence of terminal plane forming a mesial step that allows the first permanent molar to erupt into proper occlusion. **B,** Straight terminal plane with primate space; an early shift of mandibular molars into the primate space allows proper first permanent molar occlusion (early shift). **C,** Straight terminal plane without primate space; proper first permanent molar occlusion is not attained until the mandibular second primary molar exfoliates, which then allows the desirable mesial shift of the mandibular first permanent molar (late shift).

width was greater in the maxillary arch than in the mandibular arch. The increase was also greater in previously closed upper or lower primary arches than in previously spaced arches. In the mandibular arch the greatest tendency to lateral growth was noticed during the eruption of the lateral incisors, whereas in the maxillary arch it occurred during the eruption of the central incisors. A secondary spacing of the maxillary primary incisors occasionally occurred when the still undeveloped maxillary arch was widened somewhat by the eruption of the mandibular permanent central incisors. Spaced primary arches generally produced favorable alignment of the permanent incisors, whereas about 40% of the arches without spacing produced crowded anterior segments.

Bishara et al noted similar arch development changes in their study of patients from 6 weeks to 45 years of age as follows[5]:

1. Significant increases in maxillary and mandibular arch width occurred between 6 weeks and 2 years of age.
2. Although arch width increased significantly between 3 and 13 years of age, after complete eruption of the permanent teeth there was a slight decrease in the width, more in the intercanine than in the intermolar area.

3. The mandibular intercanine width was established by 8 years of age (i.e., after the eruption of the four incisors).

Therefore Bishara et al suggest that in the average patient there is no scientific basis for expanding the arches beyond the dimensions established at the time of the complete eruption of the canines and molars.

DIAGNOSTIC RECORDS AND ANALYSIS

The clinical examination should assess the patient's overall health status as well as the patient's occlusion (from both an aesthetic and a functional standpoint) and temporomandibular joint function. As for the diagnostic records that are necessary, the records obtained may be as simple as study models only, such as when treating a bilateral posterior crossbite, or as detailed as complete orthodontic records, such as when treating a 4-year-old patient with a class III skeletal malocclusion. These diagnostic records may include an eight-film series of extraoral and intraoral photographs, appropriately trimmed orthodontic study models, a full-mouth series or panoramic radiograph, lateral and anteroposterior cephalograms, and, when indicated, appropriate temporomandibular diagnostic views such as corrected axis tomograms or magnetic resonance imaging. The diagnostic records can be analyzed using many different methods. A form similar to the one used at the Indiana University School of Dentistry Pediatric Dentistry section is very helpful in composing the clinical examination and formulating the patient's diagnosis, problem list, and treatment plan summary (Fig. 27-3). Cephalometric analysis is reviewed in Chapter 26. Finally, the patient's neuromuscular growth and nasopharyngeal airway must be assessed. Patients who are obligate mouth breathers secondary to hypertrophic adenoid tissue or allergic conditions can have correspondingly poor postural relationships that can influence the developing skeletal face. Appropriate referral to the pediatrician or otolaryngologist for further assessment is warranted in these situations.

ARCH-LENGTH ANALYSIS*

Nance Analysis. Nance concluded, as a result of comprehensive studies, that the length of the dental arch from the mesial surface of one mandibular first permanent molar to the mesial surface of the corresponding tooth on the opposite side is always shortened during the transition from the mixed to the permanent dentition.[6] Nance further observed that in the average patient's mandibular arch a leeway of 1.7 mm per side exists between the combined mesiodistal widths of the

---

*The revised Hixon and Oldfather method for analyzing arch length is presented in Chapter 25.

ORTHODONTIC DIAGNOSIS, TREATMENT, AND MECHANICS PLAN

Name _____ Race ___ Sex ___ Birthdate ___ Age ___ Chart No. _____

Resident's Name: _____ Records Date: _____

1. Patient History

A. Significant Medical History: _____
_____

B. Patient's and/or Parents' Chief Complaint: _____
_____

C. Attitude Toward Treatment: _____
_____

2. Clinical Examination

A. Soft Tissue
   Profile _____ Lip Competence _____ Lip/Incisor at Rest _____ Smiling _____
   Oral Hygiene _____ Periodontal Status _____ Other _____

B. Occlusion Class: I   II   III   Division: I   II
   Overjet _____ mm   Overbite _____ mm   Midline _____ mm
   Crossbite _____
   Molar Relation: Left _____   Right _____
   Cuspid Relation: Left _____   Right _____

C. Dental Development Stage and Eruption Sequence:

D. Habits and/or Other Significant Clinical Findings:

E. TMJ and Function:
   Opening Path: Normal Deviated: _____
   Closing Path: Normal Deviated: _____
   Range of Motion: Vertical _____ mm   Protrusion: _____ mm
                        Left Deviation: _____ mm Right Deviation: _____ mm
   Joint Sounds   None   Left   Right
                   Opening   _____   _____
                   Closing   _____   _____
                   Crepitus   _____   _____
   Muscle Tenderness: None   _____
   Tongue Function: Normal   _____

3. Model Analysis   Static Tanaka and Johnston Analysis (JADA 1974)

Total M-D Width of Upper Incisors _____ mm "A"   Total M-D Width of Lower Incisors _____ mm "B"

Maxillary Arch Length Discrepancy (From $\underline{6|}$ to $\underline{|6}$)   Mandibular Arch Length Discrepancy (From $\overline{6|}$ to $\overline{|6}$)
Total Predicted Tooth Mass: Total Predicted Tooth Mass:
   [("B" ÷ 2) + 11 mm] × 2 + "A" = _____ mm   [("B" ÷ 2) + 10.5 mm] × 2 + "B" = _____ mm
Total Measured Arch Length   =   _____ mm   Total Measured Arch Length   =   _____ mm
         Difference   _____ mm   Difference   _____ mm

FIG. **27-3.** Indiana University School of Dentistry Pediatric Dentistry section "Orthodontic Diagnosis, Treatment, and Mechanics Plan" form.   *Continued*

4. Attach computerized cephalometric tracing and appropriate analysis.

5. Diagnostic and Arch Length Analysis Summary and Problem List

6. Treatment Plan or Objective Sequence

7. Mechanics Plan—Appliance Selection—Retention

8. Projected Treatment Time (With Good Compliance), Treatment Fees

9. Faculty Authorization to Start Treatment:

_____   _____

Signature   Date

FIG. **27-3, cont'd.** Indiana University School of Dentistry Pediatric Dentistry section "Orthodontic Diagnosis, Treatment, and Mechanics Plan" form.

primary mandibular canine and first and second primary molars and the mesiodistal widths of the corresponding permanent teeth, with the primary teeth being larger. This difference in the total mesiodistal width of the corresponding three primary teeth in the maxillary arch compared with the width of the three permanent teeth that succeed them is only 0.9 mm per side.

Currently the Nance arch-length analysis is seldom used, partly because the involved procedures for this analysis require a complete set of periapical radiographs. The clinical reliability of other analyses that do not use radiographs is sufficient for determining major arch-length inadequacies.

Moyers Mixed Dentition Analysis. The analysis advocated by Moyers has numerous advantages. It can be completed in the mouth as well as on casts, and it may be used for both arches.[4] The analysis is based on a correlation of tooth size; one may measure a tooth or a group of teeth and predict accurately the size of the other teeth in the same mouth. The mandibular incisors, because they erupt early in the mixed dentition and may be measured accurately, have been chosen for measurement to predict the size of the upper, as well as the lower, posterior teeth.

Tanaka and Johnston Analysis. The Tanaka and Johnston method of arch-length analysis is a variation of Moyers' analysis except that a prediction table is not needed.[7] The estimated widths in millimeters of the unerupted canines and premolars correspond to the 75% level of probability in Moyers' prediction table. The sum of the widths of the mandibular permanent incisors is measured and divided by 2. For the lower arch, 10.5 mm is added to the result and, for the upper arch, 11 mm is added to the result to obtain the total estimated widths of the canines and premolars. For example, if the width of the lower incisors is 23 mm, divide by 2 and add 10.5 mm for the lower arch. The result is 22 mm compared with 22.2 mm obtained from Moyers' table. The corresponding values for the maxillary arch are 22.5 mm according to the Tanaka and Johnston analysis and 22.6 in Moyers' table. One can then take these tooth mass predictions and compare them with the total measured arch length and obtain any redundancies or inadequacies in the arch length.

Irwin, Herold, and Richardson reviewed the various methods of mixed dentition analysis.[8] They concluded that the Hixon and Oldfather method is more accurate and any error involves a consistent underprediction of tooth size, which is of less clinical significance than the overprediction of tooth size, as seen in all the other methods. Its disadvantage is that it is more cumbersome. Moyers claimed that, for the measure of mandibular incisors alone, 95% of the dentitions of patients with a combined width of canine and premolar

teeth within 1 mm of the predicted value should be clinically acceptable.[4] Therefore the Tanaka and Johnston analysis provides significant clinical acceptability with a minimal amount of time and effort.[7]

Another particularly valuable study model analysis is the Bolton analysis.[9] This analysis addresses tooth mass discrepancies between the maxillary and mandibular arches. It can be used to compare the sum of the mesiodistal widths of the 12 maxillary teeth with that of the 12 mandibular teeth, first molar to first molar, and to compare the 6 maxillary teeth with the 6 mandibular teeth, canine to canine. The Bolton analysis ratio is as follows:

$$\text{(Sum mandibular)}/\text{(Sum maxillary)} \times 100 = \text{Tooth mass ratio}$$

For the overall ratio (12 teeth versus 12 teeth), the mean is 91.3 (±1.91)%. For the anterior ratio (6 teeth versus 6 teeth), the mean is 77.2 (±1.65)%.

When a significant discrepancy with these ratios is noted, the clinician must assess where the tooth mass problem is located and decide on the best method to resolve it. It is not always an easy matter to detect a problem. A common example is smaller than normal maxillary lateral incisors. Depending on the size of the discrepancy and the patient's overall malocclusion, two methods that might be used to resolve this problem include slenderization of the mandibular anterior teeth or bonding to increase the mesiodistal width of the lateral incisors.

PREVENTIVE MANAGEMENT OF THE DEVELOPING OCCLUSION
PLANNING FOR SPACE MAINTENANCE

Ideally, as the occlusion develops from the primary dentition through the transitional (or mixed) dentition to the permanent dentition, a sequence of events occurs in an orderly and timely fashion. These events result in a functional, esthetic, and stable occlusion. When this sequence is disrupted, however, problems arise that may affect the ultimate occlusal status of the permanent dentition. When such disruptions do occur, appropriate corrective measures are needed to restore the normal process of occlusal development. Such corrective procedures may involve some type of passive space maintenance, active tooth guidance, or a combination of both.

Miyamoto, Chung, and Yee observed the effects of the early loss of primary canines and first and second molars on malocclusion of the permanent dentition.[10] They studied 255 schoolchildren 11 years of age or older at the final examination of the permanent dentition. Malocclusion was evaluated by scoring malalignment and measuring crowding in the anterior teeth. Children who had a premature loss of one or more canines or molars more commonly received orthodontic treatment for the permanent dentition. The likelihood of needing orthodontic treatment increased with the number of prematurely lost teeth. The frequency of orthodontic treatment in children who had lost one or more primary teeth through 9 years of age was more than three times higher than in the control group. In untreated children there was no detectable relationship between the premature loss of canines and the malalignment of permanent teeth. However, the premature extraction of molars significantly affected alignment and was especially associated with major malalignment of permanent teeth. No differences in effects were observed between the loss of the first and second primary molars. Crowding of the anterior teeth was directly affected by the premature loss of primary canines.

A tooth is maintained in its correct relationship in the dental arch as a result of the action of a series of forces (Fig. 27-4). If one of these forces is altered or removed, changes in the relationship of adjacent teeth will occur and will result in drifting of teeth and the development of a space problem. There is lack of agreement regarding the frequency with which space closure will occur or a malocclusion will develop after premature loss of a primary or a permanent tooth; however, the following general factors influence the development of a malocclusion:

1. *Abnormal oral musculature.* High tongue position coupled with a strong mentalis muscle may damage the occlusion after the loss of a mandibular primary molar. A collapse of the lower dental arch

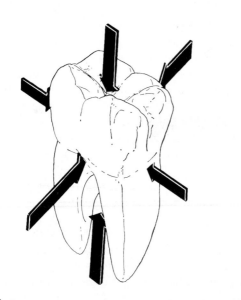

FIG. **27-4.** Forces that act on a tooth to maintain its relationship in the arch. If one of these forces were removed, as would be the case if a tooth mesial to the tooth shown were extracted, forward tipping and mesial drifting would occur.

and distal drifting of the anterior segment will result.
2. *Oral habits.* Thumb or finger habits cause abnormal forces on the dental arch and are responsible for initiating a collapse after the untimely loss of teeth.
3. *Existing malocclusion.* Arch-length inadequacies and other forms of malocclusion, particularly class II, division 1, usually become more severe after the untimely loss of mandibular primary teeth.
4. *Stage of occlusal development.* In general, more space loss is likely to occur if teeth are actively erupting adjacent to the space left by the premature loss of a primary tooth.

The following factors are important when space maintenance is considered after the untimely loss of primary teeth.

1. *Time elapsed since loss.* If space closure occurs, it usually takes place during the first 6 months after the extraction. When a primary tooth is removed and all factors indicate the need for space maintenance, it is best to insert an appliance as soon as possible after the extraction.
2. *Dental age of the patient.* The chronologic age of the patient is not as important as the developmental age. Grøn studied the emergence of permanent teeth based on the amount of root development, as viewed on radiographs, at the time of emergence.[11] She found that teeth erupt when three fourths of the root is developed, regardless of the child's chronologic age. Several studies have indicated that the loss of a primary molar before 7 years of age (chronologic) will lead to delayed emergence of the succedaneous tooth, whereas the loss after 7 years of age leads to an early emergence. The magnitude of this effect decreases with age. In other words, if a primary molar is lost at 4 years of age, the emergence of the premolar could be delayed by as much as 1 year; emergence will occur at the stage of root completion. If the same primary molar is lost at 6 years of age, a delay of about 6 months is more likely; emergence will occur at a time when root development approaches completion.
3. *Amount of bone covering the unerupted tooth.* Predictions of tooth emergence based on root development and the influence of the time of the primary tooth loss are not reliable if the bone covering the developing permanent tooth has been destroyed by infection. In such a situation the emergence of the permanent tooth is usually accelerated. If there is bone covering the crowns, it can

be readily predicted that eruption will not occur for many months; insertion of a space-maintaining appliance is indicated. A guideline for predicting emergence is that erupting premolars usually require 4 to 5 months to move through 1 mm of bone as measured on a bite-wing radiograph.

4. *Sequence of the eruption of teeth.* The dentist should observe the relationship of developing and erupting teeth adjacent to the space created by the untimely loss of a tooth. A similar situation exists if the first primary molar has been lost prematurely and the permanent lateral incisor is in an active state of eruption. The eruption of the permanent lateral incisor will often result in a distal movement of the primary canine and an encroachment on the space needed by the first premolar. This condition is frequently accompanied by a shift in the midline toward the area of the loss. In the mandibular arch a "falling in" of the anterior segment may occur and an increased overbite may result.

5. *Delayed eruption of the permanent tooth.* Individual permanent teeth are often observed to be delayed in their development and consequently in their eruption. It is not uncommon to observe partially impacted permanent teeth or a deviation in the eruption path that will result in abnormally delayed eruption. In cases of this type it is

generally necessary to extract the primary tooth, construct a space maintainer, and allow the permanent tooth to erupt and assume its normal position (Fig. 27-5).

6. *Congenital absence of the permanent tooth.* If permanent teeth are congenitally absent, the dentist must decide whether to hold the space for many years until a fixed replacement can be provided or to allow the space to close.

FACTORS RELATED TO ARCH-LENGTH ADEQUACY

Before placing space maintainers or starting tooth movement, the dentist must thoroughly evaluate arch length. This is particularly important during the primary and mixed dentition periods. Regardless of the arch-length analysis method used, several factors other than linear arch length and tooth size must be considered. First, the position of the lower incisors over basal bone must be determined. If the teeth are retroclined, one may obtain additional arch length by placing them in a more normal axial inclination. If the lower incisors are near their upper limit when measured to the mandibular plane on a cephalogram, further flaring or anterior advancement would jeopardize the periodontal support of these teeth. Also, the degree of crowding and amount of space needed to correctly align the anterior segment must be determined. Generally,

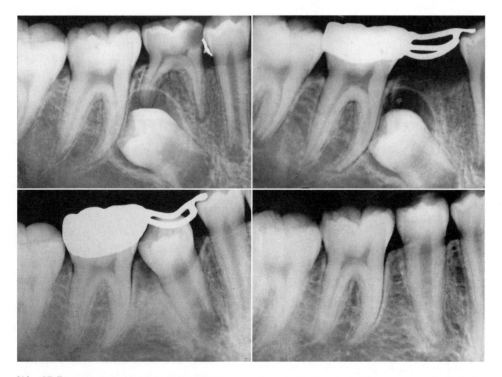

F I G. **27-5.** Extraction of the second primary molar and space maintenance were indicated because of prolonged retention of the primary tooth and partial impaction of the second premolar. The second premolar eventually erupted into its normal position.

every overlapped contact will require at least 1 mm or more of space for correction, depending on the severity of crowding.

Using radiographic measurements, prediction charts, or combinations of the two, one should determine the size of the unerupted premolars and canines. In some instances, unusually large permanent teeth will necessitate removal of teeth because of the significant tooth mass/arch-length discrepancy. The depth of the curve of Spee may also influence available arch length. According to Andrews, the ideal occlusion will have a nearly flat or very slight curve of Spee.[12] When leveled, the teeth will require more linear space than they occupied before. Generally, 1 mm of linear space is required per side for every millimeter of the depth of the curve of Spee (Fig. 27-6).

Finally, if the leeway space as described by Nance is not used, the total arch length will be decreased further as the permanent molars shift mesially. Whether this space should be maintained with holding arches depends on the space requirements as determined from an arch-length analysis. In some instances, holding leeway space may allow the permanent premolars and

canines to erupt and still provide some space to alleviate anterior crowding. If the leeway space is not held, future orthodontic treatment may require premolar extractions to allow the anterior segment to be aligned.

The available arch circumference (arch length), which is the distance from the mesial surface of the first permanent molar on one side of the arch to the mesial surface of the first permanent molar on the opposite side of the arch, is continually decreasing. Arch length decreases through the proximal wear and mesial movement of the first permanent molars at the time of the exchange of teeth. Moorrees reported that the average arch length of an individual is smaller at 18 years of age than at 3 years of age.[13] This is the result of the decrease in maxillary and mandibular dental arch length that occurs between 10 and 14 years of age, caused by the exchange of primary molars for the first and second premolars.

Barber believes that the goal should be the prevention of arch-length loss in any degree, no matter how small.[14] He points out that the combined mesiodistal widths of the primary teeth essentially equal the combined mesiodistal widths of their permanent successors in the same arch. Thus the leeway described by Nance between the combined mesiodistal widths of the primary canine, first and second molars, and their successors may be needed to allow the already erupted permanent incisors to unwind and alleviate anterior crowding in many persons.[6]

SPACE MAINTENANCE

In instances in which there is no question that permanent teeth will have to be removed to obtain a favorable occlusion, space maintenance may not be advisable; the space would need to be closed during orthodontic treatment anyway. Regardless of the possibility of future orthodontic treatment for the patient, holding space to allow the teeth to erupt and to prevent impactions is valuable. Teeth always can be removed later if necessary.

Another factor involved in space management is the developmental stage of the occlusion at the time of tooth loss. Obviously, loss of a second primary molar at 5 years of age requires different considerations than loss of the molar prematurely during the late mixed dentition period. Also, teeth erupting adjacent to the edentulous area have a greater effect on the amount of space lost than do fully erupted teeth. For example, if the first primary molar is lost during the time of active eruption of the first permanent molar, a strong forward force will be exerted on the second primary molar, causing it to tip into the space required for the eruption of the first premolar. Changes in the occlusion may extend as far as the midline after the loss of the first primary molar; a shift of the midline toward the space

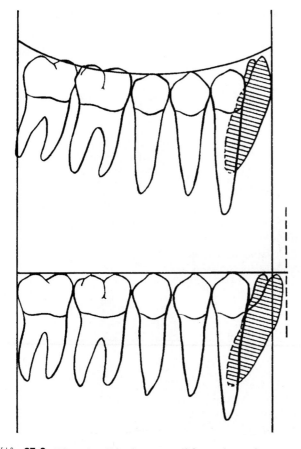

FIG. **27-6.** When leveling the curve of Spee shown here, one needs approximately 4 mm additional length (2 mm on each side), because the average depth is 2 mm.

is created by the untimely loss, and retrusion of the anterior segment on the affected side and an increased overbite may result.

Space Maintenance for the First and Second Primary Molar and the Primary Canine Area

The Band and Loop Maintainer. The space maintainer called a *band and loop* is easy and economical to make, takes little chair time, and adjusts easily to accommodate the changing dentition (Figs. 27-7 and 27-8). However, it does not restore chewing function and will not prevent the continued eruption of the opposing teeth; these may or may not be important factors, depending on the case requirements.

The stainless steel crown and loop maintainer may be used if the posterior abutment tooth has extensive caries and requires a crown restoration or if the abutment tooth has had vital pulp therapy, in which case it is

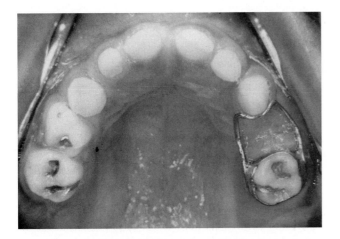

FIG. **27-7.** Trial seating of a properly fitted and designed band and loop appliance. The appliance is ready to be cemented into place.

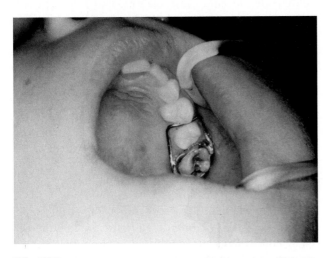

FIG. **27-8.** Band and loop maintainer. The loop is sufficiently large to allow the eruption of the permanent tooth.

desirable to protect the crown with full coverage. The steel crown should be prepared as described in Chapter 18. However, before cementation, a compound impression is made, the crown is removed from the tooth and seated in the impression, and the stone working model is prepared. A piece of 0.036-inch steel wire is used to prepare the loop. The advantages of the crown and loop maintainer are similar to those of the band and loop. Because it is difficult to remove the crown to make adjustments in the loop, some dentists prefer to adapt a band over a cemented crown restoration and construct a conventional band and loop appliance.

The loss of the second primary molar will usually have less effect on the teeth in the anterior segment than the loss of a first primary molar. However, an irregularity may develop in the permanent molar relationship. Early loss of the second primary molar is invariably followed by mesial drifting of the first permanent molar and possible impaction of the second premolar (Fig. 27-9). Also a maxillary molar often will rotate mesial in.

The space-maintaining appliances that are generally advocated when the second primary molar is lost are the band and loop and the passive lingual arch. The passive lingual arch is discussed later in the chapter. In relatively uncomplicated cases, the band and loop maintainer with the band placed on the first permanent molar can be used (Fig. 27-10). If the first primary molar is the abutment tooth, it may be lost before the time when the space-maintaining appliance can be discarded.

Loss of the primary canine is infrequently caused by dental caries but may occur at the time of the eruption of the permanent lateral incisor. When the loss of the primary canine occurs prematurely and there has been no shift in the midline or space closure, a band and loop or a lingual arch with a spur can be used. The first primary molar is the abutment tooth if a band and loop is made. If the permanent molars can be banded, the lingual arch is probably the preferred appliance.

A band and loop may require a vertical projection in which the loop contacts the abutment tooth (see Fig. 27-5). This occlusal rest can prevent tipping and can prevent the anterior portion of the loop from sliding below the proximal height of contour, which can lead to the wire's embedding in the gingival tissue several weeks or months later.

In the mixed dentition, a passive soldered lingual arch is almost always the appliance of choice in the mandibular arch, especially if the permanent mandibular incisors exhibit crowding. Also, the upper lingual arch (Nance appliance) or the lower lingual arch is the appliance of choice when bilateral space loss is present or when leeway space must be preserved. The use of unilateral and bilateral band and loop maintainers is

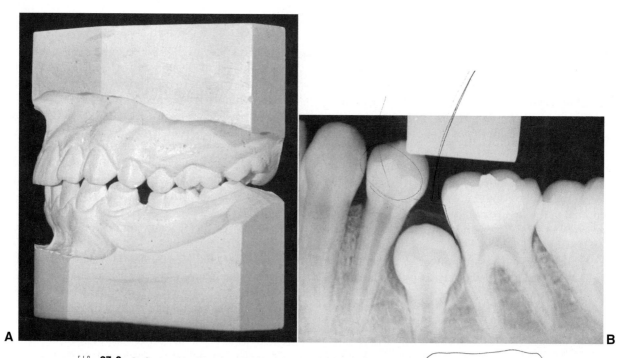

FIG. 27-9. A, Casts showing the result of the early loss of a mandibular second primary molar. **B,** Radiograph of an impacted second premolar. Space needed for the eruption of this tooth has been almost completely lost.

not indicated to manage leeway space; however, bilateral band and loop maintainers are needed before the eruption of the permanent incisors.

Loss of the Second Primary Molar Before Eruption of the First Permanent Molar

Mesial movement and migration of the first permanent molar often occurs before eruption in instances of premature loss of the second primary molar (Fig. 27-11). This is one of the most difficult problems of the developing dentition to confront the pediatric dentist. Use of a space maintainer that will guide the first permanent molar into its normal position is indicated.

The Distal Shoe Appliance. Roche has advocated a crown and band appliance with a distal intragingival extension.[15] This appliance or modifications of it may be used to maintain space or, in some instances, to influence the active eruption of the first permanent molar in a distal direction (Fig. 27-12).

Using the first primary molar as the abutment, the dentist first prepares the tooth for a stainless steel crown, which is carefully contoured and cemented. The stainless steel crown provides a desirable retentive contour for the placement of a stainless steel band, although a well-adapted band on a noncrowned tooth may be satisfactory.

The band is placed over the steel crown on the abutment tooth. A compound impression is made, the band is removed and placed in the impression, and a stone model is prepared. If the second primary molar

has not yet been removed, it is cut off the model. A hole that simulates the position of the distal root of the tooth is made in the model using a bur. If the second primary molar has been removed previously, the positioning of the tissue extension may be determined with dividers and a bite-wing radiograph. If the corresponding second primary molar is present, the correct mesiodistal width can be measured from it.

The tissue-bearing loop is next contoured with a 0.040-inch wire extending distally and into the prepared opening on the model. The free ends of the loop are soldered to the band. Next, the band and loop appliance is removed from the model and the V of the tissue extension is filled in and soldered with pieces of 0.040-inch wire. A knife edge is formed at the apex of the V if the second primary molar has previously been extracted and the extraction site has healed. Thus the maintainer may still be used, because the sharpened distal shoe may be forced through the anesthetized area of the ridge. If the appliance is delivered at the time of extraction, the intragingival extension is just polished but not sharpened.

Before final placement of the maintainer in the mouth, a radiograph of the appliance should be made to determine whether the tissue extension is in proper relationship with the unerupted first permanent molar. Final adjustments in length and contour of the shoe may be made at that time. The soft tissue has been observed to tolerate the extension of this type of

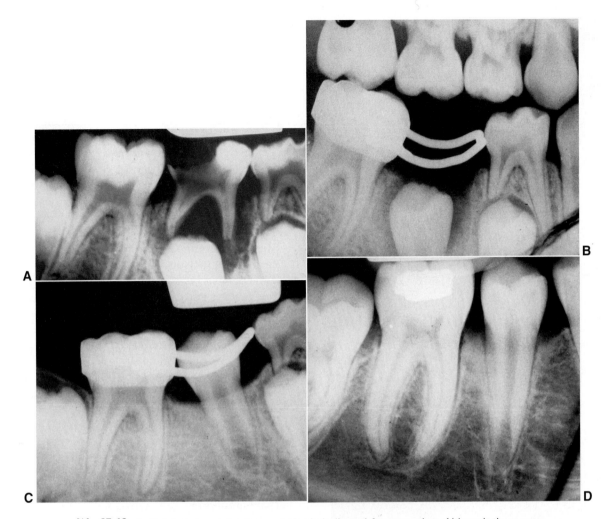

FIG. **27-10.** **A,** Pulpless second primary molar is indicated for extraction. Although there was considerable loss of bone covering the crown of the second premolar, there was concern about space loss before eruption of the tooth. **B,** A band and loop maintainer has been constructed immediately after the removal of the pulpless primary tooth. **C,** The second premolar has erupted through the loop. The maintainer may now be removed. **D,** Adequate space has been maintained in the arch of the second premolar.

appliance well, although a small metallic "tattoo" in the gingiva may result. A minimum of adjustment is required (Fig. 27-13). It is not necessary for the distal extension to be in direct contact with the permanent molar unless the tooth has already moved mesially. If the mesiodistal dimension of the second premolar has been duplicated in the appliance, the length of the loop will be correct. The depth of the intragingival extension should be about 1.0 to 1.5 mm below the mesial marginal ridge of the molar, or just sufficient to "capture" its mesial surface as the tooth erupts and moves forward. After the molar has erupted, the intragingival extension is removed. If the appliance is to be used as a reverse band and loop space maintainer, it may be necessary to add a supragingival extension to prevent the molar from tipping over the wire.

Brill describes the chairside-fabricated distal shoe appliance as an efficient and cost-effective appliance for guiding the unerupted permanent first molar into position after premature loss or extraction of the second primary molar (Fig. 27-14).[16] The data he presented indicate that success rates for this chairside-fabricated distal shoe are approximately equal to those in previous studies examining the longevity of other space maintainers.

There are several conditions that contraindicate the use of the distal shoe appliance. If several teeth are missing, abutments to support a cemented appliance may be absent. Poor oral hygiene or lack of patient and parental cooperation greatly reduces the possibility of a successful clinical result. Certain medical conditions, such as blood dyscrasias, immunosuppression, congenital

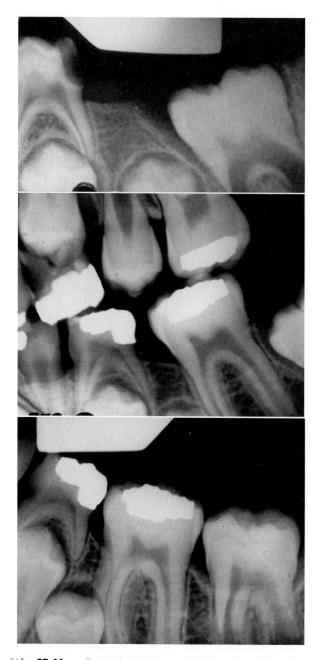

FIG. **27-11.** A sequence of three radiographs showing the untimely loss of the second primary molar and mesial movement of the first permanent molar before its eruption. Eventually there was complete closure of the space needed for the second premolar.

heart defects, history of rheumatic fever, diabetes, or generalized debilitation, almost without exception contraindicate the use of the distal shoe. The normal, healthy patient usually will have no problems with the appliance; the medically compromised patient will be placed at greater risk. Histologic studies show that the distal shoe implant never becomes totally lined

with epithelium and is associated with a chronic inflammatory response.

In cases in which use of the distal shoe is contraindicated, two possibilities for treatment exist: (1) allow the tooth to erupt and regain space later or (2) use a removable or fixed appliance that does not penetrate the tissue but places pressure on the ridge mesial to the unerupted permanent molar. Carroll and Jones have reported three cases in which a pressure appliance, removable or fixed, was used to guide the permanent molar as it erupted.[17] If several teeth are missing, the removable appliance can also be designed to restore function and prevent supereruption of opposing teeth.

Space Maintenance for the Primary and Permanent Incisor Area

Some dentists believe that space closure rarely occurs in the anterior part of the mouth, but this is not true; each case must be critically evaluated. It is important to consider the occlusion and the degree of spacing, if any, between the anterior teeth. If the anterior primary teeth were in contact before the loss or there is evidence of an arch-length inadequacy in the anterior region, a collapse in the arch after the loss of one of the primary incisors is almost certain (Fig. 27-15).

Removable Partial Dentures. Even when spacing is present, it may be desirable to construct a partial denture or a fixed appliance to reproduce a desirable esthetic appearance, to reestablish function, or to prevent abnormal speech and tongue habits. Acrylic partial dentures have been used successfully to replace maxillary anterior primary teeth (Fig. 27-16). Appliances of this type can be constructed for young children who show a degree of cooperation and interest. It is unwise to place a removable partial denture, however, if an uncontrolled dental caries problem exists or if the child's mouth will not be kept clean enough to reduce the possibility of dental caries activity.

Fixed Appliances. If a fixed appliance is required, one approach is to attach the anterior replacement teeth to a 0.040- or 0.045-inch stainless steel wire framework retained with bands or crowns on the second primary molars. If the first primary molars are present, an indirect retainer may be placed on the occlusal area to prevent the wire from flexing. One can also obtain additional stabilization by using a Nance button or covering the ridge with dental acrylic resin.

The loss of anterior permanent teeth requires immediate treatment by the dentist if intraarch changes are to be prevented. Within a few days after the loss of a tooth as a result of trauma or the extraction of a severely traumatized tooth, the teeth adjacent to the space will begin to drift, and often within a few weeks several millimeters of space will be lost. Rather than allow the extraction area to heal and regain normal contour,

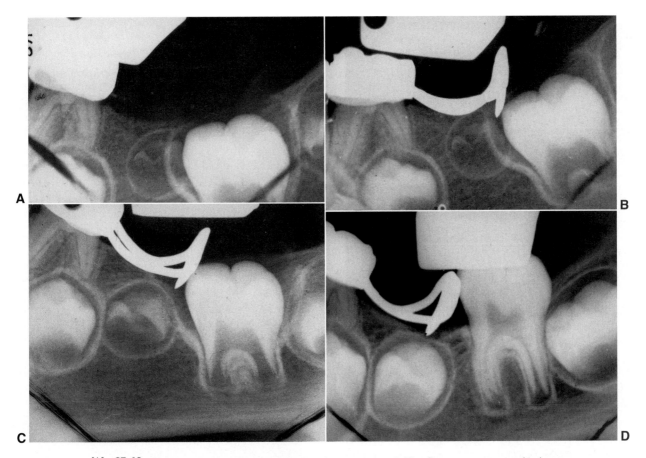

FIG. **27-12.** **A,** The second primary molar has been extracted. The first permanent molar has migrated mesially several millimeters after the extraction. **B,** Crown and band appliance with a distal shoe to guide an unerupted first permanent molar into its normal position. Notice the contour of the distal shoe to direct the first permanent molar distally and regain the lost space. **C,** Progress can be seen in the eruption of the permanent molar. **D,** The first permanent molar has erupted. The distal shoe tissue extension may now be removed. The appliance may be recemented as a reverse band and loop space maintainer, or a lingual arch appliance may be required.

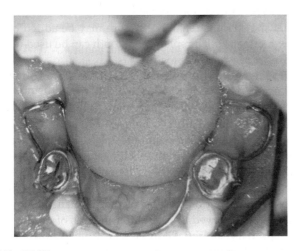

FIG. **27-13.** A modified Roche distal shoe appliance to provide bilateral space maintenance and eruption guidance for the first permanent molars. The permanent molars are erupting properly, and the intragingival extensions may be removed.

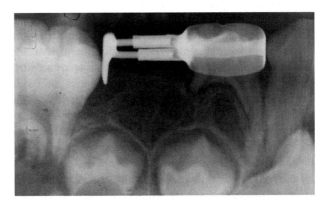

FIG. **27-14.** Radiograph of chairside-fabricated distal shoe space maintainer in place.

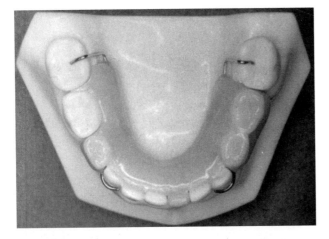

FIG. **27-19.** Acrylic partial-denture space maintainer to compensate for the untimely loss of three primary molars. The acrylic base material can be cut away to allow for the early eruption of one of the premolars before the maintainer is discarded. The acrylic may also be extended along the lingual tissues of the first permanent molars to incorporate retentive clasps for the molars if necessary.

fabrication of the acrylic extension. The acrylic will extend into the alveolus after removal of the primary tooth. The extension may be removed after the eruption of the permanent tooth. The contraindications for use of this appliance are the same as previously discussed with regard to the distal shoe appliance.

Passive Lingual Arch. The soldered lingual arch may be the space maintainer of choice after the multiple loss of primary teeth in the maxillary or in the mandibular arch (Fig. 27-22). Although it does not satisfy the requirements for restoring function, the appliance has many advantages that outweigh this fact. The use of the lingual arch essentially eliminates the problem of patient cooperation. With properly fitted bands and a well-made appliance, there should be no problems with breakage or retention and no concern about whether the child is wearing it.

On the working model a 0.036- or 0.040-inch steel wire is contoured to the arch, extending forward to make contact with the cingulum area of the incisors. In contouring the arch wire, one should allow for the path of eruption of the premolar and canines so that the arch wire will not interfere. Should this occur, the appliance will need to be remade or altered. Where possible, an ideal anterior arch form should be constructed so that the incisors have an opportunity for alignment. The arch wire should be extended posteriorly along the middle third of the lingual surface of the molar band and soldered firmly, but passively, in this position. A similarly designed lingual arch or one of the W-shaped kind can be used in the maxillary arch.

Full Dentures for Children. It is occasionally necessary to recommend the extraction of all the primary

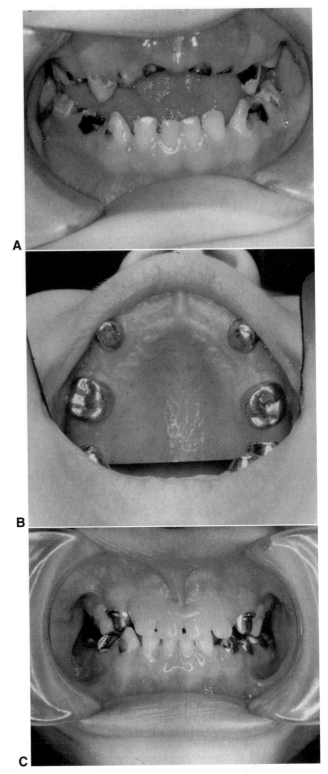

FIG. **27-20. A,** This child requires removal of the maxillary primary incisors and the first primary molars. **B,** Chrome steel crowns have been placed on the primary canines and second molars. **C,** A maxillary partial denture restores function, improves appearance, and reduces the possibility of a tongue-thrusting habit.

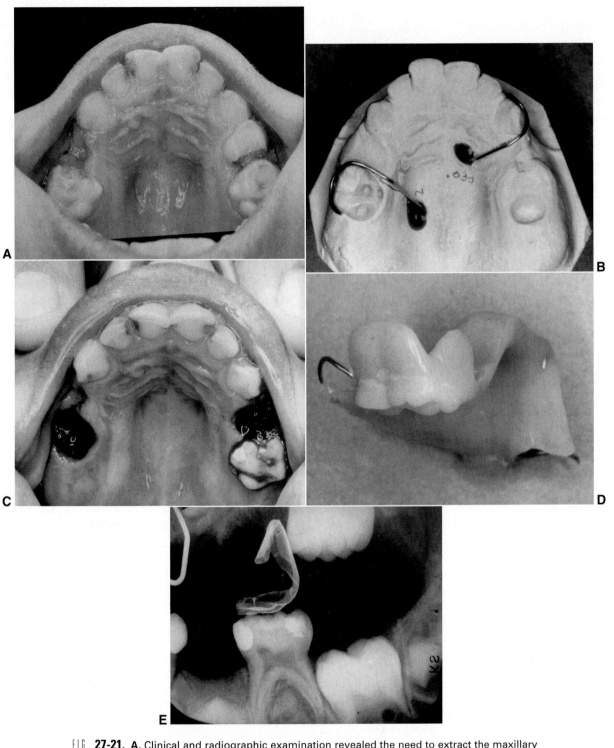

FIG. **27-21.** **A,** Clinical and radiographic examination revealed the need to extract the maxillary left first and second primary molars. The photograph is a mirror image. **B,** The teeth indicated for extraction are cut away from the stone model. A depression is made on the second molar area for the acrylic distal shoe extension. **C,** The primary teeth have been extracted in preparation for the placement of the partial denture. **D,** Acrylic distal shoe extension. **E,** Lead foil has been placed over the tissue extension to determine, with the aid of a radiograph, whether the acrylic is positioned properly to guide the eruption of the first permanent molar. *(Courtesy Dr. Paul E. Starkey.)*

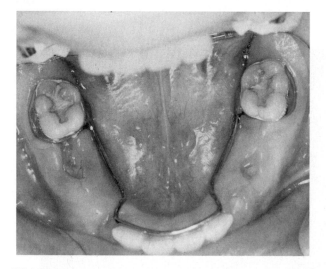

FIG. **27-22.** Mirror view of a passive mandibular soldered lingual arch immediately after cementation. *(Courtesy Dr. Theodore R. Lynch.)*

teeth of a preschool child. Although this procedure was more common in the prefluoridation era, some children even today must have all of their teeth removed because of widespread oral infection and because the teeth are unrestorable. Preschool children can wear complete dentures successfully before the eruption of permanent teeth (Fig. 27-23).

Loss of the First Permanent Molar

The first permanent molar is unquestionably the most important unit of mastication and is essential in the development of functionally desirable occlusion. A carious lesion may develop rapidly in the first permanent molar and occasionally progress from an incipient lesion to a pulp exposure in a 6-month period. The loss of a first permanent molar in a child can lead to changes in the dental arches that can be traced throughout the life of that person. Unless appropriate corrective measures are instituted, these changes include diminished local function, drifting of teeth, and continued eruption of opposing teeth.

The second molars, even if unerupted, start to drift mesially after the loss of the first permanent molar. A greater degree of movement will occur in children in the 8- to 10-year age group; in older children, if the loss occurs after the eruption of the second permanent molar, only tipping of this tooth can be expected. Although the premolars will undergo the greatest amount of distal drifting, all the teeth anterior to the space, including the central and lateral incisors on the side where the loss occurred, may show evidence of movement. Contacts will open and the premolars, in particular, will rotate as they fall distally (Fig. 27-24). There is a tendency for the maxillary premolars to move

distally in unison, whereas those in the lower arch may move separately.

When the maxillary first permanent molar loses its opponent, it will erupt at a faster rate than the adjacent teeth. The alveolar process will also be carried along with the molars and will cause problems when prosthetic replacements are needed. The treatment of patients with the loss of first permanent molars must be approached on an individual basis. A superimposed existing malocclusion, abnormal musculature, or the presence of deleterious oral habits can affect the result, as in the case of the premature loss of primary molars.

Loss of the First Permanent Molar Before the Eruption of the Second Permanent Molar. Although it is possible to prevent overeruption of a maxillary first permanent molar by placing a lower partial denture, there is no completely effective way to influence the path of eruption of the developing second permanent molar other than the use of an acrylic distal shoe extension on a partial denture as described previously. The second molar will drift mesially before eruption when the first permanent molar has been extracted. Repositioning this tooth orthodontically is possible after its eruption. However, the child must then be considered for prolonged space maintenance until the time when a more permanent tooth replacement can be inserted.

The removal of the opposing first permanent molar, even when the tooth appears to be sound and caries free, is sometimes recommended in preference to allowing it to extrude or to subjecting the child to prolonged space maintenance and eventual fixed replacement (Figs. 27-25 and 27-26).

If the first permanent molars are removed several years before the eruption of the second permanent molars, there is an excellent chance that the second molars will erupt in an acceptable position (Fig. 27-27). However, the axial inclination of the second molars, particularly in the lower arch, may be greater than normal.

The decision as to whether to allow the second molar to drift mesially or to guide it forward in an upright position may be influenced by the presence of a third molar of normal size. If there is a question regarding the favorable development of a third molar on the affected side, repositioning the drifted second molar and holding space for a replacement prosthesis is usually the treatment of choice.

Loss of the First Permanent Molar After the Eruption of the Second Permanent Molar. When the first permanent molar is lost after the eruption of the second permanent molar, orthodontic evaluation is indicated, and the following points should be considered: Is the child in need of corrective treatment other

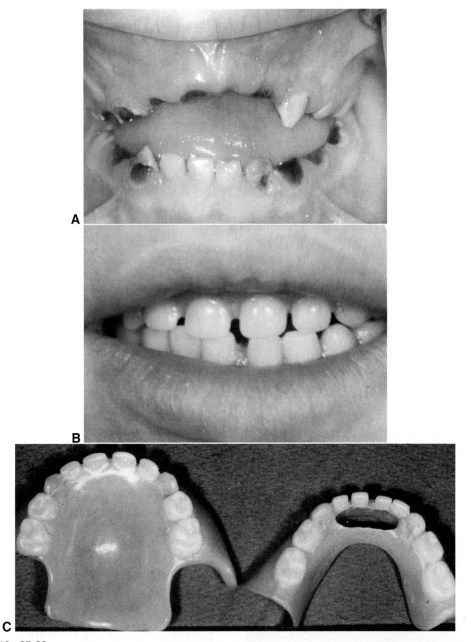

FIG. 27-23. **A,** Primary teeth have gross caries and pulpal involvement. **B,** Complete dentures were constructed after the extraction of all primary teeth. **C,** The dentures were modified after the eruption of the maxillary first permanent molars and the mandibular permanent incisors.

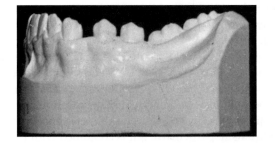

FIG. 27-24. Lower cast showing distal drifting of the premolars and mesial tipping of the second and third molars after the extraction of the first permanent molar.

than in the first permanent molar area? Should the space be maintained for a replacement prosthesis? Should the second molar be moved forward into the area formerly occupied by the first molar? The latter choice is often the more satisfactory, even though there will be a difference in the number of molars in the opposing arch. A third molar can often be removed to compensate for the difference. Without treatment the second molar will tip forward within a matter of weeks (Fig. 27-28).

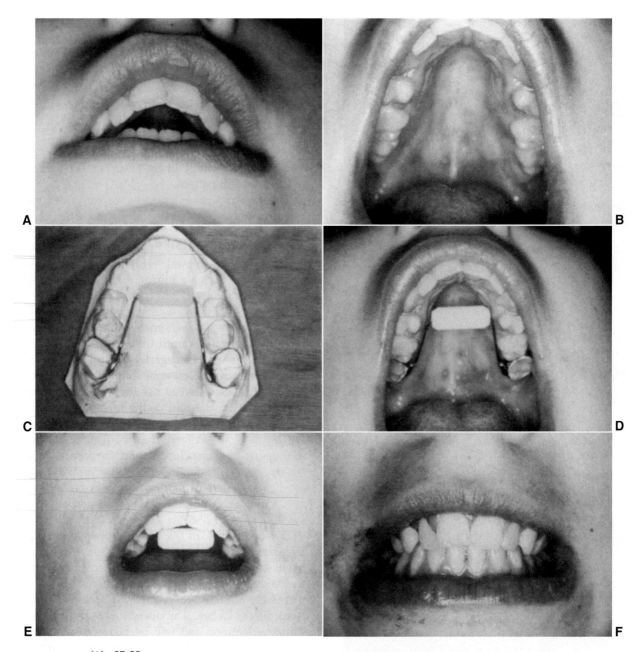

FIG. **27-33.** **A,** Anterior open bite in the mixed dentition because of thumb sucking. **B,** Palatal configuration of the patient. **C,** Appliance in place on a plaster cast. **D,** Occlusal view of the appliance cemented in place. **E,** Anterior view of the appliance in place. **F,** Correction of the anterior open bite. *(Courtesy Dr. John R. Mink. **A, B, D, E,** and **F** from Haskell BF, Mink JR: Pediatr Dent 13:83-85, 1991.)*

Traumatic occlusion with resultant stripping of the gingival tissue and pocket formation on the labial aspect of the lower tooth is a common result (Fig. 27-36). Unsightly wear facets may also develop on the incisal and labial surfaces of the involved maxillary incisors. Anterior crossbite is the result of a variety of conditions, including the following:

1. A labially positioned supernumerary tooth may cause torsiversion and lingual deflection of an incisor, which may erupt in a rotated or crossbite relationship.

2. Trauma to an anterior primary tooth may cause displacement of the developing permanent successor and eruption in crossbite. If a primary incisor is delayed in its exfoliation because of a necrotic pulp resulting from trauma or caries, the tooth may act as a foreign body and cause deflection of permanent teeth in the area (Fig. 27-37). Pulpless primary teeth often do not undergo

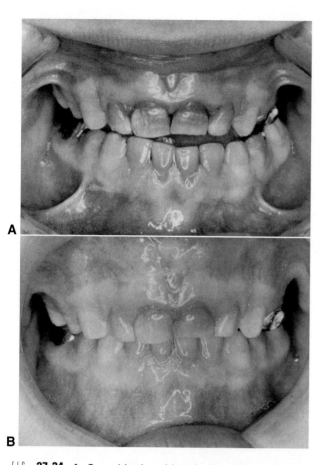

A

B

FIG. **27-34.** **A,** Open bite is evident in the primary dentition resulting from a thumb-sucking habit. **B,** The child was encouraged by the dentist to discontinue the habit. There was self-correction of the open bite when the habit was discontinued.

normal root resorption and can cause serious complications in the developing occlusion.

3. An arch-length deficiency can cause a lingual deflection of permanent anterior teeth during eruption, which is often observed in the maxillary lateral incisor area. The premature eruption of permanent canines in instances of arch-length deficiency can cause a lateral incisor to be squeezed lingually and to erupt in crossbite.

If the following conditions are present, the problem may be considered one in which uncomplicated treatment may be undertaken:

1. Sufficient room exists mesiodistally to move the tooth into its correction position.
2. The apical portion of the in-locked tooth is in relatively the same position as a tooth in normal occlusion.
3. The patient has normal occlusion in the molar and canine areas.

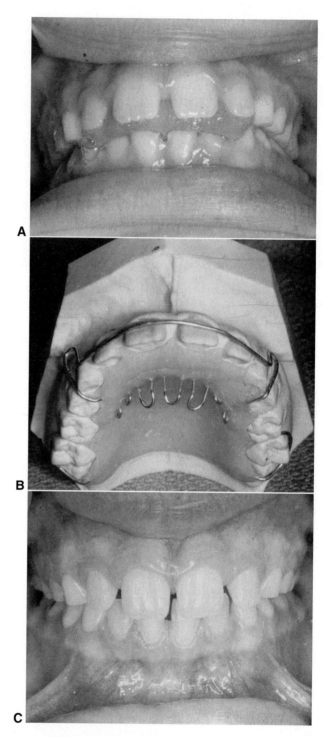

A

B

C

FIG. **27-35.** **A,** Anterior open bite resulting from a tongue-thrust habit. **B,** A removable palatal retainer was constructed to prevent the tongue from being thrust forward during the swallowing process. **C,** The tongue-thrusting habit has been overcome. The occlusion is greatly improved.

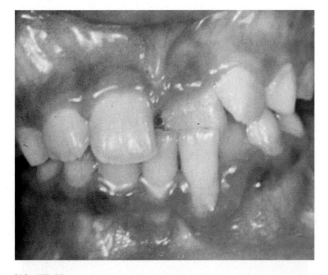

FIG. **27-36.** Untreated in-locked central incisor has resulted in stripping of the tissue, pocket formation, and a loss in arch length.

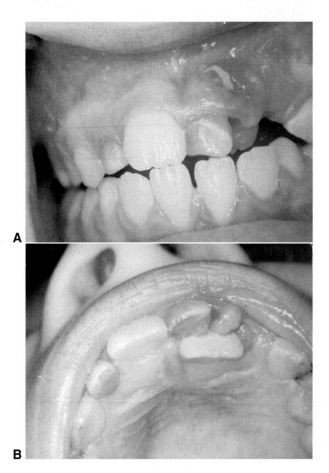

FIG. **27-37. A,** Prolonged retention of a pulpless primary incisor has resulted in lingual eruption and in-locking of permanent tooth. Notice exposed and unresorbed apex of necrotic primary incisor that has perforated the gingival tissues. **B,** Incisal view.

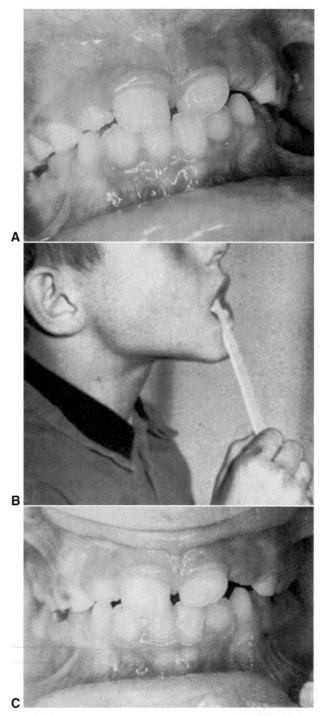

FIG. **27-38. A,** Partially erupted central incisor with a minimum degree of in-locking. A tongue blade can often be used to correct the condition successfully. **B,** Tongue blade used to exert pressure on the in-locked tooth. **C,** Correction of the in-locked condition accomplished with the aid of the tongue blade.

One of several treatment methods may be selected after an evaluation of factors such as patient cooperation, the degree of overbite that can be expected after correction, the state of the development of the occlusion, and the sequence of eruption.

Tongue Blade Therapy. In children who are cooperative and have proper encouragement and guidance at home, an anterior crossbite can be corrected with a narrow, wooden tongue blade (Fig. 27-38). Teeth in the initial state of eruption with a minimal degree of in-locking can often be repositioned within 24 hours.

The child is instructed to place the tongue blade behind the in-locked tooth and, using the chin as a fulcrum, to exert pressure on the tooth toward the labial side. This procedure should be practiced at least 5 minutes of each hour as often as possible during the day. The results of this type of therapy are often disappointing, however, because of poor cooperation of the child and parents. Tongue blade treatment is less effective if the tooth is almost fully erupted.

Lower Cemented Bite Plane. An acrylic inclined plane cemented to the lower anterior teeth is another way to reposition one or more in-locked anterior teeth. However, if a maxillary retainer may be needed, another appliance may be the best choice.

An acrylic bite plane is constructed on a stone model made from an accurate alginate impression (Fig. 27-39). Self-curing resin is applied to the model to cover the lower incisors and possibly the canines, depending on the degree of retention and stability required. An inclined plane approximately ¼ inch in length is then added, extending lingually at a 45-degree angle to the long axis of the lower incisors.

Adjustment of the plane is made before cementation. Only the in-locked tooth should be in contact with it; there should be no other tooth contacting the plane, and the plane should not touch the palatal tissue. The posterior teeth should be out of occlusion by 2 to 3 mm. This limits the time the appliance can be worn. Considerable eruption of the posterior teeth may occur within 10 days, and a tendency to an open bite in the anterior region will result. The inclined plane may be removed when the in-locked tooth has passed over the incisal edge of the lower incisors. Moreover, if the crossbite is not

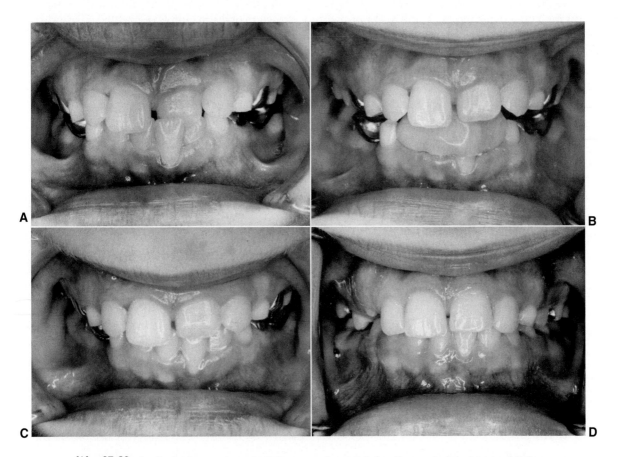

FIG. **27-39. A,** Occlusion was essentially normal except for the central incisor crossbite. **B,** A lower cemented acrylic bite plane was used to reposition the in-locked tooth. **C,** The in-locked tooth has been moved into correct position, and there is sufficient overbite to maintain the new relationship. **D,** Four years after the treatment of the crossbite. Notice the improvement in the appearance of the tissue on the labial surface of the lower left central incisor.

corrected within 7 to 10 days, a different appliance should be considered.

The physical activities of children wearing bite planes should be sharply restricted to minimize the possibility of injury to the teeth. Teeth that occlude on an inclined bite plane are especially vulnerable to avulsion or luxation from a blow to the chin.

Palatal Appliances. The use of a fixed or removable palatal appliance is indicated when one or two teeth, particularly lateral incisors, are in crossbite (Fig. 27-40). Occasionally, along with providing crossbite treatment, the palatal appliance can be used to maintain space or to correct other minor irregularities in the arch. Because good retention of this type of appliance is needed, adequate clasps or other fixation must be used. It is rarely necessary to open the bite to correct the crossbite, although in cases of deep overbite an open bite may be needed until the crossbite is corrected.

POSTERIOR CROSSBITE IN PRIMARY AND MIXED DENTITION

Crossbite in the primary dentition, involving the second molar or even all of the teeth anterior to it, is common. In a study involving 515 children 3 to 9 years of age,

Kutin and Hawes observed the prevalence of posterior crossbite in the primary and mixed dentition to be 1 in 13, or 7.7%.[30] Although often obscure, the cause of crossbite can be different in the three general types of the condition: skeletal, dental, and functional. The irregularity in the occlusion of the young child may not be clear-cut but may occur as a combination of all three types of buccal crossbite. A careful clinical examination, supplemented by occlusion models and an observation of the mandible at rest, are required for accurate diagnosis.

A posterior crossbite in the primary dentition usually is not self-corrected with continued development of the dentition. In fact, occlusal interference and resultant shift into a crossbite relationship can develop into a true skeletal defect if untreated. Kutin and Hawes discovered that posterior crossbite is not self-correcting and that untreated primary dentition crossbite is followed by mixed dentition crossbite. The treatment of crossbite in the primary dentition favors development of normal occlusion in the mixed dentition.

A *skeletal crossbite* results from a discrepancy in the structure of the mandible or maxilla. A basic discrepancy

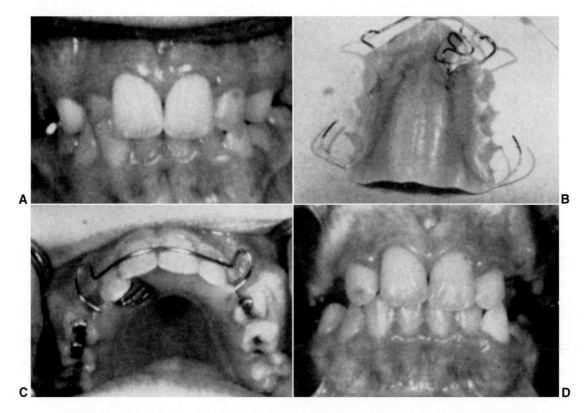

FIG. **27-40. A,** In-locked permanent lateral incisor. There was sufficient space to bring the tooth forward but a minimum amount of overbite; therefore the removable working retainer was selected. **B,** The appliance designed to correct the in-locked condition. **C,** Activation of the S-shaped wire at weekly intervals resulted in the labial movement of the in-locked tooth. **D,** The corrected occlusion at the time the appliance was discarded.

in the width of the arches may be noted. A narrow maxillary or wide mandibular arch is often associated with a buccal crossbite. The axial inclination of the molars, as viewed from the distal aspect, may show a flat occlusal plane relationship. In this situation, an appliance such as a W arch or quad helix, which primarily causes dental tipping, can be used. However, if the maxillary molars have a favorable axial inclination of the roots and crowns, dental expansion will only result in further lingual inclination of the roots and buccal tipping of the crowns. Thus use of an appliance that expands the palate and places less tipping force on the teeth is indicated (Fig. 27-41).

A *dental crossbite* results from a faulty eruption pattern; one or more of the posterior teeth erupt into a crossbite relationship. There may be no irregularity in the basal bone. After the teeth erupt, the occlusion locks them into position and drives them even further into a crossbite relationship. A low tongue position can result in the application of unequal forces to the maxillary posterior teeth and can allow these teeth to assume a crossbite relationship with the mandibular teeth. In patients who breathe through their mouths the tongue can assume a position in the floor of the mouth, which results in a muscle imbalance and subsequently a buccal crossbite.

Hershey, Stewart, and Warren report that breathing may improve in children with crossbites when the hard palate is widened to improve occlusion.[31] The beneficial effects of this procedure on occlusion and appearance are obvious, but the effects on breathing are often not noticed until the patient discovers that there is less nasal resistance and breathing is easier. Pressures such as those caused by thumb sucking and other aberrant sucking habits can modify the conformation of the

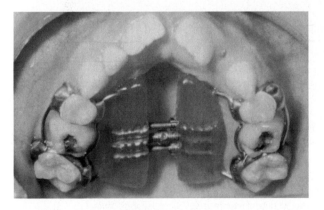

FIG. **27-41.** An acrylic jackscrew appliance with abutments on the primary and permanent first molars. This palatal expansion appliance causes less dental tipping than a solely toothborne appliance.

arch. However, they can also be directly related to the development of a crossbite.

A *functional crossbite* results from the shift of the mandible into an abnormal but often more comfortable position. The presence of a functional crossbite can be determined by observation of the relationship of the arches in the rest position. If no evidence of a discrepancy in the upper and lower midlines is seen when the mandible is at rest but a deviation of the mandible toward the side of the crossbite is noted when the teeth are brought into occlusion, the malocclusion should be considered functional. Also, when models of the upper and lower arches are examined separately, they should appear essentially symmetric. However, if there is a midline discrepancy that remains constant at the rest position and when the teeth are in occlusion, the condition is more serious and indicates a skeletal deformity requiring major orthodontic treatment.

Some functional crossbites can be corrected by reducing cuspal interference, particularly if the interference is responsible for the shift into the crossbite relationship in the canine area. Occasionally, equilibration involving a reduction of the inclined planes of the primary teeth, particularly the canines, may be all that is necessary to correct the condition. More frequently, however, the crossbite can be corrected more quickly and easily with an appliance. If examination of the occlusion reveals a developing class II or III malocclusion, the crossbite may be corrected during more comprehensive orthodontic treatment.

The time to treat a posterior crossbite is determined by several factors. If the patient is cooperative, treatment in the primary dentition is feasible. Otherwise, it is best to wait until the patient is more mature. If the permanent molars have not erupted but are no longer covered by bone, treatment should be delayed until the permanent molars can be banded. This will preclude the eruption of the molars into crossbite if the patient is treated in the primary dentition with an appliance that mainly causes dental tipping. The absence of teeth to be used for abutments also affects treatment timing and appliance design. In some instances the early loss of primary molars may require a delay of treatment until the late mixed or early permanent dentition stage.

Soldered W Arch. The soldered W lingual arch, or Porter appliance, is an efficient appliance for the correction of posterior crossbites. In some instances anterior crossbites can be corrected by extension of the arm to include the canine, laterals, and centrals. The W arch may simultaneously function as a reminder appliance in some posterior crossbites associated with thumb sucking. Preformed stainless steel bands are adapted to the most distal teeth involved in the crossbite, and a

0.036- or 0.040-inch steel wire is contoured to the arch. The wire should be free of the tissue by 1 to 2 mm, particularly in the molar loop areas, so that no impingement on the tissue will occur during activation of the wire.

Activation is correct when the appliance must be compressed 2 to 3 mm to place it on the banded teeth. The appliance is activated approximately every 3 or 4 weeks until the crossbite has been corrected (Fig. 27-42). It is cemented during active treatment and is removed only for additional activation and adjustment. The passive appliance may be used as a retainer for 4 to 6 months after active treatment. If longer periods of retention are needed, it is best to construct a conventional Hawley type of retainer.

Although the soldered W arch is a very stable appliance, its primary value is for situations that require only buccal or labial tipping of teeth. In the younger patient (3 to 5 years of age), however, some palatal expansion occurs with the W arch. The removable W arch appliance and the quad-helix appliance allow control of root angulation of the banded permanent first molars during crossbite treatment.

Cross-Elastic Technique. If only the first permanent molar is in crossbite, the condition can often be corrected by the use of cross elastics (Fig. 27-43). A hook or button is bonded (or welded onto bands) to the lingual surface of the upper molar and the buccal surface of the lower molar and the child is shown how to place the elastics on the hooks. The elastics should be changed by the child or parent each day until the crossbite has been corrected. Normally, a crossbite involving two teeth can be corrected with cross elastics in 4 to 8 weeks. If the opposing tooth is in correct arch alignment before treatment, an anchorage appliance (lingual arch or Nance) may help prevent excessive movement of that tooth. The corrected cuspal interdigitation usually holds the teeth in their new relationship, so a retentive appliance is not needed.

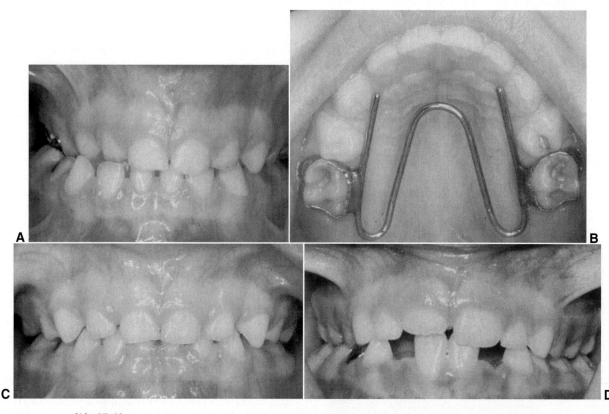

FIG. **27-42.** **A,** Buccal crossbite in the primary dentition involving the lateral incisor and all teeth posterior to it. In the rest position the dental midlines are normal, but in maximum interdigitation, as shown here, there is a 1.5-mm mandibular midline shift to the affected side. **B,** Soldered W lingual arch ready for cementation after activation and trial seating. **C,** The crossbite was corrected in 6 weeks, and the appliance was removed after 3 months of retention. Notice that the dental midlines are properly aligned. **D,** After 3 years the first permanent molars are in proper relationship and the dental midlines remain properly aligned. There is no mandibular shift during closure.

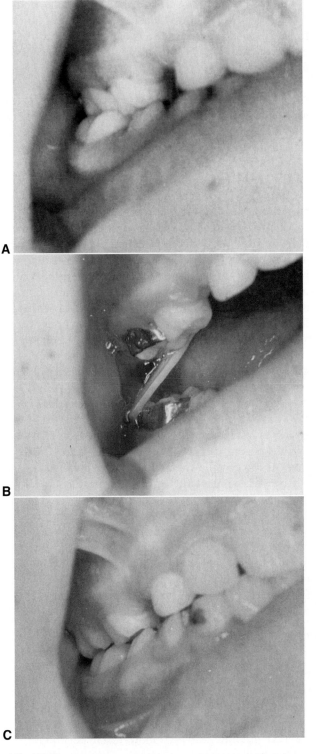

FIG. **27-43. A,** Buccal crossbite is limited to the first permanent molars on the right side. Correction of the crossbite at this time will favorably influence the eruption of the second permanent molars. **B,** Molar bands with hooks and cross elastics are being used to correct the crossbite. **C,** The molar crossbite has been corrected in a 4-week period.

PROBLEMS RELATED TO THE ERUPTION OF TEETH

A variety of eruption problems arise during the transitional dentition period. Early diagnosis and treatment may prevent a more complicated malocclusion. The dentist must be alert to these problems and complicating sequelae.

Ectopic Eruption of the First Permanent Molars. Examination of periapical and bite-wing radiographs is important before the eruption of the first permanent molars to detect ectopic eruption. A first permanent molar, in instances of otherwise ideal occlusion, may be positioned too far mesially in its eruption, with resultant resorption of the distal root of the second primary molar. The permanent molar may become completely locked and may cause the premature exfoliation of the second primary molar or make it necessary to extract the affected tooth. In some instances the ectopically erupting first permanent molar may correct itself and erupt into its normal position after causing only minor destruction of the primary molar (Fig. 27-44).

Young observed that ectopic eruption of the first permanent molar occurred 52 times in 1619 boys and girls (3% of the time).[32] The ectopic eruption occasionally occurred in more than one quadrant in the same mouth but was most often observed in the maxilla. In fact, only two ectopically erupting mandibular first permanent molars were noted. The anomaly was observed more frequently in boys (33 times) than in girls (19 times). Young further observed that 66% of the ectopically erupting molars finally erupted into their essentially normal position without corrective treatment. When the impacted first permanent molar has not erupted or is only partially erupted, the treatment of choice is watchful waiting because more than half of the teeth will eventually erupt into normal position. However, a report by Bjerklin and Kurol indicates that ectopic permanent molars of the reversible type had freed themselves by the time the patient reached 7 years of age but that only a few molars of the locked or irreversible type had freed themselves by this age.[33] According to Bjerklin and Kurol, whether the ectopic molar is reversible or irreversible can be determined fairly accurately in patients between 7 and 8 years of age.

Humphrey described a technique for correcting ectopically erupting first permanent molars.[34] A preformed steel band was adapted to the second primary molar on the affected side, and a wire was adapted and soldered to the band. An S-shaped loop was placed in the wire with a No. 139 pliers. The loop was opened slightly and was heat-treated with a match flame (950° F) before cementation of the loop (Fig. 27-45). The distal extension of the wire was placed in an opening in

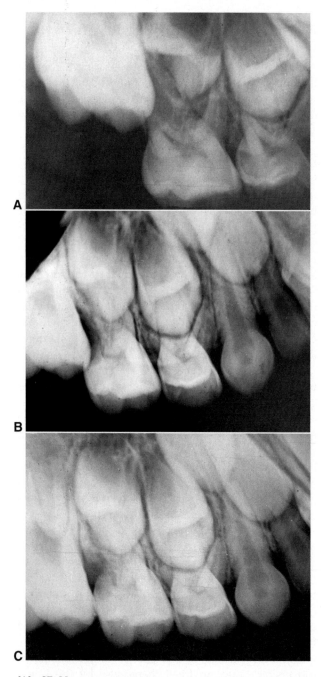

FIG. **27-44.** **A,** Ectopic eruption of a maxillary first permanent molar. There is evidence of resorption of the distal buccal tooth of the second primary molar. **B** and **C,** Subsequent radiographs show continued resorption of the primary molar but normal positioning of the first permanent molar.

the occlusal surface of the ectopically erupting molar. It was sometimes necessary to remove the appliance in 7 to 10 days for a second activation of the loop. Another useful appliance for correcting ectopic eruptions is the Halterman appliance, which is fabricated by banding the second primary molar and soldering an extension arm that runs distal to the ectopic molar.[35] A button is

bonded to the occlusal surface of the ectopic molar and an elastic power chain is attached from this button to the small hook built into the most distal aspect of the extension arm (Fig. 27-46). The power chain is changed every 2 to 3 weeks.

Occasionally the affected second primary molar is mobile as a result of resorption of its root and the forces exerted by the ectopically erupting first permanent molar. The basic design of the Humphrey or Halterman technique may be incorporated into a bilateral lingual arch if additional appliance stability is desired or if leeway space must be preserved as already mentioned.[34,35] The Halterman appliance may also be fabricated as a removable appliance (Fig. 27-47).

A helical, or Kesling, self-locking separating spring* may be used to correct an ectopically erupting permanent molar (Fig. 27-48). The spring was designed primarily for the separation of teeth before orthodontic banding but can be used to correct ectopic eruption of the maxillary and mandibular first permanent molars if there is sufficient dental development for its insertion and cross-arch anchorage is not required.

Insertion of the spring is most easily achieved by grasping the active arm of the spring adjacent to the helix with a How or Weingardt pliers. A floss loop through the helix serves as a safety device if the spring slips out of the pliers during insertion. The head of the spring is placed on the marginal ridge or near the middle of the contact area and held firmly with a cervical force while the active arm is directed below the contact point of the ectopically positioned tooth. The dentist may insert the spring from the buccal or lingual side (whichever provides the greatest access); the buccal approach is usually easier. The patient is instructed to keep the helix of the spring at the gingival margin and can adjust the helix occlusally if it impinges on the soft tissue. The spring should be left in place until the tooth has freed its contact with the adjacent tooth and is erupting in a normal manner. The patient should be seen every 5 to 6 weeks to evaluate the progress of the eruption and to reactivate the spring.

If the second primary molar is lost or extracted before the permanent molar has erupted sufficiently to band, a reverse band and loop or a distal shoe appliance may be used. If the first permanent molar has not tipped too far mesially, the distal shoe can be constructed with an inclined guiding plane to allow distal positioning of the tooth. If cross-arch anchorage is required, it can be incorporated into the appliance design.

Impacted Second Permanent Molars. Although impaction of second permanent molars occurs less frequently than impaction of first permanent molars,

---

*TP Orthodontics, Inc., LaPorte, Ind.

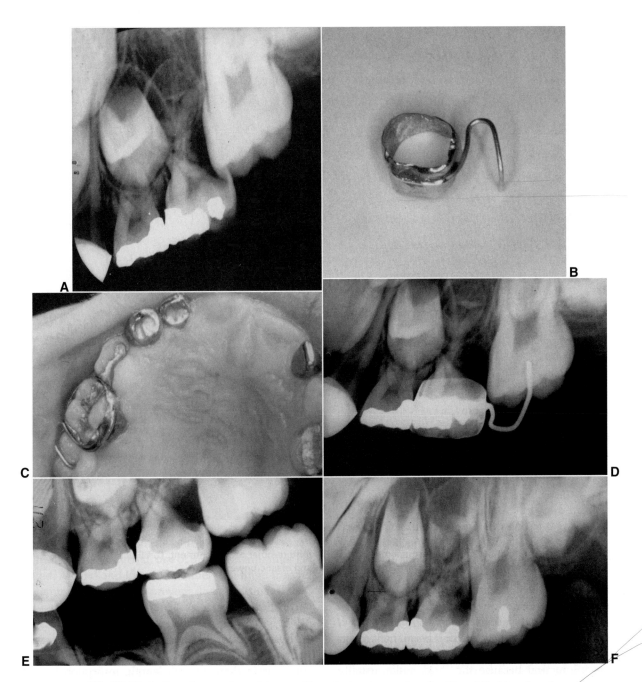

FIG. 27-45. A, Ectopic eruption of the maxillary first permanent molar. B and C, A band and S-shaped wire have been fabricated to reposition the first permanent molar. D and E, Radiographs demonstrate the distal repositioning of the first permanent molar. F, The first permanent molar has erupted into a favorable position.

when the condition occurs, it is generally in the mandibular arch. Insufficient arch length, excessive tooth mass, or an abnormal eruption path may be responsible.

Treatment goals are to upright the tooth and achieve complete eruption (Fig. 27-49). Appliances like those recommended for the correction of an ectopically erupting first permanent molar may be used. Sometimes, simply inserting an elastic orthodontic separator in the

contact area (if it is accessible) initiates uprighting. Use of a Kesling spring may also help. A spring of another design, known as the De-Impactor,* helps in uprighting many mesioangular impacted posterior teeth, particularly impacted mandibular second permanent molars.

*Arkansas Dental Products Co., West Plains, Mo.

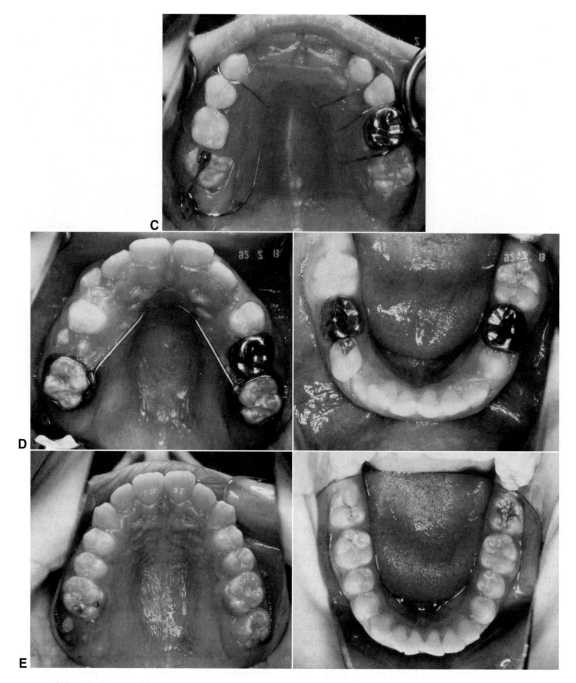

FIG. **27-47, cont'd. C,** Removable appliance in place with elastic power chain attached. **D,** Occlusal views after correction and with Nance appliance in place. **E,** Occlusal views in early permanent dentition.

from palpation of the canine crypt or from radiographs by the time the patient is 8 or 9 years of age. A delay in the eruption can allow adjacent teeth to encroach on the space needed for the canine and contributes to the impacted condition. If the maxillary permanent canine is definitely impacted, surgical intervention is indicated. However, localization of the tooth by special radiographic technique is essential. The procedure described in Chapter 5 will help in localizing the impacted tooth.

The available arch space for the canine should be compared with the size of the crown. The measurement of the opposite canine can be used, or the impacted canine can be measured directly from the radiograph. If space for the tooth is adequate and occlusion is essentially normal, the space should be maintained.

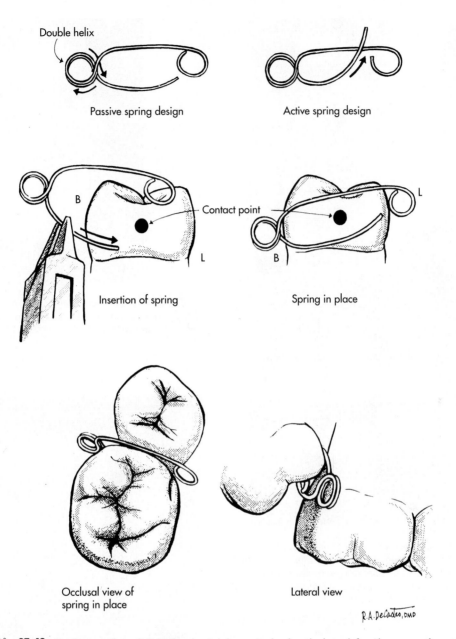

Double helix

Passive spring design   Active spring design

Contact point

Insertion of spring   Spring in place

Occlusal view of
spring in place   Lateral view

R.A.DeCastro, DMD

FIG. **27-48.** Kesling spring of 0.022-inch stainless steel wire designed for the correction of ectopically erupting permanent molars.

Surgical exposure of the impacted canine and maintenance of the pathway are normally the treatment of choice. If the primary canine is still present, it should be extracted. Sufficient soft tissue and bone should then be removed from the crown of the impaction to maintain an opening that will stimulate the eruption of the impacted tooth. A canine in deep palatal impaction may move into an in-locked position or may require orthodontic movement to bring it into a desirable relationship with other teeth.

Supernumerary Teeth and Accompanying Malocclusion

Supernumerary teeth, which result from the continued budding of the enamel organ of the preceding tooth or from excessive proliferation of cells, can be responsible for a variety of irregularities in the primary and transitional dentition. The stage of differentiation determines whether a cyst, an odontoma, or a supernumerary tooth will result. In separate studies, Stafne[39] and Schulze[40] concluded that supernumerary teeth occur in approximately 1 of 110 children. The ratio

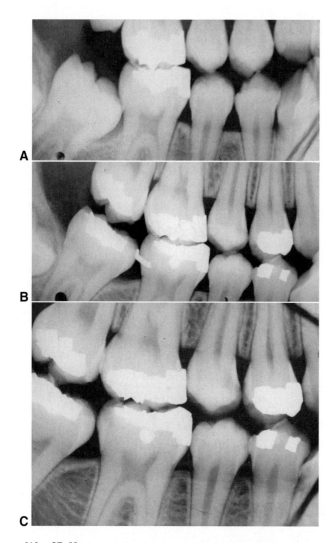

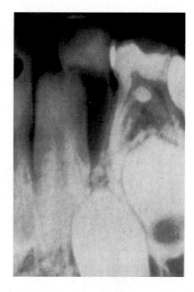

FIG. **27-50.** Premature primary canine root resorption, resulting from arch-length inadequacy and ectopic eruption of the permanent lateral incisor.

FIG. **27-49. A,** Impacted second molar. The second molar should not be extracted; instead, an attempt should be made to upright the tooth. **B** and **C,** A separating wire has been used successfully to reposition the second permanent molar. Treatment was extended over 12 months.

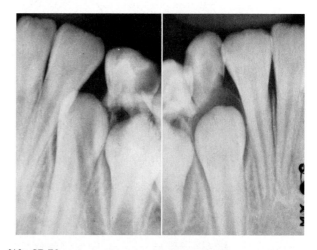

FIG. **27-51.** Primary canine has been lost prematurely on the left side of the arch. The permanent incisor has drifted distally into contact with the first primary molar. Extraction of the corresponding primary canine would have aided in maintaining symmetry in the arch.

of the prevalence in the maxilla and in the mandible is 8:1. The most common site for supernumerary teeth is the maxillary incisor area. Supernumerary primary teeth (Fig. 27-52) are apparently less common than supernumerary permanent teeth. The occurrence of supernumerary teeth in several members of the same family has been observed, which indicates a familial pattern.

Supernumerary teeth, particularly in the maxillary anterior region, may prevent the eruption of adjacent permanent teeth (Fig. 27-53) or cause their ectopic eruption (Fig. 27-54). Both conditions frequently result in an irregularity of the developing occlusion that requires treatment. If a supernumerary tooth is found,

a special radiographic technique, as described in Chapter 5, can be used to localize the tooth. The decision whether to intervene surgically or keep the tooth under observation can then be made.

Surgical Removal of Supernumerary Teeth. The surgical removal of an unerupted supernumerary tooth is the eventual course of treatment. However, if the supernumerary tooth does not interfere with the symmetric development and eruption of adjacent teeth

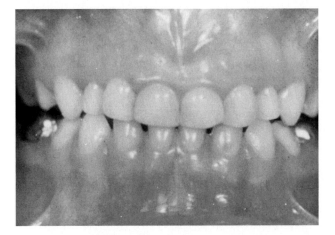

FIG. **27-52.** Supernumerary maxillary primary incisors. There may be corresponding supernumerary permanent teeth. The teeth should be counted at the time of the clinical examination so that erupted supernumerary teeth will not be overlooked.

and no evidence of the formation of a cyst exists, the correct decision may be to observe the tooth until the child is old enough to tolerate the procedure better. Many pediatric dentists and surgeons prefer to delay surgery until the permanent teeth erupt and root closure is complete, provided that no evidence is seen of a developing irregularity in the occlusion.

The delayed eruption of a maxillary incisor as a result of a midline supernumerary tooth is common. In this case, immediate surgical removal of the supernumerary tooth is recommended. During surgery, the bone and soft tissue should be removed from the incisal third of the tooth or teeth that are delayed in their eruption. If the permanent teeth are positioned extremely high, however, a prolonged period of watchful waiting may be necessary until they have migrated within the bone to a position that would allow additional surgical

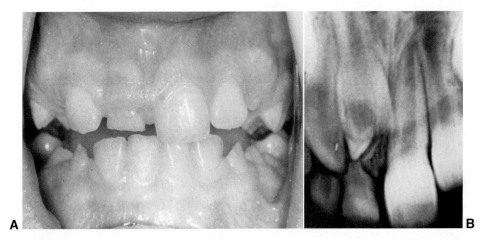

FIG. **27-53. A,** Dentition of a patient with an unerupted maxillary permanent incisor. Space closure is the result of delayed eruption. **B,** The radiograph shows a supernumerary tooth (mesiodens), which has delayed the eruption of the permanent incisor.

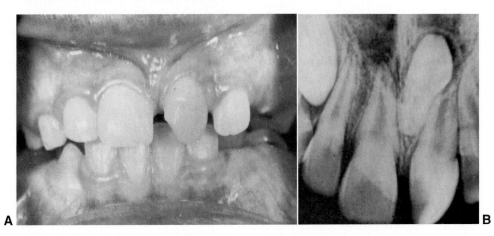

FIG. **27-54. A,** Rotation and labioversion of a maxillary anterior tooth may be caused by the presence of a supernumerary tooth. The position of this tooth increases its susceptibility to fracture. **B,** Radiograph of a well-developed midline supernumerary tooth. Surgical removal of the tooth is indicated.

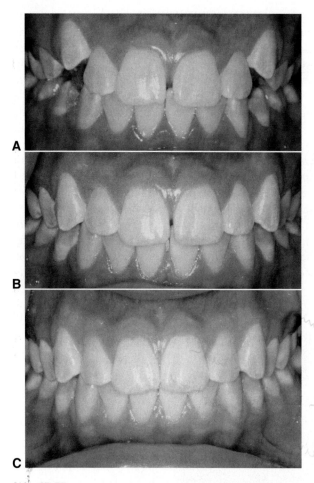

27-55. A, Diastema and highly positioned canines. No treatment was instituted. **B,** Twenty-four months later, the diastema has closed significantly and the canines are erupting into a more favorable position. **C,** Thirty-six months later, the diastema has closed completely, and the canines have assumed a near-ideal position.

intervention. An open pathway should be maintained, if possible, to hasten the eruption of the delayed tooth. A thin covering of dense scar tissue can delay eruption indefinitely.

Anterior Diastemas. Frequently parents are concerned about the anterior diastema, which is usually present during eruption of the maxillary incisors and canines. They might insist that active orthodontic treatment be started to close the space. Unless there is a valid reason to close the space early, active treatment should be postponed until the complete eruption of the permanent canines. The dentist should explain that the diastema will close as the laterals and canines erupt. After the canines erupt, the condition can be reevaluated and appropriate treatment undertaken as needed. Fig. 27-55, A, shows a patient whose parent wanted the diastema closed and was concerned about the high position of the canines. No treatment was begun.

Fig. 27-55, B, shows the extent of the diastema 24 months later. Notice that the canines are now in reasonably good alignment.

Early closure of a diastema may be required if the laterals are erupting lingually and do not have sufficient space to be moved labially into the arch. Sometimes a heavy labial frenum prevents the natural closure of a diastema. In these instances, if orthodontic closure is advocated, it should occur before surgery to reduce the chance that scar tissue will impede tooth movement. If there is sufficient arch space for the eruption of incisors and canines, it is best to delay frenum surgery until these teeth have fully erupted.

Congenitally Missing Teeth. Managing problems of congenitally missing teeth requires a complete diagnosis and thorough evaluation of arch length and occlusion. Early consultation with the orthodontist and prosthodontist may help in determining appropriate long-term care.

If one or both of the permanent maxillary laterals are missing, the dentist must decide whether to hold space for prosthetic replacements or to let the permanent canine erupt or drift mesially into the lateral incisor position. In the latter instance, limited orthodontic treatment may be needed to place the canine in the correct axial inclination before the crown is reshaped to resemble the lateral. In some instances the shape of the canine may not be favorable for its use as a lateral, even with extensive recontouring.

In the past the recommendation has been to influence eruption of the permanent canine to encourage it to erupt as close as possible to its normal position. In the case of the missing lateral incisor (Fig. 27-56), and with the advent of implants for replacement of lateral incisors, that recommendation has changed. According to Kokich, the ideal situation is to encourage the canine to erupt adjacent to the permanent central incisor.[41] After it has erupted, it can be moved distally into its normal position. When the tooth is moved distally, bone is laid down, forming an alveolar ridge with adequate buccal-lingual width to facilitate proper implant placement.

When one or more permanent premolars, usually the seconds, are congenitally missing, a thorough evaluation is needed to determine the best course of treatment. Should the space be maintained for fixed prostheses later, or should the space be closed? Many factors influence the decision and must be carefully considered. For example, if just one premolar is absent and the rest of the occlusion is esthetically and functionally sound, the treatment of choice may be prosthetics. Such treatment may maintain the most favorable occlusal relationship, even though several replacements may be required during the patient's lifetime. On the other hand, if three or four premolars are missing,

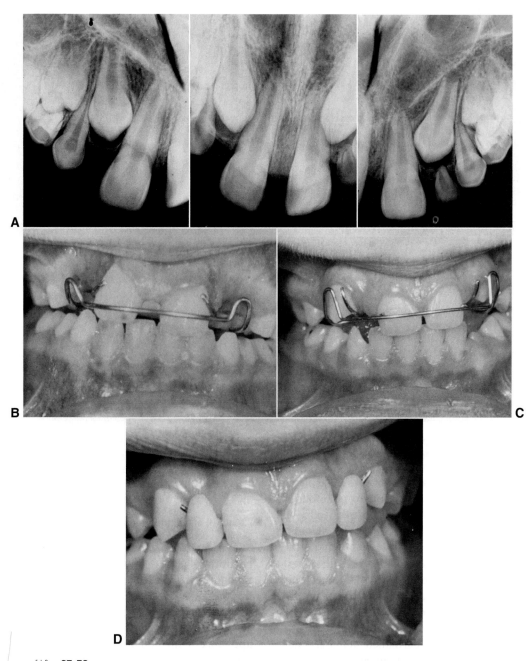

FIG. **27-56. A,** Congenital absence of permanent lateral incisors. **B,** The primary canines have been extracted, and a working appliance has been constructed to close the diastema between the central incisors. **C,** Auxiliary wires have been added to the appliance to guide the permanent canines into a more favorable position. **D,** Space has been regained for eventual fixed prostheses to replace the lateral incisors. Meanwhile the removable retainer will be worn.

orthodontic treatment may obviate the cost and need for continued prosthetic care and replacement.

In some instances the primary molar may be left intact, may be retained, and may function well for many years. In many cases, however, the larger mesiodistal width of the primary molar may cause incorrect occlusal relationships with the permanent teeth.

Sometimes, slicing the mesial and distal surfaces of the primary molar allows the proper permanent molar interdigitation, but often the bulbous, divergent roots of the primary second molar prevent the mesial movement of the permanent molar. Also, even if the permanent successor is missing, the roots of the primary molar may be resorbed, and the tooth may be lost eventually.

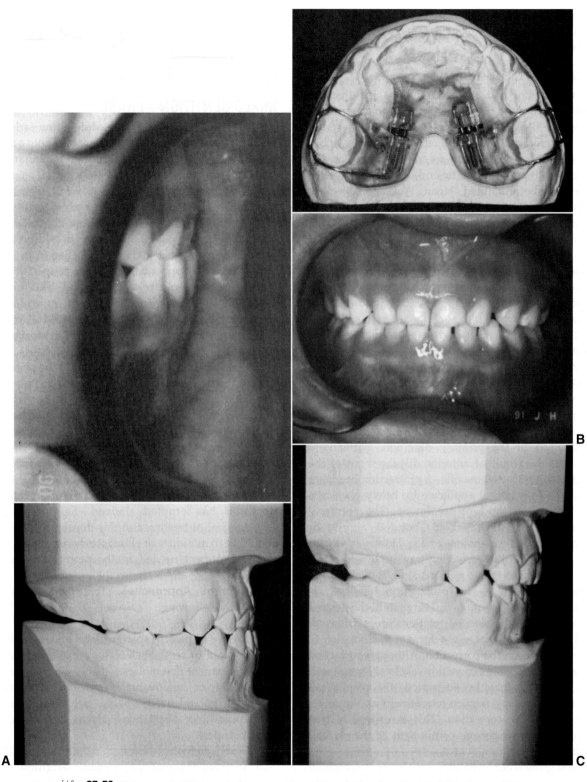

FIG. **27-59.** Primary dentition anterior crossbite with anterior functional shift of mandible. **A,** Pretreatment clinical *(top)* and model *(bottom)* view. **B,** Anterior push sagittal appliance designed to flare incisors. **C,** Posttreatment clinical *(top)* and model *(bottom)* view.

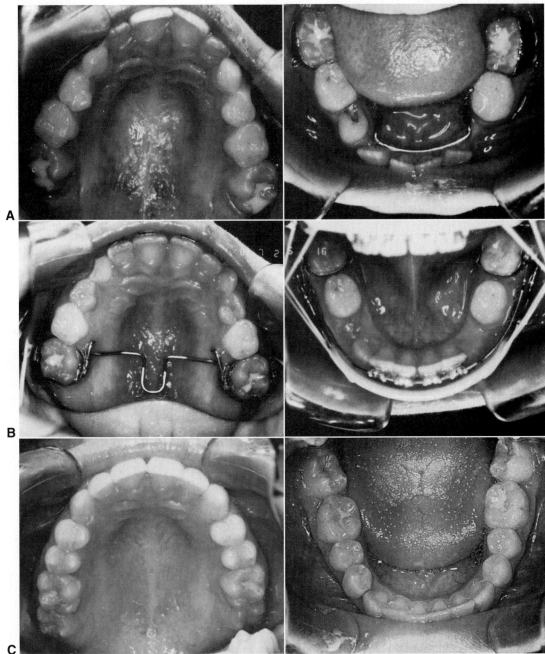

FIG. **27-60.** Patient treated with phase I orthodontics only. **A,** Pretreatment occlusal views; note tapered maxillary arch and arch-length insufficiency in the mandibular arch. **B,** Phase I treatment with fixed "2 × 4" edgewise appliances, maxillary transpalatal arch bar, and mandibular lip bumper; note arch-length development, particularly in the mandibular arch. **C,** Posttreatment occlusal views in permanent dentition without additional full edgewise bracketing.

5. Functional appliances—Frankel appliances (Fig. 27-62), Bionaters, Herbst appliances, anterior and posterior bite planes. The type of functional appliance and its design vary significantly depending on the facial growth pattern.

Of course, the patient's orthodontic diagnosis will dictate which combination of the aforementioned treatment modalities will be necessary. One pervasive philosophy in early orthodontic treatment is that the simplest biomechanical approach necessary to achieve the desired treatment outcome is the best (Fig. 27-63).

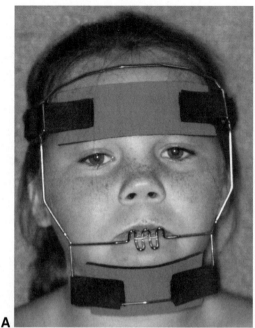

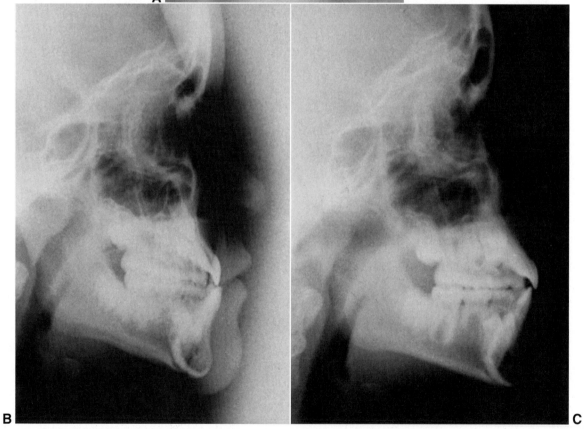

FIG. **27-61. A,** Patient with protraction headgear in place. **B,** Pretreatment lateral head plate. **C,** Posttreatment lateral head plate.

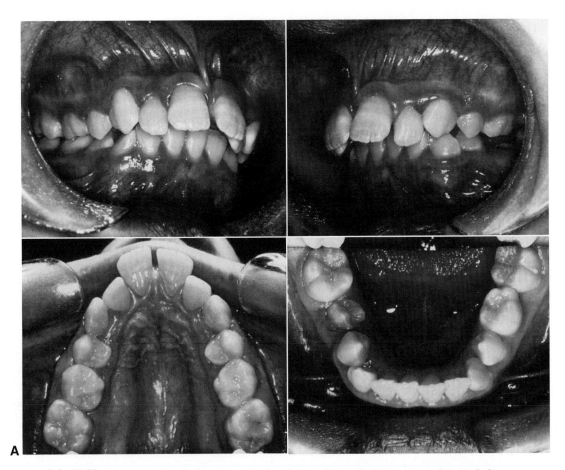

FIG. **27-62.** Dentition of patient treated with Frankel appliance. **A,** Pretreatment intraoral views.
Continued

In many cases of mixed dentition malocclusion, this routinely means the following:

1. Fixed 2 × 4 therapy to correct dental alignment and intrusion problems
2. Mandibular lingual arch or lip bumper treatment to facilitate arch development
3. Headgear therapy to address skeletal and dental vertical and sagittal problems

Often in the mixed dentition, depending on the individual patient's diagnostic assessment, significant arch development can be realized as follows:

Arch width expansion	2 mm
Leeway space maintenance or regaining	4 mm
Uprighting, tipback, or derotation of first permanent molars	2 mm
Flaring of incisors	2 mm
TOTAL	10 mm

Several different methods have been advocated for retention of the orthodontic and orthopedic effect achieved after mixed dentition treatment and until

eruption of the remaining permanent teeth *(rest phase).* They include maxillary and mandibular fixed and/or removable bilateral space maintainers (such as an upper Hawley and a lower lingual arch), custom or stock eruption guidance appliances (such as a tooth positioner), and segmented archwires with the bands and brackets remaining attached to the teeth. In patients with corrected dentofacial orthopedic problems, it is useful to continue, at night only, the use of headgear or functional appliances during this rest phase to maintain the orthopedic change.

EARLY PERMANENT DENTITION—PHASE II

Phase II of comprehensive orthodontic care again includes both orthopedic and orthodontic components. Orthopedic components might involve use of headgear or functional appliances. The orthodontic component includes the use of full, fixed, edgewise orthodontic appliances to establish as near-perfect interdental relationships as possible.

If a patient has undergone an earlier phase of comprehensive orthodontic treatment, this second phase of treatment might take as little as 12 to 18 months and

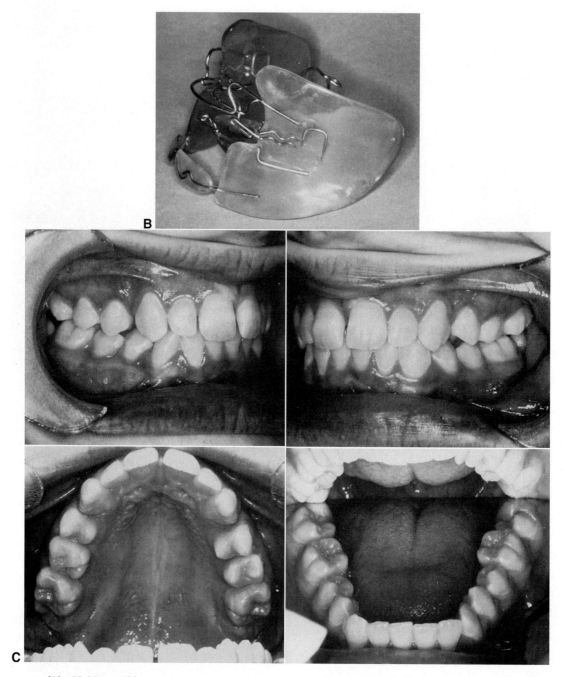

FIG. **27-62, cont'd. B,** Frankel appliance. **C,** Rest phase retention with Frankel appliance worn only at night before phase II treatment.

hopefully will involve little, if any, orthopedic components. If this is the start of comprehensive care, however, more time will be needed (Fig. 27-64). The ultimate goal of all orthodontic treatment is to establish a stable esthetic and functional result. The specific dentition goals include the six keys to normal occlusion advocated by Andrews: proper molar relationships, proper crown angulation and inclination, no rotations, tight contacts, and a flat occlusal plane.[12]

Treatment after a mixed dentition phase includes the following:

1. Space consolidation
2. Sagittal arch coordination (class II or III elastic wear)
3. Root parallelism
4. Finishing and detailing: first-, second-, and third-order archwire bends as necessary

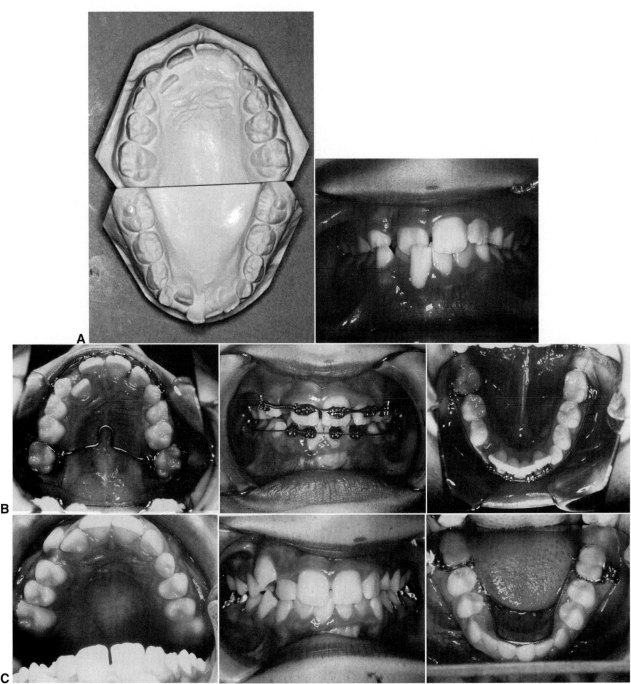

FIG. **27-63.** Typical phase I treatment. **A,** Pretreatment models and intraoral view. **B,** Phase I fixed edgewise therapy. **C,** Rest phase retention with Hawley retainer and lower lingual arch before phase II treatment.

5. Buccal or anterior segment elastic wear to establish maximum interdigitation between arches
6. Orthopedics as necessary

Certainly most of this treatment is accomplished with fixed, edgewise appliances. However, in selected patients, phase II treatment will be limited in nature, determined to be unnecessary by the dental practitioner, or unwanted by the patient and/or parent. Limited treatment can involve tooth positioners or segmented arch therapy in which only the teeth or arch segments needing attention are addressed. Occasionally the practitioner may be so satisfied with the final orthodontic

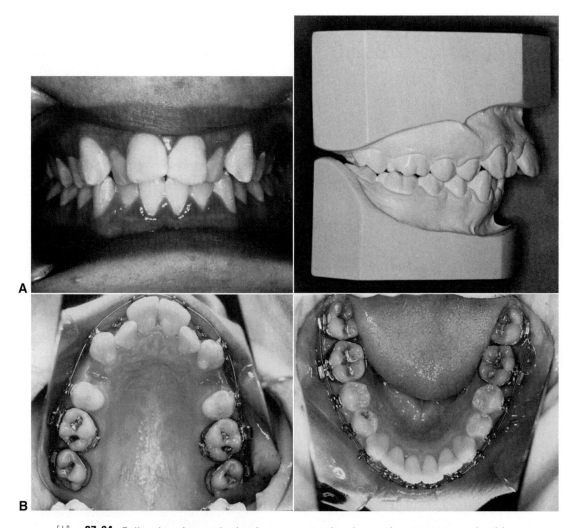

FIG. **27-64.** Full edgewise orthodontic treatment in the early permanent dentition. **A,** Pretreatment intraoral and model views; note overjet and full cusp class II occlusion. **B,** Intraoral views of uni-arch extraction treatment.

result after phase I that no further treatment is recommended. However, this is fairly uncommon. A more likely occurrence is that the patient and/or parents decide that they are satisfied with the result, even though some finishing details are needed. To avoid this event, it is necessary to stress to parents before initiating phase I treatment that most children clearly will benefit from a final period of full orthodontic appliance use (phase II). It is particularly important to allow for final tooth positioning of the permanent second molars.

Retention following this period of treatment should involve the philosophy of "retention for a lifetime." There are many different types of retention schemes; however, the following retention schedule seems to provide for stable results:

1. Maxillary and mandibular Hawley retainers are worn 24 hours a day for 4 months, followed by 8 months of wear at night only.

2. After 1 year, a reassessment is made to see if wear can be reduced to 1 or 2 nights per week, with the patient increasing wear as needed if the retainers become tight from tooth movement.

3. Wear is continued as above for "retention for a lifetime" or, at an absolute minimum, until age 21 years, at which time the craniofacial growth rate has been reduced to that of an adult.

The provision of a backup set of thin acrylic overlay retainers is a very useful way of inexpensively giving the patient an emergency set of retainers in case the Hawley retainers are lost or damaged. As an added benefit, they can be used for home bleaching of the teeth by those patients who are interested. Fixed retainers may be necessary in special circumstances and can be fabricated from 0.0175-inch braided wire, heat-treated to be dead soft. A lower canine-to-canine fixed, bonded

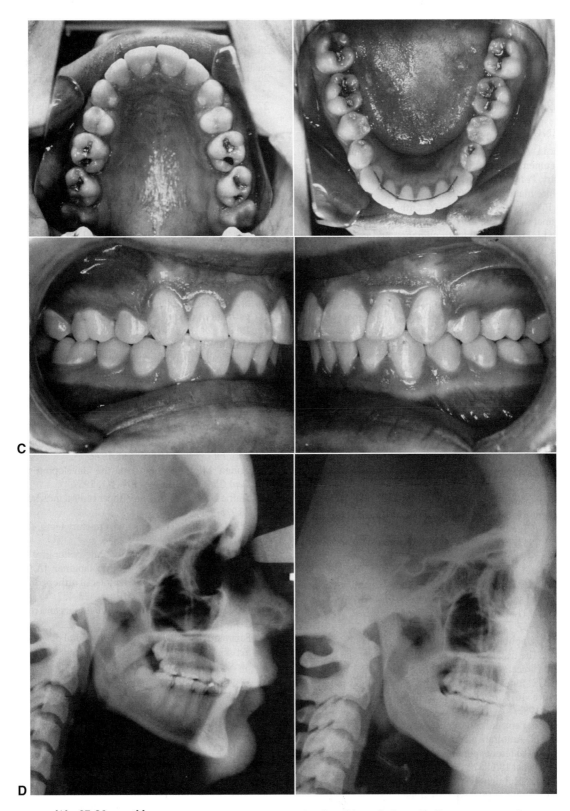

FIG. **27-64, cont'd. C,** Intraoral posttreatment occlusal and lateral views. **D,** Pretreatment and posttreatment lateral head plates; note overjet and profile improvement even though molars were left in class II position.

Multidisciplinary Team Approach to Cleft Lip and Palate Management

JAMES E. JONES

ALAN MICHAEL SADOVE

JEFFREY A. DEAN

DONALD V. HUEBENER

Cleft lip and palate, the most common of the craniofacial anomalies, are severe congenital anomalies that have an incidence of 0.28 to 3.74 per 1000 live births globally. In the United States, cleft lip and palate occur in approximately 1 in 1000 newborns. The incidence varies widely among races. Cleft lip and palate occur in about 1 in 800 white newborns, 1 in 2000 black newborns, and 1 in 500 Japanese or Navaho Indian newborns. Isolated cleft lip and palate occur in about 1 in 2000 newborns and demonstrates less racial variation. Cleft lip and palate together account for approximately 50% of all cases, whereas isolated cleft lip and isolated cleft palate each occur in about 25% of cases. Many of these congenital anomalies appear to be genetically determined, although the majority are of unknown cause or are attributable to teratogenic influences (see Chapter 6).

CLASSIFICATION OF CLEFT LIP AND PALATE

There is a tendency to conceptualize cleft lip and palate as a homogenous anomaly. If that were true, a treatment plan that would be applicable to all cases could be formulated. However, the reality is that children born with clefts vary widely in their clinical presentations (Fig. 28-1).

To standardize reporting of cleft lip and palate, the Nomenclature Committee of the American Association of Cleft Palate Rehabilitation devised a classification system that later was adopted by the Cleft Palate Association. The complexity of this system, however, has made its acceptance less than overwhelming. Veau proposed the most frequently used system.[1] He classified clefts of the lip as follows:

- Class I—a unilateral notching of the vermilion not extending into the lip
- Class II—a unilateral notching of the vermilion border, with the cleft extending into the lip but not including the floor of the nose
- Class III—a unilateral clefting of the vermilion border of the lip extending into the floor of the nose
- Class IV—any bilateral clefting of the lip, whether it be incomplete notching or complete clefting

Veau divided palatal clefts into four classes as follows (Fig. 28-2):

- Class I—involves only the soft palate
- Class II—involves the soft and hard palates but not the alveolar process

- Class III—involves both soft and hard palates and the alveolar process on one side of the premaxillary area
- Class IV—involves both soft and hard palates and continues through the alveolus on both sides of the premaxilla, leaving it free and often mobile

Veau did not include submucous clefts of the palate in his classification system. Submucous clefts may frequently be diagnosed by the following physical findings: bifid uvula, palpable notching at the posterior portion of the hard palate, and a "zona pellucida" (thin, translucent membrane). Submucous clefts of the palate may be associated with an incomplete velopharyngeal mechanism or eustachian tube dysfunction.

MULTIDISCIPLINARY CLEFT LIP AND PALATE TEAM

Children born with cleft lips and palates have many problems that need to be solved for successful habilitation. The complexity of these problems requires that numerous health care practitioners cooperate in providing the specialized knowledge and skills necessary to ensure comprehensive care. The cleft palate team concept has evolved from that need.

In an effort to address the many treatment regimes and different care protocols, the American Cleft Palate–Craniofacial Association (http://www.cleftpalate-craniofacial.org) convened a consensus conference on recommended practices for the care of patients with craniofacial anomalies. This conference produced the document "Parameters for Evaluation and Treatment of Patients with Cleft Lip/Palate or other Craniofacial Anomalies."[2] This serves as a guide for implementing the multidisciplinary approach to cleft and craniofacial care and is used by teams in the United States and Canada.

Since optimal care is best achieved by multiple types of clinical expertise, the teams may be composed of individuals in (1) the dental specialties (orthodontics, oral surgery, pediatric dentistry, and prosthodontics), (2) the medical specialties (genetics, otolaryngology, pediatrics, plastic surgery, and psychiatry), and (3) allied health care fields (audiology, nursing, psychology, social work, and speech pathology).

These care providers assess the patient's medical status and general development, dental development, facial esthetics, psychologic well-being, hearing, and speech development (Fig. 28-3). Team members must communicate effectively among themselves, with the child and parents, and with the primary care physician and dentist. Individuals on the team must respect one another's opinions and be flexible in planning and carrying out therapy. Periodic evaluation is necessary to assess the effect of previous therapy and to determine

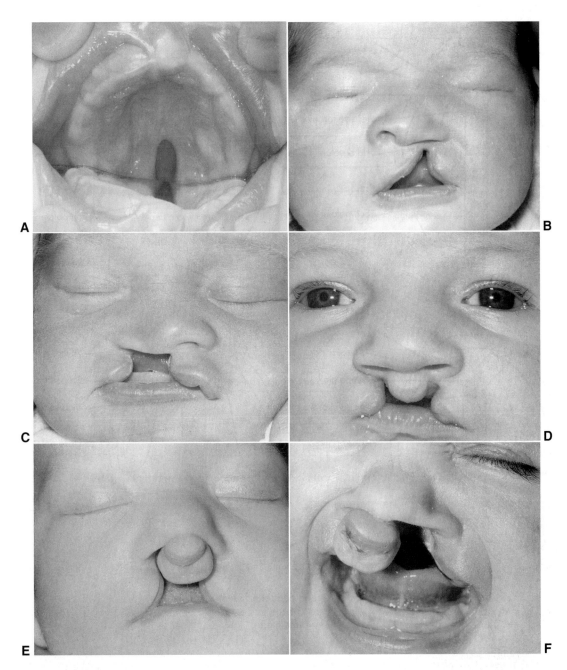

FIG. **28-1.** Various clinical presentations of cleft lip and cleft palate. (See text for descriptions of each specific type.) **A,** Isolated cleft palate (class II). **B,** Unilateral cleft of the lip (class II). **C,** Unilateral complete cleft of the lip and palate (class III). **D,** Bilateral incomplete cleft of the lip (class IV). **E,** Bilateral complete cleft of the lip and palate (class IV). **F,** Bilateral complete cleft of the lip and palate with a laterally displaced premaxillary segment (class IV).

whether an alternative approach may be necessary. A team conference immediately after patient examination is a desirable way to discuss current problems and plan timely therapy.

Whitehouse describes the clinical team as a "close, cooperative, democratic, multiprofessional union devoted to a common purpose—the best treatment of the fundamental needs of the patient."[3]

GENERAL RESPONSIBILITIES OF TEAM MEMBERS

DENTAL SPECIALTIES

The pediatric dentist is responsible for the overall dental care of the patient. Numerous dental anomalies and malocclusions occur with a cleft lip or palate. These may be attributed to the congenital clefting itself or may be secondary to the surgical correction of the primary

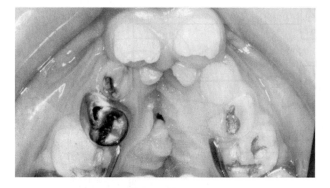

FIG. **28-6.** Palatally erupted maxillary primary lateral incisors.

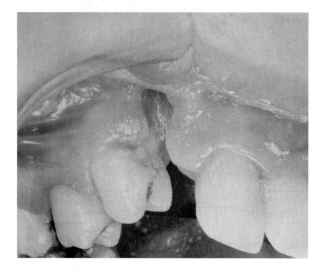

FIG. **28-7.** Maxillary right first permanent premolar adjacent to cleft defect. Notice the deficiency of mesial supporting alveolar bone.

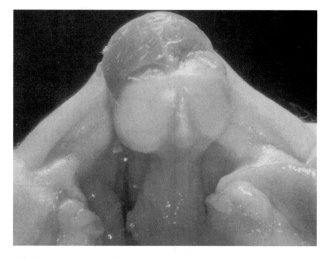

FIG. **28-8.** Bilateral complete cleft of the lip and palate with a severe anterior displacement of the premaxillary segment.

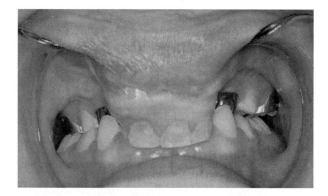

FIG. **28-9.** Bilateral complete cleft of the lip and palate demonstrating a greater than 100% overbite. Stripping of the labial attached gingiva of the mandibular central and lateral incisors is common in this presentation.

(Fig. 28-7). These teeth are susceptible to premature loss. A decrease in alveolar bone support may be accentuated when periodontal disease is present or when orthodontic appliance therapy is used indiscriminately.

7. With great frequency, permanent central incisors adjacent to an alveolar cleft erupt in a rotated position and with deviations of axial root inclination.

8. With a complete cleft of the palate and alveolus there is no longer a contiguous maxillary arch. External forces applied to the maxilla (e.g., by muscles of mastication or by the contraction of scar tissue after surgical repair of the cleft palate) can result in medial collapse of the posterior segments. A posterior crossbite may be observed unilaterally or bilaterally.

9. In an infant with a complete bilateral cleft of the lip and palate, the premaxilla is often protuberant and mobile (Fig. 28-8). There may be a greater than 100% overbite with subsequent stripping of the labial-attached gingiva overlying the mandibular incisors (Fig. 28-9). Traumatic anterior end-to-end occlusion, or an anterior crossbite, is also common.

10. In a patient with a complete unilateral or bilateral cleft of the palate, the lateral facial profile may appear noticeably convex (Fig. 28-10). This may become more perceptible as the child grows older. The appearance may be attributed to a true mandibular or pseudomandibular prognathism. In pseudomandibular prognathism, the maxilla is in spatial disharmony with the mandible. This may be caused by a retrognathic maxilla or an attenuation of the anteroposterior and vertical growth of the maxilla.

Parents are often so overwhelmed by other aspects of the cleft that they give dental care a low priority or even neglect it altogether. Preventive dental care is extremely important in these cases. The intact dental occlusion is

The orthodontist plays a key role in the diagnosis and treatment of a cleft condition by obtaining records necessary for diagnosis and treatment planning. These include cephalometric and panoramic radiographs, study models, and diagnostic photographs. Analysis of these records enables the orthodontist to describe and quantitate the facial skeleton and soft tissue deformities. Using expertise in the growth and development of the facial skeleton, this specialist can identify problem areas and, with some limitations, predict growth and development. Many team members depend on the orthodontist's analysis and quantitations of the cleft anomaly for treatment planning.

The orthodontist also provides comprehensive orthodontic care for patients. Most orthodontic care can be considered conventional, but for difficult dental configurations, innovation and imagination are required for treatment. If surgical treatment is indicated, the orthodontist works closely with the surgeon to plan the most appropriate procedure. Immediately postoperative function, esthetic result, and long-term stability are factors considered before surgery.

The ability to surgically alter skeletal relationships of the maxillomandibular complex is the basis for participation by the oral and maxillofacial surgeon on the cleft team. This specialist evaluates all patients for facial form and function and jaw position. Many patients have significant skeletal malocclusions that cannot be treated by conventional orthodontics and require surgical correction.

The surgical placement of primary and secondary alveolar cleft bone grafts is another important role of the oral and maxillofacial surgeon. These grafts aid in dental habilitation. The grafted bone supports the teeth adjacent to the cleft site and provides bone through which teeth may erupt. A detailed discussion of these grafts follows later in this chapter.

The maxillofacial prosthodontist replaces, restores, or rehabilitates orofacial structures that may be congenitally missing or malformed. Nonliving materials are used to restore and enhance form and anatomy. There is a special commitment to the oral cavity because this specialist fabricates prosthetic appliances to rehabilitate mastication, deglutition, speech, and oral esthetics.

Many patients with clefts have congenitally missing teeth or malformed teeth that may need to be removed. In these cases, masticatory function, speech, and orofacial esthetics are compromised, and successful habilitation dictates that these missing teeth be replaced to achieve as near normal a condition as possible (Fig. 28-11). The maxillofacial prosthodontist may do this with fixed or removable appliances or with a combination of the two.

Occasionally, patients demonstrate aberrant speech patterns caused by failure of the soft palate to elevate

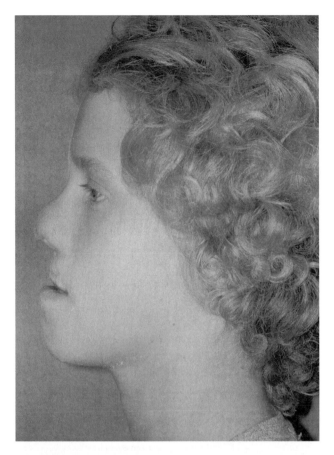

FIG. 28-10. Lateral facial profile of an adolescent boy with a repaired bilateral complete cleft of the lip and palate. Maxillary hypoplasia, secondary to the cleft defect, often produces a greatly concave lateral facial profile.

the foundation around which future orthodontic therapy takes place. For this reason, optimum dental health is essential for total habilitation of the patient. Any compromise will lead to a less than optimal result. Routine prophylaxis and fluoride treatments are mandatory. Referral for preventive dental care should be made during the first year of life. Fluoride supplements, dentifrices, and rinses are indicated if the patient lives in a nonfluoridated community. The parents and patient should be instructed in proper dental hygiene techniques, especially around the defect. Close communication between the primary care dentist and the cleft team is important to ensure the continuity of care necessary during the extended treatment of such patients. Routine periodic reports from the cleft team should be forwarded to the child's primary care dentist, especially during orthodontic or surgical treatment. Pediatric dentists often are involved in the presurgical and postsurgical treatment phase of maxillary orthopedics. Both active and passive appliances are used to bring the cleft segments into a more ideal alignment and thereby promote a more favorable initial surgical outcome.

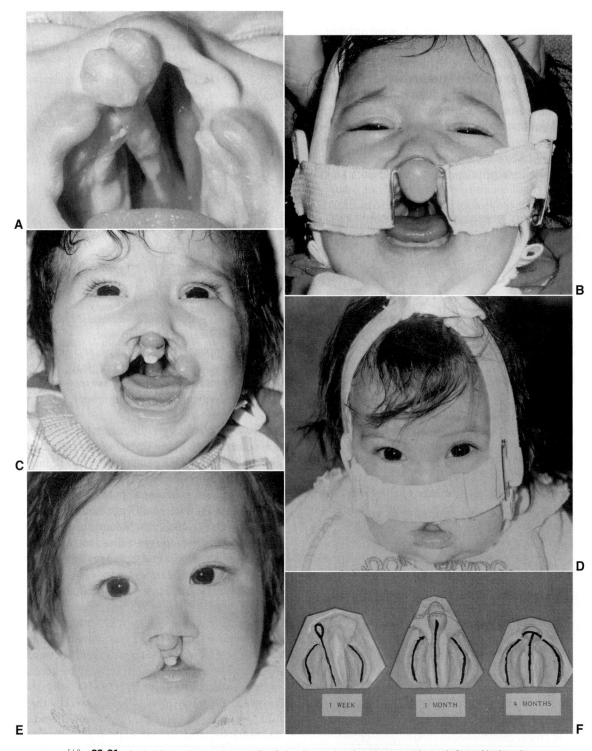

FIG. **28-21.** **A,** A bilateral complete cleft of the lip and palate in a newborn infant. Notice the severely anteriorly protruded and laterally deviated premaxillary segment. **B,** Placement of "bulb" prosthesis over the premaxillary segment; bulb is anchored to the bonnet. **C,** Patient at the end of bulb therapy to position the laterally deviated premaxillary segment to the facial midline. **D,** Strap therapy to improve the anteroposterior relationship of the protruding premaxillary segment before definitive lip closure. **E,** Premaxillary segment at the completion of strap therapy. Notice the improvement in position (compare with **A**) at this time. **F,** Sequential models at 1 week (initial presentation), 1 month (completion of bulb therapy), and 4 months (completion of strap therapy). Notice the improving position of the premaxillary segment at these various times. *(D and F from Jones JE, Lynch TR, Sadove AM: Quintessence Int 16:229–231, 1985.)*

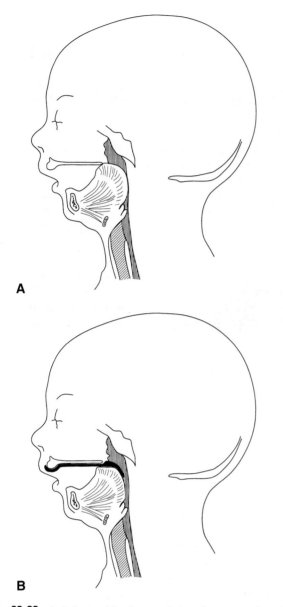

A

B

FIG. **28-22.** **A,** Infant with airway obstruction secondary to Pierre Robin sequence. Notice the closure of the oral airway related to the retroposition of the tongue. **B,** Infant with obturator in position. Notice the anterior placement of the tongue, which allows the oral airway to remain open.

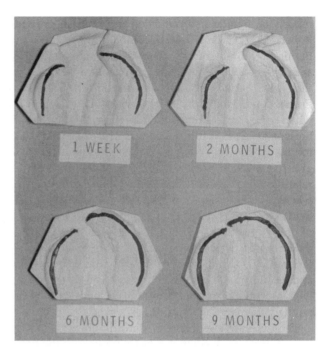

FIG. **28-23.** Sequential maxillary arch dental models demonstrating maxillary orthopedic molding in an infant with a unilateral complete cleft of the lip and palate. Notice that, as the cleft defect closes with time, lateral arch dimension is maintained, which produces optimal maxillary arch symmetry. *(From Jones JE et al: Quintessence Int 17:245–248, 1986.)*

common. It is attributed to the increased tension placed on the segments by the repaired lip. To prevent this collapse, the obturator is used to provide cross-arch stability and support. As pressure is exerted on the anterior segments of the maxilla by the repaired lip, orthopedic molding of the segments can be achieved. In unilateral cases, the force applied to the greater segment by the intact lip molds that segment around to approximate the lesser segment (Fig. 28-23). This molding is facilitated by the obturator, which provides a fulcrum around which the anterior portion of the

greater segment rotates. At the same time the appliance resists any tendency for the greater and lesser segments to collapse toward the midline. In bilateral cleft cases, the repaired lip provides further retraction at the premaxilla, positioning it between the two lateral maxillary segments. When the maxillary segments are in good alignment and abutted across the cleft sites, the patient is ready for the primary cleft bone graft. This generally occurs by 6 to 9 months of age.

Bone Grafting of Alveolar Cleft Defects. Bone grafting of alveolar cleft defects has been a confusing issue to many patients and practitioners. This stems in part from the lack of unanimity concerning terminology and technique. The following definitions, which have been reasonably accepted by practitioners, will be used in this discussion.

Primary bone grafting refers to bone-grafting procedures involving alveolar cleft defects in children younger than 2 years of age; this term implies nothing about technique. *Early secondary bone grafting* refers to bone-grafting procedures performed between 2 and 4 years of age. *Secondary bone grafting* is done between 4 and 15 years of age, and *late secondary bone grafting* refers to reconstruction of residual alveolar cleft defects in the adult.

Primary Alveolar Cleft Bone Grafting. Primary alveolar cleft bone grafting is controversial. The concept fell into disfavor in the early 1970s amid numerous

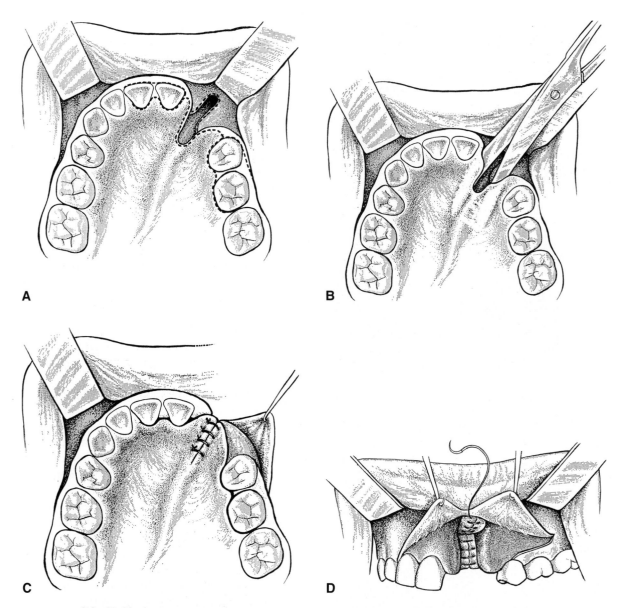

FIG. **28-30.** Technique for secondary alveolar cleft bone graft. **A,** Mucosal incisions outlined. **B,** Development of palatal mucoperiosteal flap. **C,** Closure of palatal mucosa. **D,** Closure of nasal mucosa within cleft site.

provide a stable, esthetic prosthesis is enhanced. There is often some degree of collapse of the maxillary arch form. It is possible to expand the arch after grafting, as pointed out by Boyne and Sands[21]; however, it is preferable to expand these collapsed segments to as optimal an arch form as possible before grafting. Pregraft expansion also widens the cleft site, which allows better access for nasal floor closure. After the arch expansion has occurred, the bone graft can be placed. After the graft has been incorporated, it can be expected to maintain a good arch form.

Closure of the oronasal fistula is often the most significant result of bone graft surgery, according to patients. They often have fluid regurgitation into the nose and mucus drainage from the nose into the oral cavity through the fistula. Depending on its size, the fistula can produce significant speech problems because air escapes when the patient phonates. Although closure of this fistula can be effected with only soft tissue closure, Enemark, Krantz-Simonsen, and Schramm have indicated that closure is more successful when combined with a bone graft.[22]

With a cleft maxilla the cleft extends through the piriform rim beneath the alar base of the nose. As a result, the alar base on the cleft side is often depressed because of lack of underlying bony support. Filling the cleft with bone provides underlying bony support that often elevates the alar base of the nose. Although this

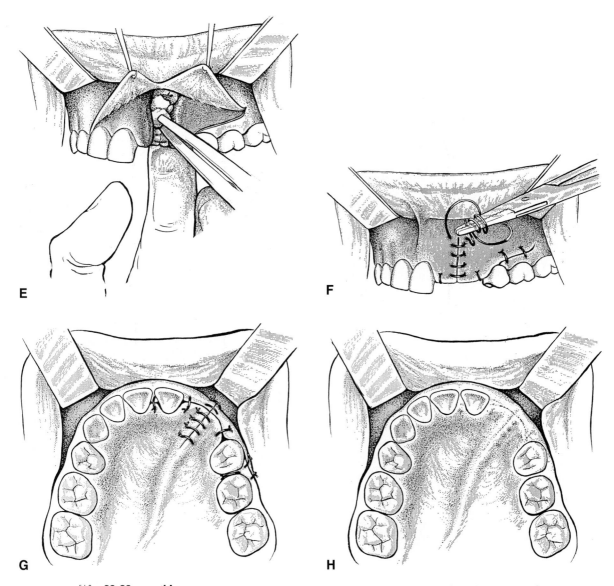

FIG. **28-30, cont'd. E,** Placement of fresh autogenous bone into the cleft defect. **F** and **G,** Reapproximation and closure of mucoperiosteal flaps. **H,** The reconstructed maxillary alveolus.

may not entirely correct any existing nasal deformity, it does provide good support over which nasal reconstructive and revision surgery can be accomplished (Fig. 28-32).

Secondary alveolar cleft bone grafting has been widely accepted. Boyne and Sands,[18] Bertz,[23] Hall and Posnick,[24] Kortebein, Nelson, and Sadove,[25] Kwon et al,[26] Troxell, Fonseca, and Osbon,[27] Enemark, Krantz-Simonsen, and Schramm,[22] and Turvey et al[20] have reported favorable results and emphasize the low morbidity rate. Success rates are generally in the 90% range. Morbidity has included pain in the donor site, dehiscence of mucosal flaps, and partial or complete loss of grafted bone. Infection in the donor or recipient sites has been rare. An unpublished survey by

Huebener indicated that secondary alveolar bone grafting (grafting performed in the mixed dentition) is routinely performed by all teams.

Secondary alveolar cleft bone grafting is an important procedure that greatly facilitates total habilitation. Not only is speech improved but dental, esthetic, and psychosocial benefits are to be gained. It is necessary again to emphasize the different objectives of primary and secondary grafting and to reiterate that they are not mutually exclusive procedures. The primary graft, over time, may satisfy some or all the objectives of secondary grafting. However, to the extent that it does not, augmenting the primary graft with particulate marrow and cancellous bone from the iliac crest may be recommended as a secondary procedure.

REFERENCES

1. Veau V: Treatment of the unilateral hairlip, *International Dental Congress Eighth Transaction*, pp 126-131, 1931.
2. Parameters for the evaluation and treatment of patients with cleft lip/palate or other craniofacial anomalies. American Cleft Palate-Craniofacial Association. Cleft Palate–Craniofacial J 30 (suppl 1), 1993, revised 2000.
3. Whitehouse FA: Treatment as a dynamic system, *Cleft Palate J* 2:16-27, 1965.
4. McNeil CK: *Oral and facial deformity*, London, 1954, Pittman.
5. McNeil CK: Congenital oral deformities, *Br Dent J* 101: 191-198, 1956.
6. Jones JE: The use and clinical effectiveness of the maxillary obturator appliance in cleft lip and palate infants: birth through six months of age, doctoral dissertation, San Jose, Costa Rica, 2003, Empresarial University.
7. Pashayan HM, McNab M: Simplified method of feeding infants with cleft palate with or without cleft lip, *Am J Dis Child* 133:145-147, 1979.
8. Hofman JP: De labiis leoporinis/von Hasen-Scharten, Heidelberg, 1686, Bergmann.
9. Robertson NRE, Jolleys A: Effects of early bone grafting in complete clefts of the lip and palate, *Plast Reconstr Surg* 42: 414-421, 1968.
10. Friede H: The vomero-premaxillary suture: a neglected growth site in midfacial development of unilateral cleft lip and palate patients, *Cleft Palate J* 15:398-404, 1978.
11. Rosenstein SW et al: The case for early bone grafting in cleft lip and cleft palate, *Plast Reconstr Surg* 70:297-302, 1982.
12. Rosenstein SW et al: The case for early bone grafting in cleft lip and palate: a second report, *Plast Reconstr Surg* 87: 644-654, 1991.
13. Rosenstein SW et al: A long-term retrospective outcome assessment of facial growth, secondary surgical need, and maxillary lateral incisor status in surgical-orthodontic protocol for complete clefts, *Plast Reconstr Surg* 111(1):1-13, 2003.
14. Huebener DV, Marsh JL: A survey of early management of cleft lip and palate—the first 18 months, unpublished data presented at the American Cleft Palate–Craniofacial Annual Meeting, 2002.
15. Rosenstein SW: Orthodontic and bone grafting procedures in a cleft lip and palate series: an interim cephalometric evaluation, *Angle Orthod* 45:227-237, 1975.
16. Grayson BH, Cutting CB: Presurgical nasoalveolar orthopedic molding in primary correction of the nose, lip, and alveolus of infants born with unilateral and bilateral clefts, *Cleft Palate Craniofac J* 38:193-198, 2001.
17. Latham RA, Kusy RP, Georgiade NG: An extraorally activated expansion appliance for cleft palate infants, *Cleft Palate J* 13:253-261, 1976.
18. Boyne PJ, Sands NR: Secondary bone grafting of residual alveolar and palatal clefts, *J Oral Surg* 30:87-92, 1972.
19. ElDeeb M et al: Canine eruption into grafted bone in maxillary alveolar cleft defects, *Cleft Palate J* 19:9-16, 1982.
20. Turvey TA et al: Delayed bone grafting in the cleft maxilla and palate: a retrospective multidisciplinary analysis, *Am J Orthod* 86:244-256, 1984.
21. Boyne PJ, Sands NR: Combined orthodontic surgical management of residual palato-alveolar cleft defects, *Am J Orthod* 70:20-37, 1976.
22. Enemark H, Krantz-Simonsen E, Schramm JE: Secondary bone grafting in unilateral cleft lip and palate patients: indications and treatment procedure, *Int J Oral Surg* 14:2-10, 1985.
23. Bertz JE: Bone grafting of alveolar clefts, *J Oral Surg* 39: 874-877, 1981.
24. Hall HD, Posnick JC: Early results of secondary bone grafts in 106 alveolar clefts, *J Oral Maxillofac Surg* 41:289-294, 1983.
25. Kortebein MJ, Nelson CL, Sadove AM: Retrospective analysis of 135 secondary alveolar cleft bone grafts, *J Oral Maxillofac Surg* 49:493-498, 1991.
26. Kwon HJ et al: The management of alveolar cleft defects, *J Am Dent Assoc* 102:848-853, 1981.
27. Troxell JB, Fonseca RJ, Osbon DB: A retrospective study of alveolar cleft grafting, *J Oral Maxillofac Surg* 40:721-725, 1982.
28. Striker G et al: Psychosocial aspects of craniofacial disfigurement: a "state of the art" assessment conducted by the Craniofacial Anomalies Program Branch, the National Institute of Dental Research, *Am J Orthod* 76:410-422, 1979.
29. MacGregor FC: Social and psychological implications of dentofacial disfigurement, *Angle Orthod* 40:231-233, 1970.

SUGGESTED READINGS

Burston WR: The early orthodontic treatment of cleft palate conditions, *Dent Pract Dent Rec* 9:41-52, 1958.

DiBiase DD, Hunter SB: A method of pre-surgical oral orthopedics, *Br Dent J* 10:25-31, 1983.

Friede H, Johanson B: A follow-up study of cleft children treated with primary bone grafting, *Scand J Plast Reconstr Surg* 8: 88-103, 1974.

Hanson JW, Murray, JC: Genetic aspects of cleft lip and palate. In Bardach J, Morris HL, editors: *Multidisciplinary management of cleft lip and palate,* Philadelphia, 1990, WB Saunders, chapter 14, pp 121-124.

Hathaway RR et al: Primary alveolar cleft bone grafting in unilateral cleft lip and palate: arch dimensions at age 8. *J Craniofac Surg* 10:58, 1999.

Hotz M, Gnoinski W: Clefts of the secondary palate associated with the "Pierre Robin Syndrome": management by early maxillary orthopedics, *Swed Dent J Suppl* 15:89-97, 1982.

Huddart AG, Ziberman Y: Presurgical treatment in the newborn cleft palate infant, *Isr J Dent Med* 26:15-19, 1977.

Huebener DV: Maxillary orthopedics. Advances in management of cleft lip and palate. In *Clinical plastic surgery,* Philadelphia, 1993, WB Saunders.

Jacobsen BN, Rosenstein SW: Early maxillary orthopedics for the newborn cleft lip and palate patient: an impression and an appliance, *Angle Orthod* 54:247-263, 1984.

Jolleys A, Robertson NRE: A study of the effects of early bone grafting in complete clefts of the lip and palate: five year study, *Br Plast Surg* 25:229-237, 1972.

Jones JE: Early management of severe bilateral cleft lip and palate in an infant, *J Dent Child* 48:50-54, 1981.

Jones JE: Self-concept and parental evaluation of peer relationships in cleft lip and palate children, *Pediatr Dent* 6:132-138, 1984.

Jones JE, Friend GW: Cleft orthotics and obturation, *Oral Maxillofac Surg Clin North Am* 3(3):517-529, 1991.

Jones JE, Kerkhof RL: Obturator construction for maxillary orthopedics in cleft lip and palate infants, *Quintessence Dent Technol* 8:583-586, 1984.

Jones JE, Lynch TR, Sadove AM: Three-dimensional premaxillary orthopedic technique for improved position and symmetry prior to cheiloplasty in bilateral cleft lip and palate, *Quintessence Int* 16:229-231, 1985.

Jones JE, Meade P, Edwards A: Treating cleft lip and palate infants, *Dent Assist* 4:20-23, 25, 1985.

Jones JE et al: Maxillary arch expansion in cleft lip and palate prior to primary autogenous alveolar bone graft surgery, *Quintessence Int* 17:245-248, 1986.

Kennedy TJ et al: The team approach to treatment of cleft lip and palate, *Am Fam Physician* 18:74-84, 1978.

Kernahan DA: The striped Y: a symbolic classification of cleft lips and palates, *Plast Reconstr Surg* 47:469-470, 1971.

Kernahan DA: On cleft lip and palate classification, *Plast Reconstr Surg* 51:578, 1973.

Maull DJ, Grayson BH, Cutting CB: Long term effects of nasoalveolar molding on three dimensional nasal shape in unilateral clefts, *Cleft Palate Craniofac J* 36:391-397, 1999.

Malson TS: Prostheses for the newborn, *J Prosthet Dent* 21:384-387, 1969.

Markowitz JA, Gerry RG, Fleishner R: Immediate obturation of neonatal cleft palates, *Mt Sinai J Med* 46:123-129, 1979.

Monroe CW et al: The correction and preservation of arch form in complete clefts of the palate and alveolar ridge, *Plast Reconstr Surg* 41:108-112, 1968.

Morris HL, Jakobi P, Harrington D: Objectives and criteria for the management of the cleft lip and palate and the delivery of management services, *Cleft Palate J* 15:1-5, 1978.

Nelson CL et al: Indiana's craniofacial anomalies team: dentists play an important role, *J Indiana Dent Assoc* 65(6):9-13, 1986.

Nelson WE, Behrman RE, Vaughan VC: *Textbook of pediatrics*, ed 12, Philadelphia, 1983, WB Saunders.

Osuji OO: Preparation of feeding obturators for infants with cleft lip and palate, *J Clin Pediatr Dent* 19(3):211-214, 1995.

Pickerell K, Quinn G, Massengill R: Primary bone grafting of the maxilla in clefts of the lip and palate, *Plast Reconstr Surg* 41:438-443, 1968.

Pruzansky S: The multidiscipline approach of the treatment of cleft palate in children, *Cleft Palate Bull* 10:99-104, 1960.

Rehrmann AH, Koberg WR, Koch H: Long term postoperative results of primary and secondary bone grafting in complete clefts of the lip and palate, *Cleft Palate J* 7:206-221, 1969.

Rosenstein SW et al: A series of cleft lip and cleft palate children five years after undergoing orthopedic and bone grafting procedures, *Angle Orthod* 42:1-8, 1972.

Rosenstein SW et al: Comparison of 2-D calculations from periapical and occlusal radiographs versus 3-D calculations from CAT scans in determining bone support for cleft-adjacent teeth following early alveolar bone grafts, *Cleft Palate J* 34:199-205, 1997.

Ross RB, MacNamera MC: Effect of presurgical infant orthopedics on facial esthetics in complete bilateral cleft lip and palate, *Cleft Palate J* 31:68-73, 1994.

Rotrick R, Black PW, Jurkiewicz MJ: Bilateral cleft lip and palate: presurgical treatment, *Ann Plast Surg* 12:105-117, 1984.

Santini R et al: Fundamental principles and appliances for the treatment of newborn children with cleft palates, *Ortodoncia* 39:5-19, 1975.

Santini R et al: Treatment of a newborn child with bilateral complete cleft palate and lateral deviation of the premaxilla: original appliance, *Ortodoncia* 39:79-83, 1975.

Williams AC, Rothman BN, Seidman LH: Management of a feeding problem in an infant with cleft palate, *J Am Dent Assoc* 77:81-83, 1968.

29

Practice Management

ANN PAGE GRIFFIN

LEE M. HARRISON, JR.

JASPER L. LEWIS, JR.

PERSONNEL SYSTEMS
Personnel Needs
Interviewing and Hiring
Orientation and Training
Wage and Benefit Administration
Performance Appraisals
Personnel Records
Dismissal
Communication
PATIENT SYSTEMS
First Appointment
Patient Flow
Preventive Program
Marketing and Practice Growth
Communications with Parents and Patients
OPERATIONAL SYSTEMS
Scheduling
Recare System
Checking of Recare Effectiveness
Broken Appointments and Purging of Patient
Charts
Production and Collections
Payment Policy
Dental Insurance and Other Third-Party Plans
Insurance Assignment
Insurance Reference Guide
Predetermination
Filing Claims
Health Insurance Portability and Accountability
Act
Pending Insurance Claims

Direct Reimbursement
Managed Care
Dental Management Companies
Fiscal Management
Billing and Accounts Receivable
Fees
Accounts Payable
Budget Setting
Practice Monitors
Daily Statistics
Monthly Statistics
Averages, Medians, and Goals in a Pediatric
Dental Practice
Production
Collections
Accounts receivable
Appointments
Average work times per week, month, and year
Treatment and hygiene minimum goals
*Example of checking recare system
effectiveness*
Typical Ratios in a Pediatric Dental Practice
Overhead
Hygiene department production
Hygiene compensation
Chairside assistants' compensation
Business staff compensation
Number of business staff
*Staff compensation including wages, payroll
taxes, and benefits*

The practice of modern dentistry requires delivery of quality care combined with adherence to excellent business principles. Dentists, traditionally trained in the art and science of dentistry, must also become skilled in techniques of sound business management. Today's practitioner must be clinically astute and knowledgeable about consumer needs and demands, government regulations, and third-party participation—aspects of dentistry not often addressed in the clinical setting of dental school.

The transition from a role of dental student or resident to business owner and manager is an enormous challenge. That transition often begins when the new-to-practice dentist enters practice and suddenly realizes that dentistry encompasses more than clinical and technical competence. A successful dentist must be concerned with many office-management concepts, including leadership, delegation, interpersonal relationships, personal style, community image, and time management, as well as the day-to-day operation and fiscal management of a business.

The primary responsibility of a dentist is to provide quality patient care. However, private practice—and, in today's environment, many school, hospital, and government dental facilities—like any other business, must make a profit to survive. The practitioner must maintain a balance between patient care and business requirements while keeping moral, ethical, legal, and professional responsibilities in proper perspective.

While maintaining this balance a dentist must provide a place where children can feel safe, loved, and well cared for; where parents can be educated about how to help their children have a lifetime of good oral health; where the staff know that they are an integral part of the practice, that they are important and appreciated, and that their opinions count; where other practitioners and health care providers feel good about referring patients or calling the office for information; where the community as a whole knows, respects, and appreciates the practice; and where changes can be made in any area needed and new, better, innovative ideas and methods can be endorsed and implemented.

Every new dentist begins practice expecting to be successful. Those satisfied with their level of achievement after several years realize that a successful dental practice is composed of three systems: personnel, patient, and operational.

PERSONNEL SYSTEMS
PERSONNEL NEEDS

A personable, professional staff is vitally important for practice success. The dentist must invest time, effort, and money to hire, train, and retain quality individuals who can be developed into a team. A team of committed professionals, working together, focused on the patients and the practice, can make the difference between an excellent and a mediocre practice. Therefore, staff development is a sound investment in any practice.

Before becoming an employer, the dentist must be aware of state and federal regulations concerning hiring; employment policies, including Occupational Safety and Health Administration (OSHA) requirements; employee records and retention; discipline; and dismissal. All employment applications and other forms used in the hiring process and employment policies described in the office manual should be reviewed by an attorney familiar with state and federal laws.

The number of employees in an office varies according to the type of practice and patient volume. Pediatric and orthodontic practices usually require more team members than other practices.

Initially, the new practitioner may need to hire only one or two staff members. If only one individual is hired at first, a second employee should be added when patient flow increases to the point that this person can no longer assist at the chair and handle the business desk (e.g., collect fees, make appointments, answer the telephone by the third ring, prepare and mail statements on time, and pursue broken appointments). The first employee, who is already knowledgeable about scheduling patients and practice flow, should move to the business desk. The second employee should serve as a full-time clinical assistant.

The third office employee may be a second clinical assistant or a dental hygienist. When the dentist treats hygiene patients more than 8 hours per week and the state practice act limits the performance of some hygiene duties by a certified dental assistant, a hygienist should be hired. This will allow the dentist to concentrate on other treatments and procedures. Depending on patient volume, the hygienist may be full time or part time. Other employees may then be added as needed.

Additional help may be gained through the use of part-time employees. These employees may *job share,* a term used to describe the splitting of a full-time position between two people, or a position may need to be filled only part time (i.e., a few hours per day or week).

The business of managing and administering a dental practice has become complex and time consuming for the dentist, even with a well-trained staff. Some larger dental practices now hire professionally educated and trained practice administrators. "The key responsibilities of a Practice Administrator could be compared to those of a Chief Executive Office (CEO) of any corporation:

1. Strategic planning and positioning—chief strategist

2. Team building—culture, positioning, performance contracts, empowerment
3. Monitoring all departments, making adjustments/changes as needed
4. Chief deal maker."[1]

Once a practice administrator is on staff, the doctors' position becomes similar to that of the chairman of the board of directors of a corporation or company, a major policy voice as well as owner of the right of refusal or veto authority. In some cases, several practices may share the services of a practice administrator.

INTERVIEWING AND HIRING

Mastery of the interviewing process is difficult but necessary. Hiring begins with attracting well-qualified applicants. Potential employees may come from personal recommendations made by current staff; area technical schools, colleges, and universities; or classified advertisements.

Interviewing becomes easier and more enlightening with repetition. The more opportunities an interviewer has to conduct interviews, the smoother and more productive the sessions. Use of a set of interview questions standardizes the process. These questions should explore the following traits: initiative, organization, and conscientiousness; effective communication; ability to work well with others; and technical or business training and the ability to apply previous training and experience to the job. If questions are skillfully posed, an applicant's answers will indicate strengths or weaknesses in these areas.

Following these steps should make the interview more effective:

1. Read the resume or job application to learn about the person before the interview. Chat a few moments to put the interviewee at ease as the interview begins.
2. Have a written set of questions that will elicit strengths or weaknesses in the four areas mentioned previously.
3. Tell the interviewee that some specific questions will be asked and notes will be taken.
4. Listen well. Note body language and eye contact, because they often speak louder than words.
5. The interviewer should talk less than 25% of the time. The purpose of the interview is to understand the applicant and his or her potential for the job. Excessive talking by the interviewer limits the time and opportunity that the applicant has to tell about personal abilities and experiences.
6. Do not help the interviewee answer questions. Let pauses happen. The applicant may be thinking during the silences, and the interviewer can see how well and how quickly the person responds.
7. Do not ask questions that can be answered with yes or no. If the interviewee begins answering yes or no, ask him or her to explain or expound on the answer.
8. Never argue with an applicant. Maintain poise and remember that the interviewer is in control.

Two of the most desirable traits in a dental team member are a warm, empathetic personality and cognitive ability, defined as aptitude for learning and capacity to draw from past experience in new situations. Several excellent instruments are on the market to measure cognitive ability and various aspects of personality and behavioral style.*

To maximize efficiency, a well-trained staff member may conduct the first interview. If the candidate is promising, employment tests, a tour of the office, an introduction to other staff members, and a brief conversation with the dentist should be a part of the first interview. References should be checked between the first and second interviews.

The second interview should include a longer conversation with the dentist and office observation or work time. The dentist should pay the applicant for time spent observing and/or working in the office. Inviting the prospective employee to work in the office for a few hours allows staff members to form an opinion about the person's potential. Likewise, the applicant will better understand office ambiance and patient flow before accepting the job.

Although the final hiring decision rests with the dentist, it is a good idea for certain key staff members to concur. Current employees significantly affect the success or failure of a newly hired staff member because they help train and interact closely with him or her.

An offer may be made after the working interview. If the applicant will not be hired following the first, second, or working interview, he or she may be told at that time or notified by mail within 1 week of either interview. If an applicant is rejected, maintain all applications, test forms, and other paperwork for at least 1 year in case a complaint is filed. If testing is part of the application and interviewing process, testing must be standardized. All applicants must be given the identical test. If an applicant is hired, be aware that all interview and employment records must be kept for the duration of employment plus 30 years.

*Examples include the following: cognitive ability testing instrument—Wonderlic Personnel Test, Wonderlic, Inc., Libertyville, Ill., www.wonderlic.com; personality and behavioral-style instruments—DiSC Classic (Personal Profile System), Inscape Publishing, Minneapolis, Minn., www.inscape.com.

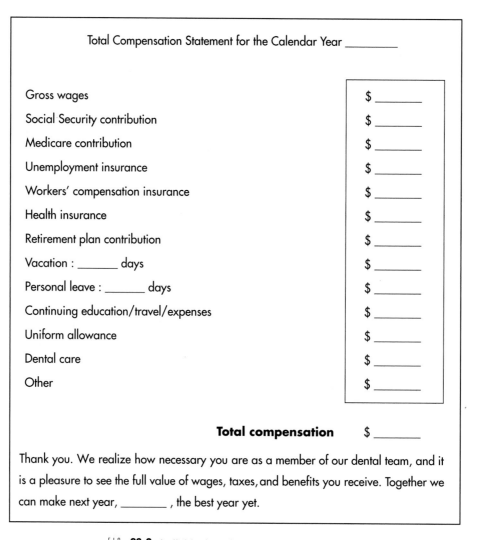

Total Compensation Statement for the Calendar Year _____

Gross wages $ _____

Social Security contribution $ _____

Medicare contribution $ _____

Unemployment insurance $ _____

Workers' compensation insurance $ _____

Health insurance $ _____

Retirement plan contribution $ _____

Vacation : _____ days $ _____

Personal leave : _____ days $ _____

Continuing education/travel/expenses $ _____

Uniform allowance $ _____

Dental care $ _____

Other $ _____

Total compensation $ _____

Thank you. We realize how necessary you are as a member of our dental team, and it is a pleasure to see the full value of wages, taxes, and benefits you receive. Together we can make next year, _____ , the best year yet.

FIG. **29-2.** Individual total compensation statement.

Employees can be expected to perform optimally only if requirements are clear. Team members must know what they are expected to do, how to do it, and what the criteria are for an acceptable or, better yet, outstanding job performance.

The purpose of performance reviews is to recognize past growth and accomplishments while setting new goals and standards of achievement. Periodic performance appraisals allow the dentist and team members to evaluate personal attributes, job strengths, and areas to be improved, so that goals for personal and professional growth can be set. Appraisals should be positive and result in better job performance and improved efficiency.

Each staff member should be evaluated according to similar criteria, including competence in performing tasks, work habits, contributions to the team, and general attitude toward patients, coworkers, the dentist, and the office. Nebulous topics, such as attitude, poor mannerisms, or personality conflicts, should be addressed by listing specific examples of positive or negative instances involving the person. Evaluation forms that can be completed by the staff member and dentist are helpful but not absolutely necessary. Simple notes about strengths, growth opportunities, and the employee's needs as they match or conflict with the needs of the practice are sufficient for the evaluation conversation. Discussing the staff member's opinion of his or her own performance often makes the appraisal more meaningful. Performance reviews must be given regularly to improve job performance and encourage personal growth. An appraisal should be given after completion of the training period and at least annually thereafter.

Job skills and work performance should be reviewed separately from salary. A conversation that combines performance review with news of a raise interferes with the staff member's concentration. An employee may be so interested in hearing about a salary increase that setting goals for performance improvement is relegated to a secondary level of importance.

During the review, strengths should be enumerated first. People listen better when they feel that the appraiser recognizes their strengths rather than only their deficiencies. Use of the term *development areas* rather than *weaknesses* when discussing areas to be improved connotes opportunity for growth.

Most people respond best when asked to concentrate on no more than three or four areas for development. Hearing about more than three or four points to be improved is overwhelming and may delay the employee's responses and improvements.

The dentist may offer to help the employee improve in certain areas through additional training, continuing-education courses, and such, and thereby give the staff member a sense of support. The dentist and staff member should agree on realistic goals to be met by a certain date, with regular discussions during the interim to evaluate progress and establish other objectives.

PERSONNEL RECORDS

Personnel records are important documents. They are a history of the employee-employer relationship, just as a patient's chart is a documentation of the patient-dentist relationship. If a problem arises with an employee (e.g., a charge of wrongful dismissal in case of termination), the record will serve as proof that the dentist correctly discharged employer responsibilities.

Records, including job application, interviewing notes, testing forms, performance appraisals, wage and benefit information, and so on, should be maintained for the duration of employment and for at least 30 years following an auxiliary's departure. Records for OSHA-mandated training must be maintained from the date the training occurred and must include dates of training, contents of the session, and the name and qualifications of the trainer. Check with your state OSHA office for information concerning the number of years that these records must be maintained. Medical and unsafe-incident records must be maintained for the duration of employment plus 30 years and include all appropriate forms with pertinent data.

Personnel records should be identical in appearance for all employees, consistently maintained, and kept confidential. A comprehensive employee record could include the following:

- Employee's name
- Address and telephone number
- Social Security number
- Completed job application and/or resume
- Employment tests given at the time of hiring
- Date of employment
- Licenses or certifications
- Completed tax forms, including federal and state income tax and Employment Eligibility Verification (I-9 form available from the Bureau of Citizenship and Immigration Services)
- Spouse's name, employer, and telephone number
- Person to contact in case of emergency
- Salary record and summary of benefits
- Training records, including OSHA training and cardiopulmonary resuscitation training
- Medical records, including injury or exposure to harmful substances; record of hepatitis inoculation or signed and dated refusal of the vaccine
- Performance appraisal forms and notes from one-on-one discussions signed and dated by the employee and the dentist
- Absentee records
- Continuing-education course records
- Record of termination, including last date of employment, the employee's letter of resignation, or notes from the dismissal conversation if the employee was fired

DISMISSAL

Dismissal of an employee is one of the most difficult tasks a dentist may face. Whereas interviewing becomes easier with experience, firing someone does not. There are, however, processes that can make a dismissal less stressful.

Dismissal usually happens because of poor attitude, incompetence in job performance, or unacceptable behavior such as patient abuse, sabotage, theft, or substance abuse on the premises. Problems arise when an employee loses interest in her or his responsibilities. Attitude and performance problems must be addressed; simply ignoring the situation will not make it go away. The dentist and staff member must discuss the problems and ways that they can be rectified. After an initial discussion with the employee, it should be absolutely clear to the employee that improved attitude and/or job skill is a requirement for continued employment. The employee and dentist should sign and date notes from the initial and subsequent meetings. A specific date by which attitudes and/or skills must improve should be set. The dentist and the staff member should meet frequently to assess improvements.

When coaching an employee who is trying but is incompetent, a combination of the following procedures may be used. The dentist should write a description of acceptable performance criteria, including skills needed for the job. It is more effective to name specific characteristics and skills needed for the particular position than to enumerate only negatives (i.e., what the person is not doing). The goal is to have the employee understand the requirements of the job, the ways that he

4. American Dental Association, Division of Legal Affairs: *Terminating the dentist-patient relationship: questions and answers,* Chicago, 1994, The Association.

5. Dunlap JE, Wagner JB: *Knowing the numbers: gain and retain control of your practice,* Tulsa, Okla, 1989, PennWell.

Suggested Readings

American Dental Association, Council on Dental Practice: *Successful dental practice: an introduction,* Chicago, 1989, The Association.

Griffin AP: Consider adding a dental health educator, *Dent Econ* 76(9):88-92, 1986.

Griffin AP, Lewis JL Jr: Dental practice considerations, *Dent Clin North Am* 4:861-875, 1995.

Guay AH: Understanding managed care, *J Am Dent Assoc* 126:425-433, 1995.

Limoli TM, Limoli TM Jr: Managed care, *RDH* 9:12-16, 1995.

Ramsey J, Ramsey I: *Budgeting basics,* New York, 1985, Watts.

The Staff of the Institute for Management: *How to prepare an employee handbook,* Old Saybrook, Conn, 1982, The Institute.

Tagiuri R: *Effective communication,* Harvard Business Review Reprint Series No 2141, Boston, 1974, Harvard College.

Wonderlic EF: *The Wonderlic Personnel Test Brochure,* Northfield, Ill, 1991, Wonderlic.

30

Community Oral Health

KAREN M. YODER

CHAPTER OUTLINE

The task of promoting optimal oral health for communities is a rewarding and daunting challenge for dental professionals, whether involved in pediatric dentistry, general practice, or dental public health. Unlike dentists in private practice, who provide services for patients one by one, dentists engaged in community oral health improvement adopt new techniques and build community partnerships to strengthen the possibilities for success for all members of the community. The rewards are great. Those who years ago fought to introduce water fluoridation can now look with pride at the dramatic difference that has occurred in oral health status. Those who are now developing innovative ways to take dental services to underserved children in rural and inner city locations will undoubtedly feel the satisfaction of having accomplished a meaningful goal.

Pediatric dentists and general dentists have the capability of enhancing the oral health of groups of people in the communities in which they practice. To fully understand dentists' role in influencing healthful public policy, developing oral health programs, and contributing to the understanding of the oral health needs of specific population groups, one must have background information on the resources, systems, and information currently available. Collaboration with dental public health professionals is a constructive way to begin a community oral health program. Understanding the role and skills of these professionals is basic to success.

Community oral health is a component of the larger field of public health. The core functions of public health at all levels of government are assessment, policy development, and assurance.[1] The *assessment* role of public health requires systematic collection and analysis of information about the health of communities. The information to be assessed includes statistics on health status and health needs, and epidemiologic data on health problems. The second core function, *policy development*, ensures healthful public policy by promoting the use of scientific knowledge in decision making about health issues and by conveying science-based information to decision makers. *Assurance*, the third core function of public health, strives to provide the services necessary to maintain the health of the community. These health services can be provided by the private or the public sector or by a coalition of sources, and should include subsidized or direct provision of necessary personal health services to those unable to pay for them.

The art and science of dental public health enables community-based approaches to oral health promotion and fosters skills necessary for the task. Dental public health is defined by the American Board of Dental Public Health as the science and art of preventing and controlling dental diseases and promoting dental health through organized community efforts. It is that form of dental practice that serves the community as a patient rather than the individual. It is concerned with the dental education of the public, with applied dental research, and with the administration of group dental care programs as well as with the prevention and control of dental diseases on a community basis.[2]

Specialists in dental public health are leaders in organizing programs to enhance community oral health and can be a resource for private practitioners interested in developing oral health programs for their communities. The fundamental attributes of the dental public health specialist include the following:

- Training as a dentist
- Demonstration of public health values, which essentially means viewing health issues as they affect a population rather than an individual and putting particular emphasis on prevention, the environment in its broadest sense, and service to the community
- Leadership characteristics, such as the ability to influence health policies and practice through research, education, and advocacy; to help articulate a vision for the profession (American Association of Public Health Dentistry); to negotiate and resolve conflicts; etc.
- Subscription to the code of ethics set down by the American Association of Public Health Dentistry

The skills that dental public health specialists can bring to program planning, implementation, and evaluation include the ability to:

- Plan oral health programs for populations
- Select interventions and strategies for the prevention and control of oral disease and promotion of oral health
- Develop resources and implement and manage oral health programs for populations
- Incorporate ethical standards into oral health programs and activities
- Evaluate and monitor dental care delivery systems
- Design and understand the use of surveillance systems to monitor oral health
- Communicate and collaborate with groups and individuals on oral health issues
- Advocate for, implement, and evaluate public health policy, legislation, and regulations to protect and promote the public's oral health
- Critique and synthesize scientific literature
- Design and conduct population-based studies to answer oral and public health questions

GUIDANCE FOR COMMUNITY-BASED PROGRAMS

HEALTHY PEOPLE 2010 NATIONAL HEALTH OBJECTIVES

For those making decisions related to community-based programs to improve oral health, *Healthy People 2010*,[3] developed by the Centers for Disease Control and Prevention, Health Resources and Services Administration, National Institutes of Health, and Indian Health Service, provides guidance in selecting which oral health issues to address. *Healthy People 2010* provides a set of measurable oral health objectives and baseline data against which program outcomes can be measured. The oral health objectives are part of a much larger document setting forth objectives for all areas of health. *Healthy People 2010* was designed to be a roadmap for improving the health of all people in the United States. Many other countries have national health objectives specific to their populations. *Healthy People 2010* targets the goals of increasing quality and years of healthy life and eliminating health disparities. It identifies 10 leading health indicators and 29 focus areas. Oral Health is focus area 21. Each component is stated in general terms and is followed by baseline data for various racial and ethnic groups. Several objectives contain subsections that specifically address children's oral health issues. The following are the oral health objectives set forth in focus area 21 of *Healthy People 2010:*

21-1. Reduce the proportion of children and adolescents who experience dental caries in their primary or permanent teeth. Target: 11%.

21-2. Reduce the proportion of children, adolescents, and adults with untreated dental decay. Targets vary by age category.

21-3. Increase the proportion of adults who have never had a permanent tooth extracted because of dental caries or periodontal disease. Target: 42%.

21-4. Reduce the proportion of older adults who have had all their natural teeth extracted. Target: 20%.

21-5. Reduce periodontal disease. Targets: gingivitis, 41%; destructive periodontal disease, 14%.

21-6. Increase the proportion of oral and pharyngeal cancers detected at the earliest stage. Target: 50%.

21-7. Increase the proportion of adults who report having had an examination to detect oral and pharyngeal cancer in the previous 12 months. Target: 35%.

21-8. Increase the proportion of children who have received dental sealants on their molar teeth. Target: 50%.

21-9. Increase the proportion of the U.S. population served by community water systems with optimally fluoridated water. Target: 75%.

21-10. Increase the proportion of children and adults who use the oral health care system each year. Target: 83%.

21-11. Increase the proportion of residents of long-term-care facilities who use the oral health care system each year. Target: 25%.

21-12. Increase the proportion of children and adolescents under age 19 years with a family income at or below 200% of the federal poverty level who have received preventive dental services during the previous year. Target: 57%.

21-13. Increase the proportion of school-based health centers that have an oral health component. No target established.

21-14. Increase the proportion of local health departments and community-based health centers, including community centers and those serving migrants and the homeless, that have an oral health component. Target: 75%.

21-15. Increase the number of states (including the District of Columbia) that have a system for recording and referring infants and children with cleft lips, cleft palates, and other craniofacial anomalies to craniofacial anomaly rehabilitative teams. Target: all states and the District of Columbia.

21-16. Increase the number of states (including the District of Columbia) that have an oral and craniofacial health surveillance system. Target: all states and the District of Columbia.

21-17. Increase the number of tribal, state (including the District of Columbia), and local health agencies that serve jurisdictions of 250,000 or more persons that have in place an effective public dental health program directed by a dental professional with public health training. No target established.

Additional objectives related to oral health are found in other focus areas of *Healthy People 2010*. The following are selected focus areas that include objectives related to oral health: Access to Quality Health Services (focus area 1), Cancer (focus area 3), Diabetes (focus area 5), Educational and Community-Based Programs (focus area 7), Health Communication (focus area 11), Heart Disease and Stroke (focus area 12), Immunization and Infectious Diseases (focus area 14), Injury and Violence Prevention (focus area 15), Maternal, Infant, and Child Health (focus area 16), Nutrition and Overweight (focus area 19), Public Health Infrastructure (focus area 23), and Tobacco Use (focus area 27).

ORAL HEALTH IN AMERICA: A REPORT OF THE SURGEON GENERAL

Understanding which populations to target in community oral health programs is basic to achieving measurable outcomes. Recent publications have given precise direction to community oral health initiatives. *Oral Health in America: A Report of the Surgeon General,*[4] released in May 2000, described the impact of oral disease on people and communities and the interrelationship of general and oral health. The report also pointed out disparities in access to oral health care among specific populations. These are the major findings of the Surgeon General's report:

- Oral diseases and disorders in and of themselves affect health and well-being throughout life.
- Safe and effective measures exist to prevent the most common dental diseases—dental caries and periodontal diseases.
- Lifestyle behaviors that affect general health such as tobacco use, excessive alcohol use, and poor dietary choices affect oral and craniofacial health as well.
- Profound and consequential oral health disparities exist within the U.S. population.
- More information is needed to improve America's oral health and eliminate health disparities.
- The mouth reflects general health and well-being.
- Oral diseases and conditions are associated with other health problems.
- Scientific research is key to achieving further reductions in the burden of diseases and disorders that affect the face, mouth, and teeth.

A 2000 report of the U.S. General Accounting Office[5] provided documentation for the Surgeon General's report on oral health and described the extent to which dental disease is a chronic problem among many low-income and vulnerable populations. Poor children have five times more untreated dental caries than children in higher-income families, and poor adults are much more likely to have lost six or more teeth to decay and gum disease than higher-income adults. Dental problems result in pain, infection, and millions of lost school days each year. National survey data showed that fewer low-income children visit the dentist on an annual basis; about 36% of 6- to 18-year-olds living at or below the federal poverty level had visited a dentist in the preceding year compared with about 71% living in families with incomes higher than 400% of the federal poverty level. Another indicator of the use of dental care by children is the prevalence of dental sealant application. The General Accounting Office document reported that the poorest children were furthest away from the national

health objectives as defined in a *Healthy People 2010*[3] goal calling for 50% of children to have sealants on permanent molars. Only 12% of children aged 6 to 14 years living at or below the federal poverty level had sealant on at least one tooth, roughly one-third the prevalence among children in higher-income families.

The report of the Surgeon General inspired the beginning of a Partnership Network Group dedicated to developing a National Oral Health Call to Action.[6] The two major goals of the call to action are (1) to eliminate oral health disparities and (2) to improve quality of life. The proposed vision is to promote general health and well-being by promoting oral health through the formation of critical partnerships at all levels. The key action elements of the national oral health call to action build on the five major components described in the Surgeon General's report on oral health and include two additional elements identified at the 2001 Partnership Network conference:

- To change perceptions regarding oral health and disease so that oral health becomes an accepted component of general health
- To accelerate the building of the scientific and evidence base and apply science effectively to improve oral health
- To build an effective health infrastructure at the local, state, and national levels that meets the oral health needs of all Americans and integrates oral health effectively into overall health
- To strengthen and expand oral health research and education capacity
- To ensure the development of a responsive, competent, diverse, and flexible workforce
- To remove known barriers between people and oral health services
- To use public-private partnerships and build on common goals to improve the oral health of those who still are affected disproportionately by oral diseases

ORAL HEALTH PROGRAM GUIDELINES

Guidance for developing community-based programs that specifically address the general and oral health needs of infants, children, and adolescents can be found in the Bright Futures publications. The Bright Futures guidelines were developed by the Maternal and Child Health Bureau of the Health Resources and Services Administration with additional program support from the Medicaid Bureau of the Health Care Financing Administration. Bright Futures publications attempt to improve health outcomes of children by enhancing health professionals' knowledge, skills, and practice of developmentally appropriate health care within the context of family and community. The guidelines are designed to foster partnerships between families, health professionals, and communities, and to increase family knowledge, skills, and participation in health promotion and prevention activities.

Bright Futures health supervision guidelines are unique and especially useful for the development of community oral health programs because they view health from a developmental perspective and describe a continuum of care as children progress through childhood milestones. Bright Futures guidelines provide practical tools and materials for technical assistance and training. The guidelines were updated and revised in 2000 to incorporate current scientific knowledge in health practice. *Bright Futures in Practice: Oral Health*[7] provides information on oral health supervision for infants, children, and adolescents; risk assessment; outcomes measurement; and improvement in the accessibility of oral health supervision. It also includes helpful information about the essential components of oral health.

COMMUNAL WATER FLUORIDATION AND NEW RECOMMENDATIONS FOR THE USE OF FLUORIDE FOR CARIES PREVENTION

The single most influential dental public health measure to date has been the fluoridation of communal water supplies. Children's and adults' oral health has improved dramatically since the introduction of water fluoridation more than 50 years ago and the use of fluoridated dentifrice. Early studies of community water fluoridation showed caries reductions of 50% to 60%. More recent estimates are lower: 18% to 40%. This decrease is probably caused by exposure to fluoride from other sources such as fluoride dentifrice. Food and beverages processed in fluoridated areas but consumed in nonfluoridated areas spread some of the benefit of fluoridation to nonfluoridated communities through a "halo" effect. Therefore the dental caries differential between fluoridated and nonfluoridated communities has decreased. Water fluoridation also reduces the disparities in caries experience among poor and nonpoor children.[8]

The Centers for Disease Control and Prevention's "Recommendations for Using Fluoride to Prevent and Control Dental Caries in the United States,"[9] published in August 2001, made it clear that the beneficial effect of fluoride is predominantly posteruptive and topical, and that, to achieve this effect, fluoride must be available in the right amount in the right place at the right time. This is a reversal of previously held beliefs. The message is slowly reaching practitioners and the public that fluoride works primarily after teeth have erupted rather than by strengthening enamel through incorporation of fluoride into the developing tooth structure. Fluoride is especially effective in preventing dental caries when low concentrations of fluoride are constantly present in the mouth in plaque and saliva. This new information refutes the traditional belief that water fluoridation is primarily beneficial for children and supports the view that water fluoridation has posteruptive benefits for adults as well. The Centers for Disease Control and Prevention strongly encourage that water fluoridation be continued and extended to more communities.

Additional Centers for Disease Control and Prevention recommendations for the use of fluoride that specifically affect children include the following:

- Parents and caregivers should be counseled regarding the use of fluoride toothpaste by young children, especially those younger than 2 years of age.
- Fluoride supplements should be prescribed judiciously (this recommendation is especially pertinent in light of the new understanding that fluoride's predominant effect is posteruptive).
- The use of fluoride toothpaste should be supervised in children younger than 6 years of age.
- An alternative source of water should be obtained for children 8 years of age or younger whose primary drinking water contains more than 2 ppm fluoride.
- The use of small amounts of fluoride toothpaste by children younger than 6 years of age should be promoted.
- A low-fluoride toothpaste should be developed for children younger than 6 years of age.
- Biomarkers of fluoride should be identified.

PROMOTION OF THE USE OF DENTAL SEALANTS IN COMMUNITY-BASED PROGRAMS

Most dental sealants are placed in private-practice dental offices, but the children at greatest risk for problems resulting from dental caries are those least likely to receive dental care in a private setting.[10] Only 18.5% of children and adolescents have at least one sealed permanent tooth.[11] In an attempt to provide sealant application for impoverished children, states and communities have initiated school-based sealant programs that use portable dental equipment (Fig. 30-1) or mobile dental vans (Fig. 30-2). The programs typically move from school to school and often target Title I schools that enroll the highest percentage of children who qualify for free and reduced-price lunches, an indicator of low income. A study conducted in Ohio among 11,191 third-graders who were eligible for the sealant program found that the use of appropriately targeted school-based programs increased the

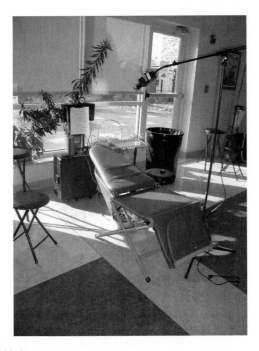

FIG. **30-1.** Portable equipment can be taken into schools and other community sites to create an instant dental clinic for application of dental sealants.

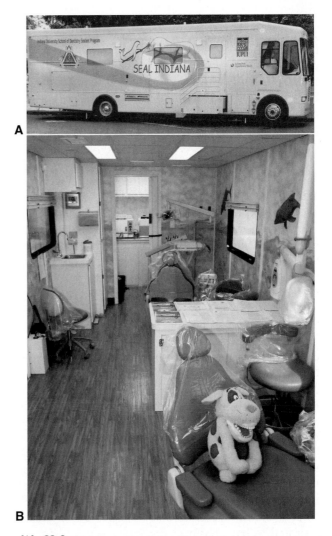

FIG. **30-2.** Mobile dental clinics allow dental sealant treatment to be taken to locations that serve children with limited access to care. **A,** Exterior view of mobile van. **B,** Interior view of mobile van.

prevalence of dental sealant use among children from low-income families and reduced the racial and income disparities in sealant prevalence among elementary school students.[12] Appropriate targeting for sealant programs includes identifying schools with a high percentage of children who are least likely to receive regular dental care and are at high risk for dental caries. A cost-effectiveness analysis of a school-based dental sealant program for children of low socioeconomic status in New York determined that, during a 5-year follow-up period, caries incidence was 6.8 among control children in another school and 2.2 in the group receiving sealant application.[13]

ASSESSMENT OF COMMUNITY ORAL HEALTH NEEDS

The completion of large-scale oral health surveys conducted by qualified dental examiners presents logistic and financial challenges; therefore, the Association of State and Territorial Dental Directors developed materials to simplify information gathering. The system materials, *Basic Screening Surveys: An Approach to Monitoring Community Oral Health*, are available through the Association of State and Territorial Dental Directors web site.[14] The information collected through this system is not intended to be used for clinical diagnosis but rather is used to monitor the specific oral health components listed in the national health objectives in *Healthy People 2010*. Screeners with

or without dental backgrounds can employ the protocol. The use of nondental professionals is advocated because, in many communities, no dental public health professionals are available but other public health professionals, such as nurses, have access to dentally underserved populations.

Useful items provided in the training materials include color photographic reference guides for screening preschool children, schoolchildren and adults; sample cover letter; sample consent form; screening criteria; advice on sampling; data-recording form; format for data entry; advice on human subjects clearance; and screener training information. This manual and accompanying videotape and computer disk are a valuable tool for communities interested in assessing the oral health status of their members.

UTILIZATION OF DENTAL SERVICES AND ACCESS TO CARE

BEHAVIOR RISK FACTOR SURVEILLANCE SYSTEM

Utilization of dental services in the United States has been tracked since 1995 by the Centers for Disease Control and Prevention through its Behavior Risk Factor Surveillance System, a national telephone survey.[15] Although useful information has been gathered, the survey has limitations because it reaches only those people who have telephones and thus eliminates some people from lower socioeconomic groups. The survey includes questions that are indicators of access to oral health services, such as: (1) Have you visited a dentist or dental clinic within the past year for any reason? (2) Have you had your teeth cleaned by a dentist or dental hygienist within the past year? (3) Have you lost six or more teeth due to decay or gum disease? Asking people if they had their teeth cleaned during the previous year provides an indicator of access to preventive services. An affirmative answer to the first question regarding dental visits for any reason identifies those who accessed dental professionals for preventive, restorative, surgical, or emergency services. It is apparent from Table 30-1 that annual utilization of dental services is clearly linked to socioeconomic factors. Race, educational level, and income are consistently strong predictors of access to oral health care: people who are white, have higher incomes, and have more education are more likely to have had a dental visit and to have received preventive services during the previous year. In 2001, 14 states included in the telephone survey a question related to dental insurance: Do you have any kind of insurance coverage that pays for some or all of your routine dental care, including dental insurance, a prepaid plan through a health maintenance organization, or a government plan such as Medicaid? Of those who responded in these 14 states, 58.77% answered yes.

PUBLIC FUNDING OF DENTAL CARE FOR UNDERSERVED CHILDREN

Medicaid. Medicaid is a program established in 1965 to provide health insurance to low-income populations. It is jointly funded by the federal and state governments, includes dental services for children, and covers one in every four children in the United States. Medicaid's Early and Periodic Screening Diagnostic, and Treatment program requires comprehensive children's health and dental services to be provided by all states. Because Medicaid is an entitlement program, enrollment must be offered to eligible children without regard to the fiscal impact on the state. Many barriers exist that deter children from receiving dental services through Medicaid, including low reimbursement rates to dentists, cumbersome claims processing, and real or perceived poor health behaviors by recipients.

State Children's Health Insurance Program. The Balanced Budget Act of 1997 amended the Social Security Act to add a new program, the State Children's Health Insurance Program, which provides access to medical care for children through age 18 who live in households with incomes of up to 200% of the federal poverty guidelines. Twenty-four billion dollars of federal funds was allocated to cofund State Children's Health Insurance Program coverage through state programs for the working poor. The program provides states with a higher federal match rate than Medicaid and allows the states to design the program. The inclusion of dental care was optional for the State Children's Health Insurance Program in each state; however, all but two states included children's dental services. States were required to involve the public in the design and implementation of the plan, as well as to ensure ongoing public participation. Many uninsured Americans are already eligible for free or low-cost public coverage through Medicaid or the State Children's Health Insurance Program but do not enroll in that coverage. Several factors that influence enrollment include size of program benefits, convenience of the enrollment process, possibility of stigma or social sense of disrespect associated with program participation, availability of information about the program, and immigration status.[16]

Children's Special Health Care Services. The Children's Special Health Care Services program helps families of children with serious chronic medical conditions obtain treatment related to their child's condition. This program provides coverage for dental services. The program is federally and state funded, and features care coordination services that help children and their families get medical and dental care. To participate in the program, the individual must be between 0 and 21 years of age and meet certain medical and financial eligibility criteria. Families with an income no greater than 250% of the federal poverty level guidelines are eligible. To meet medical eligibility criteria, the individual must have a condition that is expected to last longer than 2 years and require more health care services than would usually be needed by a child of the applicant's age. The condition must be severe enough to have caused, or be expected to cause, disability, disfigurement, or limitation of function, or to require a special diet or dependence on an assistive device. Also, in the absence of treatment, the disorder must lead to a chronic, disabling physical condition.

TABLE 30-1 2002 Behavioral Risk Factor Surveillance: Utilization of Oral Health Services National Center for Chronic Disease Prevention and Health Promotion Centers for Disease Control and Prevention

HAD TEETH CLEANED BY THE DENTIST OR DENTAL HYGIENIST IN THE PAST YEAR						VISITED THE DENTIST OR DENTAL CLINIC WITHIN THE PAST YEAR FOR ANY REASON					
RACE	MEDIAN % YES	ANNUAL INCOME	MEDIAN % YES	EDUCATION	MEDIAN % YES	RACE	MEDIAN % YES	ANNUAL INCOME	MEDIAN % YES	EDUCATION	MEDIAN % YES
		ALL 69.2%						ALL 69.2%			
White	72.1	<$15,000	48.6	<High school	47.2	White	71.8	<$15,000	49.8	<High school	47.2
Black	62.3	$15,000-24,999	56.1	High school or equivalent	64.7	Black	66.0	$15,000-24,999	56.5	High school or G.E.D.	65.1
Hispanic	65.4	$25,000-34,999	64.6	Some post-high school	72.4	Hispanic	66.4	$25,000-34,999	66.0	Some post-high school	72.8
Other	64.1	$35,000-49,999	72.3	College graduate	79.2	Other	64.3	$35,000-49,999	73.2	College graduate	80.5
Multiracial	56.2	$50,000	80.6			Multiracial	58.0	$50,000	81.6		

HEALTH INSURANCE PORTABILITY AND ACCOUNTABILITY ACT (HIPAA) OF 1996

The Health Insurance Portability and Accountability Act (HIPAA) of 1996 was signed into law by President Bill Clinton on August 21, 1996. Conclusive regulations were issued on August 17, 2000, to be instated by October 16, 2002. HIPAA requires that the transactions of all patient health care information be formatted in a standardized electronic style. In addition to protecting the privacy and security of patient information, HIPAA includes legislation on the formation of medical savings accounts, the authorization of a fraud and abuse control program, the easy transport of health insurance coverage, and the simplification of administrative terms and conditions.

HIPAA encompasses three primary areas, and its privacy requirements can be broken down into three types—privacy standards, patients' rights, and administrative requirements.

1. Privacy Standards. A central concern of HIPAA is the careful use and disclosure of protected health information (PHI), which generally is electronically controlled health information that is able to be distinguished individually. PHI also refers to verbal communication although the HIPAA Privacy Rule is not intended to hinder necessary verbal communication. The U.S. Department of Health and Human Services (USDHHS) does not require restructuring, such as soundproofing, architectural changes, and so forth, but some caution is necessary when exchanging health information by conversation.

An Acknowledgment of Receipt Notice of Privacy Practices, which allows patient information to be used or divulged for treatment, payment, or health care operations (TPO), should be procured from each patient. A detailed and time-sensitive authorization can also be issued, which allows the dentist to release information in special circumstances other than TPOs. A *written consent* is also an option. Dentists can disclose PHI *without* acknowledgement, consent, or authorization in very special situations, for example, perceived child abuse, public health supervision, fraud investigation, or law enforcement with valid permission (i.e., a warrant). When divulging PHI, a dentist must try to disclose only the *minimum necessary* information, to help safeguard the patient's information as much as possible.

It is important that dental professionals adhere to HIPAA standards because health care providers (as well as health care clearinghouses and health care plans) who convey *electronically* formatted health information via an outside billing service or merchant are considered *covered entities*. Covered entities may be dealt serious

civil and criminal penalties for violation of HIPAA legislation. Failure to comply with HIPAA privacy requirements may result in civil penalties of up to $100 per offense with an annual maximum of $25,000 for repeated failure to comply with the same requirement. Criminal penalties resulting from the illegal mishandling of private health information can range from $50,000 and/or 1 year in prison to $250,000 and/or 10 years in prison.

2. Patients' Rights. HIPAA allows patients, authorized representatives, and parents of minors, as well as minors, to become more aware of the health information privacy to which they are entitled. These rights include, but are not limited to, the right to view and copy their health information, the right to dispute alleged breaches of policies and regulations, and the right to request alternative forms of communicating with their dentist. If any health information is released for any reason other than TPO, the patient is entitled to an account of the transaction. Therefore, it is important for dentists to keep accurate records of such information and to provide them when necessary.

The HIPAA Privacy Rule determines that the parents of a minor have access to their child's health information. This privilege may be overruled, for example, in cases where there is suspected child abuse or the parent consents to a term of confidentiality between the dentist and the minor. The parents' rights to access their child's PHI also may be restricted in situations when a legal entity, such as a court, intervenes and when a law does not require a parent's consent. For a full list of patient rights provided by HIPAA, be sure to acquire a copy of the law and to understand it well.

3. Administrative Requirements. Complying with HIPAA legislation may seem like a chore, but it does not need to be so. It is recommended that you become appropriately familiar with the law, organize the requirements into simpler tasks, begin compliance early, and document your progress in compliance. An important first step is to evaluate the current information and practices of your office.

Dentists will need to write a *privacy policy* for their office, a document for their patients detailing the office's practices concerning PHI. The ADA's *HIPAA Privacy Kit* includes forms that you (the dentist) can use to customize your privacy policy. It is useful to try to understand the role of health care information for your patients and the ways in which they deal with the information while they are visiting your office. Train your staff; make sure they are familiar with the terms of HIPAA and your office's privacy policy and related forms. HIPAA requires that you designate a *privacy officer,* a person in your office who will be responsible for applying the new policies in your office, fielding complaints, and making choices involving the minimum necessary requirements. Another person with the role of *contact person* will process complaints.

A *Notice of Privacy Practices*—a document detailing the patient's rights and the dental office's obligations concerning PHI—also must be drawn up. Further, any role of a third party with access to PHI must be clearly documented. This third party is known as a *business associate* (BA) and is defined as any entity who, on behalf of the dentist, takes part in any activity that involves exposure of PHI. The *HIPAA Privacy Kit* provides a copy of the USDHHS "Business Associate Contract Terms," which provides a concrete format for detailing BA interactions.

The main HIPAA privacy compliance date, including all staff training, was April 14, 2003, although many covered entities who submitted a request and a compliance plan by October 15, 2002, were granted one-year extensions. Contact your local branch of the ADA for details. It is recommended that dentists prepare their offices ahead of time for all deadlines, which include preparing privacy polices and forms, business associate contracts, and employee training sessions.

For a comprehensive discussion of all of these terms and requirements, a complete list of HIPAA policies and procedures, and a full collection of HIPAA privacy forms, contact the American Dental Association for a *HIPAA Privacy Kit*. The relevant ADA Web site is www.ada.org/goto/hipaa. Other Web sites that may contain useful information about HIPAA are:

- USDHHS Office of Civil Rights www.hhs.gov/ocr/hipaa
- Work Group on Electronic Data Interchange www.wedi.org/SNIP
- Phoenix Health www.hipaadvisory.com
- USDHHS Office of the Assistant Secretary for Planning and Evaluation http://aspe.os.dhhs.gov/admnsimp/

Data from *HIPAA Privacy Kit*; and http://www.ada.org/prof/prac/issues/topics/hipaa/index.html.
(From Mosby's Dental Dictionary, St Louis, Mosby, 2004.)

INDEX

Page numbers followed by f indicate figures; t, tables; b, boxes.